Instructional Course Lectures Foot and Ankle

Edited by
Elly Trepman, MD
Faculty of Medicine
University of Manitoba
manuscriptsurgeon.com
Mercer Island, Washington

Co-Edited by
George A. Arangio, MD
Chief, Section of Foot and Ankle Surgery
Department of Surgery, Division of Orthopedics
Lehigh Valley Health Network
Allentown, Pennsylvania

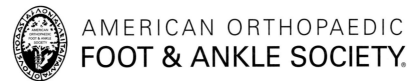

AMERICAN ORTHOPAEDIC
FOOT & ANKLE SOCIETY®

Developed with support from
American Orthopaedic Foot & Ankle Society

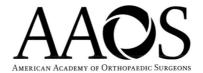

AMERICAN ACADEMY OF ORTHOPAEDIC SURGEONS

Published by the
American Academy
of Orthopaedic Surgeons
6300 North River Road
Rosemont, IL 60018

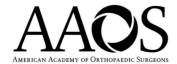

AMERICAN ACADEMY OF ORTHOPAEDIC SURGEONS

The material presented in *Instructional Course Lectures Foot and Ankle* has been made available by the American Academy of Orthopaedic Surgeons for educational purposes only. This material is not intended to present the only, or necessarily best, methods or procedures for the medical situations discussed, but rather is intended to represent an approach, view, statement, or opinion of the author(s) or producer(s), which may be helpful to others who face similar situations.

Some drugs or medical devices demonstrated in Academy courses or described in Academy print or electronic publications have not been cleared by the Food and Drug Administration (FDA) or have been cleared for specific uses only. The FDA has stated that it is the responsibility of the physician to determine the FDA clearance status of each drug or device he or she wishes to use in clinical practice.

Furthermore, any statements about commercial products are solely the opinion(s) of the author(s) and do not represent an Academy endorsement or evaluation of these products. These statements may not be used in advertising or for any commercial purpose.

Some of the authors or the departments with which they are affiliated have received something of value from a commercial or other party related directly or indirectly to the subject of their chapter.

First Edition
Copyright © 2009 by the American Academy of Orthopaedic Surgeons
6300 North River Road
Rosemont, IL 60018

ISBN 978-0-89203-632-5
Printed in the USA

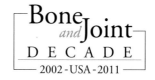

Bone *and* Joint
DECADE
2002 - USA - 2011

Editorial Board

George A. Arangio, MD or a member of his immediate family serves as a board member, owner, officer or a committee member of the American Orthopaedic Foot & Ankle Society and has stock or stock options held in Merck, London Health Sciences Centre, Pfizer, and Johnson & Johnson.

Disclosures for the other members of the Editorial Board are included with their commentaries.

Contributors

Annunziato Amendola, MD, FRCSC
Associate Professor of Orthopaedic Surgery
Department of Surgery
University of Western Ontario
London, Ontario, Canada

Jeffrey O. Anglen, MD
Chairman and Professor of Orthopaedic Surgery
Indiana University School of Medicine
Indianapolis, Indiana

Michael T. Archdeacon, MD, MSE
Director, Division of Musculoskeletal Traumatology
Associate Professor and Vice Chairman
Department of Orthopaedic Surgery
University of Cincinnati
Cincinnati, Ohio

Peter F. Armstrong, MD, FRCSC, FAAP
Director of Medical Affairs
Shriners Hospitals for Children
Shriners International Headquarters
Tampa, Florida

Judith F. Baumhauer, MD
Associate Professor of Orthopaedics
Chief, Division of Foot and Ankle Surgery
Department of Orthopaedics
University of Rochester Medical Center
Rochester, New York

Joseph Borrelli Jr, MD
Associate Professor
Chief, Orthopaedic Trauma
Department of Orthopaedic Surgery
Washington University School of Medicine
St. Louis, Missouri

James W. Brodsky, MD
Clinical Associate Professor
University of Texas Southwestern Medical Center
Director, Foot and Ankle Surgery Fellowship
Baylor University Medical Center
Dallas, Texas

Joseph A. Buckwalter, MD
Professor of Orthopaedic Surgery
Department of Orthopaedic Surgery
University of Iowa
Iowa City, Iowa

Lisa K. Cannada, MD
Assistant Professor
Department of Orthopaedic Surgery
University of Texas
Southwestern Parkland Hospital
Dallas, Texas

Rebecca Cerrato, MD
Foot and Ankle Surgery Fellow
The Institute for Foot and Ankle Reconstruction
Mercy Medical Center
Baltimore, Maryland

Stephen F. Conti, MD
Chief, Division of Foot and Ankle Surgery
Department of Orthopaedic Surgery
University of Pittsburgh School of Medicine
Pittsburgh, Pennsylvania

Michael J. Coughlin, MD
Clinical Professor, Orthopaedics
Oregon Health Science University
Portland, Oregon
Private Practice
Boise, Idaho

Haemish A. Crawford, MBChB, FRACS
Clinical and Research Fellow
Fowler-Kennedy Sports Medicine Clinic
University of Western Ontario
London, Ontario, Canada

R. Jay Cummings, MD
Chairman, Department of Orthopaedics
Nemours Children's Clinic
Jacksonville, Florida

Richard S. Davidson, MD
Associate Clinical Professor
Children's Hospital of Philadelphia
University of Pennsylvania
Philadelphia, Pennsylvania

James K. DeOrio, MD
Associate Professor
Duke Orthopaedics
Department of Orthopaedics
Duke University Medical Center
Durham, North Carolina

Frederick R. Dietz, MD
Professor of Orthopaedic Surgery
Department of Orthopaedics
University of Iowa
Iowa City, Iowa

Douglas R. Dirschl, MD
Frank C. Wilson Distinguished Professor and Chair
UNC Department of Orthopaedics
University of North Carolina
Chapel Hill, North Carolina

Mark E. Easley, MD
Assistant Professor
Department of Orthopaedics
Duke University Medical Center
Durham, North Carolina

Carol C. Frey, MD
Assistant Clinical Professor
Department of Orthopaedic Surgery
University of California, Los Angeles
Co-Director and Chief, Foot and Ankle Surgery
West Coast Sports Medicine Foundation
Manhattan Beach, California

Lowell H. Gill, MD
Private Practice
Miller Orthopaedic Clinic
Clinical Faculty
Carolinas Medical Center
Charlotte, North Carolina

Frank Gottschalk, MB.BCh, FRCSEd
Professor, Orthopaedic Surgery
Department of Orthopaedic Surgery
UT Southwestern Medical Center
Dallas, Texas

Gregory P. Guyton, MD
Assistant Professor
Department of Orthopaedics
University of North Carolina at Chapel Hill
Chapel Hill, North Carolina

David L. Helfet, MD
Orthopaedic Trauma Service
Director, Orthopaedic Trauma Center
Hospital for Special Surgery
New York Presbyterian Hospital
New York, New York

Dolfi Herscovici Jr, DO
Attending, Trauma and Foot and Ankle Service
Associate Professor, Clinical Orthopaedics
Florida Orthopaedic Institute
University of South Florida
Temple Terrace, Florida

Jeffrey E. Johnson, MD
Associate Professor
Department of Orthopaedic Surgery
Barnes-Jewish Hospital at Washington University School
    of Medicine
St. Louis, Missouri

Donald C. Jones, MD
Orthopedic Healthcare Northwest
Orthopedic Consultant
University of Oregon Athletic Department
Clinical Instructor
OHSU
Eugene, Oregon

Thomas N. Joseph, MD
Private Practice
Foot and Ankle Orthopaedics
Camden Bone and Joint
Camden, South Carolina

Harold B. Kitaoka, MD
Department of Orthopaedics
Mayo Clinic
Rochester, Minnesota

Floris P.J.G. Lafeber, PhD
Department of Rheumatology and Clinical Immunology
University Medical Centre of Utrecht
Utrecht, The Netherlands

Peter Laimans, MD
Assistant Clinical Professor
Department of Orthopaedic Surgery
University of Southern California Medical School
Los Angeles, California
Southern California Permanente Medical Group
Panorama City, California

Wallace B. Lehman, MD
Chief Emeritus, Pediatric Orthopaedic Surgery
Professor, Clinical Orthopaedic Surgery
New York University School of Medicine
Pediatric Orthopaedic Surgery
Hospital for Joint Diseases
New York University Hospital Center
New York, New York

Jeffrey A. Mann, MD
Private Practice
Oakland, California

Roger A. Mann, MD
Private Practice
Oakland, California

Arthur Manoli II, MD
Director, Michigan International Foot and Ankle Center
St. Joseph Mercy Hospital, Oakland
Pontiac, Michigan

Richard M. Marks, MD
Associate Professor
Director, Division of Foot and Ankle Surgery
Department of Orthopaedic Surgery
Medical College of Wisconsin
Milwaukee, Wisconsin

J. Lawrence Marsh, MD
Professor of Orthopaedic Surgery
Department of Orthopaedics and Rehabilitation
University of Iowa Hospitals and Clinics
Iowa City, Iowa

Richard J. Mason, MD
Orthopaedic Surgeon
Chesapeake Orthopaedics
Memorial Hospital Easton
Easton, Maryland

Craig D. Morgan, MD
Clinical Professor
University of Pennsylvania
Philadelphia, Pennsylvania

Mark S. Myerson, MD
Director, Institute for Foot and Ankle Reconstruction
Mercy Medical Center
Baltimore, Maryland

Walter J. Pedowitz, MD
Associate Clinical Professor
Department of Orthopaedic Surgery
College of Physicians and Surgeons
Columbia University
Columbia, New York

Glenn B. Pfeffer, MD
Assistant Clinical Professor
Department of Orthopaedics
University of California at San Francisco
San Francisco, California

Marco Antonio Guedes de Souza Pinto, MD
Orthopaedic Workshop of the Lar Escola Sao Francisco
Universidade Federal de Sao Paulo
Sao Paulo, Brazil

Michael S. Pinzur, MD
Professor of Orthopaedic Surgery and Rehabilitation
Department of Orthopaedic Surgery and Rehabilitation
Loyola University Medical Center
Maywood, Illinois

David A. Porter, MD, PhD
Orthopedic Foot and Ankle Specialist
Methodist Sports Medicine/The Orthopedic Specialists
Indianapolis, Indiana

E. Greer Richardson, MD
Professor of Orthopaedic Surgery
University of Tennessee
Campbell Clinic
Memphis, Tennessee

Charles L. Saltzman, MD
Professor
Department of Orthopaedic Surgery
Department of Biomedical Engineering
University of Iowa
Iowa City, Iowa

V. James Sammarco, MD
Cincinnati Sports Medicine and Orthopaedic Center
Cincinnati, Ohio

Michael S. Sirkin, MD
Assistant Professor
Chief, Orthopaedic Trauma Service
Department of Orthopaedics
New Jersey Medical School
Newark, New Jersey

Douglas G. Smith, MD
Professor
Department of Orthopaedics and Sports Medicine
Harborview Medical Center
University of Washington
Seattle, Washington

James W. Stone, MD
Assistant Clinical Professor, Orthopedic Surgery
Medical College of Wisconsin
Milwaukee, Wisconsin

Michael Suk, MD, JD, MPH
Orthopaedic Trauma Fellow
Hospital for Special Surgery
New York, New York

James P. Tasto, MD
Clinical Professor
Department of Orthopedics
University of California, San Diego
San Diego, California

C. Niek van Dijk, MD, PhD
Department of Orthopedic Surgery
AMC Hospital/University of Amsterdam
Amsterdam, The Netherlands

Peter M. van Roermund, PhD
Orthopaedics
University Medical Centre of Utrecht
Utrecht, The Netherlands

Keith L. Wapner, MD
Clinical Professor, Orthopaedic Surgery
Department of Orthopaedic Surgery
University of Pennsylvania
Philadelphia, Pennsylvania

James R. Yu, MD
Fellow
Department of Orthopedic Surgery
Barnes-Jewish Hospital at Washington University School
  of Medicine
St. Louis, Missouri

Preface

This compilation of selected chapters from past *Instructional Course Lectures* volumes is focused on advances in the treatment of conditions of the foot and ankle. This specialty volume continues the tradition of collaboration between the American Academy of Orthopaedic Surgeons (AAOS) and the American Orthopaedic Foot & Ankle Society (AOFAS) that has resulted in superb educational materials including *Orthopaedic Knowledge Update: Foot and Ankle*, *Advanced Reconstruction: Foot and Ankle*, and numerous other publications and digital productions for the practicing orthopaedic surgeon.

In this eighth year of the "Bone and Joint Decade" campaign, the AOFAS celebrates its 40th anniversary as a specialty society and continues to expand sponsorship of education and research in the areas of reconstruction, sports medicine, trauma, technology, and diabetes care. In the past, the foot and ankle had been underrepresented in orthopaedic training programs. However, as a credit to the hard work of numerous individuals, the AOFAS has grown into one of the most dynamic orthopaedic subspecialty societies serving the general orthopaedic community and their patients.

The primary goal in arranging this compilation was to provide a clinically useful and up-to-date review of selected topics for the general orthopaedic surgeon, foot and ankle subspecialist, and orthopaedic trainee. We responded to this challenge with two strategies to provide a useful and current book. First, we selected articles that included general principles that have withstood the test of time and have remained relevant and valid for the practicing clinician. Second, we worked closely with the section editors to create commentaries that included an update of pertinent studies that have appeared since the original publication date of the reprinted chapters. We anticipate that editors of the annual AAOS *Instructional Course Lectures* series will increase foot and ankle representation in future volumes.

The first section of this specialty edition of *Instructional Course Lectures* reviews foot and ankle complications of diabetes mellitus, a disease of epidemic prevalence and one of the most disabling and costly public health problems of this century. The second section about foot and ankle trauma addresses another major category of foot and ankle morbidity in developed and underdeveloped countries. The sections on sports medicine, arthroscopy, and forefoot conditions review common conditions encountered in general orthopaedic and foot and ankle practices. Finally, the sections on ankle arthrosis and deformity reconstruction highlight some of the most complex challenges confronted by foot and ankle clinicians and researchers.

The editors are grateful to the Boards of Directors of the AAOS and AOFAS for supporting this project. We thank the expert staff of the AAOS Publications and Marketing Departments, including Marilyn Fox, PhD, Lisa Moore, Kathleen Anderson, Courtney Astle, Bronwyn Barrera, and Natalie Vakhovsky for their outstanding assistance. We appreciate the time, effort, and expertise of all the authors and section editors. We dedicate this volume to the founding members of the AOFAS (Nicholas Giannestras, Nathaniel Gould, Melvin H. Jahss, Robert Joplin, Hampar Kelikian, Paul Lapidus, and Joseph Milgram) and the editors of the AOFAS peer-reviewed journal *Foot & Ankle International* (Melvin H. Jahss, Kenneth A. Johnson, Lowell D. Lutter, E. Greer Richardson, and David B. Thordarson). We hope the current volume will contribute to improved foot and ankle care and a better quality of life for our patients.

Elly Trepman, MD
George A. Arangio, MD

Contents

Section 1 The Diabetic Foot and Ankle

Section 2 Trauma

Section 6 Ankle Arthrosis

Section 7 Reconstruction of Foot and Ankle Deformity

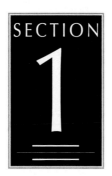

SECTION 1

The Diabetic Foot and Ankle

The Diabetic Foot and Ankle

The diabetes epidemic has become one of the major public health problems of the early 21st century. Orthopaedic surgeons play an important leadership role in the diagnosis and treatment of patients with diabetic foot and ankle disorders. Since 1999, when several of the articles in this section were published, the number of patients in the United States with diabetes mellitus has increased by 50%, from 15.7 million (5.9% of the population) to 23.6 million (7.8% of the population) in 2007. The condition remains undiagnosed in approximately 24% of patients. The increase in the number of patients with diabetes has been associated with the increase in the number of overweight and elderly people in the population.[1]

In the United States in 2007, the economic cost of diabetes exceeded $174 billion.[2] Diabetes accounted for 15 million work days absent, 120 million work days with reduced performance, and an additional 107 million work days lost because of unemployment disability attributed to diabetes. An estimated $58.3 billion was spent on inpatient hospital care and $9.9 billion on physician office visits directly attributed to diabetes. Diabetes-related hospitalizations totaled 24.3 million days.

More than 60% of nontraumatic lower limb amputations occur in people with diabetes, with approximately 71,000 nontraumatic lower limb amputations performed in these patients in 2004.[2] To help reduce the risk of ulcers that may predispose a patient to amputation, the American Orthopaedic Foot and Ankle Society has prepared a brochure with foot care instructions in multiple languages.[3]

The seven chapters in this section provide a wealth of information for treating the diabetic foot. The chapter by Brodsky reviews the important contribution of neuropathy to most diabetic foot and ankle disorders, and provides a practical overview of basic diabetic foot care. Patient history and physical examination are reviewed, including assessing neuropathy, vascular status, deformity, systemic factors such as blood sugar control and nutritional status, and local tissue factors. The evaluation and identification of the diabetic foot with vascular ischemia is important. The depth-ischemia classification of diabetic foot ulcers is an extension of the Wagner classification, which still is widely used. Deformities and associated areas of pressure are identified and managed with a combination of shoe modifications, orthotic insoles, bracing, and, in specific instances, surgical correction. More recent advances in wound care have been developed since this article was published, including suction (so-called negative pressure) wound care systems and specialized dressings, improving the success of treatment of many diabetic foot wounds.

Guyton and Saltzman provide a thorough review of the mechanisms of diabetic foot disease, including neuropathy, deformity, and vascular disease. Pathophysiologic factors are reviewed, including nutritional status, immune function, and glucose control. The lateral talar-first metatarsal angle of greater than –27° may be a predictor of ulcer formation in patients with diabetic Charcot midfoot.[4] Recent advances in treating diabetic neuro-

pathic pain have included the use of anticonvulsant drugs such as pregabalin.[5]

The pathophysiology of Charcot arthropathy is reviewed by Guyton and Saltzman, including the neurotraumatic and neurovascular mechanisms. More recent work in the characterization of Charcot arthropathy has shown that decreased bone mineral density is associated with Charcot fracture without dislocation, in contrast with normal bone mineral density with Charcot dislocation in the absence of fracture.[6]

Immunohistochemical studies of Charcot bone samples have shown increased osteoclastic bone resorption and cytokine mediators of bone resorption.[7] Inflammation associated with trauma, ulcer, infection, or surgery may be associated with cytokine activation, osteopenia, and osteolysis, possibly leading to Charcot arthropathy.[8] Recent clinical evaluations of patients with Charcot arthropathy have confirmed the potentially devastating impact of this condition on the health-related quality of life.[9,10] Earlier detection of Charcot arthropathy may be facilitated with imaging methods other than plain radiographs, such as bone scintigraphy, CT scanning, and MRI.[11]

Total contact casting is a valuable tool for treating diabetic foot ulcers and Charcot arthropathy. Conti's chapter describes the rationale, indications, contraindications, and precautions for total contact casting. A useful patient instruction sheet is included. Total contact casting remains the standard against which newer treatments are assessed; however, this treatment method is labor intensive and may be associated with complications in 30% of patients.[12] Newer methods, such as the use of a prefabricated removable walker brace and custom insole, may be successful in treating Charcot arthropathy, with a high patient satisfaction rate and safety profile.[13]

The principles of managing diabetic foot infections described in the chapter by Saltzman and Pedowitz remain relevant. More recent work has confirmed the lack of concordance between wound swab and bone cultures in diabetic foot osteomyelitis.[14,15] A recent meta-analysis has shown that MRI is the most accurate imaging modality for diagnosing osteomyelitis; however, the presence of exposed or probed bone remains useful.[16] The reliability of MRI to distinguish osteomyelitis from Charcot arthropathy is equivocal, and limited information is available on the usefulness of

gadolinium-enhanced MRI in the diabetic foot.[17] Antibiotic resistance observed with methicillin-resistant *Staphylococcus aureus* and vancomycin-resistant enterococci may be a challenging emerging clinical problem. The treatment of diabetic foot infection continues to include culture-specific antibiotics; knowledge of local resistance patterns; support from consultants in internal medicine and infectious diseases; surgical débridement; and wound care, including specialized dressings and wound suction systems.

The surgical treatment of Charcot arthropathy has continued to evolve during the decade since the publication of the chapter by Johnson. Recent advances in the surgical treatment of Charcot arthropathy have included a more detailed classification system,[18] early surgical stabilization for stage I Charcot arthropathy,[19] plantar plate and

intramedullary screw fixation of midfoot rocker-bottom deformity,[20,21] intramedullary rod fixation for ankle Charcot arthropathy,[22] and ring external fixation for correction of midfoot deformities.[23]

The chapter by Smith reviews principles and controversies in partial foot amputation including decision making about biologic healing and the functional level of amputation. The section ends with a chapter by Pinzur and associates that discusses controversies in amputation surgery such as amputation level and establishing a distal tibiofibular bone bridge in transtibial (below-knee) amputations.

Naomi N. Shields, MD
Department of Orthopaedic Surgery
University of Kansas School of Medicine
Advanced Orthopaedic Associates
Wichita, Kansas

References

1. National Diabetes Fact Sheet. Centers for Disease Control and Prevention, Department of Health and Human Services, 2007. www.cdc.gov/diabetes/pubs/pdf/ndfs_2007.pdf. Accessed June 5, 2009.

2. Diabetes Statistics: American Diabetes Association Website. http://www.diabetes.org/diabetes-statistics.jsp. Accessed June 5, 2009.

3. Trepman E, Bracilovic A, Lamborn KK, et al: Diabetic foot care: Multilingual translation of a patient education leaflet. *Foot Ankle Int* 2005;26:64-127.

4. Bevan WP, Tomlinson MP: Radiographic measures as a predictor of ulcer formation in diabetic Charcot midfoot. *Foot Ankle Int* 2008;29:568-573.

5. Arezzo JC, Rosenstock J, Lamoreaux L, Pauer L: Efficacy and safety of pregabalin 600 mg/d for treating painful diabetic peripheral neuropathy: A double-blind placebo-controlled trial. *BMC Neurol* 2008;8:33.

6. Herbst SA, Jones KB, Saltzman CL: Pattern of diabetic neuropathic arthropathy associated with the peripheral bone mineral density. *J Bone Joint Surg Br* 2004;86:378-383.

7. Baumhauer JF, O'Keefe RJ, Schon LC, Pinzur MS: Cytokine-induced osteoclastic bone resorption in Charcot arthropathy: An immunohistochemical study. *Foot Ankle Int* 2006;27:797-800.

8. Jeffcoate WJ: Charcot neuro-osteoarthropathy. *Diabetes Metab Res Rev* 2008;24(suppl 1): S62-S65.

9. Willrich A, Pinzur M, McNeil M, Juknelis D, Lavery L: Health related quality of life, cognitive function, and depression in diabetic patients with foot ulcer or amputation: A preliminary study. *Foot Ankle Int* 2005;26:128-134.

10. Sochocki MP, Verity S, Atherton PJ, et al: Health related quality of life in patients with Charcot arthropathy of the foot and ankle. *Foot Ankle Surg* 2008;14:11-15.

11. Chantelau E: The perils of procrastination: Effects of early vs. delayed detection and treatment of incipient Charcot fracture. *Diabet Med* 2005;22:1707-1712.

12. Guyton GP: An analysis of iatrogenic complications from the total contact cast. *Foot Ankle Int* 2005;26:903-907.

13. Verity S, Sochocki M, Embil JM, Trepman E: Treatment of Charcot foot and ankle with a prefabricated removable walker brace and custom insole. *Foot Ankle Surg* 2008;14:26-31.

14. Senneville E, Melliez H, Beltrand E, et al: Culture of percutaneous bone biopsy specimens for diagnosis of diabetic foot osteomyelitis: Concordance with ulcer swab cultures. *Clin Infect Dis* 2006;42:57-62.

15. Embil JM, Trepman E: Microbiological evaluation of diabetic foot osteomyelitis. *Clin Infect Dis* 2006;42:63-65.

16. Dinh MT, Abad CL, Safdar N: Diagnostic accuracy of the physical examination and imag-

ing tests for osteomyelitis underlying diabetic foot ulcers: Meta-analysis. *Clin Infect Dis* 2008;47:519-527.

17. Sella EJ: Current concepts review: Diagnostic imaging of the diabetic foot. *Foot Ankle Int* 2009;30:568-576.

18. Schon LC, Easley ME, Cohen I, Lam PW, Badekas A, Anderson CD: The acquired mid-tarsus deformity classification system: Interobserver reliability and intraobserver reproducibility. *Foot Ankle Int* 2002;23:30-36.

19. Simon SR, Tejwani SG, Wilson DL, Santner TJ, Denniston NL: Arthrodesis as an early alternative to nonoperative management of Charcot arthropathy of the diabetic foot. *J Bone Joint Surg Am* 2000;82:939-950.

20. Marks RM, Parks BG, Schon LC: Midfoot fusion technique for neuroarthropathic feet: Biomechanical analysis and rationale. *Foot Ankle Int* 1998;19:507-510.

21. Sammarco VJ, Sammarco GJ, Walker EW Jr, Guiao RP: Midtarsal arthrodesis in the treatment of Charcot midfoot arthropathy. *J Bone Joint Surg Am* 2009;91:80-91.

22. Pinzur MS, Noonan T: Ankle arthrodesis with a retrograde femoral nail for Charcot ankle arthropathy. *Foot Ankle Int* 2005;26:545-549.

23. Pinzur MS: Neutral ring fixation for high-risk nonplantigrade Charcot midfoot deformity. *Foot Ankle Int* 2007;28:961-966.

Naomi N. Shields, MD or a member of her immediate family serves as a board member, owner, officer, or committee member of Our Lady of Lourdes Rehabilitation Hospital, Ruth Jackson Orthopaedic Society, and the American Orthopaedic Foot & Ankle Society; is a member of a speakers' bureau or has made paid presentations on behalf of Arthrosurface; has received research or institutional support from Biomimetic FDA trial; and has stock or stock options held in Medical Images.

Evaluation of the Diabetic Foot

James W. Brodsky, MD

Introduction

It has been over 5 years since the last presentation of a course on the diabetic foot in the Instructional Course Lectures. In that interval, much additional knowledge, research, and practical strategies for treatment and diagnosis have evolved. The burgeoning interest in the diabetic foot has been manifested by work published in the literature of many different and diverse medical specialties, including orthopaedic surgery. The current Instructional Course on the diabetic foot was revised and expanded 4 years ago in response both to the growth in information that needs to be conveyed on this complex subject and to a rising interest among orthopaedic surgeons in surgical and nonsurgical problems of the diabetic foot.

The increasing interest of orthopaedists reflects a natural predilection of that specialty for understanding the pathology of and treating the lesions of the insensitive foot. Most of the lesions of the diabetic foot are related in some way to areas of abnormal pressure under or on the foot and/or to biomechanical abnormalities of the foot, ankle, and leg. As extremity specialists, and as specialists in the musculoskeletal system, it is gratifying to see both orthopaedic clinical practice and orthopaedic

research resources turned to the problems of the enlarging diabetic population in this and other developed countries.

In the current milieu of managed care in this country, orthopaedic surgeons are further motivated to provide comprehensive lower extremity care. The vast spectrum of disease, disorders, and injuries of the lower limb make it imperative that the principles of diabetic foot care form an integral part of our teaching literature. In this expanded format, authors expound on the diabetic foot according to the following topics: Outpatient diagnosis and management, James W. Brodsky, MD; Total contact casts, Stephen A. Conti, MD; Infections, Charles Saltzman, MD; Charcot joints, Jeffrey E. Johnson, MD; and Amputations of the foot, Douglas A. Smith, MD. My thanks to each of my fellow contributors for making this a successful teaching effort.

The Problem

Patients with diabetes have become an increasingly familiar part of the orthopaedic patient population. The number of diabetics in the United States has continued to increase, not only by virtue of increased numbers, but also as a result of greater recognition of a portion of the millions of undiagnosed patients. Estimates by

the American Diabetes Association are that the prevalence of diabetes totals 15.7 million people today (5.9% of the American population). Of these, fully one third are undiagnosed. The incidence of diabetes is high in our population as a whole, with variations noted among different ethnic and socioeconomic groups. More than half of the lower limb amputations in this country are performed in patients with diabetes. With greater longevity, the number of complications of the diabetes and the number of patients with multisystem complications continues to increase. Patients with unrelated trauma or degenerative musculoskeletal conditions are noted ever more frequently also to have diabetes and its complications. Infection, deformity, and dysfunction of the lower extremity that result from the effects of diabetes pose threats to other orthopaedic interventions. For example, patients with total knee or total hip arthroplasty are at risk from infected foot wounds because the distal lesions could seed the implants. Fractures of the ankle, even nondisplaced fractures, can become disasters of deformity and joint destruction in diabetics with peripheral neuropathy. Failure to recognize the loss of protective sensation that results from diabetic peripheral neuropathy, and, therefore, the increased risk of developing a neuropathic joint after fracture has produced countless cases of unhappy, even litigious patients. Knowledge of these complications is an important tool that enables the orthopaedic surgeon to inform the patient of the risks to the foot and ankle in diabetes. Moreover, orthopaedic surgeons are uniquely qualified to manage these complex musculoskeletal problems because of their training and experience in treating a wide range of lower limb problems and trauma, of prescribing shoes, and of comprehending the issues of gait and stability as they relate to the function of the entire lower limb. At times it can be a confusing, even a daunting, task to determine the proper specialty or combination of specialists to care for the multiple systems involved in the acutely or chronically ill patient with diabetes. These chapters on the diabetic foot should assist the reader in forming a treatment plan for patients who present with an acute diabetic foot problem.

Diabetic foot problems are estimated to account for approximately 25% of all diabetic hospital admissions. The economic impact of diabetic foot problems was estimated to reach $98 billion in the United States in 1997, representing $44 billion in actual medical costs and $54 billion in expenses related to disability and mortality. Although these statistics attempt to include the costs of lost productivity of workers with diabetes, the human impact on daily routines of family life, of work, and of recreation is truly widespread and inestimable. The American Diabetes Association noted 88 million disability days lost from work in 1997 as a result of diabetes. Early recognition of diabetic foot problems, prompt and proper diagnosis, patient education, and preventive care have been shown to be effective measures for reductions in morbidity and in cost to individuals, families, and society.[1]

Pathophysiology of the Diabetic Foot

Many factors contribute to the altered physiology and the pathologic states of the lower limb of diabetics. The major factors are neuropathy, vascular disease, deformity, immune abnormalities, gait and pressure abnormalities, local tissue factors, and systemic abnormalities.

Neuropathy

The primary cause or source of the vast majority of diabetic foot and ankle lesions, problems, and complications is diabetic peripheral neuropathy. Although they are not exclusively the effect of sensory neuropathy, most problems arise because the foot, leg, or parts thereof, are wholly or partially insensate.[2,3] Vascular disease and vascular abnormalities are common in diabetics and well recognized as a part of the complex combination of systemic influences on the feet of diabetic patients, but it is clear that most diabetic problems begin as a result of local trauma and tissue damage caused by the loss of or diminution of protective sensation. Injury to the bones and joints can occur following repetitive trauma, trivial trauma, or no recognized trauma at all. Most ulcers and infections are the result of a break in the soft-tissue envelope caused by unrecognized (unperceived) pressure.

This simple concept of the central, key role of neuropathy is frequently overlooked. Because the neuropathy cannot be reversed or ameliorated, most orthopaedic surgical and non-surgical interventions are aimed at accommodating areas of pressure and compensating for the loss of protective sensation by substituting other methods of injury prevention, such as cushioning shoewear and insoles and routines for daily inspection of feet and of shoes.

Laboratory studies have demonstrated that repetitive low-level trauma to soft tissue can produce tissue inflammation and, ultimately, tissue necrosis, if sufficient cycles of trauma were applied to the limb. Even if each repetition is well below the threshold for tissue damage, the cumulative effect exceeds that threshold, resulting in ulceration. Histologic documentation of the progressive stages of cellular infiltrates of inflammation and necrosis have been demonstrated. In the final stage, tissue necrosis leads to tissue loss, ie, ulceration.[4] The same mechanism occurs in the diabetic foot, in which pressure under or over a bony prominence may not be particularly great, but eventually leads to soft tissue loss as a result of the many repetitions of the mechanical cycle of gait.

The most dramatic component of diabetic peripheral neuropathy is the sensory loss, but there are 3 different aspects of neuropathy. These are sensory, autonomic, and motor neuropathies.

Sensory Neuropathy Sensory neuropathy is the most important of the 3 forms of peripheral neuropathy, because it is most directly related to trauma to the lower extremity. Sensory neuropathy is the most critical contributing factor to neuropathic fractures, ulcerations, and skin breakdown. The absence of protective sensation leads to small injuries, catastrophic injuries, or a cumulative set of injuries to the foot. The neuropathy typically occurs in a stocking distribution, ie, it tends to be below the knee. It is progressively more dense as the examination progresses distally on the lower limb. This is consistent with the fact that ulcerations and infections over the toes and under the metatarsals are far more common than similar lesions around the ankle.

Testing for diabetic neuropathy is critical, even if the testing is very basic. To begin, a specific history inquiring about previous neuropathic events is essential. The examination for sensation can be brief. Even in the emergency department, one can test for light touch, pinprick, and position sense. The key is first to recognize the need to include this information in the orthopaedic history and physical, and second, to document the findings in the patient's record. Failure to identify the neuropathy in a patient with a fractured ankle can have long-reaching medical and even medicolegal ramifications if the otherwise appropriately treated fracture fails to heal and drifts into a neuropathic varus or valgus deformity.

The simplest, most reproducible, and currently most widely used method of testing for neuropathy is to use the Semmes-Weinstein monofilaments.[5,6] The monofilaments are relatively inexpensive, and are easy to use. They are graded on a logarithmic scale of the pressure that the filament applies, which is a function both of the cross-sectional area of the filament and of its stiffness (Fig. 1). The thicker, stiffer monofilaments require greater force to bend them. The monofilaments, made of a plastic filament embedded in a handle, are employed by holding the monofilament perpendicular to the skin. Pressure is applied through the handle on the tip until the filament begins to bend (Fig. 2). The patient, whose eyes are closed, registers whether or not the pressure is felt, ie, it is a threshold test. A small map can be constructed of the level and pattern of sensation from the knee and the toes. Most published investigations have indicated that the ability to

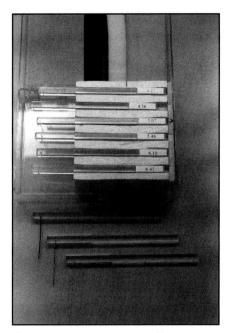

Fig. 1 Semmes-Weinstein monofilaments. Filaments are graded on a logarithmic scale. This set has a wide range.

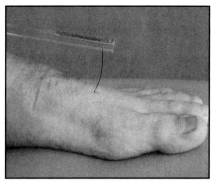

Fig. 2 Semmes-Weinstein monofilament is a threshhold test. Pressure is applied perpendicular to the skin until the filament begins to bend. The patient, with eyes closed, is asked to identify the touch of the monofilament.

feel the 5.07 monofilament correlates reasonably to a protective level of sensation in the majority of patients. However, a significant amount of work remains to be done on this subject, to refine the techniques and to define those patients who are exceptions to these guidelines. Moreover, significant variations in applied pressure occur with small variations in the angle of the filament to the skin. Despite these limitations, the Semmes-Weinstein monofilaments remain the most practical and clinically reproducible method currently available both for screening for neuropathy and for quantifying the density of peripheral neuropathy in the lower limbs of diabetics.

Autonomic Neuropathy Autonomic neuropathy is an "unseen" but very significant component of neuropathy. It is a major etiologic factor in the development of both soft-tissue and bony lesions. Autonomic neuropathy leads to abnormalities of

regulation of skin temperature and sweating. The skin of the foot becomes dry and scaly. As it stiffens, it may crack easily, opening a portal in the dermis for bacteria to enter, the first step in infection. Fissures in the typical thick calluses on the plantar surface propagate through the skin.

The autonomic neuropathy plays an important role in neuroarthropathy, or Charcot joints. This effect has been likened by some authors to the effects of a severe autosympathectomy. The resulting loss of autoregulation in blood flow causes increased flow to the area. This hyperemia has been clinically noted by numerous studies of the Charcot foot in diabetes, and documentation of the lack of ischemia has been demonstrated.[7] Weakening of the tissues is postulated to occur from this hyperemia, leading to weakening or dissolution of the periarticular tissues, followed by joint collapse.

Motor Neuropathy Motor neuropathy contributes to deformity by way of the contractures that occur as a result of the dysfunction and scarring of the intrinsic muscles of the foot. This contracture leads to claw toe deformities. As the metatar-

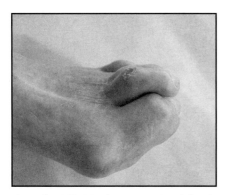

Fig. 3 The MTP joint hyperextension deformity causes increased weightbearing pressure under the metatarsal head. The associated PIP joint flexion increases pressure over the dorsum of PIP joint, where it rubs against the shoe.

sophalangeal joints hyperextend, the base of the proximal phalanx migrates proximally and depresses the distal metatarsalgia (Fig. 3). This increases the mechanical pressure under the metatarsal head, leading to the classic metatarsal "mal perforans" ulceration on the plantar forefoot. The reciprocal flexion contracture at the interphalangeal joints creates dorsal prominences that rub against the toe box of the shoe, which lead to ulceration as well. Peroneal mononeuropathy is a special form of combined motor and sensory neuropathy that occurs occasionally. A foot drop, either unilateral or bilateral, is the motor result of the lesion.

Peripheral Vascular Disease

Peripheral vascular disease, in fact, all forms of atherosclerotic cardiovascular disease, are more prevalent, more severe, and occur at an earlier age in the diabetic compared to the nondiabetic population. The distribution throughout the extremity is more diffuse, particularly in the lower limb, and it can be rapidly progressive. It affects diabetic women more than women in the population in general. The lesions occur in the large vessels of the aortoiliac and femoral regions, but also have a wide distribution and peculiar characteristics in the infrapopliteal arterial tree.

Treatment of the proximal vascular lesions is an important part of the program for healing the diabetic foot. These patients will experience major improvement in the viability of the foot once the large, proximal lesions are treated with endarterectomy or a bypass procedure. Frequently, these proximal procedures are essential to overcome the distal ischemia of the foot and ankle.

Distal lesions of the arterial tree in the lower leg are characterized by diffuse involvement of all 3 of the vessels of the popliteal trifurcation, the anterior tibial, posterior tibial, and peroneal arteries. The lumenal narrowing is ragged and widespread, unlike the limited, discrete atherosclerotic lesions in the nondiabetic with vascular occlusive disease, which seldom occur below the knee. Histologically, diabetic and nondiabetic lesions differ in the location of the calcification, which is in the intimal layer in nondiabetics, but in the media in the arteries of diabetics. The latter leads to the pipe-like radiographic appearance of vessels on plain radiographs.

Treatment of distal arterial lesions usually requires a distal bypass procedure to whichever of the vessels is patent at or below the level of the ankle. Balloon angioplasty, selectively used in some medical centers, is applicable only in cases of a relatively isolated and discrete lesion, which, as noted above, is more the exception than the rule. The distal bypass procedures frequently use in situ saphenous vein grafts in which the venous valves have been cut, avoiding the need to reverse the vein within the limb. Salvage of a foot is frequently a function of the combined teamwork of the orthopaedic and vascular surgeons, who represent only two of the members of the multidisciplinary team required to treat the diabetic patient with foot problems.

Much has been discussed about the supposed "small vessel disease" in diabetics, but the anatomic lesion of this purported condition remains unidentified, and its very existence has been challenged by more than one author.[8–10] Changes in the capillary permeability and basement membrane thickening are well described, but there is no proof of a small vessel occlusive lesion, and the connection between these capillary changes and the occurrence of infection or ulceration remains unproved.[11] Blood flow in diabetics has been demonstrated to be the same as in other patients with peripheral neuropathy from other causes. Thus the cause of diabetic ulcerations cannot scientifically be ascribed to microvascular disease. Neuropathy continues to be a sufficient and pathophysiologically accurate explanation for most lesions.

Vascular disease has a large role in the presence of pain in the lower extremity of diabetic patients with neuropathic foot disease. This is separate and distinct from the pain of Charcot joints and the pain of the neuropathy itself. Contrary to the conventional wisdom that Charcot joints present with classical "painless swelling," previous studies have documented that about half of all patients with Charcot joints present with a chief complaint of pain;[7] although the pain is not commensurate with the degree of osseous destruction, as it would be felt in a nonneuropathic patient.

Paradoxically, the peripheral neuropathy of diabetes (and other etiologies as well), which produces a loss of sensory capacity, can, at the same time, cause painful dysesthesias. The treatment of dysesthesias usually consists of medication. The most commonly employed regimen is low-dose or medium-dose amitriptylline or nortriptylline, taken at bedtime. The medication is difficult to administer and difficult to take. The dosage must be slowly increased to titrate it to the level of the patient's symptoms while minimizing the frequent side effects of drowsiness and lethargy. Other medications used include other neuroleptics, such as hydantoin or tegretol, as well as mexitilene.[12,13] Some patients obtain relief from the use of topical capsaicin-containing creams. These nonprescription derivatives of chili peppers produce a burning sensation initially, but paradoxically reduce the burning and other dysesthesias after continued use. Intractable cases require consultation with a neurologist or pain management specialist. Painful dysesthesias remain a vexing chronic problem for which no treatment is uniformly applicable or wholly successful.

Most diabetic patients with neuropathy treated by the orthopaedic surgeon have altered but not absent sensation. As noted above, both Charcot arthropathy and peripheral neuropathy can cause pain. However, the most serious cause of pain is ischemia. The doctor (the whole health care team, actually) needs to be wary of the patient who complains of a painful distal lesion on the foot, the most common example of which is the "painful ingrown toenail." In patients with neuropathic ulcerations, it is unlikely that they have sufficient sensation to report pain from the nail or other distal source. In most instances, what is mistakenly reported as a painful nail or painful ulcer is actually the pain of distal ischemia. This rest ischemia is char-

acterized by a history of pain that is felt at night, often waking the patient from sleep, and is relieved by standing, or walking about. The dependent position of the lower limb increases the arterial flow to the foot through the marginal effect of gravity. Thoughtless but aggressive nail trimmings have resulted in below-knee amputations when the pain of ischemia is unrecognized. If the vascular status of the limb is uncertain, and if there are questionable pulses or no palpable pulses, then vascular testing must be undertaken before even the simplest procedure, such as nail trimming.

Deformity

Deformity of the foot and ankle, whether gross or subtle, usually leads to an area or areas of increased bony prominence. These areas produce various problems, including localized areas of pressure, gait abnormalities, and biomechanical malalignment of the limb. The diagnosis and treatment of these deformities is one aspect of the management of the diabetic foot that is particularly within the expertise of the orthopaedic surgeon.

The most common deformity, the clawed toe, is actually a combination of flexion deformities at the interphalangeal joints and extension deformity at the metatarsophalangeal joints. The severity is a function of the stiffness and irreducibility of the deformities. While hammertoes and clawtoes occur in the nonneuropathic population, the incidence appears to be higher in diabetics. The stiffness may be a function of the duration of the diabetes, the severity of the neuropathy, or the chronic level of elevated glucose (level of control of diabetic hyperglycemia). Limited joint mobility syndrome has been described in diabetics. It affects mul-

tiple joints, is not localized preferentially to the lower limb, and is caused by stiffening of the periarticular soft tissue. This stiffening is believed to occur as a result of glycosylation of the collagen in those tissues.[14,15]

Other deformities include local prominences of a Charcot joint, equinus deformities at the ankle and/or transverse tarsal joints, and varus and valgus deformities of the hindfoot and of the ankle. Dr. Johnson discusses Charcot deformities in detail in Chapter 5. These deformities can be the result of prolonged bedrest due to other medical conditions or can be caused by peroneal mononeuropathy. An equinus contracture can obviously cause dramatic abnormalities of gait. But the equinus can also be responsible for plantar metatarsal ulcerations caused by rigid pressure on the forefoot. It is important to identify proximal deformities that increase midfoot and forefoot pressures in order to properly diagnose the source of the pressure and take appropriate therapeutic steps. Another example would be recurrent ulceration under the lateral border of the foot at the base of the fifth metatarsal, in the presence of a varus hindfoot deformity due, for example, to a Charcot deformity in the subtalar joint. Resection of the base of the metatarsal may be insufficient to relieve the pressure borne on this spot, and it may be necessary to realign the hindfoot out of the varus deformity in order to solve the forefoot problem. Still, this example remains consistent with the principle of identifying the source of the pressure in neuropathic ulcerations. That source can be local, or augmented by proximal deformity.

Identification of deformity is an integral part of comprehending the primary formula for the development of neuropathic ulceration in the diabetic foot. While mildly over-simplified, it is accurate to say that all neuropathic ulceration requires the combination of 2 factors, insensitivity (caused by neuropathy) and pressure (usually caused by bony prominences). Patients without neuropathy who have deformity, such as a hammertoe or hallux valgus, report pain, but do not ulcerate because their intact sensibility of the foot protects them by causing pain at the site of the deformity. The opposite is also true. That is, patients with peripheral neuropathy generally do not ulcerate, especially over the midfoot and forefoot, in the absence of a source of pressure, either internal or external. The internal source would be the bony prominence and the external source would be either pressure from a shoe or applied trauma to the soft tissue. Ulcerations in the plantar arch are uncommon because there is no source of pressure in this area unless the patient has a type 1 midfoot Charcot breakdown, with collapse or reversal of the bony arch.[16] Thus, the most common sites of diabetic foot ulceration in the absence of a Charcot joint are under the metatarsal heads, the medial sesamoid, the dorsum of the interphalangeal joints of the toes, the navicular tuberosity, and the base of the fifth metatarsal.

Despite the central role of mechanical pressure in the development of neuropathic ulceration, it still remains ignored or unrecognized, especially by other medical specialists who participate in the care of the diabetic foot. Reduction or elimination of pressure is a fundamental role for the orthopaedic surgeon in the diabetic foot care team. Regardless of what kind of control we exert on local or systemic factors; regardless of the types of dressings we apply, or the choice of antibiotics, if we fail to treat the underlying pressure, the ulcera-

tions will either recur or will fail to heal primarily. Orthopaedic decision making with regard to the diabetic foot often involves the decision between external pressure relief, with casts, braces, shoes, and insoles, versus internal pressure relief, with bone resection or realignment.

The notable exception to this rule is the ulceration over the heel, especially the posterior aspect of the heel. These ulcers tend to be predominantly vascular in origin. Clinical experience has shown that they respond poorly to the weight-relieving measures, such as total contact casts, that are so effective in the forefoot and midfoot; because the source is not primarily mechanical. Patients with ulcerations over any portion of the heel—posterior, sides or plantar—need expeditious vascular evaluation. The fat pad under the heel is relatively vascular tissue. When a heel ulcer occurs, frequently there is occlusion, or stenosis of the arterial branches to the heel that arise from the posterior tibial artery, and revascularization must take priority consideration.

Immune Abnormalities

Diabetics do not necessarily have an increased susceptibility to bacterial infection, but once infection is present, many diabetic patients appear to have abnormalities in combating the infection. Laboratory studies have demonstrated the altered chemotaxis of polymorphonuclear leukocytes. Capillary abnormalities affect white cell migration as well.[17]

Gait Abnormalities

Numerous studies have documented gait abnormalities and increased pressures under the feet of diabetic patients with neuropathy.[18–21] These contribute to our understanding of the etiology of ulceration in patients with advanced neuropathy, and cor-

respond to the role of pressure in the development of ulceration in neuropathic feet. More work remains to be done to investigate gait abnormalities in diabetic patients.

Local Tissue Factors

Local tissue factors are conditions that may change the nutrition or perfusion of the soft tissue. They include edema of the tissue, callus formation, fungal colonization of the skin, or hyperkeratotic lesions.

Systemic Abnormalities

Systemic factors, apart from neuropathy and vasculopathy, that affect healing of lesions of the diabetic foot include control of diabetic hyperglycemia and the nutritional status of the patient. Several authors have stated that better control of the primary abnormality of the diabetes, hyperglycemia, resulted in better healing of the wounds of the lower limb.[22] Conversely, infection, including foot infection, is commonly recognized to be a source of sudden worsening in glucose control, with erratic and marked elevation of serum glucose. The surgical literature is replete with studies that point to the need for adequate nutrition for healing of surgical wounds. The same is true for healing of diabetic ulcers. The simple indices of nutrition that indicate whether or not the patient has adequate nutrition for wound healing are total lymphocyte count of > 1500/ml, total protein > 6.2 gm/dl, and albumin > 3.5 gm/dl.[23]

Diagnosis: Practical Evaluation of the Diabetic Foot and Diabetic Patient

History

A thorough history is the first step in diagnosis of this uniquely unpredictable and diversely manifest disease. It is particularly important to include specific information needed to assess risk in the diabetic patient, including knowledge of a previous history of a neuropathic event, such as ulceration, Charcot joint, or extensive infection from minor injury. We need to know date of onset, and duration of diabetes; types of diabetes therapy, ie, insulin dependent or non-insulin dependent; duration of insulin therapy; frequency of blood glucose testing, and whether it is recorded; and visual function. Can the patient see well enough to use a glucometer, and to inspect his/her own feet and shoes? It is also helpful to inquire about flexibility (can the patient flex the hip and knee sufficiently to touch and see his/her own sole?); about mobility (use of walking aids such as crutches, walker, or wheelchair); about the distance the patient can walk, and symptoms of claudication with walking. We need to know the dates and nature of previous hospitalizations and surgeries for the feet, and the history of systemic disorders such as hypertension, renal disease, atherosclerotic heart disease, retinal surgery or corneal implants, and kidney or pancreas organ transplant. It is important to list immunosuppressive medications.

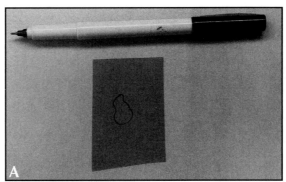
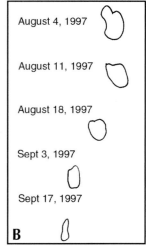

Fig. 4 A, The ulcer is traced on a clear film, and then, **B,** the ulcer outlined is traced into the chart to keep an accurate chronological record of ulcer size and shape.

August 4, 1997

August 11, 1997

August 18, 1997

Sept 3, 1997

Sept 17, 1997

Physical Examination

Examination of the foot and ankle includes the following 6 areas of concern. Vascular testing includes capillary refill, color, warmth, and hair growth. Sensory testing includes light touch, pinprick and/or position sense, and Semmes-Weinstein monofilament testing. Testing of joints checks range of motion, and looks for contractures or deformities. Tendons are tested for equinus, Achilles contracture, and flexor and extensor contractures. Bones are examined for changes in arch, unusual bony prominences, and any change in shape or orientation

of the foot. The skin is checked for breaks in the skin, onychomycosis, ingrown nails, and paronychia. Ulcerations, if present, are examined to determine site, depth, presence of granulation, exposed deep structures, surrounding cellulitis, proximal lymphangitis. Ulcers are traced onto clear film (Fig. 4, *A*) and the tracings are needed sequentially into the chart with date and orientation to give a chronologic record of ulcer size (Fig. 4, *B*).

Radiographs

Radiographs should be done standing, when possible. Standing films provide a technique that is easier to reproduce by different technologists or by the same technologist at different times. Some conditions, either local to the foot (such as a recent fracture) or systemic in the patient (poor balance, or an open plantar wound), may preclude the use of standing films. In these instances, a sitting film that places the foot plantigrade on or next to the radiographic cassette is preferable to films taken in the supine position, which have a rather unpredictable outcome. Interpretation of the films should include inspection for fractures and dislocations (either

recent or remote), deformity, Charcot joints, bone erosion in an area of a soft-tissue wound, and arterial calcification.

Vascular Studies

Laboratory evaluation of the vascular status of every diabetic patient is not necessary. Many, if not most, patients will present with strong and palpable pulses. In this situation, it is rarely necessary to incur the expense of conducting noninvasive vascular testing. However, when the patient clearly has diminished pulses, or pulses that cannot be felt at all, then vascular testing is most certainly indicated, particularly if the patient has a concurrent problem with the foot, such as a non-healing ulcer, or a progressive infection. Vascular insufficiency should be suspected in nonhealing ulcers in which appropriate pressure-relieving measures have failed to produce significant improvement. The level of vascularity necessary to maintain the uninjured foot is much less than that required to heal the injured one. That is, any trauma (such as infection, ulcers, or surgery) increases the metabolic requirements of the foot and limb. In a foot that has marginal perfusion, any trauma (including surgi-

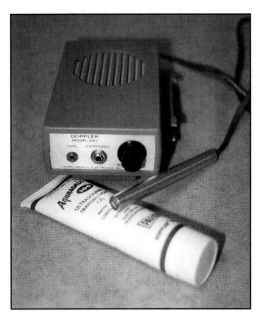

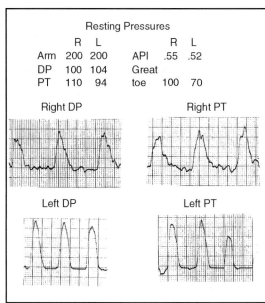

Fig. 5 Doppler arterial pulse-volume recording. (Reproduced with permission from Brodsky JW: Outpatient diagnosis and care of the diabetic foot, in Heckman JD (ed): *Instructional Course Lectures 42.* Rosemont, IL, American Academy of Orthopaedic Surgeons, 1993, pp 121–139.)

cal intervention) can push the patient over the edge of this fine balance, resulting in a nonhealing wound, or even gangrene.

Vascular evaluation usually begins with noninvasive testing. In patients who test positive and who have a clinical problem related to the arterial insufficiency (a nonhealing wound or osteomyelitis that requires debridement or partial foot amputation), consultation with a vascular surgeon is recommended. If reconstruction of the ischemia is considered, the vascular surgeon will usually order arteriography to demonstrate the lesions, their location, and severity.

There are several types of noninvasive vascular testing, but the 2 most commonly employed are arterial Doppler ultrasound and transcutaneous oxygen tension (TcPO$_2$) measurement. Multiple studies have been done evaluating both methods as predictors of amputation healing, that is, the ability to determine viable amputation levels preoperatively.[21] Fewer studies have been done evaluating these studies as predictors of healing of ulcerations. The literature suggests

that they are approximately equivalent in accuracy, although some advocates believe that the TcPO$_2$ measurement is more accurate. It is also somewhat more cumbersome and time-consuming and is somewhat temperature dependent. TcPO$_2$ measurement is not applicable distal to the midfoot, so it offers no equivalent to toe pressures with the Doppler technique. Arterial Doppler ultrasound has the advantage of being less expensive, less cumbersome, but more of an extrapolation, rather than direct data on blood flow. Arterial Dopplers are based on the assumption that flow in the vessel is proportionate to the amount of pressure required to compress the vessel to the point of occlusion. This is the same physiologic assumption on which the measurement of arterial blood pressure at the antecubital fossa is based. These blood pressures are taken in the same manner, with the exception of the use of an ultrasonic probe instead of a stethoscope. In noncalcified vessels, these assumptions are dependable, and the data is accurate relative to the established norms. The

ratio between the ultrasound-determined ankle arterial pressure and the same pressure method measuring at the antecubital fossa has been widely used. It has been referred to as the ankle-brachial index (ABI) or the ankle pressure index (API). Earlier references referred to this number as a reliable predictor of healing.[24,25] However, falsely elevated pressures are obtained when the Doppler technique is applied to the limb with arterial calcification, because greater pressures are necessary to occlude the stiffened, noncompliant vessel. Because vessel calcification is common in diabetes, it is necessary to look to additional information beyond the numbers and their ratios. Two more reliable forms of ultrasound information are toe plethysmography pressures and pulse-volume waveform recordings (Fig. 5). Toe pressures have been demonstrated to be a more accurate predictor of healing than ankle/arm ratios. Toes with an arterial pressure of 40 mm Hg or greater were shown to be most likely to heal. Below this level, healing was much less likely.[26] These pressures are measured using a small toe cuff. The vessels in the digits are less susceptible to the changes of calcification than those more proximal in the limb. Pulse volume recordings (PVRs) are tracings done on graph paper, similar to an electrocardiogram, which show the pattern of flow at a given level of ultrasound evaluation. PVRs demonstrate the quality of vessel compliance and whether or not there is pulsatile flow at a given level of the lower limb. The tracings demonstrate the pattern of the flow, which is related both to the compliance and patency of the vessel. Normal flow is triphasic (Fig. 5, *top right*) as demonstrated with the first and largest peak representing systole, the negative curve below baseline representing diastole, and the secondary smaller positive peak representing the contracture of the vessel walls. Biphasic and monophasic flow patterns demonstrate progressive loss of the normal resilience of the vessel wall (Fig. 5, *bottom left* and *right*). Both TcPO$_2$ and Doppler arterial ultrasound are screening techniques. The arteriogram is definitive, but not without its own risks, especially that of acute tubular necrosis from the contrast material. This risk is elevated if the patient is dehydrated.

The goal of vascular evaluation, and when needed, vascular reconstruction, is to provide adequate perfusion to the limb so that it can survive both injury and surgery. In nonemergent situations, revascularization by the vascular surgeon should precede orthopaedic surgery. In addition to aggressive debridement of infection and the use of partial foot amputation rather than below knee amputation where applicable, revascularization is a major factor in limb salvage surgery in the diabetic.

Laboratory Studies

Laboratory studies of the blood may be helpful in the presence of a severe

Table 1		
The depth/ischemia classification of diabetic foot lesions		
Grade	Definition	Treatment
Depth Classification		
0	The "at risk" foot. Previous ulcer, or neuropathy with deformity that may cause new ulceration	Patient education Regular examination Appropriate shoewear and insoles
1	Superficial ulceration, not infected	External pressure relief: Total contact cast, walking brace, special shoewear, etc
2	Deep ulceration exposing tendon or joint (with/without superficial infection)	Surgical debridement → wound care → pressure relief if closes and converts to grade 1 (PRN antibiotics)
3	Extensive ulceration with exposed bone, and/or deep infection: ie, osteomyelitis or abscess	Surgical debridements → ray or partial foot amputations → IV antibiotics → pressure relief if wound converts to grade 1
Ischemia Classification		
A	Not ischemic	Adequate vascularity for healing
B	Ischemia without gangrene	Vascular evaluation (Doppler, TcPO$_2$, arteriogram, etc.) → vascular reconstruction PRN
C	Partial (forefoot) gangrene of foot	Vascular evaluation → vascular reconstruction (proximal and/or distal bypass or angioplasty) → partial foot amputation
D	Complete foot gangrene	Vascular evaluation → major extremity amputation (BKA, AKA) with possible proximal vascular reconstruction

PRN, as needed; IV, intravenous; TcPO$_2$, transcutaneous oxygen pressure; BKA, below-knee amputation; AKA, above-knee amputation

(Reproduced with permission from Brodsky JW: The diabetic foot, in Mann RA, Coughlin MJ (eds): *Surgery of the Foot and Ankle*, ed 6. St. Louis, MO, Mosby Year Book, 1993, pp 1361–1467.)

infection in the foot of a diabetic. However, the white blood cell count (WBC), in particular, can be misleading in the presence of a major infection. Diabetics may fail to mount a febrile response, even in the presence of deep and extensive infection. This is even more true in the ever-increasing population of diabetics who have received kidney or combined kidney-pancreas transplants and are on life-long immunosuppressive drug regimens. When

there is clearly elevated WBC and local cellulitis, studies have documented the improvement in surgical outcome if the local and systemic parameters for infection are made to recede with wound care and intravenous antibiotics prior to performing definitive surgical resection and closing.[27]

Imaging Studies

Imaging studies can be a helpful part of the diagnostic evaluation of the diabetic foot. They should not be used routinely, but rather they are used to find occult fracture and early Charcot deformities (prior to radiographic changes), and to look for infection. Dilemmas arise, not infrequently, regarding the presence and extent of infection. It is critical to keep in mind that not all radiographic bone changes are caused by osteomyelitis. In fact, osteomyelitis is rarely seen in the diabetic foot unless there is or has been a contiguous break in the soft tissue. By contrast, diabetic osteopathy can include neuropathic fractures, spontaneous resorption of phalanges and distal portions of metatarsals, and extensive periosteal elevation along the tibia as a result of chronic venous stasis.

Cellulitis is far more common than abscess formation. If the latter is suspected, magnetic resonance imaging (MRI) is very helpful, as well as cost effective[28] for detecting deep infection. While MRI is a relatively expensive procedure, early application in suspected deep infection is a cost-saving strategy, because it can allow rapid decision-making with regard to surgical débridement. Early intervention may yield better results and reduce length of hospital stay by answering the diagnostic question.

However, it is important to understand the limitations of MRI. MRI has been shown to be extremely sensitive to changes in the bone, even more sensitive than a technetium-99 bone scan early in the disease process.[29] What the MRI has in sensitivity, it lacks in specificity with regard to imaging of the bone. Any disease process affecting the bone, or even adjacent to the bone, will cause a change in the bone signal because of edema (increased water content) of the marrow. This is not specific for osteomyelitis, which cannot be distinguished from trauma or fracture by MRI signal alone. However, in most medical centers and in the community, it is generally more cost-effective, if an occult fracture, or other bone process is suspected, to screen with a bone scan rather than with MRI. MRI is uniquely valuable in the detection and definition of the extent of soft-tissue lesions, such as abscess formation in the diabetic foot.

Once an area of suspected bone injury or occult Charcot process is identified, details of the exact nature and extent of the process should be obtained by complex motion tomography or computed tomography, which can then be directed to the area identified by the screening test. The classic example is the hot, red, swollen foot which is suspicious for abscess and appears cellulitic, in a patient who is afebrile and appears well systemically. While it is important to remember that the systemic response to infection in the extremity can often be blunted or absent in diabetic patients, the other diagnostic possibility is that this is the acute inflammation of a Charcot foot prior to the appearance of radiographic changes.

Even more confusing can be the case of a patient with a chronic Charcot foot that has collapsed, producing a bony prominence leading to ulceration. The patient presents with infection in the foot, but it is not clear whether the infection is confined to the soft tissues, or whether it involves the bone (osteomyelitis). In this situation combined, simultaneous Tc-99 bone scan and indium-labeled white blood cell scan can sometimes make this distinction.[30] However, this technique also has its drawbacks and limitations. First, it is cumbersome and time-consuming, and it requires an experienced team to administer and properly time the 2 separate administrations of radionuclides, because this is a test that spans 24 to 30 hours. Second, the interpretation of the Indium study can be frustrating or inconclusive because the low level of counts produce poor spatial resolution, and make interpretation difficult in a substantial number of cases.

Wound Classification

Wound classification of the diabetic foot began with the landmark system developed by Wagner and Meggitt at Rancho Los Amigos in the 1970s. In the Wagner-Meggitt classification,[24] there were 5 grades, which described the wound and also the condition of the entire foot. The depth of the wound, the association with infection, and the vascular status of the wound are all included in this classification. It has been the standard by which description of diabetic soft-tissue lesions could be compared throughout the world, and it is one of the most frequently cited works in the field of the diabetic foot. Because the Wagner-Meggitt classification was the earliest classification system, several other wound and foot wound classifications have emerged in recent years to advance our ability to describe the lesions and conditions of the diabetic foot, excluding, on the whole, the conditions and stages of Charcot joints.[31]

The Depth-Ischemia Classification (Table 1), a modification of the Wagner classification, has several advantages. It is simple and easy to remember, and its principles are familiar. It addresses the viability and condition of the foot by separately describing the wound and the underlying vascular status of the foot.

In the Depth-Ischemia Classification each foot is assigned a number, which represents the status or depth of the wound, and a letter, which represents the vascular status of the foot.

The justification for this is that the old Wagner classification allowed a number of confusing combinations of lesions and, in certain instances, incorrectly represented the true condition of the foot by the assigned grade. For example, if a foot had forefoot ischemia with uninfected soft tissues and a superficial ulcer under one of the lesser metatarsal heads, it is inadequately descriptive for it to be classified as a grade 1 lesion (superficial ulcer), but it is exaggerated to call it a grade 4 lesion (partial forefoot gangrene). The Depth-Ischemia classification is more concise and practical and separates the two concepts of wound severity and ischemia, which are not related, as was implied by the old classification. Moreover, in the original classification, a grade 1 lesion (superficial ulcer) clearly could be seen to progress to a grade 2 (deep ulcer) and then to a grade 3 (osteomyelitis or abscess). However, there is no logical progression from osteomyelitis (grade 3) to forefoot gangrene (grade 4). The original Wagner classification showed a reversibility between and among some lesions that was not possible, such as the reversion from grade 4 (gangrene) to grade 3 (osteomyelitis).

The Depth-Ischemia classification is represented in Table 1. There are four levels in each part of the classification. In the depth portion, grade 0 is the foot at risk. This foot has no current ulceration or wound, but is classified as at risk because of a history of a previous ulceration or because of the presence of sensory neuropathy, especially with deformity in the toes or foot.

Grade 1 is a superficial ulcer, which is neither infected nor has exposed at its base any deep structure (Fig. 6). Grade 2 is a deep ulcer, which has exposed a deep structure of tendon or joint, but not bone (Fig.

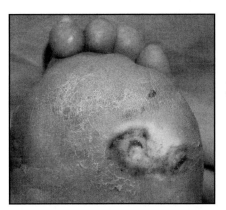

Fig. 6 Grade 1A diabetic ulcer. The wound is relatively superficial.

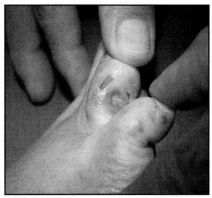

Fig. 7 Grade 2A diabetic ulcer. The proximal interphalangeal joint capsule is exposed.

7). A grade 2 lesion may or may not have superficial infection. A grade 3 lesion is extensive ulceration with exposure of the bone and/or deep infection. If the bone is palpated through the ulcer with a sterile, blunt instrument, it is grade 3, and probably has osteomyelitis[32] (Fig. 8). The deep infection can be osteomyelitis and/or abscess.

The first of the four levels in the "Ischemia" portion of the classification is grade A, which represents the foot that is not ischemic. There is sufficient vascularity for healing of the wound. No diagnostic or therapeutic vascular intervention is required. Grade B is a level of ischemia that may impair healing, but has not yet led to gangrene. This is clearly a wide band on the spectrum; but as a classification group it is justified by the corresponding treatment, vascular evaluation, and possible vascular reconstruction. A large group of lesions of the diabetic foot fall in this category. Grade C is partial gangrene of the foot. This level also requires vascular evaluation and possible reconstruction, but these feet are evaluated and treated for the best level of amputation that can be healed. This grade denotes the fact that partial foot salvage is now

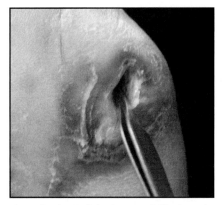

Fig. 8 Grade 3B diabetic wound. The bone is palpable at the depth of the ulcer. Radiographs demonstrate early osteomyelitis.

the best possible outcome. Grade D is complete gangrene of the foot. While this patient also requires vascular evaluation and possible proximal vascular bypass, the goal is no longer foot salvage, but rather limb salvage. Determination of the level of amputation, either above the knee amputation or below the knee amputation, is now the question.

Clinical Problems and Outpatient Treatments

Although it may seem that a host of indescribable problems assail the diabetic foot, these can be categorized into the 5 major areas, vascular disease, ulcerations, infections, Charcot

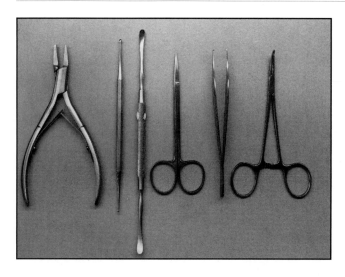

Fig. 9 Basic nail care instruments for the clinic.

Outline 1
Nail care instruments

Double-action bone rongeur
Anvil nail splitter
Freer elevator
Hemostat for nail removal
Cotton-tipped swabs
Nail currette
Pointed iris scissors and Adson's forceps
Hobby drill with sanding disks/drums

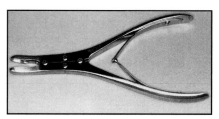

Fig. 10 Double-action rongeur for nail trimming.

joints, and amputations. These chapters on the diabetic foot reflect the design of the course itself over the last 4 years in the division of the lectures according to these subjects. Vascular disease has been discussed above. In the following lectures, Dr. Conti will discuss ulcerations, in particular the use of total contact casts in outpatient treatment; Dr. Saltzman will discuss infection and its treatment; Dr. Johnson will discuss the outpatient and inpatient management of Charcot joints; Dr. Smith discusses the criteria and techniques for amputation and foot salvage. Three treatment areas, wound care, skin and nail care, and patient education, are discussed below.

Wound Care

Innovations in the treatment of diabetic foot wounds, especially plantar ulcers, continue to be sought and found by many researchers in different fields. These innovations include the use of hyperbaric oxygen, platelet-derived and other topical wound-healing factors, and skin substitutes. A number of these new developments hold promise of improved wound healing, but as many questions have been raised as have been answered. First, what is the goal? Is it to achieve closure of a wound that otherwise would not have healed? Most uninfected wounds fail to heal because of ischemia or persistent pressure on the soft tissue. If that is the case, will a topical or local modality supercede the import of the basic principles of adequate perfusion and relief of pressure? If, as is likely, these modalities do not supercede these 2 principles, then what advantage is sought? In many

studies, the goal sought, or at least the result gained, is more rapid healing of the wound. A few excellent studies have demonstrated quicker wound healing, but data are still lacking to conclude that the reduced days or weeks of treatment represent a clinically significant improvement in outcome. While some of these modalities have succeeded in achieving more rapid wound healing, are they sufficiently better, qualitatively or quantitatively, to justify the costs, especially in this cost-conscious era? We must still investigate how long the healed feet remain healed and whether these modalities add anything to our typical prescription of shoes and insoles. On the other hand, if ease of treatment is greatly enhanced, such innovations may well prove to be keys to an overall higher level of care of the diabetic foot by all specialties of medicine.

Skin and Nail Care

Routine skin and nail care in the diabetic patient is an unglamorous but essential part of both treatment and prevention. Most of the routine work is done by a nurse, physician's assistant, or other trained medical affiliate, but the orthopaedic surgeon must still know and understand enough to direct these activities. It is essential to be willing to deal with these small problems properly in order to give both correct and complete care, and to prevent escalation of small problems to larger ones.

The basic instruments for the care of the nails in the clinic or office are shown in Figure 9 and are listed in Outline 1. The single most useful tool is a double action rongeur, such as the one depicted in Figure 10. This powerful bone-cutting instrument provides the safest method for trimming a thickened, onychomycotic nail that defies cutting with ordinary nail clippers (Fig. 11). It can generate

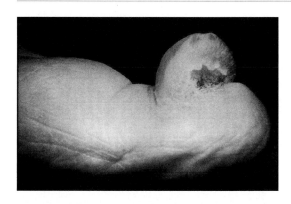

Fig. 11 A thickened, hypertrophic, onychomycotic great toe nail. (Reproduced with permission from Brodsky JW: Outpatient diagnosis and care of the diabetic foot, in Heckman JD (ed): *Instructional Course Lectures 42.* Rosemont, IL, American Academy of Orthopaedic Surgeons, 1993, pp 121–139.)

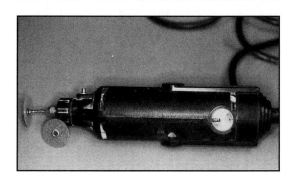

Fig. 12 Electric hobby drill for sanding down calluses and nails in diabetic patients.

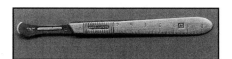

Fig. 13 The No. 17 blade, designed specifically for callus and ulcer trimming. Note the rounded shape.

sufficient force to nibble away the nail without twisting, elevating, or avulsing it. The rounded beaks protect the surrounding soft tissue and can be used to carefully push the soft tissue away. The nail should be trimmed in multiple small bites, not sheared in a single stroke. In grossly thickened nails, the nail can be thinned somewhat, as well as shortened. The edges are then smoothed with the electric sander (Fig. 12).

The electric sander is the safest instrument for smoothing and reducing calluses and nails. It works rather slowly on very thick, fungal nails; therefore, it is more efficient to trim them first. However, if the personnel doing this task are not highly skilled with the rongeur, or if the patient has severe or unreconstructable peripheral vascular disease, it is safer to use the sander alone. The primary danger is that the sanding disk can become a rotating blade when turned sideways. Sanding drums as well as disks can be used. The sander should be used on the slowest speed. When used to reduce calluses, the skin temperature should be tested intermittently with the examiner's fingertip to guard against overheating and burning the skin, because the patient may not feel it.

To trim calluses, as well as the hyperkeratotic borders of ulcers, the number 17 scalpel blade is ideally suited (Fig. 13). It has a double edge, but a rounded shape, which reduces the risk of nicking the patient. It fits a regular scalpel handle.

Autonomic neuropathy can cause the skin of the feet to be excessively dry and scaly. As the skin loses its normal compliance, it tends to crack and fissure, leading to infection. Patients with these skin problems should be instructed in the use of a skin moisturizing routine to keep the skin pliable. Various moisturizing creams and lotions are acceptable. One practical and inexpensive routine is to have the patient spread a thin layer of petroleum jelly on the feet after the shower or bath to seal in the water absorbed by the skin. Reduction of the calluses themselves also helps to prevent cracking.

In addition to routine trimming, nail care includes treatment of infected and uninfected ingrown nails. Most ingrown nails occur in the hallux. It is not the distal corner alone that becomes ingrown, rather the entire side of the nail. Infection follows ingrowing, and similarly begins along medial or lateral borders, or both. In order to cure the infection, it is necessary to decompress the area by removing the nail margin, allowing drainage. It is imperative to assure that the patient has adequate perfusion before this very distal procedure is performed. If necessary, the patient is first sent to the vascular laboratory for evaluation. Some procedures are delayed because of the newfound need for vascular reconstruction.

The anvil-type nail splitter is the ideal method for this procedure, which is usally done under digital block anesthesia. The lower jaw of the splitter is flat and separates the nail from the nail bed. The upper jaw of the splitter is triangular in cross-section and it splits the nail as it comes down on the flat lower blade (Fig. 14). The split-off section of the nail is then elevated with the blunt end of a Freer or other elevator. The nail section is removed with a clamp, and the resulting pocket is gently,

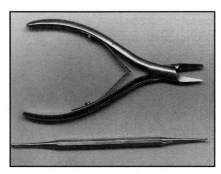

Fig. 14 Nail splitter ("nail anvil") has a flat lower jaw to slide between the nail bed and the nail plate. The upper jaw is sharp and splits the nail against the lower jaw, protecting the nail bed.

superficially explored and gently debrided with a curette to remove fibrous material, but not to remove the matrix itself. This nail splitter is safer to use than a scalpel, because it prevents laceration of the nail bed. The nail bed is a very thin layer directly over the phalanx, and bone involvement, with infection, is possible. It is safer, more effective, and more reliable to use the phenol to ablate the matrix cells than to use the curette to remove the matrix, which is seldom, if ever, complete.

If the ingrown nail is a recurring problem, in addition to removal of the nail margin, ablation of the corresponding margin of the matrix and nail bed is required. After removal of the nail under the ischemia of a digital tourniquet (made of a 2.5-inch penrose drain), phenol is applied to ablate the cells of the nail matrix and nail bed. I have found that 2 applications of 90 seconds duration is successful, with each application followed by an alcohol rinse. Prior to applying the phenol each time, the nail bed must be thoroughly dried. Application is done with cotton-tipped swabs.

Patient Education

Patient education is said to be important in all medical problems, but in the diabetic patient, it is critical. Prevention of diabetic foot problems remains the very best treatment, and the patient must take the responsibility for prevention through a self-care program. Much has been done to set the stage. Many clinics and hospitals offer diabetic education. The American Diabetes Association has great resources available for patient education and teaching. The American Association of Diabetic Educators is dedicated to the enormous task of teaching diabetic patients about all aspects of their care, including glucose testing, insulin administration, and many other parts of the disease, in addition to inspection of the feet.

We, too, must encourage a program of daily or twice daily foot and shoe inspection. Patients and/or family members must be taught to shake out shoes before donning to remove any foreign objects. They must look all around and over the feet for signs of erythema, discoloration, or breaks in the skin. Many of our patients cannot do this for themselves. They may be too stiff or arthritic to position the foot for viewing, or they may have impaired vision from diabetic retinopathy. Use of a mirror can be handy. Most often the help of a family member or friend must be enlisted. The goal is to build daily inspection into the routine of bathing and dressing. Allied medical professionals can teach these techniques to the patient.

References

1. *Diabetes: 1997 Vital Statistics*. Alexandria, VA, American Diabetes Association, 1997.

2. Delbridge L, Ctercteko G, Fowler C, Reeve TS, Le Quesne LP: The aetiology of diabetic neuropathic ulceration of the foot. *Br J Surg* 1985;72:1–6.

3. Masson EA, Hay EM, Stockley I, Veves A, Betts BP, Boulton AJ: Abnormal foot pressures alone may not cause ulceration. *Diabet Med* 1989;6:426–428.

4. Brand PW: The insensitive foot (including leprosy), in Jahss MH (ed): *Disorders of the Foot and Ankle: Medical and Surgical Management,* ed 2. Philadelphia, PA, WB Saunders, 1991, vol 3, pp 2170–2186.

5. Gelberman RH, Szabo RM, Williamson RV, Dimick MP: Sensibility testing in peripheral-nerve compression syndromes: An experimental study in humans. *J Bone Joint Surg* 1983;65:632–638.

6. Levin S, Pearsall G, Ruderman RJ: Von Frey's method of measuring pressure sensibility in the hand: An engineering analysis of the Weinstein-Semmes pressure aesthesiometer. *J Hand Surg* 1978;3A:211–216.

7. Brodsky JW, Chambers R, Kwong PK, Wagner FW: Abstract: Patterns of disintegration in the Charcot tarsus of diabetes and relation to treatment. *Foot Ankle* 1986;6:323–324.

8. Chantelau E, Ma XY, Herrnberger S, Dohmen C, Trappe P, Baba T: Effect of medial arterial calcification of O2 supply to exercising diabetic feet. *Diabetes* 1990;39:938–941.

9. Irwin ST, Gilmore J, McGrann S, Hood J, Allen JA: Blood flow in diabetics with foot lesions due to "small vessel disease." *Br J Surg* 1988;75:1201–1206.

10. LoGerfo FW, Coffman JD: Vascular and microvascular disease of the foot in diabetes. Implications for foot care. *N Engl J Med* 1984;311:1615–1619.

11. Louie TJ, Bartlett JG, Tally FP, Gorbach SL: Aerobic and anaerobic bacteria in diabetic foot ulcers. *Ann Intern Med* 1976;85:461–463.

12. Oskarsson P, Ljunggren JG, Lins PE: Efficacy and safety of mexiletine in the treatment of painful diabetic neuropathy: The Mexiletine Study Group. *Diabetes Care* 1997;20:1594–1597.

13. Stracke H, Meyer UE, Schumacher HE, Federlin K: Mexiletine in the treatment of diabetic neuropathy. *Diabetes Care* 1992;15:1550–1555.

14. Delbridge L, Perry P, Marr S, et al: Limited joint mobility in the diabetic foot: Relationship to neuropathic ulceration. *Diabet Med* 1988;5:333–337.

15. Fernando DJ, Masson EA, Veves A, Boulton AJ: Relationship of limited joint mobility to abnormal foot pressures and diabetic foot ulceration. *Diabetes Care* 1991;14:8–11.

16. Brodsky JW: The diabetic foot, in Mann RA, Coughlin MJ (eds): *Surgery of the Foot and Ankle,* ed 6. St. Louis, MO, CV Mosby, 1993.

17. Bagdade JD, Root RK, Bulger RJ: Impaired leukocyte function in patients with poorly controlled diabetes. *Diabetes* 1974;23:9–15.

18. Bauman JH, Girling JP, Brand PW: Plantar pressures and trophic ulceration. *J Bone Joint Surg* 1963;45B:652–673.

19. Boulton AJ, Betts RP, Franks CI, Newrick PG, Ward JD, Duckworth T: Abnormalities of foot pressure in early diabetic neuropathy. *Diabetic Med* 1987;4:225–228.

20. Ctercteko GC, Dhanendran M, Hutton WC, Le Quesne LP: Vertical forces acting on the feet

of diabetic patients with neuropathic ulceration. *Br J Surg* 1981;68:608–614.

21. Duckworth T, Boulton AJ, Betts RP, Franks CI, Ward JD: Plantar pressure measurements and the prevention of ulceration in the diabetic foot. *J Bone Joint Surg* 1985;67B:79–85.

22. Rayfield EJ, Ault MJ, Keusch GT, Brothers MJ, Nechemias C, Smith H: Infection and diabetes: The case for glucose control. *Am J Med* 1982;72:439–450.

23. Dickhaut SC, DeLee JC, Page CP: Nutritional status: Importance in predicting wound-healing after amputation. *J Bone Joint Surg* 1984;66A: 71–75.

24. Wagner FW Jr: Part II: A classification and treatment program for diabetic, neuropathic and dysvascular foot problems, in Cooper RR (ed): American Academy of Orthopaedic Surgeons *Instructional Course Lectures XXVIII*. St. Louis, MO, CV Mosby, 1979, pp 143–165.

25. Wagner FW Jr: The dysvascular foot: A system for diagnosis and treatment. *Foot Ankle* 1981; 2:64–122.

26. Apelqvist J, Castenfors J, Larsson J, Stenstrom A, Agardh CD: Prognostic value of systolic ankle and toe blood pressure levels in outcome of diabetic foot ulcer. *Diabetes Care* 1989;12: 373–378.

27. Bessman AN, Wagner W: Nonclostridial gas gangrene: Report of 48 cases and review of the literature. *JAMA* 1975;233:958–963.

28. Morrison WB, Schweitzer ME, Wapner KL, Hecht PJ, Gannon FH, Behm WR: Osteomyelitis in feet of diabetics: Clinical accuracy, surgical utility, and cost-effectiveness of MR imaging. *Radiology* 1995;196:557–564.

29. Yuh WT, Corson JD, Baraniewski HM, et al: Osteomyelitis of the foot in diabetic patients: Evaluation with plain film, 99mTc-MDP bone scintigraphy, and MR imaging. *Am J Roentgenol* 1989;152:795–800.

30. Splittgerber GF, Spiegelhoff DR, Buggy BP: Combined leukocyte and bone imaging used to evaluate diabetic osteoarthropathy and osteomyelitis. *Clin Nucl Med* 1989;14:156–160.

31. Pecoraro RE, Reiber GE: Classification of wounds in diabetic amputees. *Wounds* 1990; 2:65–73.

32. Grayson ML, Gibbons GW, Balogh K, Levin E, Karchmer AW: Probing to bone in infected pedal ulcers: A clinical sign of underlying osteomyelitis in diabetic patients. *JAMA* 1995; 273:721–723.

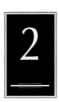

The Diabetic Foot: Basic Mechanisms of Disease

Gregory P. Guyton, MD
Charles L. Saltzman, MD

Diabetic foot disease is usually thought of in simple terms: neuropathy leads to ulceration and neuroarthropathy. However, a number of more subtle aspects are critical in the development of the disorder. For practical purposes, the diabetic neuropathy cannot be altered, but the additional causes of the disease often can be treated, tipping the balance back in favor of healing.

In the absence of large-vessel disease, diabetic foot disease is predicated on two inexorably linked factors: neuropathy and an abnormal mechanical environment. A freely floating foot will not ulcerate, and most patients with a deformed foot will not use it to the point of ulceration if sensory feedback instructs them not to do so. Both factors require closer examination.

Diabetic Neuropathy

The heterogeneous nature of diabetic neuropathy produces the variable course of diabetic foot disease. All components of the nervous system can be affected, including sensation, motor control, pain, proprioception, and autonomic functions, but, in any given patient, the mix of components that are affected determines how and when complications will develop (Fig. 1).

Somatic neuropathy is the most wide-ly recognized pattern and affects both sensory and motor components. This pattern begins with the classic "stocking-and-glove" distribution; as nerve function diminishes along the length of the axon, the longest nerves are affected first. Diminished distal sensation is the hallmark of this neuropathy, and several methods have been developed for quantification. The Semmes-Weinstein monofilaments are the easiest to apply and the most widely used.[1,2] Each monofilament is a piece of nylon line of a precise diameter that is applied end-on to the skin until the line begins to bend, providing a reproducible, metered sensory stimulus. The level of sensation for a specific patient is recorded as the smallest size of monofilament felt by the patient. Recognition of the 5.07 monofilament represents the threshold of "protective sensation"—that is, the amount of sensation required to avoid the possibility of unrecognized injury. In approximately 90% of diabetic patients who can feel the 5.07 monofilament, ulceration does not develop.[1]

The disease does not confine itself to classic patterns, however. Proximal diabetic neuropathy, also known as diabetic amyotrophy, is a relatively uncommon variant of somatic neuropathy that pri-marily affects the motor component and causes profound weakness in the proximal muscles of the lower extremity.[3] Clinically, it is more like a muscular dystrophy than a classic neuropathy. The etiology of amyotrophy is not clear, but early evidence suggests an autoimmune-mediated vasculopathy involving the vasa nervorum.

Diabetic mononeuropathy, another rare form of the disease,[4,5] is an acute event involving a single peripheral nerve at a single site, and it is believed to originate from an occlusive event or vasculitis in the microvasculature supplying the nerve. Fortunately, the clinical effects usually are self-limited, and recovery is common.

Autonomic neuropathy represents one of the most underrecognized components of the disease. Direct measurement of sympathetic nerve activity in unmyelinated postganglionic C fibers is possible with use of intraneural micro-electrodes.[6] Fagius[7] showed that sympathetic nerve impulses were absent in 64% of patients with diabetic neuropathy compared with 19% of patients who had other types of polyneuropathy. Autonomic dysfunction can manifest primarily as failure of the parasympathetic system, with a loss of heart-rate regulation and gastrointestinal motility, or as

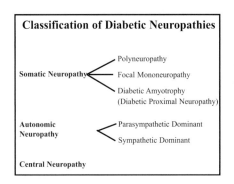

Fig. 1 Diabetic neuropathy can present in a wide variety of patterns. An individual patient may have any combination of the general syndromes listed above.

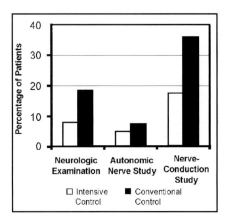

Fig. 2 The results of the Diabetes Control and Complications Trial indicated that the percentage of patients in whom abnormalities developed was significantly lower in association with intensive glucose control, according to the findings of both neurologic examination and objective nerve-conduction studies. (Adapted with permission from The Diabetes Control and Complications Trial Research Group: The effect of intensive treatment of diabetes on the development and progression of long-term complications in insulin-dependent diabetes mellitus. *N Engl J Med* 1993;329:982.)

failure of the sympathetic system, with disordered neurogenic control of blood flow. Parasympathetic or sympathetic dysfunction may predominate in any given patient.[8]

Evidence that diabetic neuropathy may extend to the central nervous system is also emerging. To date, this research has focused on diabetes-related impotence, and specific forms of cognitive dysfunction and impaired central pathways have been discovered in patients with that condition.[9-11] It is certainly possible that future research may uncover a central component that is relevant to abnormalities of the foot.

Why diabetic neuropathy has so many different clinical patterns is not at all clear. The answer must lie in the factors that cause the nerve injury itself.[12] The 1993 Diabetes Control and Complications Trial demonstrated that the progression of all components of neuropathy was clearly and directly related to glycemic control[13] (Fig. 2). Diabetes affects tissues that do not require insulin-mediated glucose transport pumps, including the retina, kidneys, and nerves, which glucose enters by diffusion. Unlike retinopathy and nephropathy, however, neuropathy originates primarily from the direct effects of glucose rather than from the indirect effects of microangiopathy.

The most commonly proposed mechanism of damage is called the "sorbitol theory." Normally, glucose is broken down, and ATP (adenosine triphosphate) is produced through the hexokinase pathway. In the presence of extremely high levels of glucose, the enzymes controlling the hexokinase pathway become saturated. The excess glucose goes into an alternative metabolic pathway and is converted to sorbitol through a series of reactions controlled by the enzyme aldose reductase. An unfortunate by-product of this "sorbitol pathway" is that the redox potential of the cell is lowered. This, in turn, impairs fatty acid metabolism, reducing axonal transport.[14] With use of aldose reductase inhibitors, which keep glucose from entering this pathway, the progression of neuropathy has been ameliorated in animal models of diabetes.[15,16]

Another commonly cited metabolic role of hyperglycemia is nonenzymatic glycosylation, a phenomenon active in a wide variety of tissues, including nerve, vascular basement-membrane, and connective tissue.[17,18] The long-term exposure of long-lived proteins, including nerve myelin, to high glucose levels eventually leads to the covalent bonding of an advanced glycation end product, disrupting protein function.[19] While the theory appears to explain the effects of diabetes on connective tissue (as will be discussed), experiments with aminoguanidine, an inhibitor of nonenzymatic glycation, have shown only mixed results in animal models of diabetic neuropathy.[20]

Recent reports also have indicated that autoimmunity may play a role, particularly in the autonomic component of diabetic neuropathy.[21,22] Vernino and associates[21] recently described autoantibodies to ganglionic acetylcholine receptors in patients with a wide variety of autonomic neuropathies, including diabetic dysautonomia. Differing roles of autoimmunity may ultimately explain a great deal of the pattern variation seen among neuropathic patients.

The Abnormal Mechanical Environment
Overuse
Static and dynamic deformities contribute to the development of diabetic foot disease, but these structural deformities are likely less important than subtle overuse. Neither extraordinarily high pressures nor abnormal shear forces are necessary to cause ulceration; ordinarily tolerable pressures lead to ulceration if the exposure is repeated too many times. This concept was first explained by Brand,[23] whose early efforts were focused not on diabetes but on leprosy. He demonstrated that "repetitive moderate stress" (as a light pressure stimulus) applied to a sensate rat forepaw at a rate of 10,000 repetitions per day could reliably lead to blistering in 1 week and to ulceration in 10 days. The initial areas of necrosis developed in the densely innervated regions of the deep layers of dermis

and underlying subcutaneous tissue. Modestly dropping the rate to 8,000 repetitions per day and pausing on weekends allowed the rats to continue indefinitely without ulceration. When denervated rat forepaws were tested, the number of repetitions that could be tolerated at any given pressure was reduced. Brand hypothesized that subtle repositioning of the forepaw by the sensate rats provided just enough intermittent mechanical relief to stave off tissue necrosis, while the insensate rats simply had no feedback telling them to do so. The same process is almost certainly at work in humans. Notably, the prevalence of ulceration is remarkably low in patients who have rheumatoid arthritis and other diseases that create severe foot deformity and locally elevated plantar pressures in the absence of neuropathy.[24]

Shear Stress

In addition to the number of loading events, the direction of loading is thought to influence the development and healing of plantar ulcers. Measuring stress parallel to the skin surface is difficult, and direct data on shear stress in the diabetic foot are sparse. However, indirect evidence for the importance of shear is highlighted by the unique anatomy of the soles and the palms. The sole of the human foot has evolved into a complex architecture of fat embedded in a network of fine, but collectively strong, collagen fibrils that span from the skin to the underlying osteotendinous structures to absorb shock and resist shear.[25] Shear has long been implicated in the development of blisters and has been shown experimentally to occur as a result of repetitive friction.[26] The interaction of sweating, sebum secretion, and the skin's coefficient of friction suggests that local biologic activity, including function of the sympathetic nervous system, influences susceptibility to blister formation from exposure to repetitive shear.[27] In diabetic patients with healed foot ulcerations, maximal shear occurs in regions of maximal vertical force.[28] Therefore, until improved shear-sensing devices with increased resolution, reliability, and speed are available, normal stress serves as a reasonable surrogate for direct measurements of shear stress.

Static Deformity

Any deformity that increases pressure on any one portion of the foot can instigate ulceration in a patient with diabetic neuropathy. In a patient with a hallux valgus deformity, an ulcer may develop along the medial border of the pronated, deviated hallux or underneath the second metatarsal head as a transfer lesion. Similarly, ulcerations may develop underneath the lateral border of the midfoot in a patient who has a varus hindfoot resulting from a mild cavovarus foot. Diabetic neuropathy can transform previously manageable foot deformities into major sources of disease. It is beyond the scope of this chapter to discuss the gamut of fixed foot deformities; however, there are two special cases in which diabetic neuropathy contributes not only to the consequences of the deformity but also to their very origin.

Claw Toes

Any lesion that denervates the intrinsic muscles of the foot while preserving the long flexors and extensors can lead to claw toes. Without the modifying force of the intrinsics to flex the metatarsophalangeal joints and extend the interphalangeal joints, the opposite deformities develop, with an extended posture of the metatarsophalangeal joints and a flexion posture of the interphalangeal joints. The anatomic principle is homologous to the clawing seen after distal nerve lesions in the upper extremity. In a convincing demonstration of this principle, Mann photographed the claw-toe deformities that resulted when force was applied to only the long flexors and extensors in a fresh cadaveric limb.[29] The motor component of diabetic neuropathy, which is often overlooked, selectively affects the intrinsic muscles of the foot while preserving the more proximally innervated long motor units.[30]

The claw-toe deformity creates several sites of increased pressure, particularly after the deformity has been present for some time and has become fixed. Ulcers can occur under the tip of the toe where it strikes the floor or over the dorsum of the proximal interphalangeal joint where it strikes the shoe (Fig. 3). In addition, dorsiflexion of the metatarsophalangeal joint causes the metatarsal fat pad to be pulled distally through its attachments to the proximal phalanx, leaving only a thin layer of tissue between the metatarsal head and the floor. This leads to increases in peak pressures under the metatarsal heads and increased risk of ulceration.[31]

Charcot Arthropathy

While the mechanical problems associated with hammer toes are subtle and slow to develop, the deformities of Charcot arthropathy can be sudden and dramatic. Neuroarthropathy is one of the most difficult and intractable sources of excess mechanical pressure in the diabetic foot and can create large osseous prominences in various locations. Ulceration and rapid progression to osteomyelitis can follow (Fig. 4). A large prospective study of risk factors for ulcerations in a population of male diabetic patients showed that the presence of Charcot arthropathy carried the highest relative risk of all of the factors examined, eclipsing even the absence of protective sensation and a history of amputation.[32]

Soft-Tissue Contractures

Diabetes acts on the foot not only through the indirect mechanisms of neuropathy but also by direct impact on the tissues themselves. Initially, high glucose concentrations lead to the formation of reversible breakdown products of glucose that bind to free amino groups on proteins. Prolonged exposure of long-lived

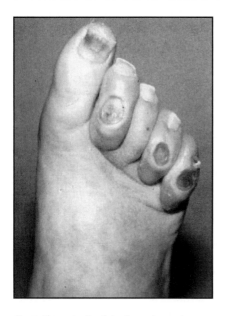

Fig. 3 Photograph of the foot of a patient with neuropathic claw toes, showing ulcerations over the prominent dorsal aspects of the proximal interphalangeal joints where the toes rubbed against the shoe.

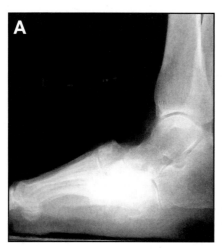
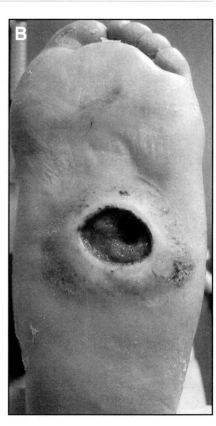

Fig. 4 A and **B,** A radiograph and clinical photograph of the foot of a patient with a midfoot ulceration from Charcot arthropathy with subsequent collapse. Osseous deformity resulting from neuroarthropathy is one of the strongest risk factors for the development of ulceration.

proteins to this environment initiates a series of poorly understood dehydrations and rearrangements, yielding an irreversibly bound advanced glycation end product, or AGE.[19] The theory that these end products are important factors is supported by the experimental finding, in animal models, that diabetic complications were prevented by the administration of aminoguanidine, a potent inhibitor of nonenzymatic glycation.[17] Collagen appears to be particularly susceptible because cross-links derived from advanced glycation end products occur along the entire length of the molecule, dramatically stiffening its construct.[17,18] Joint contractures in the hand (presumably from type I collagen involvement) are strongly correlated with such microvascular complications of diabetes as retinopathy and nephropathy.[33-35] In addition, the development of joint contracture has been shown to correlate directly with glycemic control, a result that would

be expected if the contracture were due to the nonenzymatic accumulation of advanced glycation end products.[36,37]

In a diabetic patient, progressive stiffening of the collagen-containing tissues manifests itself in a number of ways and can be implicated, in part, in the syndromes of adhesive capsulitis in the shoulder, flexor tenosynovitis about the hand and wrist, Dupuytren's contracture, and "limited joint mobility."[38] The last syndrome, consisting of multiple contractures of the small joints, originally was called "diabetic cheiropathy" and has been increasingly recognized since its original description in 1957.[39] This syndrome can be detected clinically with use of the "prayer sign," in which the patient is asked to flatten the hands together as if to pray (Fig. 5). If the patient has limited joint mobility, the combined effects of small flexion contractures at both the interphalangeal joints and the metacarpophalangeal joints do not allow the

palms to flatten and a small space is visible between the fingers.

Although easily seen in the hand, limited joint mobility has been identified in the foot as well.[40] Delbridge and associates[41] identified a substantial impairment in the subtalar range of motion in diabetic patients with a history of ulceration compared with that in control populations of both nondiabetic and diabetic subjects without a history of foot disease. Limited subtalar motion also was associated with limited joint mobility in the hand. Mueller and associates[42] found that subtalar motion in diabetic patients with a history of ulceration was diminished compared with that in controls. Fernando and associates[43] reported elevated plantar pressures in the forefoot and limited subtalar joint motion in patients who had limited joint mobility as assessed by measurements of metacarpophalangeal and interphalangeal joint motion in the hand.

In addition to capsular contractures of

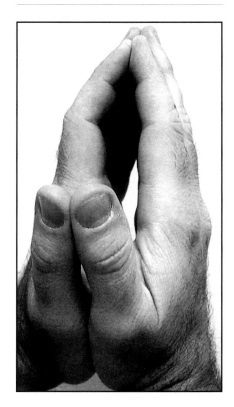

Fig. 5 A patient with diabetic cheiropathy (limited joint mobility) exhibits the "prayer sign." Subtle contractures at the interphalangeal and metacarpophalangeal joints prevent the fingers from fully opposing each other. A space is visible between the fingers when a praying posture is attempted.

the joints, increasing stiffness can occur in the motor units powering the foot. This is particularly true in the gastrocnemius-soleus complex. Yosipovitch and Sheskin,[44] in a study of neuropathic patients with leprosy, proposed that a stiff gastrocnemius-soleus complex forces the heel up earlier in the gait cycle, thus placing increased loads on the forefoot. Subsequent reports have confirmed the presence of a tight heel cord and limited ankle dorsiflexion in diabetic patients with a history of ulceration.[42,45] Lin and associates[46] successfully used percutaneous lengthening of the Achilles tendon to treat ulcers that previously had been recalcitrant to treatment with a total-contact cast alone and also found a reduced rate of ulcer recurrence after lengthening.

Similarly, Armstrong and associates[47] observed that percutaneous lengthening of the Achilles tendon reduced forefoot pressures in neuropathic diabetic patients with a history of ulceration.

Gait Abnormality

Perhaps the most compelling argument for gait abnormalities as a factor in the pathogenesis of the diabetic foot is that deformity alone still fails to explain why ulceration develops in some patients but not in others. While ulcers clearly occur at sites of high loading in some diabetic patients, the lesions never develop in a great many patients with high focal pressures.[24,32,48-50] Smith and associates[50] reported that the maximal pressures under the sites of previous ulceration in patients with a history of ulceration were higher than those in matched diabetic control patients with no history of ulceration. However, the pressure patterns were identical to those on the contralateral side, even when the contralateral foot had never had an ulcer. Veves and associates,[49] in a prospective study of 86 diabetic patients with documented high pressures in the plantar aspect of the foot, reported that ulcerations developed in 35% of the patients within 30 months, a finding that had been noted in earlier small studies as well.[24] Although that figure is substantial, it is difficult to explain why ulcerations do not develop in even more patients. While behavioral factors and shoe wear may hold much of the answer, subtle gait changes in patients with diabetic neuropathy also have been proposed as an additional etiology.

Altered proprioception and postural instability have been reported in patients with diabetic neuropathy and a history of ulceration.[51] These observations imply that, not surprisingly, posterior column function and proprioception as well as the other components of the somatic nervous system are affected in diabetic neuropathy. It is still unclear how these findings translate into abnormalities of gait. Cavanagh and associates suggested that an absence of afferent feedback during gait in neuropathic subjects leads to increased variability of gait kinematics in the sagittal plane, although the effect proved difficult to elicit when the subjects walked on a treadmill.[52,53] Other investigators have found that patients with diabetic neuropathy subtly use the hip flexors to assist in bringing the leg forward rather than pushing off with the gastrocnemius-soleus muscles,[54] have a slower overall walking speed,[55] and have increased peak plantar-flexor moments. All of these effects are due to increased passive stiffness of the gastrocnemius-soleus complex.[56] Taken as a whole, the weight of evidence in the literature suggests that there is indeed a gait abnormality in these patients, but its exact nature remains to be clearly defined.

Additional Factors

In addition to the etiologies of neuropathy and an abnormal mechanical environment seen in all patients with diabetic foot disease, there are other factors that can contribute. While these factors are certainly not universal, they may play a dominant role in some patients.

Sweat

Sweating represents a unique autonomic function in that it has a mixture of both sympathetic and parasympathetic components. Although the nerve fibers that stimulate sweat glands run with the sympathetic outflow, the fibers themselves are entirely cholinergic with the exception of a few adrenergic fibers to the palms and the soles.[57] Parasympathetic centers in the hypothalamus are ultimately responsible for the stimulation of sweat production; therefore, sweating is best viewed as a unique parasympathetic function that is anatomically segregated in the sympathetic pathways. In this way, altered sweat function represents the only clear mechanism by which failure of a parasympathetic rather than a sympathet-

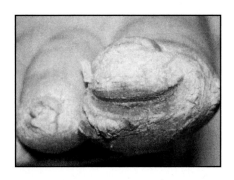

Fig. 6 The hallux of a patient with severe autonomic neuropathy. In this disorder, the normal sweat function is disrupted, resulting in dry, cracked skin that can serve as a portal for infection.

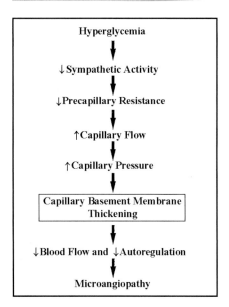

Fig. 7 A diagram representing a partial explanation of the pathogenesis of microangiopathy.

ic system can lead to disease in the diabetic foot. Sweat function can be assessed with use of the quantitative sudomotor axon reflex test (QSART), in which sweating is induced by iontophoresis of a metered dose of acetylcholine and a sweat cell is used to calculate the resultant volume of sweat produced per unit area of skin.[58] Ahmed and Le Quesne[59] found sweat production to be well below the nondiabetic control range in 75% of patients with a history of a neuropathic ulcer. A similar result was reported by Ryder and associates.[60] As the stimulation of sweating is lost, the resulting dry skin becomes scaly and fissures develop (Fig. 6). The crevices can run deep into the dermis and serve as a portal for infection. It is for this reason that long-term lubrication is an important component of preventive care of a diabetic foot.

Vascular Disease

Arteriosclerotic disease is more prevalent, occurs at an earlier age, is more diffuse, accelerates faster, and is more extensive in patients with diabetes than in patients without diabetes. Pathologically, the arterial intima and media show changes. In a diabetic patient, plaques develop circumferentially along the length of the vessel and calcification occurs within the tunica media. A commonly affected area for diabetic patients is the popliteal trifurcation and the distal runoff of these vessels. The underlying reasons for the diffuse development of diabetic angiopathy remain unclear and may be different between patients with type I and type II diabetes. Both mechanical and biologic factors have been implicated. A chronic decrease in shear stress abnormalities has been found to contribute to endothelial dysfunction in patients with hypertension, although this effect has not been demonstrated in patients with diabetes.[61]

Biologic mediators of endothelium-dependent vasodilation have been implicated in the development of diabetic macrovascular disease. The chief putative causes involve abnormalities of signal transduction mechanisms, alterations in cell-membrane fluidity that change the expression or presentation of a wide range of receptors, or changes in oxidative stress.[62] Of these potential disturbances, the strongest evidence points to an intrinsic dysfunction of nitric oxide (NO).[63] NO is an important cellular mediator that interferes with monocyte and leukocyte adhesion to the endothelium, platelet-vessel wall interaction, smooth muscle proliferation, and vascular tone, all key in the development of atherosclerosis. Chronic hyperglycemia appears to lead to the local formation of reactive oxygen species such as superoxide or hydrogen peroxide, which bind NO, reducing its local bioavailability. In addition, excessive postprandial lipidemia induces enhanced oxidative stress and a diminished action of NO.[64]

Diabetic retinopathy and nephropathy are almost entirely due to microvascular disease, and almost certainly the same microvascular disease plays a role in the development and persistence of ulcers by impairing the skin's nutritive blood flow reserve.[65] The pathognomonic histologic feature of diabetic microangiopathy is a generalized basement-membrane thickening in capillaries, arterioles, and venules.[66] The pathophysiology of microangiopathy is complex. Recent-onset diabetes is characterized by an increase in tissue blood flow that is partially normalized by glycemic control. However, as the duration of diabetes increases, microvascular blood flow decreases and autoregulation is lost.[67,68] This pattern can be observed in diverse microvascular beds, including the eye,[69] kidney,[70,71] and skin,[65,72] supporting the concept that a fundamental microvascular control mechanism is disturbed in patients with diabetes. There is now convincing evidence that the increased peripheral blood flow in patients with diabetes is due to precapillary vasodilatation[67,73,74] that leads to capillary hyperperfusion and capillary hypertension[75] (Fig. 7). The precapillary vasodilatation that appears to be instrumental in starting the process could result from a variety of different factors, including hyperglycemia, altered blood flow mechanics, vascular smooth-muscle dysfunction, or endothelial dysfunction, although autonomic neuropathy is the mostly likely initiator.[67,76] Excessive pressure stimulates the endothelial cells to produce more extracellular matrix proteins, leading to a thickening of the capillary basement membrane.[77] The formation of advanced glycation end products and the abnormal cross-linking of type IV collagen also may contribute to the process.[17-19,33-35] Capillary sclerosis ultimately results and is accompanied by limited microvascular blood flow, dysfunctional autoregulation, and impaired oxygen and nutrient exchange.

The sympathetic nervous system is known to play an important role in the control of microvascular function.[78,79] Neurogenic control of the microcirculation permits global metabolic needs to be fulfilled and is balanced with local autoregulation of the microcirculation, which reflects local tissue requirements. Dysfunctional sympathetic neurovascular control can produce a profound microcirculatory disturbance with capillary hypertension, impaired postural vasoconstriction, increased arteriovenous shunting, and abnormal inflammatory responses to tissue injury.[80-82] With time, the resulting capillary hypertension and microangiopathy can add to the pathologic process by impairing blood flow through the vasa nervorum, thereby adding an ischemic component to the neuropathy itself.[83]

Abnormal Wound Healing of Established Diabetic Ulcers

When approaching diabetic foot ulceration, the first question to be addressed is: "Why do diabetic ulcers occur?" Equally important, though, is the question: "Why don't they heal?" The answer to the second question involves some unexpected subtlety. There are several additional factors related to the wound environment itself that cannot necessarily be implicated in the creation of ulcers but that clearly act to perpetuate them once they are established.

Tissue oxygen tensions of 20 to 30 mm Hg are required for the secretion of collagen by fibroblasts, and low tissue-oxygen concentrations reduce the secretion of collagen by fibroblasts.[84] Oxygen is also necessary for energy-dependent metabolic processes, fibroblast proliferation, and epithelialization.[85-88] Normal

tissue oxygenation is also vital for combating bacterial infection, and an impaired oxygen supply increases the risk of infection.[85,86,88] Extramolecular oxygen, when reduced to superoxide, has potent bactericidal effects, and oxygen is critical to the functioning of granulocytes, which use oxygen to produce free radical oxidants to control bacteria by oxidizing cell membranes and by interfering with protein enzymatic processes.[89] White blood cells accelerate oxygen consumption during phagocytosis and intracellular killing, and their killing capacity is severely limited in low-oxygen environments.[90,91]

The degree to which tissue oxygen influences the healing of diabetic foot ulcers in the context of other intrinsic and extrinsic variables in the healing environment remains equivocal. Most randomized, controlled trials of diabetic foot ulcers have excluded patients whose transcutaneous oxygen tension ($TcPO_2$) is less than 30 mm Hg,[92,93] so that the impact of tissue oxygen levels on healing cannot be analyzed. An exception is the study by Boyko and associates,[94] who compared dry and moist dressings and reported that $TcPO_2$ on the dorsum of the affected foot was significantly higher for subjects in whom the ulcer had healed than for subjects in whom it had not healed over a 4-week period, regardless of dressing type.

If local oxygenation is poor enough to cause tissue necrosis, the negative effects are amplified and necrotic tissue is associated with wound infection.[95,96] Endotoxins that are released from dying cells can kill or injure nearby healthy cells, and high levels of endotoxins prevent fibroblasts and keratinocytes from reaching the wound site. Sapico and associates[96] reported that foot ulcers demonstrated large numbers of both aerobes and anaerobes only when necrotic tissue was present and that the density of all organisms was greater in wounds with necrotic tissue than in those without it. Robson and associates,[97] in their seminal study of

pressure ulcers, established that a bacterial level of more than 10^5 organisms per gram of tissue resulted in delayed healing. The notable exception was β-hemolytic streptococci, as a lower level of such organisms (10^3 per gram of tissue) was sufficient to produce the effect.[97] Soft-tissue or bone infection can prolong the inflammatory phase of wound healing, destroy surrounding tissue, increase protease activity, and retard epithelialization and collagen deposition. Steed and associates[98] showed that débridement may enhance the healing of diabetic foot ulcers by lowering the bacterial burden and eradicating growth-factor inhibitors from the wound environment. Therefore, débridement of necrotic tissue in an ulcer has a sound biologic basis.

Overt malnutrition, as well as subtle nutritional deficits, can affect wound repair and resistance to infection. Wound-healing abnormalities usually are associated with protein-calorie malnutrition rather than with depletion of a single nutrient,[99,100] and preliminary work by Wipke-Tevis and Stotts[101] suggested that nutritional deficiencies are present in a large proportion of patients with vascular ulcers. The data are sparser for diabetic foot ulcers, but nutrition has been implicated in the pathogenesis of the broad spectrum of chronic wounds, and it is doubtful that diabetic ulcers would be an exception.[102]

Competent immune function is vital to the wound-healing process and is necessary for the synthesis, release, and regulation of the numerous endogenous growth factors, inflammatory cells, and proliferative cells involved in wound repair. In patients with foot ulcers, the influence of chronic hyperglycemia on leukocyte function has important implications for healing.[103] Diminished chemotaxis, phagocytosis, and intracellular bacterial killing lead to impaired healing because of a less efficient inflammatory response. Even in the absence of infection, however, the altered function of neutrophils, macrophages, and lymphocytes can further limit healing by decreasing fibroblast proliferation and collagen deposition. The extent to which hyperglycemia-related immunopathy limits the healing of diabetic foot ulcers has not been delineated completely.

The role of short-term glucose control in wound healing is complex and is not fully understood. Goodson and Hung[104] demonstrated significantly reduced tensile strength and hydroxyproline content when wounds in animals with acute experimental diabetes were compared with wounds in control animals. Insulin treatment for the first 11 days following wounding corrected the hyperglycemia and improved healing. If insulin administration was not begun until the 11th postoperative day and was continued thereafter, the impaired healing was not corrected. On the other hand, Barr and Joyce[105] reported that re-endothelialization of an experimental microarterial anastomosis was slowed in rats with streptozotocin-induced diabetes and that impaired healing was not alleviated by treatment with insulin starting at the time of the operation and continuing postoperatively. Seifter and associates[106] found that supplemental vitamin A given to rats with streptozotocin-induced diabetes alleviated the impaired healing without affecting the hyperglycemia, suggesting that its effects were independent of glucose control. It has been suggested that high glucose levels interfere with cellular transport of ascorbic acid into various cells, including fibroblasts, and cause decreased leukocyte chemotaxis.[107] Glucose is similar in structure to ascorbic acid and may competitively inhibit its transport across cell membranes.[107] In the context of other intrinsic and extrinsic factors that influence the wound-healing environment of diabetic foot ulcers, the role of short-term glucose control remains uncertain.

The Special Case of Charcot Arthropathy

Neuroarthropathy, or "Charcot arthropa-
thy," is a diagnosis that predates the modern era of long-term survival with diabetes, having been first described in patients with tertiary syphilis.[108] Despite a history of 130 years in the medical literature, the disorder remains an enigma that deserves special consideration.

Shortly after publication of Charcot's original description of neuroarthropathy, a school of thought evolved that implicated repetitive, unrecognized microtrauma to the anesthetic joint as the sole etiology. In 1917, Eloesser[109] concluded, from a series of experiments on cat knees, that both an anesthetic joint and an element of trauma were required for joint destruction. In reality, he did not demonstrate the primary onset of neuroarthropathy but rather the acceleration of posttraumatic arthrosis. Similarly modern animal models have been inappropriately cited as models of Charcot arthropathy.[110] This "neurotraumatic" hypothesis entered the literature and served as the mainstream view for over half a century.[111,112] A challenge to this hypothesis is based on a number of troubling anecdotal observations that have lent support to the notion that something more than unrecognized repetitive trauma is involved. For example, Schwarz and associates[113] described a diabetic patient in whom a Charcot foot developed immediately following a surgical sympathectomy, neuropathic joints are occasionally seen in the lower extremities of paraplegic patients, and Norman and associates[114] and Knaggs[115] independently reported neuropathic arthropathy of the hip in patients managed with complete bed rest.

The origin of the alternative "neurovascular" hypothesis is commonly attributed to Leriche,[116] who noted concurrent osseous hyperemia and osseous resorption following sympathetic nerve damage. This hypothesis was concisely articulated by Watkins and Edmonds[117] as follows: "Sympathetic denervation of arterioles causes an increased blood flow,
which in turn causes rarefaction of bone, making it prone to damage even after minor trauma. Loss of sensation from somatic neuropathy, in particular reduction of pain sensation, permits abnormal stresses that would normally be prevented by pain. Relatively minor trauma can therefore cause major destructive changes in susceptible bones."

This hypothesis has been accepted, at least in part, by the authors of many studies,[117-119] for it offers an alternative explanation for some of the questions left unsolved by the neurotraumatic hypothesis. Alterations in blood flow following the sympathetic dysfunction brought on by diabetic neuropathy are well documented.[117,120] The phenomenon of "dependent rubor," in which the dependent leg is markedly engorged with blood that drains rapidly when the leg is elevated, is common in patients with neuroarthropathy (Fig. 8). Even in the absence of radiographic abnormalities, increased blood flow to bone has been demonstrated directly in the neuropathic foot by radioisotope uptake studies.[121] Some global measurements of autonomic function correlate with blood flow measurements. Uccioli and associates,[122] in a study of diabetic patients, correlated the results of a series of cardiovascular tests with the prevalence of arteriovenous shunting as assessed with use of the albumin microsphere technique. They found direct correlations between the shunt fraction (an implied measure of the effect of the sympathetic outflow on the vasculature of the foot) and two global sympathetically mediated phenomena (postural hypotension and sustained hand grip), as well as one parasympathetic phenomenon (deep-breathing heart rate variation). More directly, Young and associates[123] found evidence of autonomic dysfunction in a significantly higher proportion of patients with Charcot arthropathy than in matched neuropathic patients without arthropathy. Anecdotal evidence in support of the neurovascular

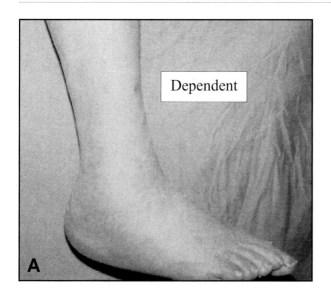
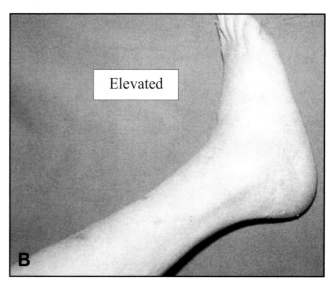

Fig. 8 Diabetic patients with autonomic dysfunction often have engorged vasculature when the foot is dependent (**A**). Disordered autoregulation allows the blood to drain rapidly when the foot is elevated, and the color of the leg fades (**B**). This phenomenon of "dependent rubor" is especially common in patients with neuroarthropathy.

hypothesis was provided by Edelman and associates,[124] who reported three patients in whom neuroarthropathy developed immediately after the restoration of blood flow by surgical revascularization. Although it was not determined if the restored blood flow was supranormal, these cases suggest that at least adequate blood flow is necessary for Charcot changes to occur.

Sympathetic denervation has been implicated in structural as well as physiologic alterations in the vasculature.[117] Kerper and Collier[125] first demonstrated foci of medial necrosis in arteries following sympathectomy in 1926, and structural changes can occur in arterial smooth muscle after long-term denervation.[126] Clinically, Edmonds and associates[127] demonstrated a strong correlation between diffuse medial vascular calcifications (Mönckeberg sclerosis) and the presence of diabetic neuropathy. This correlation is strong enough that the radiographic appearance of smooth vascular calcifications can be used as a marker for sympathetic dysfunction in the extremity (Fig. 9).

Some animal studies have also lent support to the neurovascular hypothesis.

Verhas and associates[128] noted striking correlations between increased bone blood flow (as assessed with microsphere techniques) and bone resorption in paraplegic rats. McClugage and McCuskey[129] used direct observation of marrow changes to demonstrate osseous resorption around venules in high flow–high volume states.

While the neurovascular hypothesis has gained wide acceptance in recent years, it has failed, on close examination, to provide a fundamental mechanism linking increased bone blood flow and bone resorption. There is no a priori reason why this should be so. Only McClugage and McCuskey[129] addressed the issue directly when they theorized that the hydrostatic pressure in postcapillary venules led to bone resorption. It is important to remember that other physiologic conditions (such as fracture-healing) can increase bone blood flow dramatically and lead to a net deposition of bone. For the time being, the absence of a mechanism remains the weak link in an otherwise compelling neurovascular argument.

Charcot himself initially attributed neuropathic arthropathy to the absence of

"trophic" factors supplied to the bone by the peripheral nerves. Their absence, he believed, led to rapid bone destruction and eventual dissolution of the joint in only a matter of weeks.[108] No direct evidence in support of this hypothesis has emerged, but it remains an important potential alternative. Bone does indeed have a nerve supply at the ultrastructural level, as described by Cooper.[130] Moore and associates[131] described the presence of adrenergic receptors on osteoblasts and found that beta agonists could stimulate bone resorption in vitro, although their activity in vivo remains unproven. Perhaps of greater interest, though, is the very recent evidence that osteoclasts have receptors for neuropeptides. Gough and associates[132] found up-regulated serum levels of carboxyterminal type I collagen telopeptide (a marker of osteoclast activity) in the absence of increases in serum procollagen carboxyterminal propeptide (a marker of osteoblastic bone formation) when patients with an acute Charcot arthropathy of the foot were compared with controls. Evidence is accumulating that osteoclasts express mRNA for receptors of several small neuropeptides,

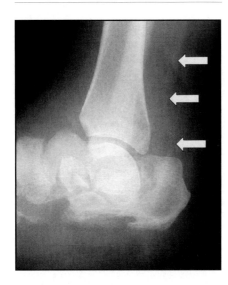

Fig. 9 Mönckeberg sclerosis (medial arterial calcification) is readily apparent on radiographs and is strongly associated with autonomic failure and Charcot arthropathy, as it was in this patient. Note the smooth, diffuse pattern of calcification (arrows) instead of the irregular intimal calcifications characteristic of common atherosclerosis.

including vasoactive intestinal peptide-1 and the related pituitary adenylate cyclase activating polypeptide,[133] both of which have been shown to down-regulate bone resorption in isolated osteoclast preparations.[134] A real possibility exists that modern molecular biology may yet prove Charcot's long-ignored neurotrophic hypothesis to be correct.

Just as in the pathophysiology of ulcers, one of the principal challenges faced by any theory of neuroarthropathy is explaining why the disease develops in some patients with apparently similar circumstances and with similar patterns of neuropathy. There are suggestions that the underlying metabolic changes in bone may in fact be more systemic than previously thought. Young and associates[123] found marked distal osteopenia on both the involved and the uninvolved sides in patients with Charcot arthropathy, and Gough and associates[132] found no difference between measurements of serum markers of bone turnover in samples drawn from the dorsal veins of involved feet and from the veins of upper extremities. Although additional work is clearly needed, both pieces of evidence suggest that there may in fact be a relatively large number of diabetic patients with a systemic disorder of bone metabolism awaiting only a relatively minor perturbation to trigger an episode of neuroarthropathy.

Summary

There remains vast truth in the statement "neuropathy causes diabetic foot pathology." However, if it were really that straightforward and if our understanding were complete, it is doubtful that ulceration and neuroarthropathy would be the public health problems that they are today. Diabetes is an insidious disease, and almost every component of the spectrum of hyperglycemic complications is active in creating foot lesions. These include dramatic alterations in all components of the peripheral nerves, the mechanical characteristics of bones and soft tissues, gait kinematics, the vasculature at both a microscopic and a macroscopic level, the immune system, and the fundamental processes of wound healing. Clinical treatments that address the biologic aspects of the problem without considering the mechanics, or vice versa, can sometimes be effective but fail to take advantage of all of the potential means to succeed. The greatest potential for future clinical advance lies in understanding and simultaneously addressing the many synergistic factors that cause both ulceration and neuroarthropathy.

References

1. Olmos PR, Cataland S, O'Dorisio TM, Casey CA, Smead WL, Simon SR: The Semmes-Weinstein monofilament as a potential predictor of foot ulceration in patients with noninsulin-dependent diabetes. *Am J Med Sci* 1995;309:76-82.

2. Pham H, Armstrong DG, Harvey C, Harkless LB, Giurini JM, Veves A: Screening techniques to identify people at high risk for diabetic foot ulceration: A prospective multicenter trial. *Diabetes Care* 2000;23:606-611.

3. Kelkar P, Masood M, Parry GJ: Distinctive pathologic findings in proximal diabetic neuropathy (diabetic amyotrophy). *Neurology* 2000;55:83-88.

4. O'Brian JT, Massey EW: Mononeuropathy in diabetes mellitus: A phenomenon easily overlooked. *Postgrad Med* 1979;65:128,130-132, 135-136.

5. Shahani B, Spalding JM: Diabetes mellitus presenting with bilateral foot-drop. *Lancet* 1969;2:930-931.

6. Vallbo AB, Hagbarth KE, Torebjork HE, Wallin BG: Somatosensory, proprioceptive, and sympathetic activity in human peripheral nerves. *Physiol Rev* 1979;59:919-957.

7. Fagius J: Microneurographic findings in diabetic polyneuropathy with special reference to sympathetic nerve activity. *Diabetologia* 1982;23:415-420.

8. Low PA, Zimmerman BR, Dyck PJ: Comparison of distal sympathetic and vagal function in diabetic neuropathy. *Muscle Nerve* 1986;9:592-596.

9. Ryan CM, Geckle MO: Circumscribed cognitive dysfunction in middle-aged adults with type 2 diabetes. *Diabetes Care* 2000;23: 1486-1493.

10. Sartucci F, Piaggesi A, Logi F, et al: Impaired ascendant central pathways conduction in impotent diabetic subjects. *Acta Neurol Scand* 1999;99:381-386.

11. Biessels GJ: Cerebral complications of diabetes: Clinical findings and pathogenetic mechanisms. *Neth J Med* 1999;54:35-45.

12. Thomas PK, Tomlinson DR: Diabetic and hypoglycemic neuropathy, in Dyck PJ, Thomas PK, Griffin JW, Low PA, Poduslo JF (eds): *Peripheral Neuropathy*, ed 3. Philadelphia, PA, WB Saunders, 1993, pp 1219-1250.

13. The effect of intensive treatment of diabetes on the development and progression of long-term complications in insulin-dependent diabetes mellitus: The Diabetes Control and Complications Trial Research Group. *N Engl J Med* 1993;329:977-986.

14. Tomlinson DR: Future prevention and treatment of diabetic neuropathy. *Diabetes Metab* 1998;24(suppl 3):79-83.

15. Shimoshige Y, Ikuma K, Yamamoto T, et al: The effects of zenarestat, an aldose reductase inhibitor, on peripheral neuropathy in Zucker diabetic fatty rats. *Metabolism* 2000;49: 1395-1399.

16. Sundkvist G, Dahlin LB, Nilsson H, et al: Sorbitol and myo-inositol levels and morphology of sural nerve in relation to peripheral nerve function and clinical neuropathy in men with diabetic, impaired, and normal glucose tolerance. *Diabet Med* 2000;17:259-268.

17. Brownlee M, Vlassara H, Kooney A, Ulrich P, Cerami A: Aminoguanidine prevents diabetes-induced arterial wall protein cross-linking. *Science* 1986;232:1629-1632.

18. Kent MJ, Light ND, Bailey AJ: Evidence for glucose-mediated covalent cross-linking of col-

lagen after glycosylation in vitro. *Biochem J* 1985;225:745-752.

19. Brownlee M: Glycation products and the pathogenesis of diabetic complications. *Diabetes Care* 1992;15:1835-1843.

20. Wada R, Sugo M, Nakano M, Yagihashi S: Only limited effects of aminoguanidine treatment on peripheral nerve function, (Na+,K+)-ATPase activity and thrombomodulin expression in streptozotocin-induced diabetic rats. *Diabetologia* 1999;42:743-747.

21. Vernino S, Low PA, Fealey RD, Stewart JD, Farrugia G, Lennon VA: Autoantibodies to ganglionic acetylcholine receptors in autoimmune autonomic neuropathies. *N Engl J Med* 2000;343:847-855.

22. Morano S, Tiberti C, Cristina G, et al: Autoimmune markers and neurological complications in non-insulin-dependent diabetes mellitus. *Hum Immunol* 1999;60:848-854.

23. Brand PW: The insensitive foot (including leprosy), in Jahss MH (ed): *Disorders of the Foot and Ankle: Medical and Surgical Management*, ed 2. Philadelphia, PA, WB Saunders, 1991, vol 3, pp 2170-2186.

24. Masson EA, Hay EM, Stockley I, Veves A, Betts RP, Boulton AJ: Abnormal foot pressures alone may not cause ulceration. *Diabet Med* 1989;6:426-428.

25. Bojsen-Moller F, Flagstad KE: Plantar aponeurosis and internal architecture of the ball of the foot. *J Anat* 1976;121:599-611.

26. Naylor PFD: Experimental friction blisters. *Br J Dermatol* 1955;67:327-342.

27. Cua AB, Wilhelm KP, Maibach HI: Frictional properties of human skin: Relation to age, sex and anatomical region, stratum corneum hydration and transepidermal water loss. *Br J Dermatol* 1990;123:473-479.

28. Pollard JP, Le Quesne LP, Tappin JW: Forces under the foot. *J Biomed Eng* 1983;5:37-40.

29. Coughlin MJ, Mann RA: Lesser toe deformities, in Coughlin MJ, Mann RA (eds): *Surgery of the Foot and Ankle*, ed 7. St Louis, MO, Mosby-Year Book, 1999, pp 320-391.

30. Negrin P, Fardin P: Multiple role of peripheral neuropathy in the pathogenesis of the so-called "diabetic foot:" Clinical and electromyographical (EMG) study of 42 cases of "mutilating acropathy." *Electromyogr Clin Neurophysiol* 1986;26:533-540.

31. Brodsky JW: The diabetic foot, in Coughlin MJ, Mann RA (eds): *Surgery of the Foot and Ankle*, ed 7. St Louis, MO, Mosby-Year Book, 1999, vol 2, pp 895-969.

32. Boyko EJ, Ahroni JH, Stensel V, Forsberg RC, Davignon DR, Smith DG: A prospective study of risk factors for diabetic foot ulcer: The Seattle Diabetic Foot Study. *Diabetes Care* 1999;22:1036-1042.

33. Jennings AM, Milner PC, Ward JD: Hand abnormalities are associated with the complications of diabetes in type 2 diabetes. *Diabet Med* 1989;6:43-47.

34. Rosenbloom AL, Silverstein JH, Lezotte DC, Richardson K, McCallum M: Limited joint mobility in childhood diabetes mellitus indi-

cates increased risk for microvascular disease. *N Engl J Med* 1981;305:191-194.

35. Arkkila PE, Kantola IM, Viikari JS, Ronnemaa T, Vahatalo MA: Limited joint mobility is associated with the presence but does not predict the development of microvascular complications in type 1 diabetes. *Diabet Med* 1996;13:828-833.

36. Silverstein JH, Gordon G, Pollock BH, Rosenbloom AL: Long-term glycemic control influences the onset of limited joint mobility in type 1 diabetes. *J Pediatr* 1998;132:944-947.

37. Arkkila PE, Kantola IM, Viikari JS: Limited joint mobility in non-insulin-dependent diabetic (NIDDM) patients: Correlation to control of diabetes, atherosclerotic vascular disease, and other diabetic complications. *J Diabetes Complications* 1997;11:208-217.

38. Rosenbloom AL, Silverstein JH: Connective tissue and joint disease in diabetes mellitus. *Endocrinol Metab Clin North Am* 1996;25: 473-483.

39. Lundbaek K: Stiff hands in long-term diabetes. *Acta Med Scand* 1957;158:447-451.

40. Campbell RR, Hawkins SJ, Maddison PJ, Reckless JP: Limited joint mobility in diabetes mellitus. *Ann Rheum Dis* 1985;44:93-97.

41. Delbridge L, Perry P, Marr S, et al: Limited joint mobility in the diabetic foot: Relationship to neuropathic ulceration. *Diabet Med* 1988;5:333-337.

42. Mueller MJ, Diamond JE, Delitto A, Sinacore DR: Insensitivity, limited joint mobility, and plantar ulcers in patients with diabetes mellitus. *Phys Ther* 1989;69:453-462.

43. Fernando DJ, Masson EA, Veves A, Boulton AJ: Relationship of limited joint mobility to abnormal foot pressures and diabetic foot ulceration. *Diabetes Care* 1991;14:8-11.

44. Yosipovitch Z, Sheskin J: Subcutaneous Achilles tenotomy in the treatment of perforating ulcer of the foot in leprosy. *Int J Lepr Other Mycobact Dis* 1971;39:631-632.

45. Bennett PJ, Stocks AE, Whittam DJ: Analysis of risk factors for neuropathic foot ulceration in diabetes mellitus. *J Am Podiatr Med Assoc* 1996;86:112-116.

46. Lin SS, Lee TH, Wapner KL: Plantar forefoot ulceration with equinus deformity of the ankle in diabetic patients: The effect of tendo-Achilles lengthening and total contact casting. *Orthopedics* 1996;19:465-475.

47. Armstrong DG, Stacpoole-Shea S, Nguyen H, Harkless LB: Lengthening of the Achilles tendon in diabetic patients who are at high risk for ulceration of the foot. *J Bone Joint Surg Am* 1999;81:535-538.

48. Frykberg RG, Lavery LA, Pham H, Harvey C, Harkless L, Veves A: Role of neuropathy and high foot pressures in diabetic foot ulceration. *Diabetes Care* 1998;21:1714-1719.

49. Veves A, Murray HJ, Young MJ, Boulton AJ: The risk of foot ulceration in diabetic patients with high foot pressure: A prospective study. *Diabetologia* 1992;35:660-663.

50. Smith L, Plehwe W, McGill M, Genev N, Yue DK, Turtle JR: Foot bearing pressure in

patients with unilateral diabetic foot ulcers. *Diabet Med* 1989;6:573-575.

51. Katoulis EC, Ebdon-Parry M, Hollis S, et al: Postural instability in diabetic neuropathic patients at risk of foot ulceration. *Diabet Med* 1997;14:296-300.

52. Cavanagh PR, Simoneau GG, Ulbrecht JS: Ulceration, unsteadiness, and uncertainty: The biomechanical consequences of diabetes mellitus. *J Biomech* 1993;26(suppl 1):23-40.

53. Dingwell JB, Ulbrecht JS, Boch J, Becker MB, O'Gorman JT, Cavanagh PR: Neuropathic gait shows only trends towards increased variability of sagittal plane kinematics during treadmill locomotion. *Gait Posture* 1999;10:21-29.

54. Mueller MJ, Minor SD, Sahrmann SA, Schaaf JA, Strube MJ: Differences in the gait characteristics of patients with diabetes and peripheral neuropathy compared with age-matched controls. *Phys Ther* 1994;74:299-313.

55. Katoulis EC, Ebdon-Parry M, Lanshammar H, Vileikyte L, Kulkarni J, Boulton AJ: Gait abnormalities in diabetic neuropathy. *Diabetes Care* 1997;20:1904-1907.

56. Salsich GB, Mueller MJ: Effect of plantar flexor muscle stiffness on selected gait characteristics. *Gait Posture* 2000;11:207-216.

57. Guyton AC (ed): *Textbook of Medical Physiology*, ed 7. Philadelphia, PA, WB Saunders, 1986, p 774.

58. Low PA, Caskey PE, Tuck RR, Fealey RD, Dyck PJ: Quantitative sudomotor axon reflex test in normal and neuropathic subjects. *Ann Neurol* 1983;14:573-580.

59. Ahmed ME, Le Quesne PM: Quantitative sweat test in diabetics with neuropathic foot lesions. *J Neurol Neurosurg Psychiatry* 1986;49:1059-1062.

60. Ryder RE, Kennedy RL, Newrick PG, Wilson RM, Ward JD, Hardisty CA: Autonomic denervation may be a prerequisite of diabetic neuropathic foot ulceration. *Diabet Med* 1990;7: 726-730.

61. Khder Y, Briancon S, Petermann R, et al: Shear stress abnormalities contribute to endothelial dysfunction in hypertension but not in type II diabetes. *J Hypertens* 1998;16:1619-1625.

62. Tooke JE: Possible pathophysiological mechanisms for diabetic angiopathy in type 2 diabetes. *J Diabetes Complications* 2000;14:197-200.

63. Cosentino F, Luscher TF: Endothelial dysfunction in diabetes mellitus. *J Cardiovasc Pharmacol* 1998;32(suppl 3):S54-S61.

64. Evans M, Khan N, Rees A: Diabetic dyslipidaemia and coronary heart disease: New perspectives. *Curr Opin Lipidol* 1999;10:387-391.

65. Rendell M, Bamisedun O: Diabetic cutaneous microangiopathy. *Am J Med* 1992;93:611-618.

66. Williamson JR, Kilo C: Vascular complications in diabetes mellitus. *N Engl J Med* 1980;302:399-400.

67. Tooke JE: Microvascular function in human diabetes: A physiological perspective. *Diabetes* 1995;44:721-726.

68. Ditzel J: Functional microangiopathy in diabetes mellitus. *Diabetes* 1968;17:388-397.

69. Sinclair SH, Grunwald JE, Riva CE, Braunstein SN, Nichols CW, Schwartz SS: Retinal vascular autoregulation in diabetes mellitus. *Ophthalmology* 1982;89:748-750.

70. Christiansen JS: Glomerular hyperfiltration in diabetes mellitus. *Diabet Med* 1985;2:235-239.

71. Parving HH, Kastrup H, Smidt UM, Andersen AR, Feldt-Rasmussen B, Christiansen JS: Impaired autoregulation of glomerular filtration rate in type 1 (insulin-dependent) diabetic patients with nephropathy. *Diabetologia* 1984;27:547-552.

72. Kastrup J, Norgaard T, Parving HH, Henriksen O, Lassen NA: Impaired autoregulation of blood flow in subcutaneous tissue of long-term type 1 (insulin-dependent) diabetic patients with microangiopathy: An index of arteriolar dysfunction. *Diabetologia* 1985;28:711-717.

73. Parving HH, Viberti GC, Keen H, Christiansen JS, Lassen NA: Hemodynamic factors in the genesis of diabetic microangiopathy. *Metabolism* 1983;32:943-949.

74. Zatz R, Brenner BM: Pathogenesis of diabetic microangiopathy: The hemodynamic view. *Am J Med* 1986;80:443-453.

75. Sandeman DD, Shore AC, Tooke JE: Relation of skin capillary pressure in patients with insulin-dependent diabetes mellitus to complications and metabolic control. *N Engl J Med* 1992;327:760-764.

76. Flynn MD, Tooke JE: Diabetic neuropathy and the microcirculation. *Diabet Med* 1995;12:298-301.

77. Riser BL, Cortes P, Zhao X, Bernstein J, Dumler F, Narins RG: Intraglomerular pressure and mesangial stretching stimulate extracellular matrix formation in the rat. *J Clin Invest* 1992;90:1932-1943.

78. Gaskell P, Burton AC: Local postural vasomotor reflexes arising from the limb veins. *Circ Res* 1953;1:27-39.

79. Renkin EM: Regulation of the microcirculation. *Microvasc Res* 1985;30:251-263.

80. Rayman G, Hassan A, Tooke JE: Blood flow in the skin of the foot related to posture in diabetes mellitus. *Br Med J (Clin Res Ed)* 1986;292:87-90.

81. Flynn MD, Hassan AA, Tooke JE: Effect of postural change and thermoregulatory stress on the capillary microcirculation of the human toe. *Clin Sci (Colch)* 1989;76:231-236.

82. Belcaro G, Nicolaides AN, Volteas N, Leon M: Skin flow the venoarteriolar response and capillary filtration in diabetics: A 3-year follow-up. *Angiology* 1992;43:490-495.

83. Fagerberg SE: Diabetic neuropathy: A clinical and histological study on the significance of vascular affections. *Acta Med Scand* 1959;345(suppl):1-80.

84. Hunt TK, Pai MP: The effect of varying ambient oxygen tensions on wound metabolism and collagen synthesis. *Surg Gynecol Obstet* 1972;135:561-567.

85. Hunt TK, Hussain Z: Wound microenvironment, in Cohen IK, Diegelmann RF, Lindblad WJ (eds): *Wound Healing: Biochemical and Clinical Aspects*. Philadelphia, PA, WB Saunders, 1992, pp 274-281.

86. Ehrlichman RJ, Seckel BR, Bryan DJ, Moschella CJ: Common complications of wound healing: Prevention and management. *Surg Clin North Am* 1991;71:1323-1351.

87. Paquet P, Lapiére CM: Causes of delayed wound healing and optimization of the patient's condition, in Westerhof W (ed): *Leg Ulcers: Diagnosis and Treatment*. Amsterdam, The Netherlands, Elsevier Science, 1993, pp 281-290.

88. Lawrence WT: Clinical management of non-healing wounds, in Cohen IK, Diegelmann RF, Lindblad WJ (eds): *Wound Healing: Biochemical and Clinical Aspects*. Philadelphia, PA, WB Saunders, 1992, pp 541-561.

89. White MJ, Heckler FR: Oxygen free radicals and wound healing. *Clin Plast Surg* 1990;17:473-484.

90. Hohn DC: Host resistance to infection: Established and emerging concepts, in Hunt TK (ed): *Wound Healing and Wound Infection: Theory and Surgical Practice*. New York, NY, Appleton-Century-Crofts, 1980, pp 264-279.

91. LaVan FB, Hunt TK: Oxygen and wound healing. *Clin Plast Surg* 1990;17:463-472.

92. Steed DL, Goslen JB, Holloway GA, Malone JM, Bunt TJ, Webster MW: Randomized prospective double-blind trial in healing chronic diabetic foot ulcers: 102 activated platelet supernatant, topical versus placebo. *Diabetes Care* 1992;15:1598-1604.

93. Steed DL: Clinical evaluation of recombinant human platelet-derived growth factor for the treatment of lower extremity diabetic ulcers: Diabetic Ulcer Study Group. *J Vasc Surg* 1995;21:71-81.

94. Boyko EJ, Ahroni JH, Stensel VL, Smith DG, Davignon DR, Pecoraro RE: Predictors of transcutaneous oxygen tension in the lower limbs of diabetic subjects. *Diabet Med* 1996;13:549-554.

95. Dhingra U, Schauerhamer RR, Wangensteen OH: Peripheral dissemination of bacteria in contaminated wounds: Role of devitalized tissue. Evaluation of therapeutic measures. *Surgery* 1976;80:535-543.

96. Sapico FL, Ginunas VJ, Thornhill-Joynes M, et al: Quantitative microbiology of pressure sores in different stages of healing. *Diagn Microbiol Infect Dis* 1986;5:31-38.

97. Robson MC, Stenberg BD, Heggers JP: Wound healing alterations caused by infection. *Clin Plast Surg* 1990;17:485-492.

98. Steed DL, Donohoe D, Webster MW, Lindsley L: Effect of extensive debridement and treatment on the healing of diabetic foot ulcers: Diabetic Ulcer Study Group. *J Am Coll Surg* 1996;183:61-64.

99. Goodson WH III, Hunt TK: Wound healing, in Kinney JM, Jeejeebhoy KN, Hill GL, Owen OE (eds): *Nutrition and Metabolism in Patient Care*. Philadelphia, PA, WB Saunders, 1988, pp 635-642.

100. Daly JM, Vars HM, Dudrick SJ: Effects of protein depletion on strength of colonic anastomoses. *Surg Gynecol Obstet* 1972;134:15-21.

101. Wipke-Tevis DD, Stotts NA: Nutrition, tissue oxygenation, and healing of venous leg ulcers. *J Vasc Nurs* 1998;16:48-56.

102. Falanga V: Chronic wounds: Pathophysiologic and experimental considerations *J Invest Dermatol* 1993;100:721-725.

103. Carrico TJ, Mehrhof AI Jr, Cohen IK: Biology of wound healing. *Surg Clin North Am* 1984;64:721-733.

104. Goodson WH, Hung TK: Studies of wound healing in experimental diabetes mellitus. *J Surg Res* 1977;22:221-227.

105. Barr LC, Joyce AD: Microvascular anastomoses in diabetes: An experimental study. *Br J Plast Surg* 1989;42:50-53.

106. Seifter E, Rettura G, Padawer J, Stratford F, Kambosos D, Levenson SM: Impaired wound healing in streptozotocin diabetes: Prevention by supplemental vitamin A. *Ann Surg* 1981;194:42-50.

107. Mann GV, Newton P: The membrane transport of ascorbic acid. *Ann N Y Acad Sci* 1975;258:243-252.

108. Charcot JM: Sur quelques arthropathies qui paraissant dépendre d'une lesion du cerveau ou de la moelle épinierè. *Arch Physiol Norm Pathol* 1868;1:161-178.

109. Eloesser L: On the nature of neuropathic affections of the joints. *Ann Surg* 1917;66:201-207.

110. O'Connor BL, Palmoski MJ, Brandt KD: Neurogenic acceleration of degenerative joint lesions. *J Bone Joint Surg Am* 1985;67:562-572.

111. Delano PJ: The pathogenesis of Charcot's joint. *AJR Am J Roentgenol* 1946;56:189-200.

112. Johnson JT: Neuropathic fractures and joint injuries: Pathogenesis and rationale of prevention and treatment. *J Bone Joint Surg Am* 1967;49:1-30.

113. Schwarz GS, Berenyi MR, Siegel MW: Atrophic arthropathy and diabetic neuritis. *AJR Am J Roentgenol* 1969;106:523-529.

114. Norman A, Robbins H, Milgram JE: The acute neuropathic arthropathy: A rapid, severely disorganizing form of arthritis. *Radiology* 1968;90:1159-1164.

115. Knaggs RL: Charcot joints, in Knaggs RL (ed): *The Inflammatory and Toxic Diseases of Bone: A Textbook for Senior Students*. Bristol, John Wright and Sons, 1926, pp 105-119.

116. Leriche R: Sur quelques maladies osseuses et articulaires d'origine vaso-motrice et sur leur traitement. *Bull et Mém Soc Nat de Chir* 1927;53:1022-1030.

117. Watkins PJ, Edmonds ME: Sympathetic nerve failure in diabetes. *Diabetologia* 1983;25:73-77.

118. Brower AC, Allman RM: Pathogenesis of the neurotrophic joint: Neurotraumatic vs. neurovascular. *Radiology* 1981;139:349-354.

119. Brooks AP: The neuropathic foot in diabetes: Part II. Charcot's neuroarthropathy. *Diabet Med* 1986;3:116-118.

120. Edmonds ME: The neuropathic foot in diabetes: Part I. Blood flow. *Diabet Med* 1986;3:111-115.

121. Watkins PJ, Edmonds ME: Autonomic neuropathy: Blood flow in the diabetic foot, in Böstrom H, Ljungstedt N (eds): *Recent Trends in Diabetes Research*. Stockholm, Sweden, Almqvist & Wiksell, 1982, pp 221-224.

122. Uccioli L, Mancini L, Giordano A, et al: Lower limb arterio-venous shunts, autonomic neuropathy and the diabetic foot. *Diabetes Res Clin Pract* 1992;16:123-130.

123. Young MJ, Marshall A, Adams JE, Selby PL, Boulton AJ: Osteopenia, neurological dysfunction, and the development of Charcot neuroarthropathy. *Diabetes Care* 1995;18:34-38.

124. Edelman SV, Kosofsky EM, Paul RA, Kozak GP: Neuro-osteoarthropathy (Charcot's joint) in diabetes mellitus following revascularization surgery: Three case reports and a review of the literature. *Arch Intern Med* 1987;147:1504-1508.

125. Kerper AH, Collier WD: Pathological changes in arteries following partial denervation. *Proc Soc Exp Biol Med* 1927;24:493-494.

126. Bevan RD, Tsuru H: Long-term denervation of vascular smooth muscle causes not only functional but structural change. *Blood Vessels* 1979;16:109-112.

127. Edmonds ME, Morrison N, Laws JW, Watkins PJ: Medical arterial calcification and diabetic neuropathy. *Br Med J (Clin Res Ed)* 1982;284:928-930.

128. Verhas M, Martinello Y, Mone M, et al: Demineralization and pathological physiology of the skeleton in paraplegic rats. *Calcif Tissue Int* 1980;30:83-90.

129. McClugage SG, McCuskey RS: Relationship of the microvascular system to bone resorption and growth in situ. *Microvasc Res* 1973;6: 132-134.

130. Cooper RR: Nerves in cortical bone. *Science* 1968;160:327-328.

131. Moore RE, Smith CK II, Bailey CS, Voelkel EF, Tashjian AH Jr: Characterization of beta-adrenergic receptors on rat and human osteoblast-like cells and demonstration that beta-receptor agonists can stimulate bone resorption in organ culture. *Bone Miner* 1993;23:301-315.

132. Gough A, Abraha H, Li F, et al: Measurement of markers of osteoclast and osteoblast activity in patients with acute and chronic diabetic Charcot neuroarthropathy. *Diabet Med* 1997;14:527-531.

133. Ransjo M, Lie A, Mukohyama H, Lundberg P, Lerner UH: Microisolated mouse osteoclasts express VIP-1 and PACAP receptors. *Biochem Biophys Res Commun* 2000;274:400-404.

134. Winding B, Wiltink A, Foged NT: Pituitary adenylyl cyclase-activating polypeptides and vasoactive intestinal peptide inhibit bone resorption by isolated rabbit osteoclasts. *Exp Physiol* 1997;82:871-886.

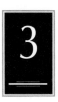

Total Contact Casting

Stephen F. Conti, MD

Introduction

In the early 1930s, Drs. Milroy Paul and Joseph Kahn, working in Ceylon, India, conceptualized the idea of using casting for trophic ulceration secondary to Hansen's disease.[1] They described an ambulatory technique to treat leprosy patients as an alternative to prolonged and expensive periods of bed rest in the hospital. In the 1960s, Paul Brand[2,3] who had worked in India in the early 1950s, adopted the same casting technique in the United States at the Gillis W. Long Hansen's Disease Center in Carville, Louisiana, to treat patients afflicted with Hansen's disease and diabetes mellitus.

Brand and his colleagues noted one significant problem with the casting technique as used in India. This problem, which was also noted by other clinicians, was that as the padding in the cast became compressed over time, it allowed the foot to move within the cast, creating new ulcers. Brand began to construct his casts without padding, in order to allow the cast material to conform exactly to the shape of the foot and leg. Currently, the term total contact cast refers to a composite, anatomically conforming, below-knee cast that is applied over minimal padding, often enclosing the toes. The use of total contact casting as an ambulatory treatment for plantar ulceration in leprosy has since been further expanded to include a variety of other conditions involving insensitivity of the feet, including diabetes mellitus, tabes dorsalis, Charcot-Marie-Tooth disease, syringomyelia and chronic alcoholism, and ulcerations due to idiopathic peripheral neuropathy. Total contact casts are also used to treat neuroarthropathy (Charcot fractures and joints) and to provide immobilization following surgery in patients with sensory neuropathy.

Pathophysiology of Foot Ulceration

A brief review of the factors that can contribute to plantar ulceration in patients with diabetes mellitus is necessary to understand the rationale behind the use of casts to treat this condition. The primary factor in the cause of diabetic foot ulceration is the presence of peripheral neuropathy, leading to diminished or absent sensation. Insensitivity allows excessive and prolonged pressures to occur over the skin, which eventually results in tissue breakdown and ulcer formation.[2,4] In addition to peripheral neuropathy, mechanical factors, such as foot deformities (including clawtoes, midfoot collapse, and hindfoot subluxation), loss of intrinsic muscle function, abnormal load distribution in the forefoot, shear forces, vascular insufficiency, poor skin quality, and infection can contribute to the formation of plantar ulcerations.[2,5,6]

Classification of Diabetic Foot Ulcerations

It is necessary to have a thoughtful classification scheme for foot ulcers in order to develop a rational treatment program and decide on the appropriate use of total contact casting. Many classification systems have been proposed. Wagner proposed a classification of foot ulcerations, which is widely accepted because of its longevity and ease of use[7] (Table 1).

Brodsky has proposed a depth/ischemia classification system that lends itself to a more refined treatment protocol[7] (Table 2). This scheme recognizes ulcer depth and circulation to the foot as separate entities rather than parts of a continuum as in the Wagner classification.

Proposed Mechanisms of Action of Casts

Four mechanisms have been proposed to explain how casts function to heal plantar ulcers. They include protection from trauma, immobilization of skin edges, reduction of edema, and reduction of pressure over the ulcers. Limb immobilization decreases the spread of local infection and, by limiting the stress on granulation tissue and skin edges, protects the foot from further trauma. In 36 to 48 hours, swelling is reduced and the resultant decrease in interstitial fluid pressure leads to improved microcirculation and, the-

Table 1
Wagner classification and recommended management

Stage	Classification	Recommendations
0	Pressure area on foot aggravated by footwear	Footwear modification
I	Open but superficial ulceration	Local treatment Footwear modification
II	Full thickness ulceration	Occlusive cast Footwear modification
III	Full thickness ulceration with secondary infection	Debridement Antibiotics
IV	Local gangrene	Antibiotics Local amputation Hyperbaric O_2
V	Extensive gangrene, entire foot	Regional amputation Antibiotics Rehabilitation

oretically, ulcer healing. Casts have been shown to reduce edema; however, this has not been correlated with improved wound healing. (Marzano R, Kay D, 1995, unpublished data.) The widely accepted rationale for how total contact casting functions to heal diabetic ulcers is that the cast reduces pressure over the wound by redistributing the weightbearing load over a greater plantar surface area.

In 1985, Birke and associates[8] reported a 75% to 84% reduction in peak pressure at the first and third metatarsal heads, respectively, when subjects walked in a cast. In this study, the right feet of 6 normal subjects were tested, using 4 relatively thick sensors, which could have possibly altered the pressures beneath them. However, because the great toe and the metatarsal head region are prone to develop ulceration in the diabetic patients[3] this simple study was significant, being the first to suggest that casts did function to reduce pressure in certain areas.

Using a more sophisticated plantar pressure measuring system, Conti and associates[6] and Martin and Conti[9] examined plantar pressures in casts in subjects with normal arches

and with midfoot collapse and rocker bottom deformity. The conclusion of these studies was that casts function by increasing the plantar weightbearing surface area, thereby lowering plantar pressures. Both short leg casts and total contact casts reduced midfoot pressure, but only total contact casts significantly lowered forefoot pressure. Neither type of cast reduced heel pressure. An average reduction of pressure over the ulcer site of 42% to 46% was achieved through casting. The authors believed that molding the cast to the bottom of the foot allows the entire sole to participate in force distribution, thereby resulting in lower pressures.

Shaw and associates[10] further refined the mechanism of reduction of forefoot pressures in total contact casts. By studying ground reaction forces, in addition to plantar pressures, they concluded that approximately one third of the total load is carried by the wall of the cast instead of being transmitted through the plantar surface. This study supports the concept that a cast that is intimately molded to the leg is better at reducing forces on the ulcer than a cast that is loosely applied. It also

highlights the potential differences between total contact casts and removable walker boots that are purported to be as effective at plantar pressure reduction.

The advantages of total contact casts over strict nonweightbearing ambulation are as follows: (1) A cast maintains the ambulatory status of the patient. Patients with diabetes, who have poor vision, balance problems, weakness, and limited cardiac reserve are significantly limited in their ability to use crutches or a walker. Also, lengthy and expensive hospital stays as well as the potential problems of prolonged bed rest can be avoided. Sedentary workers can return to their jobs without any income loss. (2) A cast reduces edema and plantar pressure. (3) A cast protects the foot from further trauma. (4) A cast requires less patient compliance than nonweightbearing crutch ambulation. There is no need for daily dressing changes or specialized wound care.

The disadvantages and/or complications of total contact casting are as follows: (1) Prolonged immobilization in a cast can cause joint stiffness and muscle atrophy. Diabetic tissue is normally less pliable, due to nonenzymatic glycosylation of collagen, and the superimposed stiffness from the cast can be significant. (2) Poor cast application and removal can cause new ulceration and skin breakdown. This can be minimized by using a skillful cast application technique and by regular monitoring at frequent office follow-up visits. Even with proper precautions, skin abrasion[11,12] and fungal infection have been reported. New skin breakdown can be treated by discontinuing use of the cast for a few days until the new ulcer has healed. Fungal infection, reported in 15% of all casted patients, can be treated with local application of antifungal cream after the cast is no longer needed. Rarely is casting interrupted due to fungal infection. (3) Because the casts have little padding, cast saw cuts can occur during removal. It is crucial to prevent this complication by using meticulous technique. Health care personnel should have special instruction on proper cast removal.

Pathophysiology of Neuroarthropathic Fractures

The second major indication for total contact casting is in the treatment of acute Charcot fractures secondary to diabetic neuropathy. Again, an understanding of the pathophysiology of Charcot fractures is necessary to conceptualize the role of total contact casts in their treatment. In 1936, William Jordan[13] first described the occurrence of neuropathic arthropathy of the foot and ankle in diabetic patients. Many similar reports have followed.[14–16] The prevalence of neuropathic arthropathy in patients with diabetes mellitus has been reported in the literature to be from 0.08% to 7.5%.[17–19] The most common areas of neuroarthropathy are the midfoot and hindfoot.[20,21]

Newman[22] stated that the earliest changes in neuroarthropathic joints occurred in the soft tissue surrounding the joints. In those cases of neuropathic osteoarthropathy that do not begin with spontaneous fractures, he postulated that gross neuropathic changes in the ligaments were responsible for spontaneous dislocation of the foot. Ligaments and joint capsules are thought to be stretched by the abnormal stress applied to the joint, leading to hypermobility, eventual joint dislocation, and subsequent fragmentation. Hyperemic resorption through osteoclastic activities can alter ligamentous insertion into the bone and

may be another contributing factor for dislocation. Multiple other factors appear to contribute to the development of bone and joint destruction in patients with diabetes mellitus;[23] however, a detailed discussion of all these factors is beyond the scope of this chapter.

Norman and associates[24] also classified neuropathic joints as acute or chronic, based on the suddenness of their onset and speed of development. The acute phase of neuropathy

is often precipitated by minor trauma and is characterized by swelling, erythema, a local increase in temperature, joint effusion, ligament laxity, and bone resorption. Early clinical and radiographic signs may resemble those of osteoarthritis and infection. The similarity between infection and neuroarthropathy can delay the diagnosis and treatment of early subluxation, especially when radiographs are normal. The early recognition and immobilization of the neuroarthro-

Table 2
The depth/ischemia classification of diabetic foot lesions

Grade	Definition	Treatment*
Depth Classification		
0	The "at risk" foot. Previous ulcer, or neuropathy with deformity that may cause new ulceration	Patient education Regular examination Appropriate shoewear and insoles
1	Superficial ulceration, not infected	External pressure relief: Total contact cast, walking brace, special shoewear, etc
2	Deep ulceration exposing tendon or joint (with/without superficial infection)	Surgical debridement → wound care → pressure relief if closes and converts to grade 1 (PRN antibiotics)
3	Extensive ulceration with exposed bone, and/or deep infection: ie, osteomyelitis, or abscess	Surgical debridements → ray or partial foot amputations → IV antibiotics → pressure relief if wound converts to grade 1
Ischemia Classification		
A	Not ischemic	Adequate vascularity for healing
B	Ischemia without gangrene	Vascular evaluation (Doppler, TcPO$_2$, arteriogram, etc.) → vascular reconstruction PRN
C	Partial (forefoot) gangrene of foot	Vascular evaluation → vascular reconstruction (proximal and/or distal bypass or angioplasty) → partial foot amputation
D	Complete foot gangrene	Vascular evaluation → major extremity amputation (BKA, AKA) with possible proximal vascular reconstruction

PRN, as needed; IV, intravenous; TcPO$_2$, transcutaneous oxygen pressure; BKA, below-knee amputation; AKA, above-knee amputation

(Reproduced with permission from Brodsky JW: The diabetic foot, in Mann RA, Coughlin MJ (eds): *Surgery of the Foot and Ankle*, ed 6. St. Louis, MO, Mosby Year Book, 1993, pp 1361–1467.)

pathic foot must be the goal of any treatment algorithm.

Radiographic Staging and Treatment of Neuropathic Joints

Eichenholtz[25] described 3 distinct radiologic stages of neuroarthropathy. These are (1) stage of development, (2) stage of coalescence, and (3) stage of reconstruction.

The stage of development represents an acute, destructive period associated clinically with joint effusion, soft-tissue edema, subluxation, intra-articular fractures, and fragmentation of bone. This stage is usually induced by minor trauma and aggravated by persistent ambulation on an insensitive foot. The process induces a hyperemic response, leading to bone resorption and progressive deterioration. Clinically, this may present with painless, unilateral warmth and swelling, with normal radiographs. It may continue for as little as a few hours or as long as several weeks before there is radiographic evidence of joint fragmentation. Early recognition is imperative for successful treatment, because aggressive cast immobilization can prevent late deformity. Nonweightbearing total contact casting should be initiated during the acute phase of the disease.

The second stage, the stage of coalescence, can be identified clinically by a lessening of edema, reduction of skin temperature, resorption of fine debris, and healing of fractures. This phase indicates the beginning of the reparative phase. Partial weightbearing total contact casting is the recommended treatment in this phase. The use of a bivalved ankle-foot orthosis (AFO) or Charcot restraint orthotic walker (CROW) brace is an alternative.

In the third and final stage, the stage of reconstruction, further repair and remodeling of the bone takes place. This stage can be recognized clinically by the absence of edema and local warmth and radiographically by increased bone density and sclerosis. At this stage, it is recommended to wean the patient into a double upright calf lacing brace with appropriate total contact orthoses and soft leather depth shoes with rocker soles. Depending on joint stability, the patient may remain in the brace indefinitely or move to footwear alone. Chronic or late neuropathic bone and joint changes are problematic but can be managed effectively with shoe modifications and, in selective cases, by reconstructive surgery.

Indications for Total Contact Casts

There are 3 indications for total contact casts. The first is ambulatory treatment of uninfected superficial forefoot and midfoot plantar ulcerations, including Wagner grade 1 and 2 ulcers or Brodsky grade 1 ulcers. Heel ulcers are often the result of ischemia combined with osteomyelitis, and because total contact casts do not unload the heel, casting is not indicated for plantar heel ulcerations. Deeper ulcers with exposed tendon or bone require surgical debridement and local wound care to convert them to superficial ulcers before total contact casting is undertaken. Casting is not recommended for dorsal foot or leg ulcers. The second indication is for treatment of Eichenholtz stage 1 or 2 neuroarthropathic fractures, and the third is for postoperative immobilization, following either open reduction and internal fixation of acute foot or ankle fractures or reconstructive surgery for late deformity.

Contraindications for Total Contact Casts

The 4 absolute contraindications are as follows: (1) Deep infection in the form of deep abscess, osteomyelitis or gangrene should not be casted. Excessive drainage from the ulcer is clinical justification to assess for underlying osteomyelitis or abscess. Antibiotic therapy and bed rest or nonweightbearing on the limb until the acute infection has subsided has been recommended.[25] If the ulcer is deeper than it is wide, it should be surgically debrided and opened to allow the deeper layers to heal and prevent premature superficial healing. (2) Poor skin quality is a contraindication to casting. Patients who are on chronic corticosteroids or those with stasis ulcers are most likely to develop skin breakdown with total contact casting. (3) Severe arterial insufficiency is another contraindication. Although most diabetic patients have some atherosclerotic vascular insufficiency, only those with pregangrenous feet are at risk of developing a catastrophic ischemic event from the circular bandage of the cast. A clinical examination suggesting ischemia, ankle/brachial index less than 0.45, Doppler toe pressures less than 30 mm Hg, or a transcutaneous pressure of oxygen ($TcPO_2$) less than 30 warrant special attention. (4) The final absolute contraindication is poor patient compliance. Patients who are unable to keep regularly scheduled follow-up visits and are unable to follow the cast precautions and instructions should not be casted.

In addition to these absolute contraindications there are 2 relative contraindications. (1) Fluctuating edema of the limb, which occurs, for example, in some dialysis patients, may be a relative contraindication for total contact casting. Total uniform contact between the cast and the limb is the essential element to success. If the limb becomes loose in the cast, shear forces caused by movement of skin in the cast can delay healing or cause skin breakdown. (2) The use of total contact casting in blind, ataxic, or obese patients is another relative contraindication. Some additional precautions or alternative methods of therapy may be necessary to prevent falls.

Cast Application

There is no universally accepted technique or single method of applying a total contact cast that is exclusively effective. In fact, multiple variations on the themes that follow are successful. The goal is to obtain an intimate fit of the cast around the foot and leg through meticulous molding. One method of doing this is to apply plaster directly to the skin without padding. However, as noted previously, standard short leg casts made of 3 layers of padding have been shown clinically and experimentally to reduce plantar pressure and allow acceptable rates of ulcer healing. Another controversy is over foot position in the cast, the question being whether a patient with a forefoot ulcer should be casted in slight dorsiflexion in an attempt to further unload that area during ambulation. Finally, the physician must decide whether to leave the toes exposed or enclose them in the cast. The claimed advantage of open toes is the ability to check circulation and for evidence of erythema. The more obvious disadvantages are that the toes are unprotected and exposed to trauma, objects may find their way into the cast through the opening, and the possibility of iatrogenic ulcer formation is increased. This last complication is of significant practical concern. Finishing the cast at the metatarsal heads can allow the end of the cast to press on the dorsal surface of the foot as it is forced down during the end of midstance and toe-off, and this pressure can cause ulceration in some patients.

Wound assessment is the first step in cast application. The ulcer surface may require mechanical debridement of the exudate that sometimes covers it. This is best accomplished with a sterile cotton swab or gauze sponge. Use of antiseptics that contain iodine, alcohol, or peroxide is not indicated, because these substances are toxic to granulating tissue and can delay wound healing. Antibiotic soaps, which are rinsed off with saline after use, can be used for this purpose. Usually, sharp debridement of the ulcer base is performed. The hypertrophic marginal callus that forms around the ulcer should be sharply excised until this area is level with the adjacent normal skin. Theoretically, pressure on the callused area during weightbearing will cause marginal ischemia that will delay wound healing. After the callous is trimmed, the ulcer may then be covered with a sterile nonadhesive dressing and one or two 2 × 2-in gauze sponges.

Skin preparation is accomplished by first washing the skin with mild soap and water if necessary. A hypoallergenic moisturizer is then applied to the skin everywhere except at the web spaces between the toes, which have an antifungal powder applied sparingly as needed. Single 2 × 2-in gauze sponges are then placed between the toes (Fig. 1). A square piece of foam padding is positioned around the toes and trimmed (Fig. 2). For midfoot ulcers, the foam is placed around the toes only. In patients with forefoot ulcers, the foam is extended proximally just behind the metatarsal heads to create a well under the metatarsal heads once the cast is applied, allowing pressure reduction. Next, the leg is wrapped with a single layer of 3 or 4-inch cast padding from the tibial tubercle to just beyond the tips of the toes, with each layer overlapped by

50%. A 0.25-in thick strip of medical grade felt is cut approximately 4 cm wide and positioned from just distal to the tibial tubercle to just proximal to the ankle joint along the crest of the tibia. Additional 0.125-in thick felt strips, made by splitting the 0.25-in felt in half, are positioned over the medial and lateral malleoli (Fig. 3).

Traditional casting technique would then involve molding a single layer of conforming plaster wrap over the entire leg, followed by 2 layers of fiberglass casting tape. The toes are completely enclosed (Fig. 4). Patients then remain nonweightbearing for 24 hours, to allow the plaster to dry thoroughly, after which they are allowed to ambulate. Using plantar pressure analysis, it has been shown that equivalent plantar pressure reductions are achieved by simply wrapping the leg with the fiberglass tape without the plaster underlayer (unpublished data). Intimate molding, especially through the longitudinal arch and around the leg, is stressed in both techniques (Fig. 5). A rocker bottom cast boot is attached to aid in gait, to protect the bottom of the cast, and to keep the cast clean. Patients can then leave the office ambulating weightbearing as tolerated if their condition permits. If the patient has a significant amount of swelling, the involved extremity is elevated for 10 minutes prior to cast application. I prefer to cast the foot with the ankle in a neutral position relative to the leg regardless of the site of the ulcer, because slight dorsiflexion or plantarflexion makes walking in the cast difficult. Plantarflexion can cause increased pressure on the anterior edge of the cast just below the knee or along the shin, producing a secondary ulcer.

Postcasting Care

Most patients are brought back after 5 to 7 days for the first cast change.

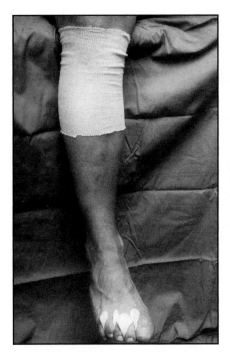

Fig. 1 After debridement of the ulcer and preparation of the skin, the stockinette is applied to the proximal leg and the gauze sponges placed between the toes.

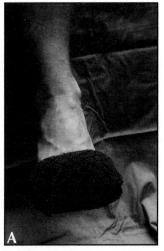
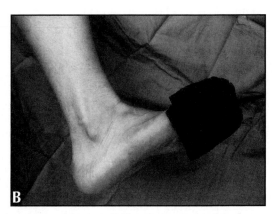

Fig. 2 A, A piece of foam is cut and placed around the toes. B, The plantar aspect of the foam is beveled just proximal to the metatarsal heads.

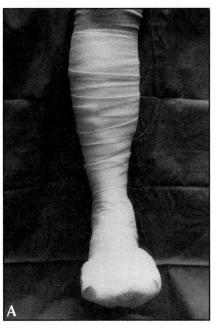
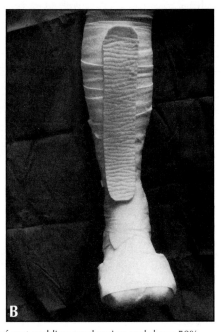

Fig. 3 A, The leg is wrapped with a single layer of cast padding overlapping each layer 50%. B, An anterior felt pad is positioned over the tibial crest. The foam absorbs the pressure of the anterior cast against the leg as the patient walks over the cast from midstance to toe-off.

Rapid edema reduction can make the cast loose, resulting in possible skin irritation or ulceration. Patients are brought back every 2 weeks thereafter for cast changes. Specific precautions and cast care instructions are reinforced at each visit. A handout is used to remind patients about the details of cast care (see Appendix). In the case of plantar ulcerations, casting is discontinued when the ulcer is healed and appropriate footwear is available to the patient. For casts used to treat Charcot fractures, the casting is discontinued when edema is reduced, the temperature difference between the 2 feet is within 2°C (no perceptible difference to the examiner), and radiographs show consolidation and healing of fractures.

Appropriate footwear must be available to patients immediately after cast removal. The basic principles in the pedorthic management of plantar ulcers are the even distribution of plantar pressure by transfer from areas of high pressure, such as metatarsal heads, to areas of lower pressure; shock absorption; reduction of friction and shear by limitation of tissue motion; and accommodation of deformities.[26] Prescription footwear should not be considered a primary treatment for ulcers, rather such care is intended as a long-term management technique for maintaining healed areas and preventing further ulceration.

Shoe modifications should be done according to the needs of the patient.

Important characteristics for shoes used in the pedorthic management of plantar ulcers include: a long medial counter to control the heel and medial arch, a Blucher opening to allow easy entry into the shoe, a shock-absorbing sole to reduce impact shock, and a low heel to decrease pressure on the metatarsal heads and the toes.

External shoe modifications include the rocker sole, the shape and position of which varies according to the patient's specific foot problems, and sole flares and stabilizers. A flare is an extension to the heel and/or sole of the shoe, and it can be placed medially or laterally to stabilize hindfoot, midfoot, or forefoot instability. An extended offset heel is an additional extension added to the side of the shoe, including both the sole and upper, to stabilize severe hindfoot or midfoot instabilities. The addition of an extended steel shank in the rocker sole can further prevent the shoe from bending, limiting toe and midfoot motion and aiding in propulsion on toe-off. Total contact orthoses are very effective in the distribution and transfer of plantar pressure and in reduction or elimination of weightbearing from problem areas. Custom-made shoes are indicated only for extremely severe deformities and for feet that cannot be fit with depth shoes, even with extensive modifications.

Alternatives to Total Contact Casting

Currently, total contact casting remains the gold standard for the treatment of diabetic foot ulceration. Some alternatives to total contact casting that have been reported in the literature will be discussed.

Standard below knee walking casts have been used to promote healing of neuropathic plantar ulcers in patients with diabetes and Hansen's disease since the 1930s. Reduction of plantar

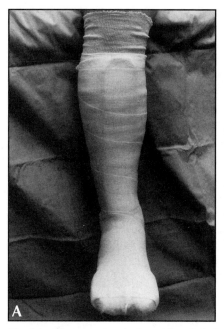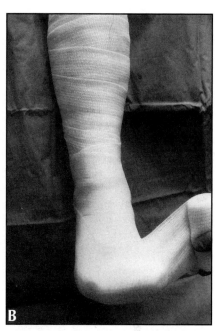

Fig. 4 A, After wrapping the leg with a single layer of gauze the fiberglass casting material is wrapped around the leg. The first layer should be applied and molded to the leg and arch area as it is hardening. This increases the contact of the skin with the cast and promotes all the functions of the cast. **B,** The toes are included in the fiberglass wrapping.

pressure over the ulcer site is the goal. Pollard and Le Quesne[27] demonstrated that conventional walking casts reduce plantar foot pressure. Birke and associates[8] demonstrated equal plantar distribution in short leg casts and total contact casts. Conti and associates[6] have shown that the 2 types of casts are similar; however, they warned that compression over time of the multilayered cast padding in a standard cast may significantly alter those results. They also felt that casts made of fiberglass without plaster were as efficacious as more traditional plaster and fiberglass composite casts. Huband and Carr[28] demonstrated ulcer healing in 12 patients using standard short leg walking casts. They showed that plaster or fiberglass casting tape was equally efficacious. The open toe design of a standard cast may predispose to iatrogenic dorsal foot ulceration and foreign body entrance into

the cast and, therefore, the closed toe design of the total contact cast is superior. As with total contact casting, a standard walking cast is indicated only for the management of patients with superficial forefoot or midfoot plantar ulcerations. Heel ulcers are not unloaded by either cast.

The bivalved AFO walker or the CROW brace[29] is a total contact orthosis that approximates the fit of a well-molded plaster cast. Conventional AFO braces had been used after cast treatment prior to the development of the CROW. Persistent anterior edema with the AFO was managed with the addition of an anterior shell. However, patients had difficulty fitting the brace into a shoe. This lead to the development of the full foot enclosure. In the CROW, a custom foot orthosis is manufactured to accommodate for bone deformity. A rocker bottom sole facilitates ambulation, and a ventilation hole is

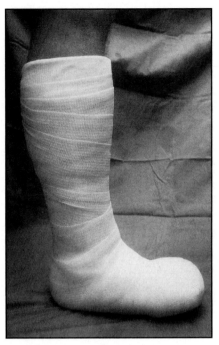

Fig. 5 Final view of total contact cast.

provided for increased comfort. The anterior and posterior shells make the CROW easy to wear. They are primarily used for patients who have a plantar ulcer associated with fluctuating edema in the foot and leg or in patients who are being weaned from a total contact cast following treatment for neuroarthropathy. The CROW continues to control edema, allows ambulation, and provides satisfaction to the patient. Few reports are available describing successful treatment with the CROW.

A commercial prefabricated walking brace[7] can be used for both diabetic ulcer care and in the management of neuroarthropathy. Diabetic ulcers must be protectively padded and closely monitored. The typical posttrauma cam walker can be modified with pads and used for this purpose. Recently, a new design in cast bracing has become available that has a closed padded heel. The fixed ankle heel control type cast brace may be modified for use in diabetic foot

ulcers. This cast brace is designed to control heel position and foot motion. With this device, use of a custom-made insole is necessary for satisfactory ulcer treatment and prevention. The cast braces offer an advantage over plaster type casts in that they may be removed for wound care, and they allow easy, frequent inspection of suspected infections. They also provide better hygiene and greater patient comfort. Disadvantages include lack of objective quantification of plantar pressure reduction. Also, because the device cannot achieve an intimate contour with the leg, it cannot unload the foot as effectively as a total contact cast.

The IPOS postoperative shoe (IPOS, Niagara Falls, NY) can be used to treat patients with superficial plantar forefoot ulcers. It is designed with 10° of dorsiflexion and a heel that is elevated 4 cm to avoid any forefoot contact with the ground. The distal edge of the shoe ends at the proximal metatarsals. Needleman[30] reported 77% of patients with Wagner grade 1 and 2 forefoot ulcers healed in an average of 8 weeks and there was a 78% compliance rate. The advantages include expected high patient compliance, ability for bipedal ambulation, ability to evaluate the foot frequently for infection, and relatively low cost. This treatment method may be more acceptable to patients who live long distances from the treating physician and who would find regular cast changes to be burdensome. Disadvantages include problems with balance and the potential for forming new ulcers on other parts of the foot due to increased load and the fact that it is indicated only for forefoot ulcerations.

Discussion

Diabetes mellitus and its complications represent a significant expense

to the health care system. The concept of disease state management includes teaching patients and physicians to use appropriate resources to prevent many of these complications. Preventing and healing neuropathic plantar ulcerations can be frustrating, time consuming, and expensive. Questions of efficacy and cost of treatment become important in this disease. There are questions about the cost of healing foot ulcers versus amputation. Costs following the successful healing of plantar ulcerations have also been raised. In a report[31] in 1995, the total cost to the system was calculated for 3 years following the successful healing of a foot ulcer either by nonsurgical treatment or amputation. The total cost for patients who were without ischemia who healed their ulcer primarily was $16,100. The total cost for the same period in patients who underwent major amputation to heal their ulcer was $63,100. It would seem that healing a plantar ulceration and salvaging a limb results in a cost savings over amputating the limb even after the acute treatment is over.

Sinacore and associates[32] described the effectiveness of total contact casting in their reports of patients who had chronic plantar ulcers for an average of 11 months (ranging from 1 week to 13 years) despite other forms of treatment, such as daily dressing changes, antibiotic therapy, frequent callus shaving and debridement, and multiple skin grafts. They noted healing in 82% of 33 ulcers after an average of 44 days in a total contact cast. Helm and asssociates[33] reported a 73% rate of healing in 22 patients, with an average time to healing of 38 days. Boulton and associates[11] found healing in 100% of 7 patients treated with a total contact cast for an average of 6 weeks. Walker and associates[34] reported a 71% healing rate in an average of 35.8 days in a series of 77 diabetic patients with neuropathic ulceration of the foot. Myerson and associates[35] confirmed the effectiveness of total contact casting in their series of 71 neuropathic ulcers of the foot in 66 patients. They reported 64 of 71 (90%) ulcers were healed at a mean of 5.5 weeks (range 1 to 14 weeks). Mueller and associates,[12] in their first reported controlled clinical trial study, described an ulcer healing rate of 90% (19 of 21 patients) with a mean time of healing of 42 ± 29 days (range 8 to 91 days). The combined results of these studies yield an average rate of successful healing of 84.3% in an average time of 39.9 days in the cast.

Time to healing has been shown to vary depending on the site of the ulcer. The time period for the healing of plantar ulcers on the forefoot by total contact casting varies from ulcers elsewhere on the foot. Walker and associates[34] reported in their study that forefoot ulcers (metatarsal heads and toe) healed in an average of 30.6 days compared to nonforefoot ulcers (dorsum of the foot, heel, plantar arch, ankle, medial aspect of the metatarsal and toe, or transmetatarsal amputation sites) which healed in an average of 42.1 days. My experience is comparable, in that forefoot ulcerations treated by total contact casting take relatively less time to heal compared to the nonforefoot ulcerations.

Although most ulcers are the result of neuropathy, the evaluation of the vascular status of the limb plays an important role in the overall management of foot ulcers in patients with diabetes mellitus. In addition to small-vessel disease, there is a significant incidence of large-vessel disease, especially below the level of the trifurcation of the popliteal artery. Sinacore and associates[32] suggested

that total contact casting was effective even for ischemic ulcers. A report by Laing and associates[36] contradicts that belief. They treated 36 diabetic patients with neuropathic ulcers, 28 healed in an average of 6.3 weeks. Eight of the ulcers failed to heal. Six of these were in ischemic limbs, with average Doppler Ankle/Brachial (A/B) index of 0.61 (range 0.44 to 0.81). By contrast, the average A/B index in the healed diabetic ulcers was 1.2 (range 0.7 to 2). Myerson and associates[35] found that most ulcers will heal in a reasonable period of time regardless of the marginal pressure indices on Doppler testing. They recommend vascular consultation only for those patients who have marginal circulation and fail to heal after an appropriate time in a total contact cast. I believe that all painless neuropathic ulcers should receive a trial of total contact casting prior to vascular evaluation. The only exceptions are obvious painful, ischemic ulcers or those that have severe ischemia with gross trophic changes suggesting impending gangrene. Alternative healing strategies should be employed pending vascular evaluation. Vascular insufficiency should be considered in cases of recalcitrant ulcerations.

There are several other reasons for failure of an ulcer to heal with total contact casting. Patient noncompliance due to absence of pain in the feet is often a factor. Although casting is an ambulatory treatment option, patients are asked to restrict their activity to one-third normal while in the cast. Appropriate counseling is often all that is necessary to achieve compliance. Severe deformity that is not accommodated by the cast is another problem. This is especially common in the case of midfoot collapse. Exostectomy, Achilles tendon lengthening, or more extensive reconstructions may be necessary to

reduce excessive pressures. Underlying osteomyelitis, especially in the forefoot and heel, is also a reason for failure of casting. Excessive drainage is often the only clinical clue to the diagnosis. Appropriate radiologic testing can confirm the diagnosis and assess the extent of the infection. Antibiotics may suppress the drainage temporarily. Occasionally, the physician may prescribe antibiotics and casting, which allows an ulcer to close, only to find that the entire foot has become cellulitic. An expeditious workup for osteomyelitis should be undertaken in this situation. Patients who are casted and have dormant osteomyelitis will often heal superficially, but breakdown occurs soon after casting is discontinued.[4,37]

Recurrent ulceration is usually caused by noncompliance with prescription footwear or by failure of footwear to reduce pressure. Significant deformity may not be sufficiently unloaded in the shoe. Plantar pressure measurement made in the shoe may help to assess if footwear is optimal. Helm and associates[38] in a 6-year research project, found that patient compliance and deformities secondary to Charcot changes were the major causes for ulcer recurrence. They reported a recurrence rate of 19.4% in their study of 102 patients. Myerson and associates[35] described a recurrence rate of 31.1% in their study of 71 neuropathic ulcers. We have used an inshoe pressure-measuring device for several years and have found that 50% of recurrent ulcerations can be prevented by modifying the footwear based on the test results.

Current research is investigating the role of topical wound healing agents on ulcer healing. The use of platelet-derived growth factor has been found effective in 3 separate published clinical trials.[39–41] These studies demonstrated that the combination of aggressive revascularization and debridement, infection control and unloading of plantar ulcers, along with the use of PDWHF (platelet-derived wound-healing factor), was effective in ulcer healing. However, the role of PDWHF apart from other aspects of an overall wound-healing regimen is not entirely clear. Results of 2 other clinical trials that used recombinant growth factors in patients with pressure sores and split thickness skin grafts have been recently published.[23,42] To date, there have been no other published studies on recombinant growth factors and diabetic ulcer healing. The next logical step in ulcer healing will be to combine FDA approved growth factor preparations with removable ambulatory pressure relieving devices. Care must be taken to evaluate these devices fully before use. Currently, total contact casting is the gold standard by which all other devices must be assessed.

References

1. Khan JS: Treatment of leprous trophic ulcers. *Leprosy India* 1939;11:19–21.

2. Brand PW: The insensitive foot (including leprosy), in Jahss MH (ed): *Disorders of the Foot*. Philadelphia, PA, WB Saunders, 1982, vol 2, pp 1266–1286.

3. Brand PW: The diabetic foot, in Ellenberg M, Rifkin H (eds): *Diabetes Mellitus: Theory and Practice*, ed 3. New Hyde Park, NY, Medical Examination Publishing, 1983, pp 829–849.

4. Bauman JH, Girling JP, Brand PW: Plantar pressures and trophic ulceration: An evaluation of footwear. *J Bone Joint Surg* 1963;45B: 652–673.

5. Coleman WG, Brand PW, Birke JA: The total contact cast: A therapy for plantar ulceration of the insensitive feet. *J Am Podiatry Assoc* 1984;74:548–552.

Appendix
Total Contact Cast Instructions

You have had a total-contact cast applied to your foot for the purpose of healing the ulcer (sore) on your foot. These ulcers do not heal because of the extremely high pressures on the sole of the foot during walking. The cast was made to decrease the pressure on the ulcer, thereby allowing the ulcer to heal. In addition to the pressure relief, the cast is designed to be very snug fitting, with the toes enclosed for protection.

For the total contact cast to be effective, you must know how to take care of your cast. The following is a list of what to do and not to do.

Do not bear weight or walk on your cast until you are told to do so by the person putting the cast on your foot.

We recommend you limit your walking and standing to one third of the normal daily routine or walking distance.

Never use the cast to strike or hit objects. Dents, cracks or softened areas of the cast may cause excessive pressure on your foot in the cast and should be reported immediately.

Keep the cast dry at all times. Water will destroy your cast. Sponge bathing is recommended instead of showering while in your cast. Use a rubberized short leg disposable sleeve to protect the cast when bathing. DO NOT submerge your cast in water. If the cast does become wet, dry it immediately with a towel or hair dryer set to "cool". If it rains, cover the cast with a plastic bag.

Your cast may be inconvenient, and you may have difficulty sleeping. This is not uncommon. You may try wrapping the cast in a towel or placing it on a pillow while in bed.

After you have been wearing the cast several days, perspiration and dirt may cause itching of the skin inside the cast. This is common. You must ignore it. Do not stick pencils, coat hangers, or other objects in the cast to scratch the skin.

Inspect the entire cast daily. Look and feel for deep cracks or soft spots on the cast. use a small hand mirror to inspect the sole of the cast or have a family member check the sole of the cast.

Never attempt to remove your cast by yourself.

Removing Your Cast

We have a specially designed saw to remove the cast with little discomfort. It should be removed only by a health care professional. After removal, your skin may be flaky and dry, and your joint may feel stiff. Apply a thick cream or oil for several days to moisten and soften the skin.

You will need to have your specially made shoes ready to wear immediately after the cast is removed to prevent your foot form getting another ulcer.

Warning Signs

If any of the following signs or symptoms occur call (physician phone number).

Excessive swelling of the leg or foot if the cast becomes too tight.

The cast becomes too loose and your leg can move up or down in the cast greater than 1/4 inch.

The cast has any deep cracks or soft spots.

Any drainage of pus or blood on the outside of the cast. This will appear brownish or dark yellow.

Any foul-smelling odor from the cast.

You experience any excessive tenderness in your groin or the casted foot.

Any excessive leg pain or annoying pressure in the ankle or foot which will not go away.

You notice any sudden onset of fever or an unusual elevation in your blood sugar. We highly recommend daily self-monitoring of your blood glucose during casting if you are not already doing so.

If any of the above conditions exist, do the following:

Notify appropriate professional personnel at once.

Do not walk on your cast. Keep your leg elevated.

Use crutches or a walker and keep the casted foot off the ground until seen by professional personnel.

6. Conti SF, Martin RL, Chaytor ER, Hughes C, Luttrell L: Plantar pressure measurements during ambulation in weightbearing conventional short leg casts and total contact casts. *Foot Ankle Int* 1996;17:464–469.

7. Brodsky JW: The diabetic foot, in Mann RA, Coughlin MJ (eds): *Surgery of the Foot and Ankle*, ed 6. St. Louis, MO, Mosby-Year Book, 1993, vol 2, pp 977–957.

8. Birke JA, Sims DS Jr, Buford WL: Walking casts: Effect on plantar foot pressures. *J Rehabil Res Dev* 1985;22:18–22.

9. Martin RL, Conti SF: Plantar pressure analysis of diabetic rockerbottom deformity in total contact casts. *Foot Ankle Int* 1996;17:470–472.

10. Shaw JE, Hsi WL, Ulbrecht JS, Norkitis A, Becker MB, Cavanagh PR: The mechanism of plantar unloading in total contact casts: Implications for design and clinical use. *Foot Ankle Int* 1997;18:809–817.

11. Boulton AJ, Bowker JH, Gadia M, et al: Use of plaster casts in the management of diabetic neuropathic foot ulcers. *Diabetes Care* 1986;9:149–152.

12. Mueller MJ, Diamond JE, Sinacore DR, et al: Total contact casting in treatment of diabetic plantar ulcers: controlled clinical trial. *Diabetes Care* 1989;12:384–388.

13. Jordan WR: Neuritic manifestations in diabetes mellitus. *Arch Intern Med* 1936;57:307–366.

14. Clohisy DR, Thompson RC Jr: Fractures associated with neuropathic arthropathy in adults who have juvenile-onset diabetes. *J Bone Joint Surg* 1988;70A:1192–1200.

15. Clouse ME, Gramm HF, Legg M, Flood T: Diabetic osteoarthropathy: Clinical and roentgenographic observations in 90 cases, *Am J Roentgenol Radium Ther Nucl Med* 1974;121:22–34.

16. Sinha S, Munichoodappa CS, Kozak GP: Neuro-arthropathy (Charcot joints) in diabetes mellitus: Clinical study of 101 cases. *Medicine* 1972;51:191–210.

17. Bailey CC, Root HF: Neuropathic foot lesions in diabetes mellitus. *N Engl J Med* 1947;236: 397–401.

18. Forgacs S: Clinical picture of diabetic osteoarthropathy. *Acta Diabetol Lat* 1976;13: 111–129.

19. Pogonowska MJ, Collins LC, Dobson HL: Diabetic osteopathy. *Radiology* 1967;89:265–271.

20. Anania WC, Rosen RC, Wallace JA, Weinblatt MA, Gerland JS, Castillo J: Treatment of diabetic skin ulcerations with povidone-iodine and sugar: Two case reports. *J Am Podiatr Med Assoc* 1985;75:472–474.

21. Holstein P, Larsen K, Sager P: Decompression with the aid of insoles in the treatment of diabetic neuropathic ulcers. *Acta Orthop Scand* 1976;47:463–468.

22. Newman JH: Spontaneous dislocation in diabetic neuropathy: A report of six cases. *J Bone Joint Surg* 1979;61B:484–488.

23. Robson MC, Phillips LG, Thomason A, Robsosn LE, Pierce GF: Platelet-derived growth factor BB for the treatment of chronic pressure ulcers. *Lancet* 1992;339:23–25.

24. Norman A, Robbins H, Milgram JE: The acute neuropathic arthropathy: A rapid, severely disorganizing form of arthritis. *Radiology* 1967;90:1159–1164.

25. Eichenholtz SN (ed): *Charcot Joints*. Springfield, IL, Charles C Thomas, 1966.

26. Chantelau E, Breuer U, Leisch AC, Tanudjaja T, Reuter M: Outpatient treatment of unilateral diabetic foot ulcers with "half shoes." *Diabet Med* 1993;10:267–270.

27. Pollard JP, Le Quesne LP: Method of healing diabetic forefoot ulcers. *Br Med J* 1983;286:436–437.

28. Huband MS, Carr JB: A simplified method of total contact casting for diabetic foot ulcers. *Contemp Orthop* 1993;26:143–147.

29. Morgan JM, Biehl WC III, Wagner FW Jr: Management of neuropathic arthropathy with the Charcot Restraint Orthotic Walker. *Clin Orthop* 1993;296:58–63.

30. Needleman RL: Successes and pitfalls in the healing of neuropathic forefoot ulcerations with the IPOS postoperative shoe. *Foot Ankle Int* 1997;18:412–417.

31. Apelqvist J, Ragnarson-Tennvall G, Larsson J, Persson U: Long-term costs for foot ulcers in diabetic patients in a multidisciplinary setting. *Foot Ankle Int* 1995;16:388–394.

32. Sinacore DR, Mueller, MJ, Diamond JE, Blair VP III, Drury D, Rose SJ: Diabetic plantar ulcers treated by total contact casting: A clinical report. *Phys Ther* 1987;67:1543–1549.

33. Helm PA, Walker SC, Pullium G: Total contact casting in diabetic patients with neuropathic foot ulcerations. *Arch Phys Med Rehabil* 1984;65:691–693.

34. Walker SC, Helm PA, Pullium G: Total contact casting and chronic diabetic neuropathic foot ulcerations: Healing rates by wound location. *Arch Phys Med Rehabil* 1987;68:217–221.

35. Myerson M, Papa J, Eaton K, Wilson K: The total contact cast for management of neuropathic plantar ulceration of the foot. *J Bone Joint Surg* 1992;74A:261–269.

36. Laing PW, Cogley DI, Klenerman L: Neuropathic foot ulceration treated by total contact casts. *J Bone Joint Surg* 1992;74B: 133–136.

37. Levin ME: Medical evaluation and treatment, in Levin ME, O'Neal LW (eds): *The Diabetic Foot*. St. Louis, MO, CV Mosby, 1983, pp 1–60.

38. Helm PA, Walker SC, Pullium GF: Recurrence of neuropathic ulceration following healing in a total contact cast. *Arch Phys Med Rehabil* 1991;72:967–970.

39. Fylling CP, Knighton DR, Gordinier RH: The use of a comprehensive wound care protocol including topical growth factor therapy in treatment of diabetic neuropathic ulcers, in Ward J, Goto Y (eds): *Diabetic Neuropathy*. Chichester, England, John Wiley & Sons, 1990, pp 567–578.

40. Knighton DR, Ciresi K, Kiegel VD, Schumerth S, Butler E, Cerra F: Stimulation of repair in chronic, nonhealing, cutaneous ulcers using platelet-derived wound healing formula. *Surg Gynecol Obstet* 1990;170:56–60.

41. Knighton DR, Fylling CP, Fiegel VD, Cerra F: Amputation prevention in an independently reviewed at-risk diabetic population using a comprehensive wound care protocol. *Am J Surg* 1990;160:466–471.

42. Brown GL, Nanney LB, Griffen J, et al: Enhancement of wound healing by topical treatment with epidermal growth factor. *N Engl J Med* 1989;321:76–79.

Diabetic Foot Infections

Charles L. Saltzman, MD
Walter J. Pedowitz, MD

Scope of the Problem

Trivial infections in diabetic feet can have disastrous effects. The monetary and human impact of these infections is staggering. The infected foot is one of the most common causes of admission of diabetic patients to the hospital, often requiring prolonged care. Infection is also a major pathway to ultimate amputation. The incidence of amputation in patients with diabetes is approximately 5%, 40 times that of the nondiabetic population.[1]

Pathophysiology

The pathophysiology of diabetic foot infection is complex. Patients with long-standing disease and multiple secondary complications are most prone to develop serious infections. Once initiated, both host and microbiologic factors impact the aggressiveness of the infection. The host factors that have been shown to result in an increased risk of amputation are diabetes mellitus for longer than 10 years, chronic hyperglycemia, impaired vision or joint mobility (required to perform preventive foot care), lack of knowledge about preventive foot care, increasing age, nephropathy, single/widowed/separated or divorced persons, alcohol use, nonwhites, males, and a history of previous amputation. Events leading to serious, limb-threatening infections typically involve an initial episode of minor trauma (eg, shoe-related repetitive pressure, accidental cuts or wounds, thermal trauma, and/or decubitus ulceration), cutaneous ulceration, and failure to heal. Other causal factors found to impact the outcome of a local foot infection are edema, impairing cutaneous blood flow; noncompliance in medical recommendations; negligent self-care; and inadequate social support.

The etiology of foot ulcers is clearly multifactorial, including neuropathy, vascular disease, infection, delayed wound healing, and, sometimes, development of gangrene. In large studies, the absence of protective sensation has been found to be the primary related factor for the development of ulcers and infection. The absence of protective sensation typically causes a distal, symmetric, "stocking" distribution of sensory loss mostly confined below the knees. Patients may initially experience a constant burning type of pain, which is worse at night. With further progression of the sensory neuropathy, they may develop unrecognized injury, ulceration, fracture, and foot deformity.

Concomitant with the development of sensory neuropathy, many patients also acquire either motor and/or autonomic neuropathy. The motor neuropathy manifests itself with claw-toe deformities caused by atrophy of the foot intrinsic muscles. Claw-toe deformities expose bony prominences on the dorsum of the toe to increased pressure from normal shoe wear. They also result in migration of the metatarsal fat pad, with plantar loss of cover of the metatarsal heads, loss of toe weightbearing during terminal stance, and increased pressure on exposed metatarsal heads. Some patients will also develop mononeuropathies causing focal deficits, such as foot drop from an anterior tibial mononeuropathy, recurrent ankle sprains from peroneal weakness, or flatfoot deformity from posterior tibialis denervation.

Although less prevalent, autonomic neuropathy can create vexing epidermal problems from diminished sweating. This may result in the drying of epidermal keratin, cracking and fissuring of noncompliant skin, and increased susceptibility to infection. Arteriovenous shunting secondary to autonomic neuropathy further compromises the ability of skin to heal minor ulcerations and deliver antibiotics peripherally.

The vascular disease that occurs secondary to diabetes mellitus usually involves all 3 major arterial supplies to the leg and foot. Decreased blood flow compromises the host's ability to heal and fight infection. Furthermore, these patients often have decreased local immune response. Basement membrane thickening has been proposed as a basic factor responsible for hampering leukocyte migration to the infection site. Laboratory studies show that phagocytic activity is impaired by hyperglycemia, and that neutrophils do not function properly in this environment.

In summary, the host factors that result in clinically significant diabetic foot infections are complex. Due to sensory neuropathy, visual or physical impairments, and frequent social isolation, many patients fail to recognize ulceration or infection early on. Lack of vascular nutrition, either due to autonomic arteriovenous shunting or from vascular insufficiency, further confounds the ability of the host to fight infection. The cellular response is often weak and insufficient to successfully eradicate invading microbiologic flora. Malnutrition, hyperglycemia, decreased peripheral microvasculature, anaerobic metabolism, and poor wound healing all help to create a hospitable environment for the bacteria.[2]

Infectious Agents

Most often, infections of the diabetic foot are polymicrobial. On average, 3 to 5 organisms are cultured from the moderately to severely infected foot. The type of organism(s) present may be gram-positive cocci and/or gram-negative rods, and anaerobes, with the latter seen more often in infections of increasing severity. The gram-positive organisms include *Staphylococcus aureus, Staphylococcus epidermidis,* group B *Streptococcus,* and *enterococci.* The gram-negative organisms may include *Proteus, Escherichia coli* or *Pseudomonas.* Among the anaerobes, *Bacteroides* is the most common infecting agent.[2]

Diagnosis of Cellulitis and/or Osteomyelitis

A complete history and physical examination are essential first steps. Local signs of infection, including erythema, swelling, and purulent drainage, should be noted. Foul-smelling drainage usually suggests an anaerobic infection. The examiner should try to probe to bone, using a sterile cotton swab. In this setting, the ability to probe to bone has an 80% positive predictive value of underlying osteomyelitis. The scope of the work-up depends on the level of clinical infection, but it usually includes obtaining a set of vital signs, temperature, a spot glucose test, and a white blood cell count with differential. These results must be interpreted with caution, because absence of fever or leukocytosis may be the result of diabetic immunosuppression, which can hide the serious underlying nature of the disease. Two thirds of patients with limb-threatening infection do not demonstrate fever of greater than 100° F. Half do not demonstrate leukocytosis.

Ulcers can be classified in various ways.[1,2–4] Probably the most common method used is that proposed by Wagner. In this classification scheme, ulcers are graded from 0 to 5 according to the depth of the ulcer, whether there is exposed tendon or bone, and whether there is an abscess or gangrene present. This system may be good to help guide surgical decisions, but it is not particularly helpful for clinical microbiologic purposes.

A more relevant system for guiding therapy is based on determining the aggressiveness of infection in the limb. Infections are classified as mild, moderate, or severe. Mild infections involve superficial ulceration, purulent discharge, minimal/absent cellulitis, and no osteomyelitis or systemic toxicity. Moderate-to-severe infec-

tions (potentially limb-threatening) involve ulcerations to deep tissues, purulent discharge, cellulitis, systemic toxicity, and mild-to-moderate necrosis, with or without osteomyelitis. Severe (potentially life-threatening) infections involve ulceration to deep tissues; purulent discharge; cellulitis; systemic toxicity, including septic shock, marked necrosis, or gangrene; and bacteremia, with or without osteomyelitis. Some of the moderate-to-severe infections that may require emergent surgical intervention are crepitant anaerobic cellulitis, non-clostridial/clostridial myonecrosis, or synergistic necrotizing fasciitis. This system of classifying infections according to whether they are local, limb-threatening, or life-threatening (mild, moderate, or severe) is helpful in determining appropriate treatment.

Culture/Biopsy

Our understanding of the need for culture or biopsy continues to evolve. Superficial cultures are rarely of value. Deep tissue cultures correlate poorly with superficial cultures, which tend to over-represent pathogens. The general consensus is to avoid superficial cultures.

The importance and need for deep cultures has changed with the emergence of better and more broad-spectrum antibiotics. Culture-specific treatment has not been shown to have better results than empiric treatment with broad-spectrum coverage. At present, it seems reasonable to perform bone biopsies or deep cultures at the time of surgical treatment, or in situations in which empiric therapy is failing. If empiric therapy results in an improved clinical condition, the authors recommend continuing that therapy rather than changing to a more culture-specific and narrower-spectrum antibiotic, because there are notorious problems with false-negative cultures in diabetic foot infections.

Imaging

The two clinical indications for imaging the diabetic foot are osteomyelitis and abscess formation. Osteomyelitis takes 10 to 21 days to become apparent on plain films, because a period of time is required before there is enough bone resorption to be radiographically apparent. In a diabetic patient with a poor vascular blood supply, bone resorption can take a considerably longer time than in a patient with an adequate blood supply.[5]

More sophisticated imaging modalities include the use of a technetium-labeled bone scan combined with indium-111 leukocyte scans, or magnetic resonance imaging (MRI) investigations. Because of the relative ease of use, MRI has become far more popular than the combined scan approach. Compared to the nuclear medicine scans, MRI will better delineate anatomy, especially abscess cavities and marrow involvement. MRI scans, however, tend to over-represent the amount of involved bone, and surgeons must be cautious when deciding the extent of osteomyelitis based on an MRI scan alone. Johnson and associates[6] have advocated the use of the indium-labeled scans to follow up negative plain films because the indium scan will not be false-positive from Charcot osteoarthropathy (as will the MRI), and when the indium scan is negative, the clinician can feel comfortable that there is little likelihood of ongoing infection.

Treatment

Most ulcers in diabetic patients are not infected, but are rather due to tissue necrosis from unrecognized elevated pressure.[1,2] Ulcers can occur anywhere on the foot. Plantar ulcers are best treated with total contact casting. Reports on total contact casting for plantar ulceration in noninfected diabetic feet are extremely encouraging. Within 5 weeks, 90% of ulcers will heal.[7]

For mild infections, patients usually are treated as outpatients with oral antibiotic coverage for *Staphylococcus aureus*, *Staphylococcus epidermidis*, and *Streptococcus*. Many different medications can be used. The most common ones are dicloxacillin, first-generation cephalosporins, clindamycin, and amoxicillin-clavulanic acid. The patient is brought back in 2 to 3 days for reevaluation. If the patient is not responding, the medication should be changed to another oral agent. If the condition is getting worse, the clinician may consider switching to IV therapy. Typically, mild infections are treated with local wound care, using wet-to-dry dressing changes or Silvadene, and pressure relief modalities, such as the use of crutches, custom-made orthotics with cut-outs, postoperative shoes with the forefoot removed, or healing sandals. After a 2 to 3 week course of antibiotics, if the infection is completely abated, the antibiotics are usually discontinued.

Moderate infections that are limb threatening are often caused by a synergistic combination of gram-positive and gram-negative aerobes and anaerobes. At the present time, to effectively treat these problems, IV antibiotics are required. The most common strategies are to use ampicillin-sulbactam, ticarcillin-clavulanate, piperacillin-tazobactam, or a fluocinolone with clindamycin (for penicillin-allergic patients). If present, abscesses are drained or excised, and necrotic bone is debrided. All patients should be assessed for the potential need for distal revascularization. The length of the IV course is typically 4 to 6 weeks, unless all infected bone and tissue has been removed. Recently, the earlier switch from IV therapy to an oral fluocinolone has been recommended.[8] More studies on the value of the newer oral fluocinolone are needed before a major change in treatment strategy can be advised.

For severe infections, the clinician must stabilize the patient and debride, drain, or amputate the infected part as is clinically necessary. In life-threatening infections, broad-spectrum antibiotics should be used. Imipenem-cilastatin is one of the more-powerful broad-spectrum antibiotics that can be used in this setting. Similarly, a combination of vancomycin, metronidazole, and aztreonam can be considered. If ampicillin-sulbactam is initiated, it should be started with an aminoglycoside to cover aggressive gram-negative organisms. If the patient is not responding to the regimen, an infectious disease consultation may be necessary.

Surgical Treatment of Infection

Appropriate antibiotics are no substitute for proper wound care and adequate surgical debridement. Patients with moderate-to-severe infections should receive early and aggressive drainage and debridement of all necrotic tissue. If the infection has significantly destroyed the function of the foot and/or endangers the patient's life, guillotine amputation to control sepsis may be indicated.

Some basic rules help in most circumstances. These rules include: (1) Debride all necrotic tissue and do not leave any dead tissue behind. (2) All surfaces should be bleeding at the end of the operation. (3) Check the histopathology of residual margins for evidence of residual infection. (4) If the initial debridement is uncertain, pack the wound open and repeat the surgery within a few days, if necessary. (5) Try to achieve an eventual closure, even if it means removal of more bone. (6) When closed, wound edges must be well perfused.

Postoperatively, the foot should not be allowed to dangle for excessive periods of time to avoid potential complications of venous stasis and wound dehiscence. The failure of a wound to heal may indicate vascular compromise. Reevaluate and restore circulation, if possible. If not possible, resect back to a viable level. These wounds heal slowly; in general, the sutures should be left in at least 3 weeks.

Improved results in the care of the diabetic foot have resulted from an aggressive approach to wound management, antibiotic coverage, revascularization when necessary, improved perioperative management, and a general team approach to the care of the patient. Relapses are more common in the diabetic foot than for other infections, and the clinician must attempt to educate the patient and the family about how to avoid unrecognized injury and how to recognize the early signs of infection.

References

1. Grayson ML: Diabetic foot infections: Antimicrobial therapy. *Infect Dis Clin North Am* 1995;9:143–161.

2. Frykberg RG, Veves A: Diabetic foot infections. *Diabetes Metab Rev* 1996;12:255–270.

3. Hass DW, McAndrew MP: Bacterial osteomyelitis in adults: Evolving considerations in diagnosis and treatment. *Am J Med* 1996;101:550–561.

4 van der Meer JW, Koopmans PP, Lutterman JA: Antibiotic therapy in diabetic foot infection. *Diabet Med* 1996;13(suppl 1):S48–S51.

5. Newman LG: Imaging techniques in the diabetic foot. *Clin Podiatr Med Surg* 1995;12:75–86.

6. Johnson JE, Kennedy EJ, Shereff MJ, Patel NC, Collier BD: Prospective study of bone, indium-111-labeled white blood cell, and gallium-67 scanning for the evaluation of osteomyelitis in the diabetic foot. *Foot Ankle Int* 1996;17:10–16.

7. Smith AJ, Daniels T, Bohnen JM: Soft tissue infections and the diabetic foot. *Am J Surg* 1996;172:7S–12S.

8. Lipsky BA, Baker PD, Landon GC, Fernay R: Antibiotic therapy for diabetic foot infections: Comparison of two parenteral-to-oral regimens. *Clin Infect Dis* 1997;24:643–648.

Surgical Treatment for Neuropathic Arthropathy of the Foot and Ankle

Jeffrey E. Johnson, MD

Nonsurgical treatment with use of a total-contact cast followed by appropriate bracing and footwear is the so-called gold standard for the treatment of most neuropathic (Charcot) fractures and dislocations of the foot and ankle. However, surgical treatment is indicated for chronic recurrent ulceration, joint instability, or, in some instances, pain that has not responded to nonsurgical treatment. Acute fractures may also be treated surgically if the patient is seen before demineralization of bone and inflammation of soft tissue have occurred. The goals of surgical treatment are to preserve function with the aid of appropriate footwear or bracing and to avoid the need for amputation. These goals are achieved through restoration of the contour or alignment of the affected segment of the foot and ankle. Despite the potential for major surgical complications, successful limb salvage and reconstruction was achieved in 124 (87%) of 143 patients in 8 clinical series.[1–7]

Natural History and Clinical Presentation

Neuropathic (Charcot) osteoarthropathy is a noninfective, destructive lesion of a bone and joint resulting from a fracture or dislocation, or both, in a patient who has peripheral neuropathy. Diabetes is the most com-

Table 1		
Classification System of Eichenholtz[10]		
Stage	Radiographic Features	Clinical Features
I—Dissolution	Demineralization of regional bone, periarticular fragmentation, dislocation of joint	Acute inflammation (easily confused with infection): swelling, erythema, warmth
II—Coalescence	Absorption of osseous debris in soft tissues, organization and early healing of fracture fragments, periosteal new-bone formation	Less inflammation, less fluctuation in swelling, increased stability at fracture site
III—Resolution	Smoothing of edges of large fragments of bone, sclerosis, osseous or fibrous ankylosis	Permanent enlargement of foot and ankle, fixed deformity, minimum daily swelling or activity-related swelling, normalization of skin temperature

(Adapted with permission from Johnson JE: Surgical reconstruction of the diabetic Charcot foot and ankle. *Foot Ankle Clin* 1997;2:39–40.)

mon cause of these deformity-causing fractures in the United States, and they were reported in 101 (0.1%) of 68,000 patients who had diabetes mellitus.[8] There are an estimated 16 million diabetic individuals in the United States.[9] Because of improvements in the treatment of diabetes, diabetic patients are living longer. Therefore, neuropathic arthropathy, a late effect of peripheral neuropathy of the foot and ankle, continues to be a problem that is seen in orthopaedic practices.

Frequently, a Charcot fracture or dislocation is caused by a minor acute injury, such as a sprain of the ankle or foot, or by an overuse syndrome resulting from repetitive minor injuries. However, it may also be the

result of an acute traumatic event, such as a fall from a height or a motor-vehicle accident.

The etiology and pathophysiology of neuropathic destruction of bones and joints are poorly understood. However, the stages of bone and joint destruction, followed by fracture-healing and remodeling, were described by Eichenholtz.[10] The Eichenholtz classification is based on the characteristic clinical and radiographic changes that occur with neuropathic destruction or fracture of a joint over time and is therefore a temporally based classification. As shown in Table 1, these changes progress from the acute phase (dissolution), through the healing phase

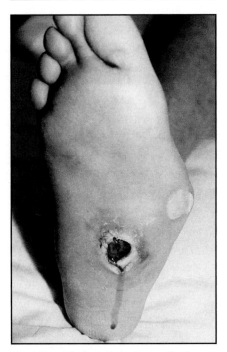

Fig. 1 The right foot of a patient with Charcot arthropathy who had collapse of the midfoot and abduction of the forefoot after a fracture-dislocation of the midfoot, which resulted in ulceration of the medial and plantar aspects of the foot.

(coalescence), to the resolution phase. The timing and selection of a reconstructive procedure for a patient who has a neuropathic joint should be made with a clear understanding of the natural history of a Charcot joint and the temporal stage of the neuropathic process. Different classifications for the characteristic patterns of neuropathic destruction of bones and joints have been described by other investigators.[11-13] An understanding of these patterns is helpful when making the diagnosis and planning treatment for patients who have occult neuropathy.

Deformities of the foot and ankle resulting from a neuropathic fracture or dislocation cause difficulty with shoe-fitting and marked alteration in the load applied to various parts of the plantar surface of the foot during weightbearing. These changes lead to an increased propensity for ulceration in high-pressure areas (Fig. 1). These ulcers may become a portal of entry for bacteria and thus may result in superficial or deep infection. A deformity may also be associated with joint instability, which is accentuated by weightbearing, especially with involvement of the hindfoot or ankle. These changes result in loss of the plantigrade position of the foot and the development of progressive varus, valgus, equinus, or calcaneus deformity.

Nonsurgical Treatment
Nonsurgical treatment is indicated for most Charcot deformities of the foot and ankle. Most deformities are treated with immobilization in a total-contact cast to allow healing and stabilization of the fracture. If the ankle or hindfoot joints are involved, prolonged immobilization in an ankle-foot orthosis for 12 to 18 months, or indefinitely, is often indicated. Involvement of the midfoot and forefoot is typically treated with appropriate extra-depth footwear and custom total-contact inserts.

Surgical Treatment
Surgical treatment is indicated when a patient has a severe deformity of the foot and ankle that is not amenable to management with a custom brace or custom footwear, marked instability (usually involving the hindfoot and ankle), or recurrent ulceration. A markedly unstable Charcot joint may be associated with pain; however, unlike painful osteoarthrosis, a painful Charcot joint is rarely the sole reason for surgical treatment.

The Goals of Surgery
One goal of surgical treatment of a Charcot foot and ankle is to restore the stability and alignment of the foot and ankle so that footwear and a brace can be worn. For most patients who have a deformity that is severe enough to necessitate surgical treatment, a partial amputation of the foot or a below-the-knee amputation is usually the only alternative treatment option. Therefore, an additional goal of surgical intervention is to prevent the inevitable amputation of a limb that is destined to have recurrent ulceration.

Patients who have a moderate-to-severe deformity resulting from neuropathic arthropathy need special footwear with custom total-contact inserts and, sometimes, a custom brace to prevent recurrent ulceration and progressive deformity. Therefore, the decision is not between surgery or the use of prescription footwear and bracing but rather between surgery followed by prescription footwear and bracing or prescription footwear and bracing alone. Therefore, surgery is indicated primarily to make these patients better candidates for prescription footwear and bracing. Although some patients who have a solid fusion after a realignment arthrodesis may eventually be weaned from the ankle-foot orthosis, weaning is an unrealistic goal for many patients and may lead to recurrent ulceration or stress fractures of the tibia.[14]

Timing of Surgery
Surgical treatment of a Charcot foot is usually carried out in the quiescent (resolution) phase of the fracture pattern (Eichenholtz stage III) after the use of a cast, prescription footwear, or a brace, or all 3, have failed. An acute fracture associated with neuropathic arthropathy may be treated with open reduction and fixation if treatment is performed early, before neuropathic inflammation of the soft tissue occurs and while bone stock is still sufficient for rigid fixation. However, most

patients are not seen for treatment early enough for this approach. When the acute (dissolution) phase (Eichenholtz stage I) has begun, the demineralization of regional bone and swelling make surgical management of the fracture difficult, leading to a higher rate of failure of fixation, recurrent deformity, and infection.

An ulcer of the foot that is associated with a neuropathic deformity is treated, until it has healed (if possible), with use of a total-contact cast so that the incision for the reconstructive procedure may be made through intact skin to reduce the possibility of postoperative infection. If underlying osteomyelitis is suspected in association with a neuropathic fracture, imaging with a combined technetium-99m bone scan and indium-111-labeled white blood cell scan with use of the dual-window technique helps to confirm or rule out this suspicion.[15,16] If osteomyelitis is present, it is treated with appropriate debridement and antibiotic therapy until the wound has healed and the infection has resolved. Then, the choice with regard to surgical or nonsurgical treatment of the remaining deformity can be made.

Treatment of an Acute Fracture Associated With Neuropathic Arthropathy

The most important factor in the successful treatment of an acute fracture in a patient who has neuropathic arthropathy is the recognition of the fact that the patient has a severe peripheral neuropathy. A series of small monofilament nylon rods (Semmes-Weinstein monofilaments) can be used to determine the severity and location of the sensory neuropathy.[17] If sensory testing with Semmes-Weinstein monofilaments shows loss of protective sensation, it is important to alter the typical treatment regimen to help prevent subsequent Charcot

destruction of the joint. It is also important to warn the patient about the potential risk of Charcot involvement of the joint, whether or not surgical treatment of the fracture is undertaken.

The first step in the treatment of an acute fracture is to determine whether it is associated with neuropathic changes (that is, Eichenholtz stage I) or with peripheral neuropathy but not yet with neuropathic changes. This differentiation often can be made on the basis of the medical history. For example, when a patient has had a relatively minor injury followed by several days or weeks of erythema and swelling and has a displaced fracture on presentation, the fracture is usually treated as an Eichenholtz stage I injury with use of a total-contact cast. However, a patient with severe diabetic peripheral neuropathy who has sustained an acute displaced fracture may be managed with the same orthopaedic principles as would be followed for a patient who does not have neuropathy (if seen acutely), except that a higher rate of complications would be expected and a prolonged postoperative period of nonweightbearing and immobilization in a total-contact cast followed by use of a brace would be indicated. If treatment after the fixation of a fracture does not include rigid external immobilization and a prolonged period of nonweightbearing, the fixation may fail before the fracture has healed (Fig. 2).

Acute fractures of the ankle, talus, or midfoot may be treated with use of the same indications for open reduction and internal fixation, assuming that the patient is medically fit, the vascular status is adequate, there is minimum swelling, and the skin is in good condition. Patients who have an acute fracture that is already Eichenholtz stage I, with early de-

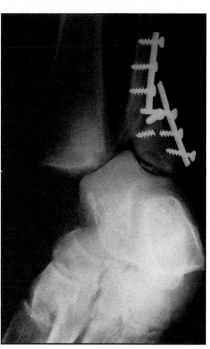

Fig. 2 Postoperative radiograph, made 4 weeks after open reduction and internal fixation of a fracture of the distal part of the fibula with injury of the deltoid ligament, demonstrating valgus displacement and failure of the plate and screws in the fibula. The patient had been managed with a prefabricated removable brace for postoperative immobilization and was allowed toe-touch weightbearing.

mineralization and soft-tissue inflammation, are poorer candidates for surgical treatment. Internal fixation of an ankle fracture is augmented by the addition of 1 or 2 Steinmann pins across the ankle and subtalar joints to prevent hardware failure and joint deformity (Fig. 3). The pins are cut off below the level of the plantar skin and are removed 6 to 8 weeks postoperatively at the time of a cast change.

It is important to extend the duration of immobilization for a fracture in a patient with peripheral neuropathy to approximately double the normal period of time that a patient without neuropathy would be non-

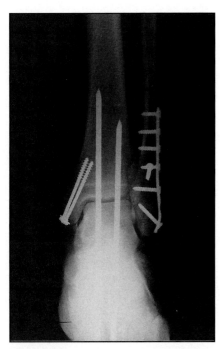

Fig. 3 Anteroposterior radiograph showing percutaneously placed smooth Steinmann pins that were used to augment the internal fixation of a bimalleolar fracture of the ankle until the fracture healed.

weightbearing. Therefore, a patient with neuropathy who has a typical fracture of the ankle is managed with nonweightbearing for approximately 3 months (compared with 6 weeks for a patient without neuropathy), and a cast is worn until approximately 4 to 5 months after the injury, at which time the patient is able to walk while wearing a weightbearing cast and the fracture has united. A brace is then worn for 1 year after the injury to prevent late development of a Charcot joint. A patient who is doing well 12 to 18 months after the injury may be weaned from the brace and subsequently managed with use of extra-depth footwear with custom-molded total-contact inserts. During this period, the patient is carefully monitored for the development of a Charcot joint.

The prolonged duration of immo-bilization in this protocol may be excessive for patients in whom a Charcot joint is not destined to develop. However, there are no known factors that predict which fracture will progress to a Charcot joint in a patient who has a neuropa-thy. Therefore, in order to prevent severe deformity, it seems prudent to manage every patient who has loss of protective sensation as if a Charcot joint will develop.

Types of Reconstructive Procedures for Neuropathic Deformity
Ostectomy

The midfoot is the most common location for neuropathic destruction.[18] The apex of the rocker-bottom defor-mity of the foot that results from this neuropathic destruction is a frequent cause of recurrent ulceration because of the prominence at the apex in the sole of the foot. The most common surgical procedure to treat a neuro-pathic deformity that causes recurrent ulceration and difficulty with foot-wear is the removal of the osseous prominence on the medial, lateral, or plantar aspect of the foot.

The first step in the surgical treat-ment of any neuropathic deformity is to obtain closure of the overlying ulcer, if possible, so that the incision to remove the osseous prominence can be made through intact skin. An alternative technique is to excise the ulcer through a plantar, longitudinal, elliptical incision made directly over the prominence. However, this tech-nique exposes a large amount of underlying cancellous bone to the open ulcer with a potential for bacte-rial colonization of the underlying superficial bone.

A preferred method (Fig. 4) is to obtain closure of the ulcer with a series of total-contact casts so that the incision can be made through intact skin on the medial or lateral border of the foot closest to the osseous promi-nence.[11,19] The skin incision is made as a full-thickness flap down to the osseous prominence. A periosteal ele-vator is used to separate the overlying soft tissue from the protuberant bone. A small power saw or an osteotome is used to resect the bone surface, which is then rasped to provide a smooth broad surface in the weightbearing area. Major tendon attachments, such as the peroneus brevis, anterior tibial tendon, posterior tibial tendon, and Achilles tendon, should be preserved and reattached to bone if they are detached. Resection of a large promi-nence in the medial part of the mid-foot involving the medial cuneiform should include reattachment of the anterior tibial tendon through holes drilled into the remaining bone. Many patients have a coexistent contracture of the Achilles tendon, and percuta-neous lengthening of the Achilles ten-don is frequently performed at the time of plantar ostectomy.[20]

The skin is closed over a suction drain, which is left in place for 24 hours with a compression splint. The next day, a total-contact cast is applied to stabilize the soft tissues, promote wound healing, and allow the patient limited weightbearing. It is especially important to avoid excessive bone re-section in the midfoot, where removal of the plantar ligaments may cause progression of the rocker-bottom de-formity. An ostectomy of the plantar aspect of the midfoot is more success-ful when the neuropathic deformity is stable in the sagittal and transverse planes.

The sutures are removed when the incision has healed, usually 2 to 3 weeks after the procedure. At the time of 1 of the cast changes, a mold of the foot is made for a total-contact insert so that the appropriate foot-wear and a custom insert will be

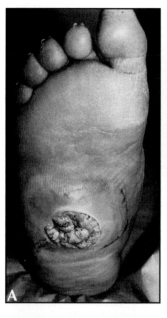
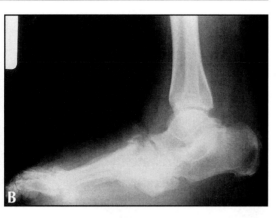
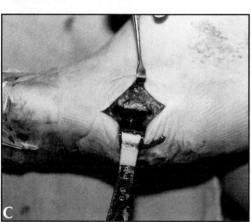
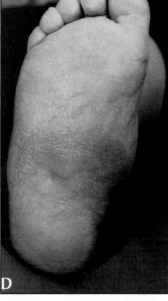

Fig. 4 A patient who had a chronic recurrent plantar ulcer beneath a rocker-bottom deformity. **A,** Photograph of the plantar aspect of the foot, made before treatment with a total-contact cast, which allowed the ulcer to heal before ostectomy. **B,** Lateral radiograph demonstrating a neuropathic rocker-bottom deformity of the midfoot with a large plantar prominence. Note the equinus position of the hindfoot secondary to contracture of the Achilles tendon. **C,** Intraoperative photograph demonstrating the incision, made lateral to the healed ulcer, for the resection of the plantar prominence, which was a portion of the cuboid bone. Percutaneous lengthening of the Achilles tendon was also performed. **D,** Postoperative photograph made 6 months after the plantar ostectomy, demonstrating the healed ulcer. Postoperatively, the patient was managed with a double-upright calf-lacer ankle-foot orthosis attached to an extra-depth shoe with a custom total-contact insert.

ready for use when healing has occurred and the cast is removed.

Realignment and Arthrodesis

Severe Charcot deformity or instability of the foot and ankle is treated with realignment of the involved joint and stabilization by arthrodesis (Fig. 5). Most patients considering this surgery have had a failure of treatment with a brace and special footwear, and amputation is the only other reasonable option for treatment. The goal of surgery is to restore the alignment and stability of the foot so that the patient can use a brace and special footwear. This surgery is not intended to substitute for appropriate footwear or use of a brace.

The contraindications to arthrodesis include: (1) infection of the soft tissue or bone except when the arthrodesis is performed as a staged procedure after the infection has been treated, all osteomyelitic bone has been resected, and the soft tissues have healed; (2) a fracture that is in the acute (dissolution) phase of the neuropathic disease process (Eichenholtz stage I); (3) uncontrolled diabetes or malnutrition; (4) peripheral vascular disease; (5) insufficient bone stock to obtain rigid fixation; and (6) the inability of the patient to comply with the postoperative regimen (because of mental illness).

Technique Preoperatively, a total-contact cast is used until the acute phase of the Charcot fracture process has subsided and the skin is intact. Extensive longitudinal incisions are used with full-thickness skin flaps to bone. If the deformity is mild to moderate and is limited to the ankle and subtalar joints, tibiotalocalcaneal arthrodesis may be performed through a posterior approach.[21] For correction of a severe deformity, exposure is enhanced by making medial and lateral incisions over the ankle rather than a posterior incision. Bone is resected to allow correction of the deformity and to provide apposition of stable bleeding bone surfaces to promote successful fusion. A contracture of the Achilles tendon is corrected with percutaneous lengthening especially when a midfoot or hindfoot arthrodesis is performed. Autologous bone grafting is used to fill any defects and to provide both an intra-articular and an extra-articular arthrodesis when

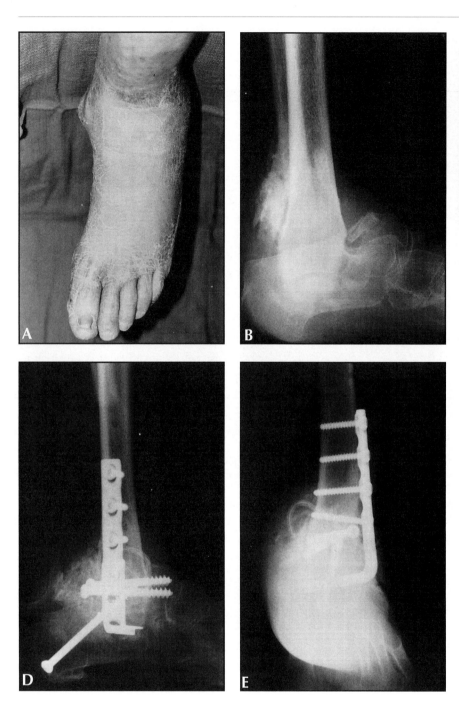

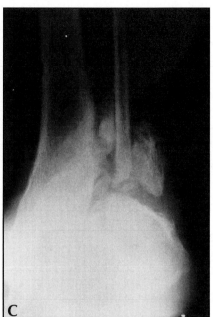

Fig. 5 A patient who had neuropathic arthropathy with marked valgus deformity of the hindfoot. **A,** Preoperative photograph showing a subcutaneous prominence of the medial malleolus with impending breakdown of the skin. **B,** Lateral radiograph demonstrating a neuropathic fracture-dislocation of the hindfoot with dissolution of the body of the talus. **C,** Anteroposterior radiograph demonstrating lateral subluxation and valgus angulation of the hindfoot with neuropathic fragmentation of the distal part of the fibula. **D,** Lateral radiograph made after open reduction, realignment, and tibiocalcaneal arthrodesis through lateral and medial incisions. The distal part of the tibia is fused to the anterior part of the calcaneus. Note the fixation of the talar head and neck to the anterior aspect of the distal part of the tibia. **E,** Anteroposterior radiograph made after the tibiocalcaneal arthrodesis, demonstrating fixation with a 4.5-mm titanium blade-plate.

possible. Morcellized pieces of resected tibial and fibular bone may also be used when bone grafting is needed primarily for extra-articular application. Large, threaded Steinmann pins, compression blade-plates, or custom intramedullary rods are used in whatever combination provides adequate rigid internal fixation (Figs. 6 and 7).

Use of a plate on the plantar aspect of the medial column of the midfoot has been advocated to enhance the rigidity of an arthrodesis of the midfoot.[22] External fixation provides adequate stability, but positioning of the foot and ankle is more difficult with an external fixator; such fixation is reserved for patients who have an

open wound and need osseous stabilization. Problems at the pin sites may also force early removal of the fixator, leading to nonunion or malunion.

Long-term immobilization is crucial for achieving union. In general, the duration of immobilization after an arthrodesis for patients who have neuropathic arthropathy is twice as long as that for patients who do not have neuropathic arthropathy. The postoperative regimen includes 3 months of nonweightbearing in a total-contact cast followed by 1 to 2 months in a weightbearing total-contact cast. The patient then is managed with a bivalved ankle-foot orthosis with a rocker sole added to the footplate until the use of footwear and a definitive brace is possible. Bracing is continued for 12 to 18 months postoperatively, as in the treatment of a neuropathic fracture. After an arthrodesis of the midfoot, an extra-depth shoe with an extended steel shank and a rocker sole may be used if there is little swelling and the fusion is solid. For patients who have involvement of the hindfoot and ankle, this type of shoe is attached either to a double-upright calf-lacer or a patellar-ligament-bearing ankle-foot orthosis (Figs. 8 and 9). A custom-molded polypropylene ankle-foot orthosis may be used inside a shoe with a rocker sole if the deformity of the foot is not severe.

When there is a severe deformity of the foot, it is preferable to use whatever shoe-and-foot-orthosis combination accommodates the foot deformity and then to have the shoe attached to a double-upright brace. A custom-molded polypropylene ankle-foot orthosis that extends into the foot region takes up space in the shoe and may not adequately accommodate a severe deformity of the foot, thereby causing a recurrent ulcer. After an arthrodesis of the midfoot, hindfoot, or ankle, use of a brace is necessary for at least the first 12 to 18 months, to allow complete healing and a return to weightbearing. Arthrodesis of the ankle, hindfoot, or midfoot at the level of the talonavicular joint is prone to either recurrent Charcot changes at adjacent joints or stress fractures[14] and should be protected with use of a brace indefinitely. After an arthrodesis

of the midfoot distal to the level of the talonavicular joint, stability of the site is provided with use of an extra-depth shoe with a total-contact insert, an extended steel shank, and a rocker sole.

The choice of whether to wean a patient from the ankle-foot orthosis at 12 to 18 months after an arthrodesis depends on multiple factors, including union and stability at the site of the arthrodesis, the location of the arthrodesis, and the reliability as well as the activity level of the patient. After an arthrodesis of the hindfoot involving the tibiotalocalcaneal joint, active patients may be prone to stress fractures in the distal part of the tibia when a brace is not used for strenuous activities because the foot acts as a long, rigid lever arm that places stresses on the tibia[14] (Fig. 7).

Results of Reconstruction of a Charcot Joint
The rates of union reported after arthrodesis of the foot and ankle for

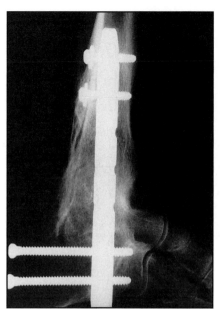
Fig. 6 Lateral radiograph made 7 months after a tibiotalocalcaneal arthrodesis through a posterior approach, showing fixation with a retrograde locked intramedullary nail.

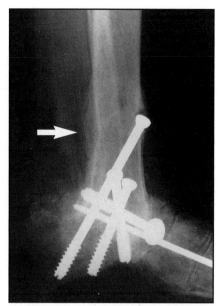
Fig. 7 Radiograph made after a tibiotalocalcaneal arthrodesis that was stabilized with multiple partially threaded cannulated screws augmented with a single threaded Steinmann pin. Note the healed stress fracture (arrow) through the proximal screw-hole in the tibia, which had occurred when the patient walked without a brace 7 months postoperatively. The fracture was treated for 12 weeks with a total-contact cast followed by resumption of the use of a brace. This stress fracture might have been prevented by the insertion of a more distal screw, avoiding the crest of the tibia, and if the patient had complied better with the postoperative use of the brace.

the treatment of neuropathic deformity in 143 patients in 8 clinical series averaged 70% (range, 54% to 100%).[1-7] However, the goal of achieving a stable foot on which a brace or a shoe, or both, could be worn was attained for 87% (124) of the patients after the initial surgical procedure, regardless of whether or not a solid union or a stable nonunion had been achieved.[1-7] Complications that may lead to failure of the procedure and necessitate a repeat procedure include a deep wound infection, an unstable nonunion, and a malunion.

Although authors of earlier reports

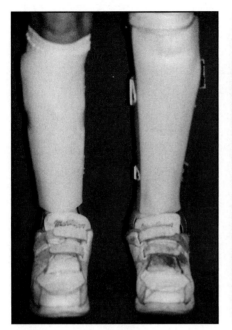 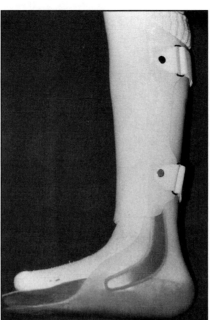

Fig. 8 The 2-piece polypropylene clamshell-type ankle-foot orthosis used for immobilization of an Eichenholtz stage-II or stage-III neuropathic fracture or after arthrodesis of the hindfoot for the treatment of a neuropathic deformity.

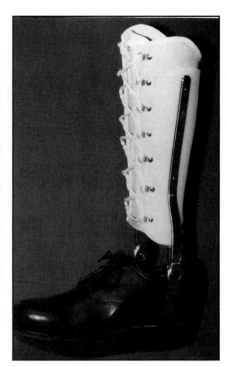

Fig. 9 Double-upright modified calf-lacer ankle-foot orthosis attached to an extra-depth shoe with an extended steel shank and a rocker sole. This style of orthosis is used when there is a severe deformity of the foot that needs to be accommodated by specialized footwear.

have expressed caution with respect to the performance of an arthrodesis for the treatment of neuropathic arthropathy,[6,23] modern techniques of internal fixation and prolonged immobilization have substantially increased the rate of union and decreased the rate of complications. The rate of satisfaction with these procedures is high, in large part because pain is not a major factor.[1,2,4,5,24] Most patients are grateful if the ability to walk in an appropriate shoe or brace is restored and an amputation is avoided.

In a recent study, 32 arthrodeses were performed for the treatment of neuropathic deformities of the foot and ankle; the series included 27 feet (25 patients) (unpublished data, 1996). Five of these procedures had been preceded by an initial attempt at realignment arthrodesis; 2 were repeat arthrodeses, and 3 were plantar ostectomies. Including the reoperations, 26 (96%) of the 27 feet were eventually rendered stable and the

patient was able to wear a brace. The goals of surgery were not met in 1 patient, who developed a deep infection requiring transtibial amputation.

The Dilemma Concerning Reconstructive Procedures in Patients Who Have Charcot Arthropathy

Because of the technical difficulty involved in managing patients who have Charcot arthropathy as well as the potential complications and the prolonged duration of treatment that is required, some practitioners may offer an amputation rather than reconstruction to treat a neuropathic deformity that does not allow use of a brace. Previous studies on energy expenditure according to level of amputation have demonstrated that the more distal the level of the amputation, the less energy expended during walking.[25] Therefore, it would be logical that a patient with a Charcot deformity who has been managed

with reconstruction would expend less energy during walking and may have a higher level of function than would a patient who has been managed with an amputation, especially a patient who has limited cardiovascular reserves.

Perhaps the most compelling reason for limb salvage is the long-term uncertainty about the status of the other foot. Peripheral vascular disease or an ulcer on the contralateral foot may lead to a deep wound infection, necessitating an amputation in the future. Reconstruction instead of amputation for the treatment of a neuropathic deformity in a patient who is a candidate for reconstruction may allow the patient to avoid eventual bilateral amputation.

Overview

Reconstruction of the Charcot foot and ankle is a valuable technique for the management of a patient who has a severe deformity that cannot be treated with use of appropriate footwear and a brace. The goals of surgery are to allow the patient to wear a shoe and a brace and to prevent amputation. Despite complications, the overall rate of success is more than 80%.[1-7] Stability and appropriate alignment are more important than union for achieving a successful result. Meticulous handling of the soft tissues and rigid internal fixation with use of bone-grafting are important parts of the surgical technique. Prolonged immobilization is necessary. Limb salvage with realignment and arthrodesis of a severely deformed foot and ankle allows most patients to avoid amputation and probably provides a more functional limb. Use of these surgical indications and techniques results in a high degree of patient satisfaction.

References

1. Alvarez RG, Barbour TM, Perkins TD: Tibio-calcaneal arthrodesis for nonbraceable neuropathic ankle deformity. *Foot Ankle Int* 1994;15: 354–359.

2. Bono JV, Roger DJ, Jacobs RL: Surgical arthrodesis of the neuropathic foot: A salvage procedure. *Clin Orthop* 1993;296:14–20.

3. Early JS, Hansen ST: Surgical reconstruction of the diabetic foot: A salvage approach for midfoot collapse. *Foot Ankle Int* 1996;17:325–330.

4. Papa J, Myerson M, Girard P: Salvage, with arthrodesis, in intractable diabetic neuropathic arthropathy of the foot and ankle. *J Bone Joint Surg* 1993;75A:1056–1066.

5. Sammarco GJ, Conti SF: Surgical treatment of neuroarthropathic foot deformity. *Foot Ankle Int* 1998;19:102–109.

6. Stuart MJ, Morrey BF: Arthrodesis of the diabetic neuropathic ankle joint. *Clin Orthop* 1990; 253:209–211.

7. Tisdel CL, Marcus RE, Heiple KG: Triple arthrodesis for diabetic peritalar neuroarthropathy. *Foot Ankle Int* 1995;16:332–338.

8. Sinha S, Munichoodappa CS, Kozak GP: Neuro-arthropathy (Charcot joints) in diabetes mellitus. *Medicine* 1972;51:191–210.

9. American Diabetes Association: *Diabetes: 1996 Vital Statistics.* Alexandria, VA, American Diabetes Association, 1996, p 13.

10. Eichenholtz SN (ed): *Charcot Joints.* Springfield, IL, CC Thomas, 1966.

11. Brodsky JW, Rouse AM: Exostectomy for symptomatic bony prominences in diabetic Charcot feet. *Clin Orthop* 1993;296:21–26.

12. Cofield RH, Morrison MJ, Beabout JW: Diabetic neuroarthropathy in the foot: Patient characteristics and patterns of radiographic change. *Foot Ankle* 1983;4:15–22.

13. Harris JR, Brand PW: Patterns of disintegration of the tarsus in the anaesthetic foot. *J Bone Joint Surg* 1966;48B:4–16.

14. Mitchell JR, Johnson JE, Collier BD, Gould JS: Stress fracture of the tibia following extensive hindfoot and ankle arthrodesis: A report of three cases. *Foot Ankle Int* 1995;16:445–448.

15. Johnson JE, Kennedy EJ, Shereff MJ, Patel NC, Collier BD: Prospective study of bone, indium-111-labeled white blood cell, and gallium-67 scanning for the evaluation of osteomyelitis in the diabetic foot. *Foot Ankle Int* 1996;17:10–16.

16. Schauwecker DS, Park HM, Burt RW, Mock BH, Wellman HN: Combined bone scintigraphy and indium-111 leukocyte scans in neuropathic foot disease. *J Nucl Med* 1988;29: 1651–1655.

17. Mueller MJ: Identifying patients with diabetes mellitus who are at risk for lower-extremity complications: Use of Semmes-Weinstein monofilaments. *Phys Ther* 1996;76:68–71.

18. Brodsky JW: The diabetic foot, in Mann RA, Coughlin MJ (eds): *Surgery of the Foot and Ankle,* ed 6. St. Louis, MO, Mosby-Year Book, 1993, pp 877–958.

19. Johnson JE: Surgical reconstruction of the diabetic Charcot foot and ankle. *Foot Ankle Clin* 1997;2:37–55.

20. Myerson MS, Henderson MR, Saxby T, Short KW: Management of midfoot diabetic neuroarthropathy. *Foot Ankle Int* 1994;15:233–241.

21. Russotti GM, Johnson KA, Cass JR: Tibiotalocalcaneal arthrodesis for arthritis and deformity of the hind part of the foot. *J Bone Joint Surg* 1988;70A:1304–1307.

22. Schon LC, Marks RM: The management of neuroarthropathic fracture-dislocations in the diabetic patient. *Orthop Clin North Am* 1995; 26:375–392.

23. Cleveland M: Surgical fusion of unstable joints due to neuropathic disturbance. *Am J Surg* 1939;43:580–584.

24. Myerson MS, Alvarez RG, Brodsky JW, Johnson JE: Symposium: Neuroarthropathy of the foot. *Contemp Orthop* 1993;26:43–64.

25. Pinzur MS, Gold J, Schwartz D, Gross N: Energy demands for walking in dysvascular amputees as related to the level of amputation. *Orthopedics* 1992;15:1033–1036.

Principles of Partial Foot Amputations in the Diabetic

Douglas G. Smith, MD

Introduction

Lower extremity amputations are performed because of gangrene, severe infection, ischemia, or severe deformity of the diabetic foot. In the years 1988 to 1992 there were an estimated 130,000 amputations performed each year in the United States. This number comes from the National Hospital Discharge Survey's (NHDS) estimate of 110,000 amputations annually, the Department of Veterans Affairs Hospital's estimate of 17,000 amputations annually, and the unknown, but lesser number estimated from the military, private charitable, and Indian Health Services Hospitals.[1] Even though persons with diabetes represent only about 3% of the total US population, 51% of the discharge diagnosis for amputation also listed the diagnosis of diabetes. Using this number, approximately 65,000 individuals with diabetes undergo lower extremity amputations per year.[1]

Table 1 shows the estimated breakdown by surgical amputation level of the percentage of lower extremity amputations performed for persons with and without diabetes, based on

the NHDS data. Many physicians believe that the rate of transfemoral amputations has decreased dramatically in the last 20 years, but statistics from the NHDS indicate that overall, more transfemoral amputations are done each year than transtibial amputations. The data do show that in persons with diabetes the ratio of transtibial to transfemoral amputations is slightly more favorable, but closer than many expect[1] (Table 1).

Decision Making

In diabetes, tissue loss, deep infection, especially osteomyelitis, chronic ulceration, or ischemia are the

most frequent reasons for amputation. The preoperative evaluation of these patients includes the clinical examination and evaluation of the tissue quality, level of tissue necrosis from infection, perfusion, nutrition, immune status, and functional abilities. Preoperative screening tests to directly or indirectly measure perfusion can be helpful, but no single test is 100% accurate. Clinical judgment is still an extremely important factor in preoperative assessment of diabetic patients. Although much attention is given to circulation, perfusion pressures, and oxygen diffusion, blood flow is not the only issue.

Table 1
Lower extremity amputations by amputation level and presence of diabetes (NHDS 1989-92)[20]

Amputation Level	Diabetes		No Diabetes		Total	
	No.	%	No.	%	No.	%
Toe	21,671	40.3	12,427	24.1	34,098	32.3
Foot/ankle	7,773	14.5	2,967	5.8	10,740	10.2
Transtibial	13,484	25.1	11,048	21.4	24,527	23.3
Knee disarticulation	704	1.3	778	1.5	1,482	1.4
Transfemoral	8,612	16.0	20,028	38.8	28,640	27.2
Hip/pelvis	87	0.2	386	0.7	473	0.5
Not specified	1,378	2.6	3,971	7.7	5,349	5.1
Total	53,709	100.0	51,605	100.0	105,309	100.0

This chapter was adapted with permission from Smith DG: Principles of partial foot amputations in the diabetic. *Foot Ankle Clin* 1997;2:171–186.

If blood flow to the involved extremity is poor and cannot be improved with angioplasty or vascular bypass, then partial foot amputation is not feasible. Attention needs to be directed at choosing the wisest proximal amputation for that particular patient's clinical situation and rehabilitation goals. For the diabetic patient who is a candidate for partial foot amputation, either the patient with adequate perfusion to the foot, or the patient with reconstructable vascular disease, the surgeon needs to ask the question: "Is this foot worth saving?" All too often, after the patient has already undergone vascular bypass surgery, the team realizes that the foot is not really salvageable and a higher level amputation is required. Some of the other factors besides blood flow that are extremely important in the decision process include the soft-tissue envelope, deformities, sensation, contractures, and rehabilitation goals.

The question regarding the soft-tissue envelope is, "Will the ulcer heal, will it stay healed, or will new ulcers form?"

Deformities, including claw toes, bunion deformity, peritalar subluxation, Charcot collapse, and other bony prominence can impact new ulcer formation and function.[2] "Can these deformities be corrected?"

Regarding sensation, the surgeon must ask, "Is there any sensation to protect the foot after salvage? Are shoe modifications available that might help protect the foot without sensation?"

Contractures, such as Achilles tendon, knee, and toe contractures are common. "How will the contractures impact the function and durability of the salvaged foot? Can the contractures be corrected?"

Questions about rehabilitation goals are: "Does or will the patient

ambulate? How will the patient transfer safely? Can this patient use special devices or a prosthesis safely?"

The answers to these questions, whether to proceed with an amputation, and at what level the amputation should be performed, should be considered for every patient during the decision-making process.

Most of the Time: The Goal is to Salvage Part of the Foot

Patients with partial foot amputations require less energy to ambulate than if amputation was performed at the transtibial or transfemoral levels.[3] Even in patients who are marginal ambulators, the improved ability to transfer independently can make a tremendous difference in lifestyle. Often it is not whether a person ambulates with a prosthesis that makes the difference between returning home or requiring nursing supervision, but rather whether they can transfer safely and independently. Most physicians underemphasize the importance of independent transfer ability.

Occasionally: The Most Distal Amputation is Not the Wisest Amputation

Occasionally it is predicted that the patient will function better with the higher level amputation. Special conditions that warrant this radical type of thinking might include nonambulatory patients, patients with spasticity, and patients with severe contractures. For nonambulatory patients, the goals are not simply to obtain wound healing, but to minimize complications, improve sitting balance, transfers, and nursing care. Thus, occasionally, a more proximal amputation might more successfully meet all of the goals. A good example is the bedridden patient with a knee-flexion contracture, who might be

better served with a knee disarticulation than a below-knee amputation, even if the biologic factors are present to allow the more distal amputation to heal.

Another example is the patient with a severe equinovarus deformity of the ankle presenting with an ulcer down to bone over the fifth metatarsal head from walking on the lateral border of the foot. A ray amputation without correction of the ankle deformity will result in rapid recurrent ulceration. Either the deformity must be corrected, or a transtibial amputation considered. Preoperative assessment of the patient's potential to be a prosthetic user, the specific needs to maintain independent transfers, or the best weight distribution for seating can also help direct level selection and postoperative rehabilitation wisely.

Surgical Level

The surgical amputation level must be the balance of biology and function. Outline 1 lists considerations in determining the biologic healing level, and the functional level. The biologic healing level is determined to try and predict the most distal amputation level that has a reasonable probability to heal. The functional level is the amputation level at which the patient will probably function best. Occasionally, if the clinical examination, ischemic index, transcutaneous oxygen tension measurement ($TcPO_2$), temperature of the skin, or nutrition indicate that there is little chance of distal wound healing, then biology determines the surgical level and one must do a very high amputation, even if only a toe or forefoot is infected and gangrenous.

Multiple surgeries in the elderly are not desirable. It is not acceptable to have the attitude that we can try the distal amputation, even if there is no reasonable chance of healing, and can amputate higher next time. Each surgery will decrease nutritional reserves and decrease the chance of wound healing. The longer patients are in bed, the more deconditioned they become, and the harder it is to rehabilitate and resume walking. The more surgeries, the higher the risk of problems such as deep venous thrombosis, pulmonary embolism, pneumonia, urinary tract infections, infected intravenous sites, and skin pressure sores. Careful selection of the initial amputation level is essential.

Comments on Adjuncts for Evaluation and Decision Making

Doppler ultrasound blood pressure assessment is the most readily available objective measurement of limb blood flow and perfusion. Arterial wall calcification increases the pressure needed to compress these vessels, often giving an artificially elevated reading. Low pressures are indicative of poor perfusion. Normal and high pressures can be confusing because of vessel wall calcification, and are not predictive of normal perfusion or of wound healing. Digital vessels are not usually calcified, and toe blood pressures appear to be more predictive of healing than ankle pressures.[4,5]

$TcPO_2$ are noninvasive and becoming more readily available in many vascular laboratories.[6] These tests measure the partial pressure of oxygen diffusing through the skin with a special temperature-controlled oxygen electrode. The ultimate reading is based on several factors, including the oxygen delivery to the tissue, the oxygen use by the tissue, and the diffusion of the gas through the skin. Cellulitis and edema can increase use and decrease diffusion, thereby giving lower values. Caution in interpretation of $TcPO_2$ during acute cellulitis or edema is warranted. Also, a

---

Outline 1
Considerations in determining functional and biologic healing

Biologic Healing Level
Trying to predict the most distal level that has a reasonable chance to heal
1. Clinical examination
2. Skin temperature–a line of demarcation is often an excellent indicator of healing level
3. Tissue quality–all necrotic and infected tissue must be removed
4. Nutrition–often accessed by using albumin and total lymphocyte count
5. Ischemic index = arm BP/ankle BP
6. Toe blood pressure–70 to 80 mm Hg is normal
7. $TcPO_2$ = transcutaneous pressure of oxygen at that site, a measure of oxygen delivered to the skin; swelling, cellulitis, venous stasis skin changes will all lower toe $TcPO_2$

Functional Level
The amputation level the patient will function the best with
1. Previous level of ambulation
2. Intelligence
3. Cognitive skills
4. Motivation
5. Cardiopulmonary capacity
6. Spasticity or contractures
7. Rehabilitation goals

BP, blood pressure

---

paradoxical response of $TcPO_2$ to warming on the plantar foot skin has been recently reported, and warrants caution in interpreting plantar foot $TcPO_2$ values.[7] $TcPO_2$ has been shown to be statistically accurate in predicting amputation healing, but false negatives still exist, and many patients' measurements fall into a gray zone for predicting healing.

Xenon 133 skin clearance has been used successfully in the past to predict healing of amputations, but the preparation of the xenon 133 gas/saline solution and the application of this test are highly technician dependent, expensive, and time consuming. A small amount of prepared xenon 133/saline solution is injected intradermally at various sites, and the rate of washout is monitored by gamma camera. After conducting a prospective trial, one previously enthusiastic author is no longer convinced of xenon 133's predictive value, and believes that $TcPO_2$ and $TcPCO_2$ are more predictive and readily available.[8]

Arteriography has not been helpful in predicting successful healing of amputations, and this invasive test is probably not indicated solely for the purpose of level selection. Arteriography is indicated if the patient is truly a candidate for arterial reconstruction or angioplasty.

Nutrition and immunocompetence have been shown to correlate directly with amputation wound healing. Many laboratory tests are available to assess nutrition and immunocompetence, and some are quite expensive. Albumin and total lymphocyte count (TLC) are readily available and inexpensive screening parameters. Several studies have shown increased healing of amputations in dysvascular patients who had a serum albumin level of at least 3.0 or 3.5 grams/deciliter, and TLC > 1,500 cells per cubic millimeter.[9,10] Preoperative nutritional screening is recommended to allow nutritional improvement preoperatively, or consideration of a higher level amputation.

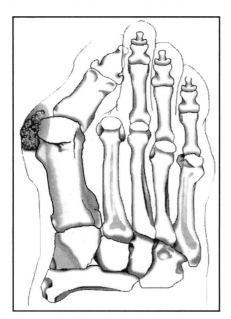

Fig. 1 Hallux valgus deformity following second toe amputation. (Reproduced with permission from the Prosthetics Research Study, Seattle, WA.)

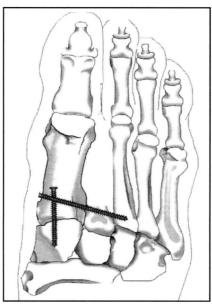

Fig. 2 Second ray amputation with screw fixation to narrow the foot. (Reproduced with permission from the Prosthetics Research Study, Seattle, WA.)

Activity level, ambulatory potential, cognitive skills, and overall medical condition must be evaluated to determine if the most distal level is really appropriate for the patient. In patients who are likely to remain ambulatory, the goal is to achieve healing at the most distal level that can be fit with a prosthesis, and to successful rehabilitate the patient. Recent series of diabetic patients demonstrate that successful wound healing can be achieved in 70% to 80% of these patients at the below-knee or more distal amputation levels. This is in sharp contrast to 25 years ago when, because of a fear of wound failure, surgeons elected to perform 80% of all lower extremity amputations at the above-knee level.

Foot Amputation Levels
Toe Amputations
Toe amputations are common, accounting for 24% of all amputations

in diabetic patients.[1] The importance of obtaining successful wound healing and minimizing complications from this often minimized procedure cannot be underestimated. Technically, toe amputations can be performed with side-to-side or plantar-to-dorsal flaps to use the best available soft tissue. The bone should be shortened to a level that allows adequate soft-tissue closure without tension, either disarticulated or metaphyseal. Durable, tension-free soft-tissue padding is much more important than the amount (if any) of phalangeal bone that remains.

In great toe amputations, if the entire proximal phalanx is removed, the sesamoids will often retract, exposing the keel-shaped plantar surface of the first metatarsal to weightbearing. This can lead to high local pressures, callous formation, and ulceration. The sesamoids can be stabilized in position for weightbearing by leaving the base of the proxi-

mal phalanx intact or by tenodesis of the flexor hallucis brevis tendon.

Beware of isolated second toe amputations, because severe hallux valgus deformity of the first toe commonly results (Fig. 1). There is no single solution for every patient. This deformity may possibly be prevented by second ray amputation, first metatarsophalangeal fusion, or considering amputation of both the first and second toes. I prefer second ray amputation and surgical narrowing of the foot with screw fixation when possible (Fig. 2). For the metatarsophalangeal joint level amputation, transferring the extensor tendon to the capsule can help to elevate the metatarsal head and maintain an even distribution for weightbearing. Prosthetic replacement is not required after toe amputations. However, custom-molded insoles and extra-depth shoes are indicated for diabetic patients who have required toe amputation.

Ray Amputations
A ray amputation removes the toe and all or some of the corresponding metatarsal. Isolated ray amputations can be durable; however, multiple ray amputations, especially in dysvascular patients, can narrow the foot excessively. After ray amputation, the body weight must be born by the remaining metatarsal heads. The amount of force that is borne by one or more of the remaining metatarsal heads can increase dramatically. This increased pressure can lead to new areas of callus and ulceration.

Surgically, it is often difficult to close the ray amputation wounds primarily. More skin is usually required than is readily apparent. Instead of closing these wounds under tension, it is usually advisable to leave a portion of the wound open and allow secondary healing, or to consider a transmetatarsal amputation.

The fifth ray amputation has been the most useful of all the ray amputations (Fig. 3). Plantar-lateral ulcers around the fifth metatarsal head are common, and often lead to exposed bone and osteomyelitis. A fifth ray amputation allows the entire ulcer to be excised and the wound closed primarily. A racquet-shaped incision is used to remove the fifth toe and the ulcer, a straight lateral incision extends toward the base of the fifth metatarsal to allow division of the fifth metatarsal near the base. The base of the fifth metatarsal is preserved to keep the attachment of the peroneus brevis tendon. If the entire fifth metatarsal needs to be excised, the peroneus brevis tendon is reattached locally to help preserve eversion of the foot.

All viable skin is retained because, as stated previously, more skin is usually required than is apparent. In the first or fifth ray amputations, any redundant skin helps by providing more padding of the remaining medial or lateral border of the foot, and this skin should be retained. In general, for more extensive involvement of the foot, which would require multiple-ray amputations, a transverse amputation at the transmetatarsal level will be more durable. Prosthetic requirements after ray amputations include extra-depth shoes with custom-molded insoles.

Midfoot Amputations
The transmetatarsal and Lisfranc amputations are reliable and durable. Surgically, a healthy, durable soft-tissue envelope is more important than a specific bone length. The bones should be shortened to allow soft-tissue closure without tension, rather than transected at a specific predetermined anatomic bone level. A long

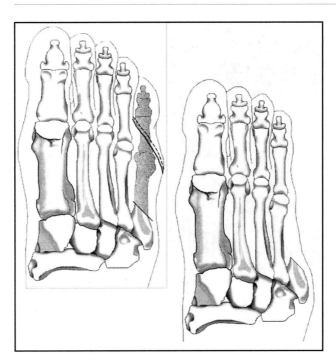

Fig. 3 Fifth ray amputation for fifth metatarsal head ulcer. (Reproduced with permission from the Prosthetics Research Study, Seattle, WA.)

plantar flap is preferable, but equal dorsal and plantar flaps work well and are often the only available option, especially for metatarsal head ulcers.

Muscle balance around the foot should be carefully evaluated preoperatively with specific attention to heel cord tightness, anterior tibialis, posterior tibialis, and peroneal muscle strength. Midfoot amputations significantly shorten the lever arm of the foot; therefore, Achilles tendon lengthening is almost always necessary (Fig. 4). Tibial or peroneal muscle insertions should be reattached locally if their attachments are released during bone resection.

The Achilles tendon lengthening is usually done using 3 percutaneous hemitendon sections. The distal and proximal cuts transect the medial half of the tendon, and the middle cut transects the lateral half of the tendon. Gentle force lengthens the tendon. In theory, this placement of cuts leaves the Achilles tendon with a more lateral attachment and tendency against the varus, which can occur

following midfoot amputations.

Postoperative casting prevents deformities, controls edema, and speeds rehabilitation. The foot should be casted in 5° to 10° of dorsiflexion. Prosthetic requirements can vary widely. During the first year following amputation, many patients benefit from an ankle-foot orthosis with a long foot plate and a toe filler. This orthosis should be worn at all times, except when bathing, in order to prevent an equinus deformity from developing. Later, a custom in-shoe orthotic device with a toe filler can be used with an extra-depth shoe for some patients.

Hindfoot Amputations
A Chopart amputation removes forefoot and midfoot, saving only the talus and calcaneus. Rebalancing procedures are required to prevent equinus and varus deformities. Complete Achilles tenotomy and transfer of the anterior tibialis, extensor digitorum longus, or peroneal tendons through a drill hole in the talus or calcaneus

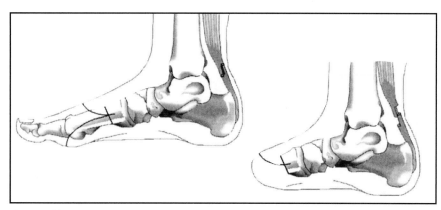

Fig. 4 Midfoot amputation and Achilles tendon lengthening. (Reproduced with permission from the Prosthetics Research Study, Seattle, WA.)

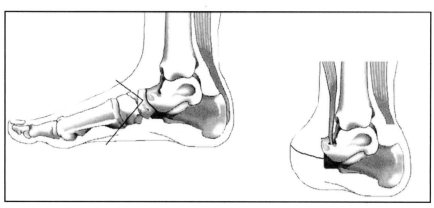

Fig. 5 Hindfoot amputation with anterior tibialis tendon transfer and Achilles tendon tenotomy. (Reproduced with permission from the Prosthetics Research Study, Seattle, WA.)

are an important part of this rebalancing (Fig. 5). Postoperative casting is also a must in order to prevent the strong tendency towards equinus. If a deformity can be prevented, patients with both a Chopart and a Syme's amputation prefer the Chopart level.

The Boyd hindfoot amputation is a talectomy and calcaneotibial arthrodesis after forward translation of the calcaneus. The Pirogoff hindfoot amputation is a talectomy with calcaneotibial arthrodesis after vertical transection of the calcaneus through the midbody, and a forward rotation of the remaining posterior process of the calcaneus under the tibia. These latter 2 amputations are done mostly in children to preserve length and growth centers, prevent heel pad migration, and improve socket suspension.[11] These amputation levels have generally not been used for patients with diabetes. The added length often complicates prosthetic fitting, compared to a Syme's amputation.

The hindfoot prosthesis for a Chopart amputation requires more secure stabilization than a midfoot prosthesis, in order to keep the heel from pistoning during gait. An anterior shell usually must be added to an ankle foot orthosis- (AFO-) style prosthesis, or, alternatively, a posterior opening socket prosthesis can be used. The ability to laminate a foot plate of carbon fiber directly to the undersurface of the prosthetic socket can now result in a hindfoot prosthesis with minimal added height. However, with this construct there is no room to add a heel cushion, and some patients find this prosthesis too rigid at heel strike. The ankle region of this prosthesis remains very bulky and cosmetically dissatisfying to some patients. For patients whose main goals are to maintain independent transfers, the hindfoot amputations can be a very good level. For patients who ambulate with higher functional activity, a more proximal amputation, such as the Syme's or transtibial amputation, might be wiser.

Partial Calcanectomy

Partial calcanectomy, which involves excision of the posterior process of the calcaneus, should be considered an amputation of the back of the foot. In select patients with large heel ulceration or calcaneal osteomyelitis, this can be a very functional alternative to a below-knee amputation.[12] The local soft-tissue flap requires that the foot have reasonable good perfusion for healing and durability.

Surgically, the ulcer is excised, and longitudinal extensions of the incision up along the Achilles tendon and distally onto the plantar aspect of the foot allow access to dissect the posterior process of the calcaneus and the insertion of the Achilles tendon. The entire posterior process of the calcaneus is removed from the posterior edge of the posterior facet of the subtalar joint along a straight line to the inferior corner of the calcaneocuboid joint. All necrotic Achilles tendon is debrided, and no reattachment of this tendon is usually possible because of the extent of debridement (Fig. 6). Removing this large bony prominence allows for fairly large soft-tissue defects to be closed primarily over suction drainage. Splinting the foot in the equinus position relaxes the soft tissues and keeps tension off the closure during healing. Long-term equinus deformity is not a problem because of the Achilles tendon resection.

Discussing this procedure with patients as an amputation of the back of the foot helps emphasize the cosmetic and functional deformity. Because the posterior process of the calcaneus and the Achilles tendon attachment are both removed, a rigid AFO-style partial foot prosthesis with a cushion heel is required.

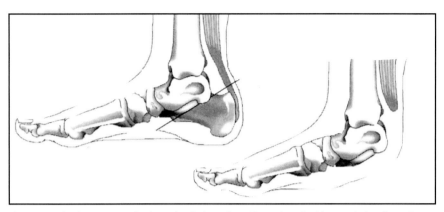

Fig. 6 Partial calcanectomy for large heel ulceration. (Reproduced with permission from the Prosthetics Research Study, Seattle, WA.)

Syme's Amputations

The Syme's amputation is an ankle disarticulation in which the calcaneus and talus are removed while carefully dissecting on bone to preserve the heel skin and fat pad to cover the distal tibia.[13–15] The malleoli must be removed and contoured. Controversy exists as to whether to remove the malleoli initially or at a second-stage operation 6 to 8 weeks later. An advantage of 2 stages might be improved healing in dysvascular patients. Disadvantages include the second surgical procedure and a delay in rehabilitation because of the inability to bear weight until after the second stage. I believe that with careful surgical technique, the Syme's amputation can be performed safely in 1 stage, even for diabetic patients.[16]

A late complication of the Syme's amputation is the posterior and medial migration of the fat pad. Options to stabilize the fat pad include tenodesis of the Achilles tendon to the posterior margin of the tibia through drill holes; transferring anterior tibialis and extensor digitorum tendons to the anterior aspect of the fat pad; or removing the cartilage and subchondral bone to allow scarring of the fat pad to bone, with or without pin fixation. My preference is to perform tenodesis of the Achilles tendon to the

posterior tibia[17] (Fig. 7). Careful casting postoperatively can also help keep the fat pad centered under the tibia during healing.

The Syme's amputation is an end-bearing level. Retaining the smooth, broad surface of the distal tibia and the heel pad allows direct transfer of weight from the end of the residual limb to the prosthesis. Below-knee or above-knee amputations do not allow this direct transfer of weight. Because of the ability to end bear, the amputee can occasionally ambulate without a prosthesis in emergency situations, or for bathroom activities. The socket design can take advantage of this end bearing to optimize a comfortable fit with a lower socket profile proximally.

The Syme's prosthesis is wider at the ankle level than a below-knee prosthesis. This cosmetic concern is occasionally bothersome. Use of newer materials and surgical narrowing of the malleolar flair have lessened this concern. Because of the low profile of some newer elastic response feet, the Syme's amputee can now benefit from energy-storing technology. Sockets do not need the high contour of a patellar-tendon bearing design because of the end-bearing quality of the residual limb.

The socket can be windowed either posteriorly or medially if the limb is bulbous, or a flexible socket-within-a-socket design can be used if the limb is less bulbous. Because of the tibial flare, the Syme's socket is usually self suspending.

Transtibial Amputations

The transtibial amputation is the most commonly performed major limb amputation. The long posterior flap technique has become standard, and good results can be expected even in a majority of dysvascular patients.[18] Anteroposterior, sagittal, and skewed flaps have all been described and are occasionally useful in specific patients. The level of tibial transection should be as long as possible between the tibial tubercle and the junction of the middle and distal thirds of the tibia, based on the available healthy soft tissues. Historically, it was taught that the tibia should always be transected 6 inches (15 cm) from the knee joint line, but the trend in recent years is toward longer transtibial amputations. Amputations in the distal third of the tibia should be avoided, because they have poor soft-tissue padding and are more difficult to fit comfortably with a prosthesis.

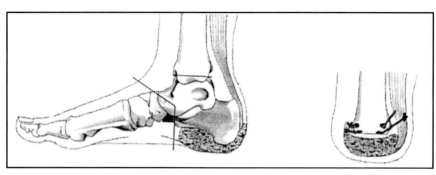

Fig. 7 Syme's amputation and stabilization of the heel pad with Achilles tenodesis to the tibia. (Reproduced with permission from the Prosthetics Research Study, Seattle, WA.)

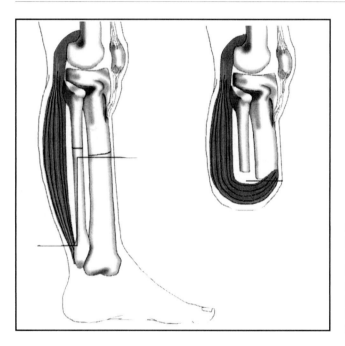

Fig. 8 Below-knee amputation with long posterior flap technique. (Reproduced with permission from the Prosthetics Research Study, Seattle, WA.)

The surgical goals are a cylindrically shaped residual limb with muscle stabilization, distal tibial padding, and a nontender and nonadherent scar. The long posterior flap length is equal to the diameter of the limb at the level of bone transection plus 1 cm. The fibula is transected 1 to 2 cm shorter than the tibia. The sural nerve should be identified, drawn down 5 to 10 cm, resected, and allowed to retract, to avoid a painful neuroma in the posterior flap. The posterior fascia should be myodesed to periosteum or to drill holes in the tibia to prevent retraction (Fig. 8).

Distal tibiofibular synostosis, the Ertl procedure, is not commonly performed. The principle, to create a broad bone mass terminally to improve the distal end-bearing property of the limb, is rarely achieved. The complication of a painful nonunion can be difficult to treat. Distal tibiofibular synostosis may be indicated in a wide traumatic diastasis to improve stabilization of the bone and soft tissues, but it is rarely indicated in dysvascular or diabetic patients.

The transtibial amputation is especially well suited to rigid dressings and immediate postoperative pros-

thetic management.[19,20] Protocols for weightbearing in these casts continue to be debated. My protocol for diabetic patients is to apply a cast in the operating room, but not initiate weightbearing until after the first cast change at 5 to 7 days. This first cast functions to help prevent knee flexion contractures, to decrease pain, and to control edema. If wound healing appears to be progressing well at the first cast change, a pilon and foot are added to the second cast, and 20 to 30 lbs of weightbearing is begun. The cast is changed weekly, and the weightbearing is advanced to 100 lbs over 4 weeks. After 4 to 6 weeks of casting, the first prosthesis is fabricated. The socket on this first prosthesis often needs to be changed 1 or 2 times in the first year, as atrophy of the residual limb occurs.

Pain Issue

Phantom sensation, a sense that all or some of the amputated part is still present, is very common following amputation.[21] This phantom sense is usually not bothersome to the patient, especially in diabetic patients with neuropathy. True phantom pain, a sensation in the amputated part that is described using words descriptive of pain, is fortunately rare. I believe that real phantom pain occurs less often in diabetic patients than in patients with traumatic amputations. The study of phantom pain is extremely interesting, and new research suggests that mechanisms designed to block the pain pathways around the time of amputation surgery do reduce the need for opioid medication in the hospital period, and may decrease the incidence of chronic phantom pain.[8,22–25]

When pain remains a serious problem, the best management is nonsurgical. Local physical measures, including massage, cold, and exercise are often effective. Other measures, such as acupuncture and regional sympathectomy, may under given circumstances have a place in therapy when the pain is intractable. Although transcutaneous electrical nerve stimulators (TENS) have been used with moderate short-term success, it is rare to see a patient who has continued to use a TENS unit for more than 1 year. Pharmacologic treatment has been reasonably successful with several oral agents, including amitriptyline, carbamazepine, dilatin, and, more recently, mexiletine. The appropriate use of an intravenous lidocaine challenge has been shown to be predictive of a favorable response to oral mexiletine. Unfortunately, we have not found good indicators to predict who will respond to treatment with amitriptyline, carbamazepine, or dilatin. Psychologic support can be beneficial, particularly when personality problems seem to accentuate the occurrence of pain. The individual needs patience and reassurance that the discomfort will improve over time, especially when a supportive social environment is present.

Summary

Unfortunately, amputation surgery is still a very important part of the treatment for diabetic foot problems. The decision-making process must be done thoughtfully, remembering that blood flow is not the only issue. Many factors enter into the decision to perform a partial foot amputation or to perform a more proximal level amputation. Adherence to good surgical principle, proven techniques, and gentle soft-tissue handling can make the difference between a successful and durable amputation or continued complications and frustrations.

Acknowledgment

A special thank you to Kathleen J. Ponto for providing the illustrations.

References

1. Reiber GE, Boyko EJ, Smith DG: Lower extremity foot ulcers and amputations in diabetes, in National Diabetes Data Group (eds): *Diabetes in America*, ed 2. Bethesda, MD, NIH, 1995.

2. Smith DG, Barnes BC, Sands AK, Boyko EJ, Ahroni JH: Prevalence of radiographic foot abnormalities in patients with diabetes. *Foot Ankle Int* 1997;18:343–346.

3. Waters RL, Perry J, Antonelli D, Hislop H: Energy cost of walking of amputees: The influence of level of amputation. *J Bone Joint Surg* 1976;58A:42–46.

4. Bone GE, Pomajzl MJ: Toe blood pressure by photoplethysmography: An index of healing in forefoot amputation. *Surgery* 1981;89:569–574.

5. Ramsey DE, Manke DA, Sumner DS: Toe blood pressure: A valuable adjunct to ankle pressure measurement for assessing peripheral arterial disease. *J Cardiovasc Surg (Torino)* 1983;24:43–48.

6. Burgess EM, Matsen FA III, Wyss CR, Simmons CW: Segmental transcutaneous measurements of PO2 in patients requiring below-the-knee amputation for peripheral vascular insufficiency. *J Bone Joint Surg* 1982;64A:378–382.

7. Smith DG, Boyko EJ, Ahroni JH, Stensel VL, Davignon DR, Pecoraro RE: Paradoxical transcutaneous oxygen response to cutaneous warming on the plantar foot surface: A caution for interpretation of plantar foot TcPO$_2$ measurements. *Foot Ankle Int* 1994;16:787–791.

8. Malone JM, Anderson GG, Lalka SG, et al: Prospective comparison of noninvasive techniques for amputation level selection. *Am J Surg* 1987;154:179–184.

9. Dickhaut SC, DeLee JC, Page CP: Nutritional status: Importance in predicting wound-healing after amputation. *J Bone Joint Surg* 1984;66A:71–75.

10. Pinzur M, Kaminsky M, Sage R, Cronin R, Osterman H: Amputations at the middle level of the foot: A retrospective and prospective review. *J Bone Joint Surg* 1986;68A:1061–1064.

11. Greene WB, Cary JM: Partial foot amputations in children: A comparison of the several types with the Syme amputation. *J Bone Joint Surg* 1982;64A:438–443.

12. Smith DG, Stuck RM, Ketner L, Sage RM, Pinzur MS: Partial calcanectomy for the treatment of large ulcerations of the heel and calcaneal osteomyelitis: An amputation of the back of the foot. *J Bone Joint Surg* 1992;74A:571–576.

13. Harris RI: The history and development of Syme's amputation. *Artif Limbs* 1961;6:4,443.

14. Harris RI: Syme's amputation: The technique essential to secure a satisfactory end-bearing stump: Part I. *Can J Surg* 1963;6:456–469.

15. Harris RI: Syme's amputation: The technique essential to secure a satisfactory endbearing stump: Part II. *Can J Surg* 1964;7:53–63.

16. Pinzur MS, Smith D, Osterman H: Syme ankle disarticulation in peripheral vascular disease and diabetic foot infection: The one-stage versus two-stage procedure. *Foot Ankle Int* 1995;16:124–127.

17. Smith DG, Sangeorzan BJ, Hansen ST Jr, Burgess EM: Achilles tendon tenodesis to prevent heel pad migration in the Syme's amputation. *Foot Ankle Int* 1994;15:14–17

18. Pinzur MS, Gottschalk F, Smith D, et al: Functional outcome of below-knee amputation in peripheral vascular insufficiency: A multicenter review. *Clin Orthop* 1993;286:247–249.

19. Burgess EM, Romano RL, Zettl JH (eds): *Management of Lower-Extremity Amputations: Surgery, Immediate Postsurgical Prosthetic Fitting, Patient Care.* Washington, DC, Prosthetic and Sensory Aids Service, Veterans Administration, 1969.

20. Mooney V, Harvey JP Jr, McBride E, Snelson R: Comparison of postoperative stump management: Plaster vs. soft dressings. *J Bone Joint Surg* 1971;53A:241–249.

21. Melzack R: Phantom limbs. *Sci Am* 1992;266:120–126.

22. Bach S, Noreng MF, Tjellden NU: Phantom limb pain in amputees during the first 12 months following limb amputation, after preoperative lumbar epidural blockade. *Pain* 1988;33:297–301.

23. Elizaga AM, Smith DG, Sharar SR, Edwards WT, Hansen ST Jr: Continuous regional analgesia by intraneuralh block: Effect on postoperative opioid requirements and phantom limb pain following amputation. *J Rehabil Res Dev* 1994;31:179–187.

24. Fisher A, Meller Y: Continuous postoperative regional analgesia by nerve sheath block for amputation surgery: A pilot study. *Anesth Analg* 1991;72:300–303.

25. Malawer MM, Buch R, Khurana JS, Garvey T, Rice L: Postoperative infusional continuous regional analgesia: A technique for relief of postoperative pain following major extremity surgery. *Clin Orthop* 1991;266:227–237.

Controversies in Lower Extremity Amputation

Michael S. Pinzur, MD
Frank Gottschalk, MB.BCh, FRCSEd
Marco Antonio Guedes de Souza Pinto, MD
*Douglas G. Smith, MD

Abstract

Using the experience gained from taking care of World War II veterans with amputations, Ernest Burgess taught that amputation surgery is reconstructive surgery. It is the first step in the rehabilitation process for patients with an amputation and should be thought of in this way. An amputation is often a more appropriate option than limb salvage, irrespective of the underlying cause. The decision making and selection of the amputation level must be based on realistic expectations with regard to functional outcome and must be adapted to both the disease process being treated and the unique needs of the patient. Sometimes the amputation is done as a life-saving procedure in a patient who is not expected to walk, but more often it is done for a patient who should be able to return to a full, active life. When considering amputation, the physician should establish reasonable goals when confronted with the question of limb salvage versus amputation, understand the roles of the soft-tissue envelope and osseous platform in the creation of a residual limb, understand the method of weight bearing within a prosthetic socket, and determine whether a bone bridge is a positive addition to a transtibial amputation.

The Lower Extremity Assessment Project (LEAP) has provided objective outcome data on patients with mutilating limb injuries.[1] Five hundred sixty-nine consecutive patients with mutilating limb injuries treated at eight academic trauma centers provided objective observational outcome data relative to limb salvage and amputation. One hundred forty-nine patients underwent lower-extremity amputation during the course of their care. This ongoing study is providing a realistic understanding of the less-than-favorable results associated with both limb salvage and amputation. Much of what has been learned from LEAP can be applied to the care of patients with a nontraumatic amputation.

A reasonable functional goal should be established before an ex-tremity amputation is performed. The goals for a young individual who is going to reenter the workforce after a traumatic amputation are very different from those for an elderly debilitated patient with diabetes who has a limited life expectancy. Before surgery is performed, four issues need to be addressed, so as to create a needs assessment:

1. If the limb is salvaged, will the functional outcome be better than it would be after an amputation and fitting of a prosthetic limb? This question needs to be addressed regardless of whether the patient has a mutilating limb injury, a diabetic foot infection, a tumor, or a congenital anomaly.

2. What is a realistic expectation following treatment? The realistic expected functional outcome is the average functional outcome for patients with the same comorbidities and level of amputation; it is not the best possible outcome.

3. What is the cost of care? This cost goes beyond resource consumption. Can the patient and his or her family afford the multiple operations and the time off from work necessary to accomplish limb sal-

*Douglas G. Smith, MD or the department with which he is affiliated has received research or institutional support from Otto Bock.

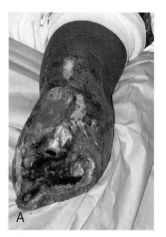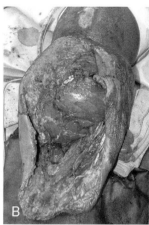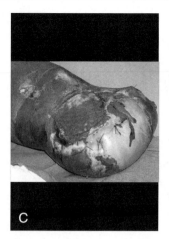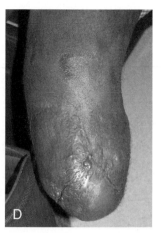

Figure 1 **A,** Photograph taken at the time that a young, active male patient first returned to the operating room following a traumatic amputation. **B,** The remaining gastrocnemius muscle was used to create a cushioned soft-tissue envelope. The skin was degloved and did not survive. **C,** Following the use of vacuum-assisted wound management, there was an adequate base for split-thickness skin grafting. **D,** The residual limb 18 months following the injury. A silicone suspension liner within the prosthetic socket was used to compensate for the split-thickness skin graft over the residual anterior aspect of the tibia.

vage, or are they best served by amputation and fitting of a prosthetic limb?

4. What are the risks? Limb-salvage surgery for any diagnosis is riskier than an amputation. When a patient has had an infection in an ischemic limb, the risk of recurrent infection and sepsis is far lower when the limb is removed than when it is retained.

Once these issues have been addressed, the patient and the surgical team generally have sufficient data to support the decision-making process.

When performing an amputation as a reconstructive effort after trauma, infection, tumor, or vascular insufficiency, one should strive to create optimal residual limb length without osseous prominences; reasonable function in the joint proximal to the level of the amputation to enhance prosthetic function; and a durable soft-tissue envelope. Although new prosthetic technology allows compensation for a suboptimal soft-tissue envelope, it is well

accepted that amputees fare better with a durable soft-tissue envelope and fare worse when the skin is adherent to bone or there is a split-thickness skin graft in areas of high pressure or shear.[2,3] Therefore, muscles should be secured to bone to prevent retraction. When possible, full-thickness myocutaneous flaps should be used, with muscle cushioning in areas of high pressure and shear (Figure 1).

Disarticulation Compared With Transosseous Amputation

The more distal the level of lower extremity amputation, the better the walking independence and functional outcome, unless the quality of the residual limb creates so much discomfort that it negates the potential benefits of limb-length retention. Therefore, the amputation should be done at the most distal level that will result in a functional residual limb. Efforts to create a functional residual limb should take into account the method of weight

bearing (load transfer) and the tissues available to create a soft-tissue envelope.

The best residual limb cannot duplicate the unique weight-bearing properties of a normal foot. The foot has multiple bones and articulations that function as a shock absorber at heel strike, a stable platform during stance phase, and a "starting block" for stability at push-off. The multiple bones and joints allow positioning of the durable plantar soft-tissue envelope in an optimal orientation for accepting load. An amputee has, in place of a foot, a residual limb that must tolerate weight bearing (load transfer) with the socket of a prosthesis.

When the amputation is through a joint (disarticulation), the load transfer can be accomplished directly; that is, there is end-bearing. When the amputation is done through the bone (transosseous), the load transfer must be accomplished indirectly by the entire residual limb, through a total-contact socket of the prosthesis, as weight bearing on the end of the residual limb is too painful. Disarticulation allows dissipation of the load over a large surface area of less stiff metaphyseal bone. With a well-constructed soft-tissue envelope to cushion the residual osseous platform, the direct-transfer prosthetic socket need only suspend the prosthesis. This differs from transosseous amputation at the transtibial or transfemoral level, where the surface area of the end of the bone is small and the diaphyseal bone is less resilient. The end of the bone must be "unweighted" by dissipating the load over the entire surface of the residual limb. This indirect load transfer requires a durable and mobile soft-tissue envelope that can tolerate the shearing forces associated with weight bearing. The socket fit becomes crucial. When a patient loses weight, the residual limb tends to bottom out, and painful end-bearing or tissue breakdown develops. Patients who gain weight are not able to fit the limb into the prosthesis. The choice of disarticulation or transosseous amputation must be individualized for each patient.

Transtibial (Below-the-Knee) Amputation

The standard transtibial prosthetic socket is fabricated with the knee in approximately 10° of flexion, to unload the distal part of the tibia and optimally distribute the load. Load transfer is accomplished by distributing the load over the entire surface area of the residual limb, with a concentration over the anteromedial and anterolateral areas of the tibial metaphysis.

Mutilating limb injuries frequently disrupt the interosseous membrane, disengaging the relationship between the tibia and fibula.

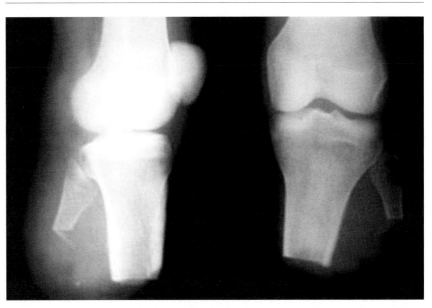

Figure 2   AP and lateral plain radiographs of a patient with an unstable fibula caused by disruption of the interosseous membrane by a transtibial amputation. The short, unstable fibula is not able to serve as an efficient platform for weight bearing. The abducted residual distal part of the fibula also creates an osseous prominence that interferes with prosthetic limb fitting. (Reprinted with permission from Pinzur MS, Pinto MA, Schon LC, Smith DG: Controversies in amputation surgery. *Instr Course Lect* 2003;52:448.)

This loss of integrity of the interosseous membrane prevents the fibula from participating in normal load transfer. In other situations, the residual fibula may become unstable following transtibial amputation because of loss of the integrity of the interosseous membrane or as a result of loss of the integrity of the proximal tibiofibular joint even without an obvious traumatic disruption.

Individuals with instability of the residual fibula following transtibial amputation can have pain because of several causes. When the residual limb is compressed within the prosthetic socket, the residual fibula may angulate toward the tibia with prolonged weight bearing. The result is a conical, pointed residual limb, which tends to bottom out during prolonged weight bearing. The conical residual limb acts as a wedge, leading to painful end-bearing and soft-tissue breakdown over the terminal tibia. When the residual limb is short, or the interosseous membrane has been disrupted, the residual fibula can be abducted as a result of unopposed action of the biceps femoris muscle[4,5] (Figure 2). These alterations of the load-bearing platform become accentuated in younger, more active amputees, with higher demand, or with prolonged activities.[6,7]

During World War I, Ertl[8] proposed the creation of an osteoperiosteal tube, derived mostly from tibial periosteum, and affixing it to the fibula to create a stable residual limb. Following World War II, his concept was successfully introduced in the United States by Loon,[4] Deffer,[9] and others.[10] Arthrodesis, or bone bridging, of the distal parts of the tibia and fibula has recently become a controversial topic, with

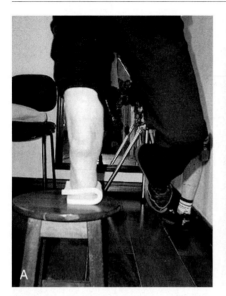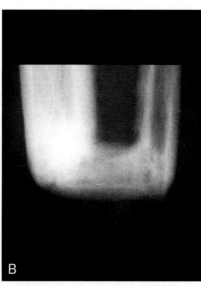

Figure 3 **A,** This patient was able to stand directly on the residual limb because he had a stable platform for weight bearing following the creation of an Ertl bone bridge between the distal parts of the tibia and fibula. (Reprinted with permission from Pinzur MS, Pinto MA, Schon LC, Smith DG: Controversies in amputation surgery. *Instr Course Lect* 2003;52:449.) **B,** Radiograph obtained 1 year following the creation of the bone bridge.

both ardent supporters and strong detractors. Recent investigations suggest that the technique may provide a potential benefit for an active amputee by creating a stable platform with an enhanced surface area for load transfer[5,11,12] (Figure 3). Most supporters suggest that the technique should be reserved for younger, more active amputees who will benefit from the potentially enhanced functional residual limb and are more able to tolerate the increased morbidity risk associated with the additional surgery necessary to obtain the bone bridge.

The surgery can also be performed as a late reconstruction for active amputees with residual limb pain that appears to be associated with an unstable or disengaged residual fibula. These patients may have a conical end-bearing residual limb, usually with pain at the end of the residual limb and occasionally with tissue breakdown. Others may have pain along a prominent or unstable fibula. On examination, the fibula usually can be felt to be unstable.

The operation involves use of a long posterior myocutaneous flap. For the average 6-ft (1.8 m)-tall patient, the optimal residual tibial length should be a minimum of 10 to 12 cm to create an adequate weight-bearing platform, but it should not be longer than 15 to 18 cm. (An excessively long residual limb requires the prosthetic socket to be put into full extension. This leads to increased distal pressure, increased end-bearing, and more stump failures.) The fibula is divided 4 cm distal to the tibia to allow the creation of the bone bridge. Care is taken to maintain as many muscular attachments to the distal aspect of the fibula as possible. One centimeter of the fibula is removed at the level of the distal tibial cut to allow rotation of the vascularized bone. A notch is made in the lateral cortex of the residual tibia to accept the rotated fibu-

lar segment. Stability can be obtained by suturing the fibular segment through drill holes or with screw fixation (Figure 3, *B*).

The transferred fibular segment used between the distal parts of the fibula and tibia can be supplemented with a vascularized periosteal sleeve taken from the tibia, as described by Ertl.[8] The periosteum on the anterior surface of the tibia, which is quite thick, is raised from the tibia distal to the level of the tibial transection. When the periosteum is raised, it is important to keep it attached proximally and to take a thin slice of cortical bone with it. This almost guarantees that the periosteum obtained has maintained its vascular supply. A 1-in (2.5-cm) osteotome is used to raise the periosteum and the thin slice of cortical bone. The periosteal sleeve is sutured over the rotated fibular segment. The periosteal graft alone has also been used in place of the fibula, but we have no experience with that technique and do not recommend it.

The anterior aspect of the distal surface of the tibia is beveled, and a durable, full-thickness myocutaneous flap is repaired to the anterior aspect of the tibia through drill holes or by suturing the posterior gastrocnemius fascia to the anterior periosteum of the residual tibia and the anterior compartment fascia.

When the surgery is performed as a late reconstruction or if there is no distal part of the fibula with which to create the bone bridge, a tricortical iliac crest bone graft is wedged between the terminal residual tibia and fibula after the inner surfaces of both have been prepared with a burr (Figure 4).

Postoperative Care

A rigid plaster dressing is applied to protect the residual limb and to con-

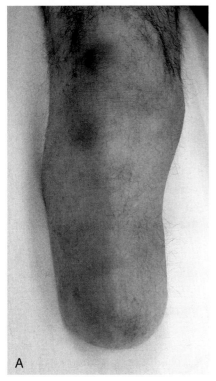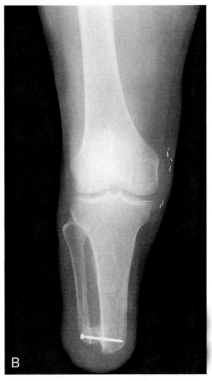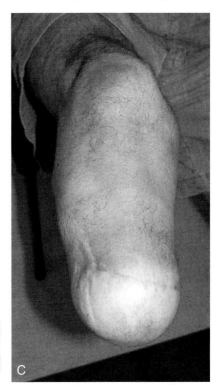

Figure 4 **A,** An active patient with a transtibial amputation reported pain in the distal part of the residual limb after prolonged activity. The conical shape of the residual limb allowed it to wedge into the prosthetic socket, creating painful end-bearing. **B,** Radiograph obtained 1 year after a successful bone bridge procedure with a tricortical iliac crest bone graft placed between the fibula and tibia. **C,** The more square shape of the residual limb created an excellent platform for load transmission. The residual limb no longer bottomed out in the prosthesis, providing better comfort with weight bearing.

trol postoperative swelling. Another option is to use elastic bandages for a compressive dressing, but these need to be put on carefully so as not to produce a pressure sore. This is especially important when a patient has a peripheral neuropathy. Our experience has been that if the patient has pain at the end of the stump or in the stump shortly after surgery, it is caused by a local problem and the dressing needs to be changed, but pain that seems to be in the distal, amputated part of the limb is the so-called phantom limb phenomenon. Phantom sensation is a normal response after an amputation that usually resolves. Telling the patient before the surgery that they will have phantom sensations tends to de-

crease anxiety about this phenomenon.

Weight bearing with a temporary prosthesis is initiated when the residual limb appears capable of tolerating weight bearing. Pain with weight bearing lasts longer for patients who have had a bone bridge reconstruction than it does for those without a bone bridge. The pain may last for 6 to 9 months and seems to resolve as the bone bridge heals. It is assumed that the site of healing between the fibula and tibia remains tender until the bone becomes solid. The pain should be treated nonsurgically unless there is a sign of inadequate placement of the graft or sutures. Usually, the patient can be fitted for a prosthesis, but he or she

may not be able to bear full weight until the tenderness resolves.

Skin Flap for Transtibial (Below-the-Knee) Amputation
Load transfer following transtibial amputation appears to be enhanced when the residual limb has a large osseous surface area covered with a durable soft-tissue envelope composed of a well-cushioned mobile muscle mass and full-thickness skin. This desired result is best achieved through use of a long posterior myofasciocutaneous flap. Despite the fact that the standard posterior flap for transtibial amputation is satisfactory for most patients, retraction of the flap over time can lead to a troublesome pressure point overlying the anterior aspect of

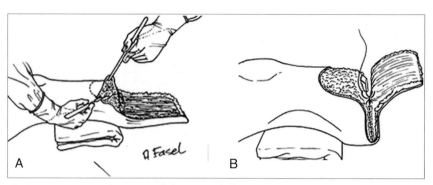

Figure 5 Artist's drawings of the extended posterior myocutaneous flap. **A,** The long posterior flap is several centimeters longer than the traditional posterior flap. **B,** A corresponding amount of proximal skin is removed to advance the suture line proximal to the anterior aspect of the distal tibial region. (Reprinted with permission from Assal M, Blanck R, Smith DG: Extended posterior flap for transtibial amputation. *Orthopaedics* 2005;28:544.)

the distal part of the residual tibia. The standard transtibial amputation technique, popularized by Burgess and associates,[13] often places the surgical incision directly over that portion of the residual tibia. This raises the potential for adherent scarring of the skin to that part of the tibia or for inadequate cushioning of this region during weight bearing. When the anterior aspect of the distal part of the residual tibia is not sufficiently padded, there is an increased likelihood of localized discomfort, blistering, or tissue breakdown associated with the normal pistoning that occurs between the residual limb and the prosthetic socket during normal walking. An extended posterior flap appears to prevent these potential morbidities by providing improved cushioning and comfort even for individuals who are capable of only limited activity.[14] The encouraging results of this relatively simple modification support the well-accepted notion that an optimal residual limb should be composed of a sufficient osseous platform and a durable and cushioned soft-tissue envelope.[11]

The extended posterior flap is created by increasing the length of the standard posterior flap by several centimeters (Figure 5). The posterior myocutaneous flap is created and the osseous cuts are performed in the traditional manner. The myocutaneous flap is generally created from the gastrocnemius muscle and overlying skin, with removal of the soleus muscle belly in all but very thin patients. Care is taken in the handling of the transected nerves to avoid the development of sensitive, painful neuromas. It is advised to avoid clamping of the nerves before transection to avoid the pain so frequently encountered following crushing injuries. The nerves should be dissected proximal to the level of the bone transection, with use of gentle traction with a sponge, and then they are transected with a fresh scalpel blade. This allows the inevitable terminal neuroma to be cushioned within bulky muscle. To avoid a bulbous stump, the posterior and lateral compartment muscles (except the gastrocnemius) should be transected at the level of the transected tibia. Anterior skin is removed to allow proximal attachment of the muscle flap and proximal placement of the wound scar. A myodesis of the posterior muscle flap to the tibia can

be performed through drill holes. The posterior gastrocnemius fascia is secured to the transected anterior compartment fascia and tibial periosteum with horizontal mattress sutures (Figure 6). A rigid plaster dressing is applied, and prosthetic fitting is initiated when the residual limb appears capable of weight bearing.

Transfemoral (Above-the-Knee) Amputation

Transfemoral amputation is performed less frequently than in the past, but it is still necessary in some patients with severe vascular disease, a neoplasm, infection, or trauma in whom reconstruction at a more distal level is not feasible.[15,16] The energy expenditure for walking, even on a level surface, by an individual with a transfemoral amputation has been shown to be as much as 65% greater than that for similar, able-bodied individuals.[17,18] Energy expenditure can be minimized by a properly performed above-the-knee amputation.

The anatomic alignment of the lower limb has been well defined. The mechanical axis lies on a line from the center of the femoral head through the center of the knee to the center of the ankle. In normal two-limbed stance, this axis measures 3° from the vertical axis and the femoral shaft axis measures 9° from the vertical axis.[19] The femur is normally oriented in relative adduction, which allows the hip stabilizers (the gluteus medius and minimus) and abductors (the gluteus medius and the tensor fasciae latae) to act on it to reduce the lateral motion of the center of mass of the body, producing an energy-efficient gait (Figure 7).

In most individuals who have undergone a transfemoral amputation, the mechanical and anatomic align-

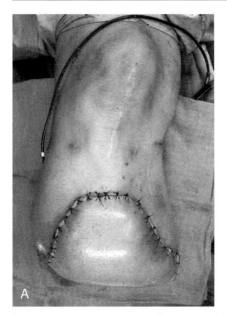 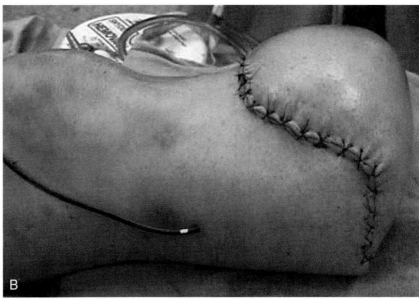

Figure 6 The appearance of an extended posterior flap immediately after closure. The bulbous end will shrink and smooth contours will develop with time. **A**, AP view. **B**, Lateral view.

ment is altered as a result of disruption of the adductor magnus insertion at the adductor tubercle and the distal part of the linea aspera.[20] This allows the residual femur to drift into abduction as a result of the unopposed action of the hip abductors. Many patients who have undergone a transfemoral amputation encounter difficulties with prosthetic fitting due to inadequate muscle stabilization at the time of the amputation.[21] The unstable femur disrupts the relationship between the anatomic and mechanical axes of the limb. The abductor lurch, so common after transfemoral amputation, is a consequence of the unopposed action of the intact hip abductors. This dynamic deformity overcomes the capacity of even modern prostheses to compensate.

Traditional transfemoral amputation is done by suturing the femur flexors to the extensors—that is, creating a myoplasty—while ignoring the adductors that contribute to stability of the residual femur.[22] When

the adductors are not anchored to bone, the hip abductors are able to act unopposed, producing a dynamic flexion-abduction deformity. This deformity prepositions the femur in an orientation that is not conducive to efficient walking.[23,24] The retracted adductor muscles lead to a poorly cushioning soft-tissue envelope, further complicating prosthetic fitting.[25]

The cross-sectional area of the adductor magnus is three to four times larger than that of the adductor longus and brevis combined. It has a moment arm with the best mechanical advantage. Transection of the adductor magnus at the time of amputation leads to substantial loss of cross-sectional area, a reduction in the effective moment arm, and loss of up to 70% of the adductor pull.[20,25] This results in overall weakness of the adductor force of the thigh and subsequent abduction of the residual femur (Figure 7). The decrease in overall limb strength is due to (1) a reduction in muscle mass at the time

of the amputation, (2) inadequate mechanical fixation of the remaining muscles, and (3) atrophy of the remaining muscles.[26,27]

MRI has demonstrated a 40% to 60% decrease in muscle bulk after a traumatic transfemoral amputation. Most of the atrophy is in the adductor and hamstring muscles, whereas the intact hip abductors and flexors show smaller changes, ranging from 0% to 30%.[28,29] As much as 70% atrophy of the adductor magnus has been found. The amount of atrophy correlates with the length of the residual limb, and this atrophy is most likely due to loss of the muscle insertion.

Electromyographic studies of residual limbs following transfemoral amputation have revealed normal muscle phasic activity; however, the active period of the retained muscles appears to be prolonged.[29] The electrical activity of sectioned muscles varies, depending on whether the muscles have been reanchored and on the length of the residual fe-

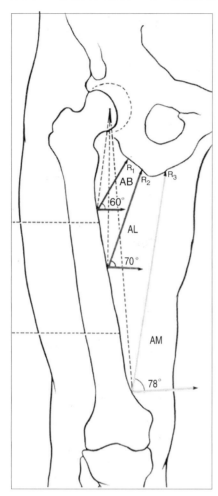

Figure 7 Diagram of the resultant forces of the adductor muscles. The relative insertion sites of the abductors are indicated. The shorter the residual femur, the weaker the limb. AB = adductor brevis muscle, AL = adductor longus muscle, AM = adductor magnus muscle.

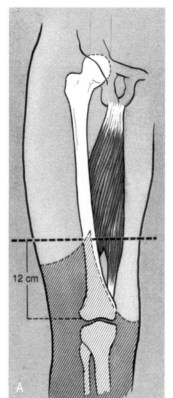
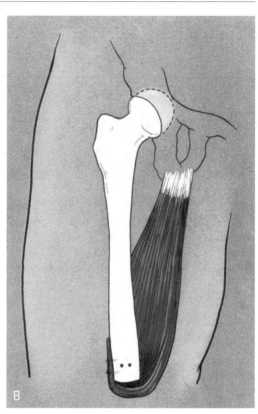

Figure 8 Adductor myodesis method of transfemoral amputation. **A,** Skin flaps and proposed bone cut. The osseous transection is optimally created at 5 in (12.5 cm) proximal to the knee joint, but it can be more proximal if necessary. **B,** The adductor magnus tendon is secured to the residual femur through drill holes in the lateral cortex. (Reprinted with permission from Gottschalk F: Transfemoral amputation: Surgical management, in Smith DG, Michael JW, Bowker JH (eds): *Atlas of Amputations and Limb Deficiencies*, ed 3. Rosemont, IL, American Academy of Orthopaedic Surgeons, 2004, p 537-538.)

mur. Furthermore, asymmetric gait has been related to residual limb length, and lateral bending of the trunk has been correlated directly with atrophy of the hip stabilizing muscles.[30]

All of these findings indicate the need to preserve the hip adductors and hamstrings. Preservation of a functional adductor magnus helps to maintain the muscle balance between the adductors and abductors by allowing the adductor magnus to maintain its power and retain the mechanical advantage for positioning the femur. Preservation is best accomplished with a myodesis. The patient is positioned supine with a sandbag under the buttocks to avoid performing the myodesis with the hip in a flexed position and thus producing an iatrogenic hip flexion contracture. A tourniquet is generally not necessary for patients with peripheral vascular disease. Depending on the size of the patient, a standard, or a sterile, tourniquet can be used when the transfemoral amputation is being performed because of a traumatic injury or a tumor and normal femoral vessels can be expected.

Equal anterior and posterior flaps should be avoided, as such flaps place the suture line under the end of the residual limb, making prosthetic fitting more difficult and adequate muscular padding less likely. A long medial-based myofasciocutaneous flap is dependent on the vascular supply from the obturator artery, which generally has less severe vascular disease and is thus preferred[31] (Figure 8). The flap configuration may need to be modified, to preserve residual limb length, when an amputation is done after trauma or because of neoplastic disease. The tendon of the adductor magnus is detached. The femoral vessels are identified in Hunter's canal and are ligated. The major nerves should be dissected 2 to 4 cm proximal to the proposed bone cut, gently retracted, and sectioned with a new sharp blade. The quadriceps is detached just proximal to the patella, with retention of some of its tendinous portion. The smaller muscles, including the sartorius and gracilis and the more posterior group of hamstrings (biceps femoris, semitendinosus, and semimembranosus) should be transected 2 to 2.5 cm longer than the proposed bone cut to facilitate the anchoring of those muscles in bone.

The femur is then transected with an oscillating power saw 12 to 14 cm proximal to the knee joint to allow sufficient space for the prosthetic knee joint. Drill holes are made in the distal end of the femur to anchor the transected muscles. The adductor magnus is attached to the lateral cortex of the femur while the femur is held in maximum adduction. This allows appropriate tensioning of the anchored muscle. The hip is positioned in extension for reattachment of the quadriceps to the posterior part of the femur, and the remaining hamstrings are anchored to the posterior area of the adductor magnus or the quadriceps.[32]

Postoperative Care

A soft compression dressing with a mini-spica wrap above the pelvis is used in the early postoperative period. Because the residual limb is relatively short, it is difficult to maintain a rigid plaster dressing. Range of motion exercises and early walking are encouraged. Preparatory prosthetic fitting can be initiated as soon

as the residual limb appears capable of accepting the load associated with weight bearing. This varies with individual patients and the experience of the rehabilitation team.

Summary

An amputation should be considered the first step in the rehabilitation of a patient for whom reconstruction of a functional limb is not possible. Care should be taken to create a residual limb that can optimally interact with a prosthetic socket to create a residual limb-prosthetic socket relationship capable of substituting for the highly adaptive end organ of weight bearing. A well-motivated patient in whom the amputation is done well and who is taught how to use the prosthesis will be able to return to most activities.

References

1. Bosse MJ, MacKenzie EJ, Kellam JF, et al: An analysis of outcomes of reconstruction or amputation after leg-threatening injuries. *N Engl J Med* 2002;347:1924-1931.

2. Gottschalk F: Transfemoral amputation: Biomechanics and surgery. *Clin Orthop Relat Res* 1999;361:15-22.

3. Pinzur MS: New concepts in lower-limb amputation and prosthetic management. *Instr Course Lect* 1990;39:361-366.

4. Loon HE. Below-knee amputation surgery. *Artif Limbs.* 1962;6:86-99.

5. Pinto MA, Harris WW: Fibular segment bone bridging in trans-tibial amputation. *Prosthet Orthot Int* 2004;28:220-224.

6. Hoaglund FT, Jergesen HE, Wilson L, Lamoreux LW, Roberts R: Evaluation of problems and needs of veteran lower-limb amputees in the San Francisco Bay Area during the period 1977-1980. *J Rehabil R D* 1983;20:57-71.

7. Legro MW, Reiber GD, Smith DG, del Aguila M, Larsen J, Boone D: Prosthesis evaluation questionnaire for persons with lower limb amputations: Assessing prosthesis-related quality of life. *Arch Phys Med Rehabil* 1998;79:931-938.

8. Ertl J: Uber amputationsstumpfe. *Chirurg* 1949;20:218-224.

9. Deffer PA. Ertl osteoplasty at Valley Forge General Hospital (interview). Committee on Prosthetic-Orthotic Education. Newsletter Amputee Clinics 1969;1.

10. Murdoch G (ed): Prosthetic and orthotic practice, based on a conference held in Dundee, June, 1969. London, UK, Edward Arnold, 1970, pp 52-56.

11. Pinzur MS, Pinto MA, Saltzman M, Batista F, Gottschalk F, Juknelis D: Health-related quality of life in patients with transtibial amputation and reconstruction with bone bridging of the distal tibia and fibula. *Foot Ankle Int* 2006;27:907-912.

12. Pinzur MS, Pinto MA, Schon LC, Smith DG: Controversies in amputation surgery. *Instr Course Lect* 2003;52:445-451.

13. Burgess EM, Romano RL, Zettl JH, Prosthetic Research Study: The management of lower-extremity amputations: Surgery, immediate postsurgical prosthetic fitting, patient care. Washington, DC, US Government Printing Office, 1969. Available at: http://www.prs-research.org/htmPages/Reference/BibRefs.html#text. Accessed March 13, 2007.

14. Assal M, Blanck R, Smith DG: Extended posterior flap for transtibial amputation. *Orthopedics* 2005;28:542-546.

15. Van Niekerk LJ, Stewart CP, Jain AS: Major lower limb amputation following failed infrainguinal vascular bypass surgery: A prospective study on amputation levels and stump complications. *Prosthet Orthot Int* 2001;25:29-33.

16. Jensen JS, Mandrup-Poulsen T, Krasnik M: Wound healing complications

following major amputations of the lower limb. *Prosthet Orthot Int* 1982; 6:105-107.

17. Volpicelli LJ, Chambers RB, Wagner FW Jr: Ambulation levels of bilateral lower-extremity amputees: Analysis of one hundred and three cases. *J Bone Joint Surg Am* 1983;65: 599-605.

18. Gonzalez EG, Corcoran PJ, Reyes RL: Energy expenditure in below-knee amputees: Correlation with stump length. *Arch Phys Med Rehabil* 1974;55:111-119.

19. Long IA: Normal shape-normal alignment (NSNA) above-knee prosthesis. *Clin Prosthet Orthot* 1985; 9:9-14.

20. Gottschalk FA, Kourosh S, Stills M, McClellan B, Roberts J: Does socket configuration influence the position of the femur in above-knee amputation? *J Prosthet Orthot* 1990;2:94-102.

21. Waters RL, Perry J, Antonelli D, Hislop H: Energy cost of walking of amputees: The influence of level of amputation. *J Bone Joint Surg Am* 1976; 58:42-46.

22. Hagberg K, Branemark R: Consequences of non-vascular transfemoral amputation: A survey of quality of life, prosthetic use and problems. *Prosthet Orthot Int* 2001;25: 186-194.

23. Barnes RW, Cox B: *Amputations: An Illustrated Manual*. Philadelphia, PA, Hanley and Belfus, 2000, pp 103-117.

24. Sabolich J: Contoured adducted trochanteric-controlled alignment method (CAT-CAM): Introduction and basic principles. *Clin Prosthet Orthot* 1985;9:15-26.

25. Hungerford DS, Krackow KA, Kenna RV (eds): *Total Knee Arthroplasty: A Comprehensive Approach*. Baltimore, MD, Williams and Wilkins, 1984, pp 34-39.

26. Gottschalk FA, Stills M: The biomechanics of trans-femoral amputation. *Prosthet Orthot Int* 1994;18:12-17.

27. Thiele B, James U, Stalberg E: Neurophysiological studies on muscle function in the stump of above-knee amputees. *Scand J Rehabil Med* 1973;5: 67-70.

28. James U: Maximal isometric muscle strength in healthy active male unilateral above-knee amputees, with special regard to the hip joint. *Scand J Rehabil Med* 1973;5:55-66.

29. Jaegers SM, Arendzen JH, de Jongh HJ: Changes in hip muscles after above-knee amputation. *Clin Orthop Relat Res* 1995;319:276-284.

30. Jaegers SM, Arendzen JH, de Jongh HJ: An electromyographic study of the hip muscles of transfemoral amputees in walking. *Clin Orthop Relat Res* 1996;328:119-128.

31. Jaegers SM, Arendzen JH, de Jongh HJ: Prosthetic gait of unilateral transfemoral amputees: A kinematic study. *Arch Phys Med Rehabil* 1995; 76:736-743.

32. Pinzur MS, Bowker JH, Smith DG, Gottschalk F: Amputation surgery in peripheral vascular disease. *Instr Course Lect* 1999;48:687-691.

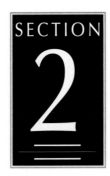

SECTION

2

Trauma

Trauma

Foot and ankle trauma is routinely managed by general orthopaedic surgeons and subspecialists in orthopaedic foot and ankle surgery and trauma care. Severe damage often ensues because the energy of the injury is dissipated through small bones and joints with a limited soft-tissue envelope. Advancements in surgical techniques and equipment are expected to lead to better outcomes. The chapters in this trauma section review general treatment principles and some troublesome injury patterns.

The chapter by Baumhauer and Manoli reviews the principles for managing severe trauma to the foot and ankle, including the initial evaluation of neurovascular status, wounds, and bone and joint injuries. Decisions are discussed regarding limb salvage or amputation, the management of open fractures, fracture stabilization with internal or external fixation, compartment syndrome, soft-tissue management, and postoperative care. The extent of soft-tissue damage may change over the first several days and a full understanding of the overall injury may not be readily apparent before complete surgical débridement. Baumhauer and Manoli emphasize the goal of achieving a functional, stable, painless, plantigrade foot that fits into a shoe or brace. They review general approaches to the initial and definitive fixation of the different regions of the foot and ankle and emphasize the goals of restoring articular surfaces, alignment, and muscle balance.

There is controversy and ongoing investigation regarding the choice of limb salvage or primary amputation in patients with severe traumatic lower extremity injuries. A recent small comparative study of unilateral traumatic amputation and limb salvage showed better quality of life and pain scores in the amputees.[1] A multicenter study of 545 patients with severe lower extremity trauma showed a higher risk for complications in patients electing limb salvage compared with amputation; complications included wound infection, dehiscence, osteomyelitis, nonunion, malunion, and prominent hardware.[2] In military patients with severe ballistic lower extremity injuries, the Mangled Extremity Severity Score may not be a reliable aid in deciding the appropriateness of amputation or limb salvage.[3] Many patients with severe foot and ankle trauma also may have more proximal injuries that may affect outcome. Limb salvage for severe (grade III) open distal tibial fractures with foot fractures may be associated with poor outcomes including marked psychosocial and physical disabilities.[4] Open metatarsal fractures may heal if there is less soft-tissue injury (grade I or II) but may result in amputation if there is more extensive soft-tissue injury (grade IIIB).[5]

Circular external fixation is being used more frequently after severe foot and ankle trauma and may provide stability to protect a free tissue flap and prevent equinus contracture.[6] In a recent study, free-flap coverage was successfully used for grade IIIB open calcaneal fractures; however, 72% of patients had residual pain or degenerative changes.[7] Other studies of open calcaneal fractures suggest that acceptable functional results can be obtained in some patients (average American Orthopaedic Foot and Ankle Society Ankle-Hindfoot Scores, 71 to 78 points).[8,9]

Compartment syndrome of the foot also is undergoing study. An MRI study described 10 distinct foot compartments in normal feet;[10] however, a cadaver study showed only 3 distinct compartments from the hindfoot to midfoot and no distinct myofascial compartments in the forefoot.[11] The measurements of compartment pressures in feet with an acute unilateral calcaneal fracture have shown higher compartment pressures (medial, central, and lateral compartments) in fractured compared with nonfractured feet.[12] In some instances, important clinical findings such as severe, uncontrollable pain may support judicious compartment release regardless of the results of compartment pressure measurements.

Distal tibial plafond (pilon) fractures are severe injuries associated with a high frequency of soft-tissue complications, loss of function, and posttraumatic arthritis.[13] The chapter by Helfet and Suk describes a minimally invasive method for treating pilon fractures to minimize soft-tissue compromise and devascularization of fracture fragments. This method consists of initial fibular internal fixation and spanning tibial external fixation, delaying definitive tibial fixation pending the resolution of soft-tissue swelling, reduction and fixation of the distal tibial articular fragments with fluoroscopy and indirect reduction or limited open reduction, percutaneous plate fixation of the articular segment to the diaphysis, and metaphyseal bone grafting.

The more recently published chapter about pilon fractures by Marsh and associates reviews classification systems, the importance of the soft tissues, and the diverse range of treatment options for this complex and potentially devastating injury. Treatment options include temporary spanning external fixation followed by internal plate fixation or external fixation (spanning or not spanning the ankle joint) with limited internal fixation.

Since the publication of the chapters by Helfet and Suk and by Marsh and associates, another study of pilon fracture treatment confirmed better clinical results with fibular fixation than without fibular fixation.[14] Another study demonstrated acceptable results for treating pilon fractures in most patients with minimally invasive percutaneous plate fixation.[15] In addition, treating pilon fractures with an oblique extension to the diaphysis can be facilitated with a small fragment, diaphyseal antiglide plate.[16] Ilizarov ring external fixation of pilon fractures may achieve similar treatment outcomes as the technique of staged external fixation and subsequent open reduction and internal fixation.[17] However, another study showed that delayed union occurred more frequently when a spanning external fixator was used for definitive treatment compared with a two-stage internal fixation method.[18] When direct reduction is required, medial and lateral incisions can be used;[19] alternatively, a lateral approach may protect the soft-tissue envelope and provide satisfactory visualization.[20]

Severe open pilon fractures with segmental metaphyseal bone loss may be salvaged with initial débridement and external fixation, subsequent internal fixation and placement of antibiotic beads, and delayed bone grafting.[21] Nevertheless, open fractures have worse outcomes than closed fractures, and posttraumatic arthrosis after a pilon fracture may cause progressive deterioration with time.[22] Highly comminuted pilon fractures may be nonreconstructable; possible treatment options include primary ankle arthrodesis with a cannulated blade plate.[23]

The chapter by Herscovici and associates reviews three important, complex foot and ankle injuries: pronation-external rotation ankle fractures, syndesmotic injuries, and talar neck fractures. The clinical features, pathoanatomy, radiography, and factors leading to malreduction are discussed. Although this chapter was originally published in early 2009, other current studies are available. In pronation-external rotation ankle fractures, the height of the fibular fracture may correlate with syndesmotic instability documented with intraoperative evaluation.[24] A recent postoperative CT study of syndesmosis injuries showed that the frequency of syndesmosis malreduction may be decreased, but not eliminated, by direct intraoperative syndesmosis visualization.[25] Fiber-wire fixation of the syndesmosis may be associated with soft-tissue irritation and granuloma formation, necessitating removal of the fiber-wire in some instances.[26]

Fractures of the talar neck are associated with high rates of morbidity and complications. Malreduction of talar neck fractures contributes to the development of both ankle and subtalar posttraumatic arthrosis. Herscovici and associates carefully identify errors in technique and fixation that contribute to malreduction, and provide tips to avoid these errors. A recent cadaver study of simulated talar neck fractures confirmed that displacement and rotation may be underestimated by plain radiography and CT studies,[27] and a low threshold for intraoperative visualization of the fracture may be indicated.

Lance M. Silverman, MD
President, Silverman Ankle and Foot
Edina, Minnesota

Elly Trepman, MD
Faculty of Medicine
University of Manitoba
manuscriptsurgeon.com
Mercer Island, Washington

References

1. Tekin L, Safaz Y, Göktepe AS, Yazýcýoðlu K: Comparison of quality of life and functionality in patients with traumatic unilateral below knee amputation and salvage surgery. *Prosthet Orthot Int* 2009;33:17-24.

2. Harris AM, Althausen PL, Kellam J, Bosse MJ, Castillo R, Lower Extremity Assessment Project (LEAP) Study Group: Complications following limb-threatening lower extremity trauma. *J Orthop Trauma* 2009;23:1-6.

3. Brown KV, Ramasamy A, McLeod J, Stapley S, Clasper JC: Predicting the need for early amputation in ballistic mangled extremity injuries. *J Trauma* 2009;66(suppl 4):S93-S98.

4. Debnath UK, Maripuri SN, Guha AR, Parfitt D, Fournier C, Hariharan K: Open grade III "floating ankle" injuries: A report of eight cases with review of literature. *Arch Orthop Trauma Surg* 2007;127:625-631.

5. Hoxie S, Turner NS, Strickland J, Jacofsky D: Clinical course of open metatarsal fractures. *Orthopedics* 2007;30:662-665.

6. Lowenberg DW, Sadeghi C, Brooks D, Buncke GM, Buntic RF: Use of circular external fixation to maintain foot position during free tissue transfer to the foot and ankle. *Microsurgery* 2008;28:623-627.

7. Ulusal AE, Lin CH, Lin YT, Ulusal BG, Yazar S: The use of free flaps in the management of type IIIB open calcaneal fractures. *Plast Reconstr Surg* 2008;121:2010-2019.

8. Loutzenhiser L, Lawrence SJ, Donegan RP: Treatment of select open calcaneus fractures with reduction and internal fixation: An intermediate-term review. *Foot Ankle Int* 2008;29:825-830.

9. Oznur A, Komurcu M, Marangoz S, Tasatan E, Alparslan M, Atesalp AS: A new perspective on management of open calcaneus fractures. *Int Orthop* 2008;32:785-790.

10. Reach JS, Amrami KK, Felmlee JP, Stanley DW, Alcorn JM, Turner NS: The compartments of the foot: A 3-tesla magnetic resonance imaging study with clinical correlates for needle pressure testing. *Foot Ankle Int* 2007;28:584-594.

11. Ling ZX, Kumar VP: The myofascial compartments of the foot: A cadaver study. *J Bone Joint Surg Br* 2008;90:1114-1118.

12. Kierzynka G, Grala P: Compartment syndrome of the foot after calcaneal fractures. *Ortop Traumatol Rehabil* 2008;10:377-383.

13. Harris AM, Patterson BM, Sontich JK, Vallier HA: Results and outcomes after operative treatment of high-energy tibial plafond fractures. *Foot Ankle Int* 2006;27:256-265.

14. Lee YS, Chen SW, Chen SH, Chen WC, Lau MJ, Hsu TL: Stabilisation of the fractured fibula plays an important role in the treatment of pilon fractures: A retrospective comparison of fibular fixation methods. *Int Orthop* 2009;33:695-699.

15. Bahari S, Lenehan B, Khan H, McElwain JP: Minimally invasive percutaneous plate fixation of distal tibia fractures. *Acta Orthop Belg* 2007;73:635-640.

16. Dunbar RP, Barei DP, Kubiak EN, Nork SE, Henley MB: Early limited internal fixation of diaphyseal extensions in select pilon fractures: Upgrading AO/OTA type C fractures to AO/OTA type B. *J Orthop Trauma* 2008;22: 426-429.

17. Bacon S, Smith WR, Morgan SJ, et al: A retrospective analysis of comminuted intra-articular fractures of the tibial plafond: Open reduction and internal fixation versus external Ilizarov fixation. *Injury* 2008;39:196-202.

18. Koulouvaris P, Stafylas K, Mitsionis G, Vekris M, Mavrodontidis A, Xenakis T: Long-term results of various therapy concepts in severe pilon fractures. *Arch Orthop Trauma Surg* 2007;127:313-320.

19. Chen L, O'Shea K, Early JS: The use of medial and lateral surgical approaches for the treatment of tibial plafond fractures. *J Orthop Trauma* 2007;21:207-211.

20. Grose A, Gardner MJ, Hettrich C, et al: Open reduction and internal fixation of tibial pilon fractures using a lateral approach. *J Orthop Trauma* 2007;21:530-537.

21. Gardner MJ, Mehta S, Barei DP, Nork SE: Treatment protocol for open AO/OTA type C3 pilon fractures with segmental bone loss. *J Orthop Trauma* 2008;22:451-457.

22. Chen SH, Wu PH, Lee YS: Long-term results of pilon fractures. *Arch Orthop Trauma Surg* 2007;127:55-60.

23. Bozic V, Thordarson DB, Hertz J: Ankle fusion for definitive management of non-reconstructable pilon fractures. *Foot Ankle Int* 2008;29:914-918.

24. van den Bekerom MP, Haverkamp D, Kerkhoffs GM, van Dijk CN: Syndesmotic stabilization in pronation external rotation ankle fractures [published online ahead of print April 2, 2009]. *Clin Orthop Relat Res.*

25. Miller AN, Carroll EA, Parker RJ, Boraiah S, Helfet DL, Lorich DG: Direct visualization for syndesmotic stabilization of ankle fractures. *Foot Ankle Int* 2009;30:419-426.

26. Willmott HJ, Singh B, David LA: Outcome and complications of treatment of ankle diastasis with tightrope fixation [published online ahead of print July 20, 2009]. *Injury.*

27. Chan G, Sanders DW, Yuan X, Jenkinson RJ, Willits K: Clinical accuracy of imaging techniques for talar neck malunion. *J Orthop Trauma* 2008;22:415-418.

Lance M. Silverman, MD or a member of his immediate family has stock or stock options held in AMAG Pharmaceuticals, Momenta Pharmaceuticals, and Resolxyx Pharmaceuticals. Elly Trepman, MD or a member of his immediate family serves as a committee member of the American Orthopaedic Foot & Ankle Society; has received royalties from USANA Health Sciences; serves as an Independent Associate of USANA Health Sciences, an employee of the University of Manitoba; and has stock in USANA Health Sciences.

Principles of Management of the Severely Traumatized Foot and Ankle

Judith F. Baumhauer, MD
Arthur Manoli II, MD

Introduction

Traumatic injury of the foot and ankle has several injury mechanisms that produce both bone and soft-tissue disruption requiring a vast array of treatment options. Several treatment principles help guide the surgeon toward the eventual goal of a functional, stable, painless plantigrade foot.

Ten percent to 17% of patients with a severely traumatized limb have associated life-threatening injuries;[1,2] therefore, initial resuscitation efforts with standardized trauma protocols are of primary importance.[3] A patient history that records comorbid conditions affecting life or limb viability is essential. A more specific limb-injury history is investigated. This includes the preinjury status of the limb, such as the patient's occupational demands and recreational and functional activity levels, as well as the time and mechanism of injury, initial care, and any delay of treatment.

Preoperative Evaluation

A thorough evaluation of the traumatized limb is not always possible in the emergency department. The lighting often is poor and the pain control inadequate. In addition, the emotional patient and family interaction are distractions that may disrupt the process of making objective management decisions. The emergency department, therefore, is the staging area to triage and resuscitate patients for a more detailed secondary survey in the operating room.

An emergency department examination of the foot and ankle consists of a bilateral determination of foot sensation, particularly the plantar aspect, as well as palpation of the dorsalis pedis and tibialis posterior pulses, noting their presence or absence and amplitude differences between the limbs. If the pulses are not palpable, then assessment of proximal pulses (femoral/popliteal) and Doppler examination are needed.[4,5] The severity of the soft-tissue injury should be noted, documenting the extent of lacerations

and soft-tissue damage on a foot-and-ankle figure in the patient's chart. Probing deep wounds is deferred to the operating room. Exposed or disrupted tendons or joint articulations are noted. The degree of contamination is recorded. Often patients are unable to move the ankle or toes because of the severity of pain; therefore, the absence of motion alone does not indicate motor unit injury and may not be helpful in the initial assessment of a severely traumatized foot and ankle.

After a record is made of all lacerations, a sterile dressing is applied to the wounds. Multiple wound exposures outside the operating room increase the risk of hospital-acquired wound infections.[6-8] In the past, recommendations were made to obtain wound cultures at the time of evaluation in the emergency department.[9,10] Lee,[11] however, found little correlation between the initial wound culture results and subsequent infecting organisms. Emergency department wound cultures are therefore of little value.

A portion of this chapter has been adapted with permission from Baumhauer JF: Mutilating injuries, in Myerson MS (ed): Foot and Ankle Disorders. *Philadelphia, PA, WB Saunders, 2000, pp 1245-1264.*

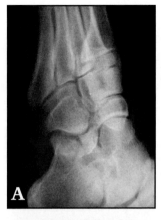
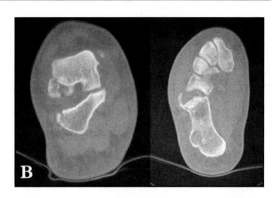
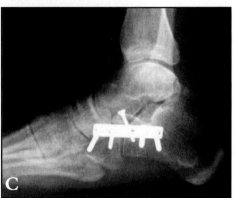
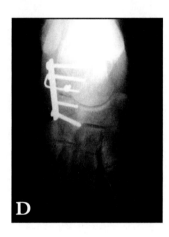

Fig. 1 A, Lateral radiograph of anterior process fracture of calcaneus. **B,** Axial (left) and frontal (right) CT images of the hindfoot demonstrating an impaction of the distal calcaneus and cuboid, with joint incongruity. Postoperative lateral (**C**) and AP (**D**) radiographs of the impaction fracture with an interfragmentary screw and bridge plating across the calcaneocuboid joint. Bone grafting was performed. The bridge plate was removed at 3 months.

Before a plaster splint is placed to immobilize the extremity, radiographic examination of the foot and ankle out of plaster is advisable to evaluate bony injury: 14-cm × 17-cm cassette films of the tibia and fibula in two planes should be obtained to assess the entire tibia and fibula as well as the knee and ankle joints. These views help identify remote fractures caused by rotation, axial load, or a direct blow. In a skeletally immature patient, contralateral foot and ankle radiographs can aid in distinguishing between skeletal injury and physeal injuries. CT is helpful for evaluating the degree of bone injury and displacement in the mid-foot and hindfoot (Figs. 1 and 2).

The use of antibiotic treatment in open fractures has been clearly demonstrated to decrease infection rates.[6,7,9,10,12-21] In their study of 1,104 open fractures, Patzakis and Wilkins[22] concluded that the rate of infection increased when antibiotics were first administered more than 3 hours after injury. The type of antibiotic chosen should provide broad coverage for gram-positive organisms and gram-negative rods.[1,12,23-25] Typically, a first-generation cephalosporin is used for grade I open fractures, and an aminoglycoside is added for grades II and III.[6,10,13,26] Gross soil contamination necessitates the addition of penicillin for the coverage of *Clostridium* organisms.[6,9,14,19,27] The recommended duration of antibiotic treatment ranges from 2 to 3 days, with most authors suggesting reinstitution of a 3-day course with each surgical manipulation.[6,7,9,14,15,26,28,29] Routine tetanus prophylaxis also is given.[30]

Limb Salvage Versus Amputation

After the preoperative evaluation, the severity of injury should be discussed with the patient and family. The choice between limb salvage and primary amputation is preferably made at this stage. As multiple authors have commented, protracted limb-salvage attempts may serve only as a demonstration of technical advances in medicine while leaving the patient physically, emotionally, psychologically, and financially in ruin.[2,31-35] Therefore, the surgeon's enthusiasm for limb-salvage procedures must be tempered by the expectations and the functional demands of the injured patient. Amputation should be considered as a positive step toward minimizing overall morbidity in severe injuries and not as a failure of treatment.[35]

Several studies have attempted to identify factors predictive of eventual amputation[2,36-38] (Table 1). A recent study[39] was unable to validate the clinical usefulness of lower extremity injury–severity scoring systems in predicting amputation. Treatment plans based on these grading systems, particularly with respect to amputation, need to be tailored with clinical judgment.

The potential economic impact of limb salvage on the health care system and the patient is significant. Bondurant and associates[31] compared the medical and economic impact of delayed versus primary amputations after severe open fractures of the lower extremity. They reported an

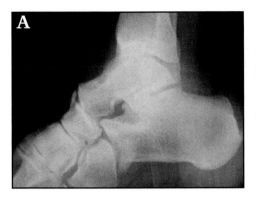
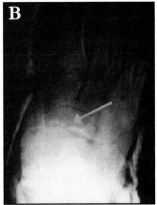
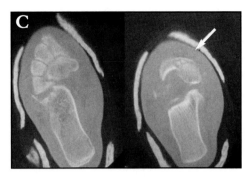

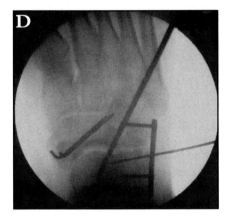
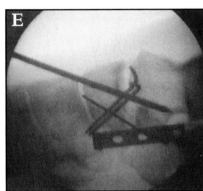

Fig. 2 A, Lateral radiograph demonstrating incongruity of the talonavicular joint and a dorsal bone fragment from the navicular. **B,** AP radiograph depicting a comminuted navicular fracture (arrow) and talonavicular incongruity. **C,** Axial CT images illustrating distal calcaneal impaction fracture at the calcaneocuboid joint (left) and comminuted displaced navicular fracture (right, arrow). AP **(D)** and lateral **(E)** fluoroscopic images of the foot with percutaneous K-wire stabilization of the navicular, bridge plating of the calcaneocuboid joint with bone grafting of the calcaneus and K-wire stabilization, and talonavicular immobilization with K-wire placement to aid in fracture healing. The bridge plate and K-wires were removed at 3 months.

approximately 50% decrease in medical costs with primary amputation compared with delayed amputation. Hansen[33] speculated there may be between 4,000 and 8,000 grade IIIC tibial fractures each year. Extrapolating the $25,000 in hospital costs saved by each primary amputation in this patient population, as much as $100,000,000 to $200,000,000 per year could be saved in hospital costs by performing appropriate primary amputations. Additional factors not considered in this study include the reduction in morbidity and earlier return to gainful employment with primary amputation.

The outcomes of partial foot amputation after trauma have been less commonly studied.[40] Two factors that appear to increase the functional impairment after partial foot amputation are trauma proximal to the ampu-

Table 1
Factors That Influence Outcome and Possible Amputation in Patients With Severe Foot and Ankle Injury

Duration and severity of limb ischemia
Patient age
Presence of shock
Energy of the injury
Degree of contamination (soil)
Nerve disruption
Open or closed injury (Gustilo open-fracture grading system)
Fracture grade, type, level(s)
Delay in fracture fixation
Elevated compartment pressures
Level and type of arterial injury
Delay of revascularization
Injury severity score/associated injuries
Comorbid medical conditions (diabetes mellitus; immunocompromised patients)
Transport time; use of pneumatic antishock garment
Experience of the receiving hospital (trauma center versus community hospital)
Steroid use
Malnutrition
Premature wound closure
Delayed soft-tissue coverage
Operating room time greater than 2 hours
Multiple wound exposures outside the operating room

tation level and a poorly performed amputation with soft-tissue instability, poor durability, and musculotendinous imbalance. Traditional partial foot amputations include digit, ray, transmetatarsal, Lisfranc's (tarsometatarsal), Chopart's (calcaneocuboid-talonavicular), and Syme's (ankle disarticulation) levels. For a successful outcome, extreme attention to detail is needed in performing the amputation, balancing the soft tissues to prevent equinus contractures or equinovarus malalignment, and handling tissue meticulously to avoid delayed wound healing. In traumatic injuries, creative soft-tissue local flap coverage may allow primary closure of wounds while allowing a more distal amputation level. The more distal the amputation level, the less necessary are bracing and shoe modification for ambulation, and the lower the energy needs and oxygen demands.[41]

When primary limb salvage is considered, the goals of surgery need to be carefully identified. The optimal result is a pain-free, functional, plantigrade foot that fits into a conventional shoe or brace. Elements required for the successful outcome of limb salvage include an adequate blood supply to the limb, sufficient bone and joint stability to provide for adequate muscle and tendon function, and a durable soft-tissue envelope to withstand the peak pressures and shear forces of weight bearing.

Initial Trauma Management

All open injuries are treated as surgical emergencies. Surgical intervention should be implemented as soon as possible. A delay in surgical irrigation and débridement of more than 8 hours has been shown to increase the infection rate.[6,7,26,38] Most literature supports the view that the severity of injury parallels the infection rate.[1,6,7,21,22,42-44] This correlation can

be attributed to several factors. The more severe injuries have a greater degree of soft-tissue damage, blood loss, and potential vascular compromise, which increases the amount of necrotic tissue and hypoxic zone of injury. A lower bacterial count is needed to produce an infection in this tissue environment than in a less severe injury.[16,20,22,45]

In a study of more than 1,000 open tibial fractures, Gustilo and Anderson[7] recommended the use of copious amounts of pulsed lavage irrigation, in addition to a thorough débridement of nonviable soft tissue and bone during each surgical event. The wounds should be reevaluated and débrided every 48 to 72 hours until they are devoid of any contaminated or nonviable tissue. The use of antibiotics within the pulsed irrigation has not been proved to be effective in decreasing wound infection rates compared with sterile saline irrigation.[21,46] The use of a tourniquet, electrocautery, and epinephrine are known to increase local soft-tissue ischemia and necrosis; therefore, these are not recommended in open fracture care.[6,10,47]

Fluorescein, a phenolphthalein dye that fluoresces when exposed to ultraviolet light,[48,49] has been used to determine skin viability. The fluorescein is injected systemically and the skin edges are viewed under ultraviolet light. With an intact capillary system, the skin will fluoresce and is considered viable. However, hypersensitivity reactions to the dye have been reported.[48-51] Flourescein use in acute trauma is not recommended.

Stabilization of Fractures and Joints of the Foot and Ankle

After thorough irrigation and débridement, stabilization of the fracture fragments is undertaken. Reduction and stabilization of the fracture fragments

with anatomic restoration of joint surfaces optimize the local conditions for wound healing, leading to decreased infection rates. Realignment and stabilization of the bones and joint surfaces also reduce swelling and eliminate abnormal soft-tissue motion and irritation, thus decreasing trauma to the adjacent neurovascular structures and improving microcirculation within the zone of injury. A less edematous soft-tissue envelope increases the efficacy of cellular and humeral defenses, decreasing infection rates.[44,52] Fracture stabilization allows early patient mobilization, thereby improving pulmonary status and decreasing the incidence of venous congestion and thrombosis while enhancing early rehabilitation.[6,23,26,46,47] Early joint mobility has been shown to improve cartilage nutrition and decrease joint stiffness.[53,54]

With significant soft-tissue trauma, isolated preliminary stabilization through the use of an external fixator to maintain length, stabilize the soft tissues, improve fracture alignment, and maintain joint reduction through ligamentotaxis may be particularly prudent during the acute swelling phase, when additional incisions may compound the zone of injury. The definitive fixation should be done as soon as possible and is dictated by the status of the soft tissues and the need for additional dissection. The principles to follow include careful soft-tissue handling with skin hooks or the retraction of flaps with sutures to avoid additional wound necrosis. The widest possible skin bridges are recommended between incisions, usually 5 cm for the dorsum of the foot and 7 cm at the ankle. Subcutaneous dissection is avoided and full-thickness flaps are raised. Care is taken to avoid denuding the bone fragments of their blood supply by excessive soft-tissue stripping.

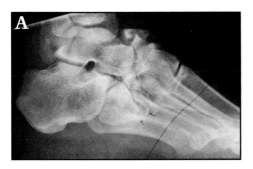

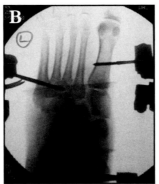

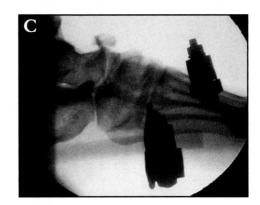

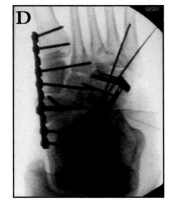

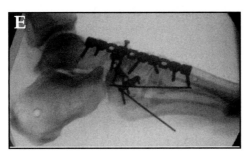

Fig. 3 A, Lateral radiograph of severely comminuted navicular, cuboid, and cuneiform fractures with joint incongruity. AP **(B)** and lateral **(C)** radiographs illustrating the placement of external fixator pins in the first and fifth metatarsals and calcaneus to maintain column length and alignment. AP **(D)** and lateral **(E)** radiographs revealing definitive fixation of complex midfoot fractures, with bridge plating from the first metatarsal to talus to maintain medial column length, and supplemental interfragmentary screw fixation. Miniplate fixation of the cuboid was performed to maintain lateral column length. Bridge plates were removed at 3 months.

The individual hardware recommendations for fracture stabilization depend on the location of the fracture (forefoot, midfoot, or hindfoot), as well as on the degree of comminution. Displaced extra-articular phalangeal fractures, metatarsal fractures, and phalangeal dislocations can be stabilized with Kirschner wires (K-wires) placed either longitudinally or in a crossed configuration.[55,56] Dorsal or plantar displacement of individual metatarsal heads relative to the adjacent metatarsal heads will alter the weight bearing on the plantar foot and create painful callosities.[56,57] These should be reduced. Interarticular phalangeal base fractures or metatarsal head fractures usually are secondary to crush injuries. Provided the toe is well aligned, percutaneous fixation with K-wires or external splint immobilization may be used.[55,56] A crush mechanism creates a severe soft-tissue injury, often leading to significant loss of motion of the small joints in the toes. Additional dissection for anatomic reduction may contribute to more loss of motion as well as the potential for additional wound problems.[58]

If the injury is in the midfoot and hindfoot, the concept of columns of the foot should be considered.[59] The columns of the foot are defined as medial (talonavicular, naviculomedial cuneiform, and first tarsometatarsal joints), middle (second and third tarsometatarsal joints, middle and lateral cuneiform articulations), and lateral (fourth and fifth tarsometatarsal and calcaneocuboid articulations). Maintenance of alignment and length of each of the columns preserves the length:tension ratio for the musculotendinous units and places the appropriate tension on the static soft-tissue structures. In addition, maintaining proper geometric relationships allows the biomechanically complex interrelated articulations of the midfoot, hindfoot, and ankle to function properly.

The fixation of tarsometatarsal fracture-dislocations has been extensively reported.[59-65] For a successful outcome, anatomic restoration of the joint surfaces and articular alignment with screw fixation are recommended. A variety of screw patterns has been suggested. Each emphasizes the need to recognize the fracture pattern, the extent of tarsometatarsal joint injury, and the associated disruption of intercuneiform and cuneiform-navicular relationships. Radiographic guidelines aid in the identification of this injury and are helpful in the intraoperative determination of an adequate reduction.[66-69] In complex injuries to the midfoot, intraoperative clinical assessment of joint stability when the foot is subjected to manual stress may reveal a

Table 2
Compartments of the Foot

Compartment	Muscle/Tendon
Calcaneal compartment	Quadratus plantae
Medial compartment	Abductor hallucis
	Flexor hallucis brevis
Lateral compartment	Abductor digiti minimi pedis
	Flexor digiti minimi brevis pedis
Superficial compartment	Flexor digitorum brevis
	Lumbricales pedis (4)
	Tendons of flexor digitorum longus
Adductor compartment	Adductor hallucis
Interosseous compartment (1)	Interossei
	dorsales pedis
Interosseous compartment (2)	plantares
	dorsales pedis
Interosseous compartment (3)	plantares
	dorsales pedis
Interosseous compartment (4)	plantares
	dorsales pedis
	plantares

more severe injury than is apparent on plain radiographs and also aids in planning screw placement.

The range of motion of the tarsometatarsal joints is small.[70] Hansen[71] suggested that the loss of motion of the flat joints of the midfoot (intertarsal and tarsometatarsal joints) has little effect on overall foot function. Therefore, despite extensive midfoot trauma, even with some bone loss, an external fixator or bridging plates and screws spanning the involved segments that maintain the proper tension and spatial relationship between static and dynamic structures may produce a foot in which late reconstruction can provide a satisfactory long-term outcome.

The hindfoot comprises the talonavicular, calcaneocuboid, and subtalar joints. These articulations join coupled motion segments that play an important role in foot mechanics and determine how the foot meets the floor. When possible, bone and corresponding articulations are anatomically reduced and rigidly fixed. Approaches and fixation for each of these individual hindfoot bones have been described.[55,71] When extensive comminution precludes anatomic repair, reestablishment of the columns of the foot in both length and hindfoot height is necessary. The use of an external fixator with limited internal fixation, by means of K-wires, screws, or bridging plate fixation, with removal in 3 to 4 months, can aid in achieving these goals (Fig. 3). Circular external fixator frames allow correction of the triplanar alignment of the foot as well as the establishment of height and length. With the exception of displaced fractures that cause excessive pressure and lead to soft-tissue compromise requiring emergency stabilization, delaying the definitive fixation of foot fractures until the acute soft-tissue swelling stage has dissipated has been suggested.

If an external fixator is not used, smooth K-wires can be placed across the affected joints of the hindfoot to maintain joint congruity (Fig. 2). In severe injuries, the soft-tissue structures supporting the joint, including the dorsal and plantar ligaments and capsular structures, are disrupted, leading to joint subluxation or dislocation. The K-wires can be left outside the skin and pulled in the early postoperative period (4 to 6 weeks).

Primary arthrodesis for severe complex injuries of the foot and ankle is an option when the joint surfaces cannot be reconstructed. Primary arthrodesis of the subtalar joint has been recommended for isolated, severely comminuted calcaneal fractures.[27,72] In severe complex foot and ankle injuries involving not only the hindfoot but also the midfoot, primary arthrodesis is a less attractive option because it will lead to a stiff, nonaccommodative foot at multiple segmental levels. It should be remembered that the goals in treating acute foot trauma are, if possible, to reestablish the intricate articular relationships and the height and length of segments, not to attempt a reconstructive salvage technique in the acute injury setting.

Typical ankle fracture patterns can be stabilized by AO treatment methods,[73,74] that is, by open reduction and internal fixation of the fracture fragments and reestablishment of the ankle mortise. With comminuted distal tibial articular fractures—pilon fractures—the principles of reduction and fixation as reported by Rüedi and Allgöwer[75,76] are appropriate: reestablishment of fibular length and rotation, reduction and fixation of the distal tibial articular surface, bone grafting of metaphyseal defects, and buttress stabilization of the medial aspect of the tibia. Although earlier AO recommendations included anatomic reduction and fixation with plates and screws, currently limited internal fixation of the articular portion of the distal tibia with interfragmentary screws is preferred.[77-80] An external fixator is placed to maintain length, provide ligamentotaxis, and function as the medial buttress to avoid late varus angulation. With a hybrid or ring fixator, the wires can be placed through larger articular fragments for reduction and stabilization, limiting the exposure necessary for interfragmentary lag screws.[81]

Compartment syndrome of the calf is a well-recognized entity, but less attention has been given to the evaluation and treatment of compartment syndrome of the foot. There are nine compartments of the foot[82,83] (Table 2). The current recommendations for evaluation include multistick compartmental pressure measurements. With calcaneal fractures, the calcaneal compartment should be measured.[83] Absolute pressure readings of more than 30 mm Hg are an indication for fascial releases. In a hypotensive patient, 10 to 30 mm Hg less than the diastolic blood pressure may be indicative of a compartment syndrome. Two dorsal incisions and one medial incision will provide exposure of all compartments.[82-84]

After emergent irrigation and débridement, fracture and joint stabilization, and compartment pressure assessment and treatment, the soft-tissue structures of the foot need to be repaired. Failure to repair the long tendons of the foot and ankle may result in biomechanical malalignment and poor foot function because of an unopposed functioning agonist. If possible, primary repair of the tendons crossing the ankle should be done. If tendon substance is lost, then either tenodesis to an adjacent tendon, as is done with the peroneus brevis and longus tendons, or appropriate bracing is done postoperatively. Delayed reconstructive tendon procedures can be done to balance the function of the foot and ankle. Soft-tissue coverage of defects should be done within the first 5 to 10 days after injury.[6,7,9,14,28,48]

Postoperative Care

After significant trauma, the foot and ankle need to be held in the plantigrade position to avoid soft-tissue and joint contractures. This can be accomplished through the use of a plaster cast; however, this makes care of soft-tissue wounds difficult. An external fixator allows the wounds to be examined and the dressings changed as needed. The external fixator can be modified to include pins into the first metatarsal or fifth metatarsal or both to allow the ankle to be brought into dorsiflexion. An alternative option is the use of an outrigger foot plate applied to the external fixator. Care must be taken to examine the plantar skin frequently because these foot plates can apply excessive pressure to the plantar aspect of the foot, causing localized pressure sores and skin necrosis.

References

1. Edwards CC, Simmons SC, Browner BD, Weigel MC: Severe open tibial fractures: Results treating 202 injuries with external fixation. *Clin Orthop* 1988;230:98-115.

2. Lange RH, Bach AW, Hansen ST Jr, Johansen KH: Open tibial fractures with associated vascular injuries: Prognosis for limb salvage. *J Trauma* 1985;25:203-208.

3. Committee on Trauma, American College of Surgeons: *Advanced Trauma Life Support Student Manual*. Chicago, IL, American College of Surgeons, 1989.

4. Keeley SB, Snyder WH III, Weigelt JA: Arterial injuries below the knee: Fifty-one patients with 82 injuries. *J Trauma* 1983;23:285-292.

5. McCabe CJ, Ferguson CM, Ottinger LW: Improved limb salvage in popliteal artery injuries. *J Trauma* 1983;23:982-985.

6. Gustilo RB, Merkow RL, Templeman D: The management of open fractures. *J Bone Joint Surg Am* 1990;72:299-304.

7. Gustilo RB, Anderson JT: Prevention of infection in the treatment of one thousand and twenty-five open fractures of long bones: Retrospective and prospective analyses. *J Bone Joint Surg Am* 1976;58:453-458.

8. McAndrew MP, Lantz BA: Initial care of massively traumatized lower extremities. *Clin Orthop* 1989;243:20-29.

9. Patzakis MJ: Management of open fracture wounds. *Instr Course Lect* 1987;36:367-369.

10. Patzakis MJ: Management of open fractures. *Instr Course Lect* 1982;31:62-64.

11. Lee J, Goldstein J, Madison M, Chapman MW: The value of pre- and post-debridement cultures in the management of open fractures. *Orthop Trans* 1991;15:776-777.

12. Antrum RM, Solomkin JS: A review of antibiotic prophylaxis for open fractures. *Orthop Rev* 1987;16:246-254.

13. Dellinger EP, Caplan ES, Weaver LD, et al: Duration of preventive antibiotic administration for open extremity fractures. *Arch Surg* 1988;123:333-339.

14. Gustilo RB: Current concepts in the management of open fractures. *Instr Course Lect* 1987;36:359-366.

15. Gustilo RB: Management of infected fractures. *Instr Course Lect* 1982;31:18-29.

16. Merritt K: Factors increasing the risk of infection in patients with open fractures. *J Trauma* 1988;28:823-827.

17. Patzakis MJ, Harvey JP Jr, Ivler D: The role of antibiotics in the management of open fractures. *J Bone Joint Surg Am* 1974;56:532-541.

18. Patzakis MJ: The use of antibiotics in open fractures. *Surg Clin North Am* 1975;55:1439-1444.

19. Tsukayama DT, Gustilo RB: Antibiotic management of open fractures. *Instr Course Lect* 1990;39:487-490.

20. Weigelt JA, Haley RW, Seibert B: Factors which influence the risk of wound infection in trauma patients. *J Trauma* 1987; 27:774-781.

21. Wilkins J, Patzakis M: Choice and duration of antibiotics in open fractures. *Orthop Clin North Am* 1991;22:433-437.

22. Patzakis MJ, Wilkins J: Factors influencing infection rate in open fracture wounds. *Clin Orthop* 1989;243:36-40.

23. Chapman MW: Role of bone stability in open fractures. *Instr Course Lect* 1982; 31:75-87.

24. Dziemian AJ, Herget CM: Physical aspects of primary contamination of bullet wounds. *Mil Surg* 1950;106:294-299.

25. Fischer MD, Gustilo RB, Varecka TF: The timing of flap coverage, bone grafting, and intramedullary nailing in patients who have a fracture of the tibial shaft with extensive soft-tissue injury. *J Bone Joint Surg Am* 1991;73:1316-1322.

26. Gustilo RB: Management of open fractures and complications. *Instr Course Lect* 1982;31:64-75.

27. Sanders R, Fortin P, DiPasquale T, Walling A: Operative treatment in 120 displaced intraarticular calcaneal fractures: Results using a prognostic computed tomography scan classification. *Clin Orthop* 1993;290: 87-95.

28. Gustilo RB, Mendoza RM, Williams DN: Problems in the management of type III (severe) open fractures: A new classification of type III open fractures. *J Trauma* 1984;24:742-746.

29. Sanders R, Swiontkowski M, Nunley J, Spiegel P: The management of fractures with soft-tissue disruptions. *J Bone Joint Surg Am* 1993;75:778-789.

30. Gustilo RB: Management of open fractures, in Gustilo RB, Gruninger RP, Tsukayama DT (eds): *Orthopaedic Infection: Diagnosis and Treatment*. Philadelphia, PA, WB Saunders, 1989, pp 87-117.

31. Bondurant FJ, Cotler HB, Buckle R, Miller-Crotchett P, Browner BD: The medical and economic impact of severely injured lower extremities. *J Trauma* 1988;28:1270-1273.

32. Hansen ST Jr: Overview of the severely traumatized lower limb: Reconstruction versus amputation. *Clin Orthop* 1989; 243:17-19.

33. Hansen ST Jr: Editorial: The type-IIIC tibial fracture: Salvage or amputation. *J Bone Joint Surg Am* 1987;69:799-800.

34. Lange RH: Limb reconstruction versus amputation decision making in massive lower extremity trauma. *Clin Orthop* 1989;243:92-99.

35. Myerson M: Soft-tissue trauma: Acute and chronic management, in Mann RA, Coughlin MJ (eds): *Surgery of the Foot and Ankle*, ed 6. St Louis, MO, Mosby-Year Book, 1993, vol 2, pp 1367-1410.

36. Gregory RT, Gould RJ, Peclet M, et al: The mangled extremity syndrome (M.E.S.): A severity grading system for multisystem injury of the extremity. *J Trauma* 1985;25:1147-1150.

37. Howe HR Jr, Poole GV Jr, Hansen KF, et al: Salvage of lower extremities following combined orthopedic and vascular trauma: A predictive salvage index. *Am Surg* 1987; 53:205-208.

38. Johansen K, Daines M, Howey T, Helfet D, Hansen ST Jr: Objective criteria accurately predicting amputation following lower extremity trauma. *J Trauma* 1990; 30:568-573.

39. Bosse MJ, MacKenzie EJ, Kellam JF, et al: A prospective evaluation of the clinical utility of the lower-extremity injury-severity scores. *J Bone Joint Surg Am* 2001;83: 3-14.

40. Millstein SG, McCowan SA, Hunter GA: Traumatic partial foot amputations in adults: A long-term review. *J Bone Joint Surg Br* 1988;70:251-254.

41. Zachary LS, Heggers JP, Robson MC, Smith DJ Jr, Maniker AA, Sachs RJ: Burns of the feet. *J Burn Care Rehab* 1987;8:192-194.

42. Dellinger EP, Miller SD, Wertz MJ, Grypma M, Droppert B, Anderson PA: Risk of infection after open fracture of the arm or leg. *Arch Surg* 1988;123:1320-1327.

43. Franklin JL, Johnson KD, Hansen ST Jr: Immediate internal fixation of open ankle fractures: Report of thirty-eight cases treated with a standard protocol. *J Bone Joint Surg Am* 1984;66:1349-1356.

44. Rittmann WW, Schibli M, Matter P, Allgower M: Open fractures: Long-term results in 200 consecutive cases. *Clin Orthop* 1979;138:132-140.

45. Swiontkowski MF: Criteria for bone debridement in massive lower limb trauma. *Clin Orthop* 1989;243:41-47.

46. Phillips TF, Contreras DM: Timing of operative treatment of fractures in patients who have multiple injuries. *J Bone Joint Surg Am* 1990;72:784-788.

47. Allgower M, Border JR: Management of open fractures in the multiple trauma patient. *World J Surg* 1983;7:88-95.

48. Papa J, Myersen MS: Soft tissue coverage in the management of foot and ankle trauma: Part 1. *Contemporary Orthopaedics* 1991;22:509-519.

49. Ziv I, Zeligowski A, Mosheiff R, Lowe J, Wexler MR, Segal D: Split-thickness skin excision in severe open fractures. *J Bone Joint Surg Br* 1988;70:23-26.

50. Kalisman M, Wexler MR, Yeschua R, Neuman Z: Treatment of extensive avulsions of skin and subcutaneous tissues. *J Dermatol Surg Oncol* 1978;4:322-327.

51. McCraw JB, Myers B, Shanklin KD: The value of fluorescein in predicting the viability of arterialized flaps. *Plast Reconstr Surg* 1977;60:710-719.

52. Wray JB: Factors in the pathogenesis of non-union. *J Bone Joint Surg Am* 1965; 47:168-173.

53. Mitchell N, Shepard N: Healing of articular cartilage in intra-articular fractures in rabbits. *J Bone Joint Surg Am* 1980;62:628-634.

54. Salter RB, Simmonds DF, Malcolm BW, Rumble EJ, MacMichael D, Clements ND: The biological effect of continuous passive motion on the healing of full-thickness defects in articular cartilage: An experimental investigation in the rabbit. *J Bone Joint Surg Am* 1980;62:1232-1251.

55. DeLee JC: Fractures and dislocations of the foot, in Mann RA, Coughlin MJ (eds): *Surgery of the Foot and Ankle*, ed 6. St Louis MO, Mosby-Year Book, 1993, vol 2, pp 1465-1703.

56. Shields NN, Valdez RR, Brennan MJ, Johnson EE, Gould JS: Metatarsal fractures and dislocations and Lisfranc's fracture-dislocations, in Gould JS (ed): *Operative Foot Surgery*. Philadelphia, PA, WB Saunders, 1994, pp 399-420.

57. Blodgett WH: Injuries of the forefoot and toes, in Jahss MH (ed): *Disorders of the Foot*. Philadelphia, PA, WB Saunders, 1982, vol 2, pp 1449-1462.

58. Johnson VS: Treatment of fractures of the forefoot in industry, in Bateman JE (ed): *Foot Science*. Philadelphia, PA, WB Saunders, 1976, pp 257-265.

59. Myerson MS, Fisher RT, Burgess AR, Kenzora JE: Fracture dislocations of the tarsometatarsal joints: End results correlated with pathology and treatment. *Foot Ankle* 1986;6:225-242.

60. Arntz CT, Veith RG, Hansen ST Jr: Fractures and fracture-dislocations of the tarsometatarsal joint. *J Bone Joint Surg Am* 1988;70:173-181.

61. Goossens M, De Stoop N: Lisfranc's fracture-dislocations: Etiology, radiology, and results of treatment. A review of 20 cases. *Clin Orthop* 1983;176:154-162.

62. Licht NJ, Trevino SG: Lisfranc injuries. *Tech Orthop* 1991;6:77-83.

63. Myerson M: The diagnosis and treatment of injuries to the Lisfranc joint complex. *Orthop Clin North Am* 1989;20:655-664.

64. Resch S, Stenström A: The treatment of tarsometatarsal injuries. *Foot Ankle* 1990;11:117-123.

65. Trevino SG, Baumhauer JF: Lisfranc injuries, in Myerson M (ed): *Current Therapy in Foot and Ankle Surgery*. St Louis, MO, BC Decker, 1993.

66. Foster SC, Foster RR: Lisfranc's tarsometatarsal fracture-dislocation. *Radiology* 1976;120:79-83.

67. Goiney RC, Connell DG, Nichols DM: CT evaluation of tarsometatarsal fracture-dislocation injuries. *AJR Am J Roentgenol* 1985;144:985-990.

68. Norfray JF, Geline RA, Steinberg RI, Galinski AW, Gilula LA: Subtleties of Lisfranc fracture-dislocations. *AJR Am J Roentgenol* 1981;137:1151-1156.

69. Stein RE: Radiological aspects of the tarsometatarsal joints. *Foot Ankle* 1983;3: 286-289.

70. Klaue K, Hansen ST, Masquelet AC: Clinical, quantitative assessment of first tarsometatarsal mobility in the sagittal plane and its relation to hallux valgus deformity. *Foot Ankle Int* 1994;15:9-13.

71. Hansen ST Jr: Foot injuries, in Browner BD, Jupiter JB, Levine AM, Trafton PG (eds): *Skeletal Trauma: Fractures, Dislocations, Ligamentous Injuries*. Philadelphia, PA, WB Saunders, 1992, vol 2, pp 1959-1991.

72. Myerson MS: Primary subtalar arthrodesis for the treatment of comminuted fractures of the calcaneus. *Orthop Clin North Am* 1995;26:215-227.

73. Lauge-Hansen N: Fractures of the ankle: II. Combined experimental-surgical and experimental-roentgenologic investigations. *Arch Surg* 1950;60:957-985.

74. Müller ME, Allgöwer M, Schneider R, Willenegger H (eds): *Manual of Internal Fixation: Techniques Recommended by the AO Group*, ed 2. Berlin, Germany, Springer-Verlag, 1979.

75. Rüedi TP, Allgöwer M: Fractures of the lower end of the tibia into the ankle-joint. *Injury* 1969;1:92-99.

76. Rüedi TP, Allgöwer M: The operative treatment of intra-articular fractures of the lower end of the tibia. *Clin Orthop* 1979;138:105-110.

77. Bonar SK, Marsh JL: Unilateral external fixation for severe pilon fractures. *Foot Ankle* 1993;14:57-64.

78. Bone L, Stegemann P, McNamara K, Seibel R: External fixation of severely comminuted and open tibial pilon fractures. *Clin Orthop* 1993;292:101-107.

79. Saleh M, Shanahan MD, Fern ED: Intra-articular fractures of the distal tibia: Surgical management by limited internal fixation and articulated distraction. *Injury* 1993;24:37-40.

80. Tornetta P III, Weiner L, Bergman M, et al: Pilon fractures: Treatment with combined internal and external fixation. *J Orthop Trauma* 1993;7:489-496.

81. Murphy CP, D'Ambrosia R, Dabezies EJ: The small pin circular fixator for distal tibial pilon fractures with soft tissue compromise. *Orthopedics* 1991;14:283-290.

82. Manoli A II, Weber TG: Fasciotomy of the foot: An anatomical study with special reference to release of the calcaneal compartment. *Foot Ankle* 1990;10:267-275.

83. Myerson M: Diagnosis and treatment of compartment syndrome of the foot. *Orthopedics* 1990;13:711-717.

84. Santi MD, Botte MJ: Volkmann's ischemic contracture of the foot and ankle: Evaluation and treatment of established deformity. *Foot Ankle Int* 1995;16:368-377.

Minimally Invasive Percutaneous Plate Osteosynthesis of Fractures of the Distal Tibia

David L. Helfet, MD
Michael Suk, MD, JD, MPH

Abstract

Fractures of the distal tibia are notoriously difficult to treat, and traditional methods of fixation are often fraught with soft-tissue complications. With recent emphasis on meticulous handling and preservation of the soft-tissue envelope, minimally invasive percutaneous plate osteosynthesis has become a safe and reliable method of treating these fractures. This technique involves conventional open reduction and internal fixation of the fibula and spanning external fixation of the tibia until the soft-tissue swelling subsides. Subsequently, limited open reduction and internal fixation of displaced articular fragments is performed through small incisions based on CT evaluation. This is followed by minimally invasive percutaneous plate osteosynthesis of the tibia, in which the plafond is attached to the tibial shaft using a variety of commercially available plates.

Fractures of the distal tibia involving the weight-bearing articular surface and metaphysis are notoriously difficult to treat.[1-14] In 1905, Lambotte called such fractures "fractures de l'epiphyse"[3,15] and was perhaps the first to perform an open reduction and internal fixation to treat this type of fracture. In 1911, Destot introduced the term pilon ("hammer").[1,16] In 1950, Bonin used the term plafond ("ceiling")[17] to describe the region of metaphyseal impaction caused by the talus as it is driven up into the tibial articular surface. And most recently, in 1971, Ruoff and Snider[18] coined the term "explosion fracture" to describe the potential complexity of fractures of the distal tibia. Disturb-

ingly, 10% to 30% of these are open fractures, and most are associated with other injuries.[2,15,19,20] Additionally, the degloving and crushing of the skin that can accompany such injuries frequently leads to necrosis and further complicates treatment.[4,5,16,19,21,22]

Historical Treatment
In 1963, the AO group introduced four principles of open reduction and internal fixation to treat intra-articular fractures of the distal tibia: (1) reestablishment of fibular length and stabilization of the lateral column, (2) reconstruction of the articular surface of the tibia, (3) placement of metaphyseal bone graft, and (4) stabilization of the medial tibia using a plate. Al-

though good to excellent results are frequently reported for closed, low-energy fractures, high-energy and open fractures are accompanied by complications. Poor results, skin slough, wound dehiscence, and infection often are associated with increased fracture severity.[5,7,8,18,19,23-28]

To improve on the poor results traditionally associated with open reduction and plate and screw fixation, minimally invasive techniques were developed to include limited internal and hybrid external fixation.[29] Other investigators have also endorsed the concept of limited surgery to treat severe pilon injuries.[15,25,29-31] From a desire to produce minimal additional insult at surgery, modern biologic principles have evolved that emphasize meticulous soft-tissue dissection, limited stripping of fracture fragments, indirect reduction techniques, and adequate fixation.[9,20,21,32]

Minimally Invasive Percutaneous Plate Osteosynthesis
Minimally invasive percutaneous plate osteosynthesis was developed in response to disappointing results following traditional methods of surgical stabilization of fractures of

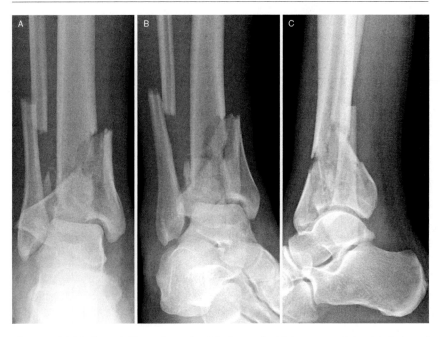

Figure 1 AP (**A**), lateral (**B**), and mortise (**C**) views of a high-energy, right-sided closed pilon fracture sustained by a 39-year-old man who fell 14 feet from a ladder.

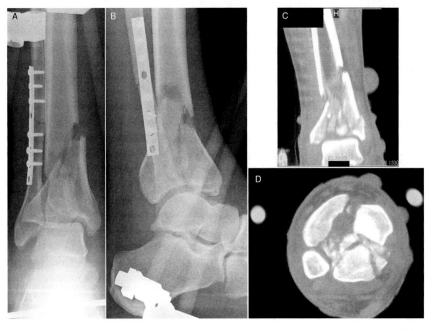

Figure 2 AP (**A**) and lateral (**B**) views after open reduction and internal fixation of the fibula fracture and application of the spanning external fixator of the patient as described in Figure 1. Coronal (**C**) and transverse (**D**) CT scans are shown.

tibia fractures include open fractures, displaced intra-articular tibial pilon fractures with sufficient medial soft-tissue coverage to allow percutaneous plating and articular reconstruction, low-energy ankle fractures associated with significant soft-tissue compromise, and unstable metaphyseal/diaphyseal fractures that are located too distally for stabilization with an intramedullary nail.

Surgical Technique

Management of patients with distal tibia fractures includes rapid skeletal stabilization on the day of admission to the hospital with the placement of a triangular ("delta") external fixator from the tibia to the calcaneus. Early placement of an external frame enhances recovery of the soft-tissue envelope and assists in the restoration of length. Two 4.5-mm or 5.0-mm Schanz screws are placed in the anterior aspect of the tibia proximal to the fracture, and a centrally threaded transfixion pin is placed through the tuberosity of the calcaneus in a medial to lateral direction. Two carbon fiber rods are used to connect the Schanz screws, thus completing the triangle. Manual traction is applied to achieve a closed reduction of alignment, length, and rotation through ligamentotaxis before the pin to bar clamps are tightened. For additional stability in the plane of the calcaneal pin, an additional 4.5-mm Schanz pin can be applied to the midfoot across the medial and middle cuneiforms.

If a fibular fracture is present, concurrent open reduction and internal fixation is performed with either a one third tubular plate or a 3.5-mm conventional or locked combination plate (LCDCP or LCP, Synthes, Paoli, PA). Early reduction of the fibular fracture provides lateral stability to the construct and serves as a

the distal tibia and the complications also introduced by the newer methods of limited internal and external fixation.[27] The percutaneous plating technique is advantageous because it minimizes soft-tissue compromise and devascularization of the fracture fragments. Indications for using minimally invasive percutaneous plate osteosynthesis to treat distal

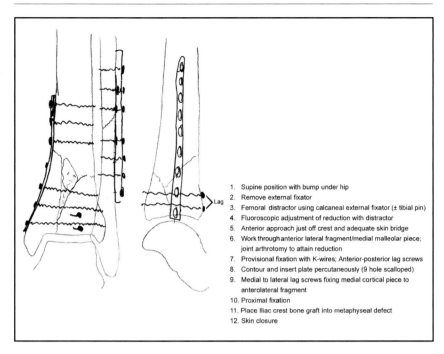

1. Supine position with bump under hip
2. Remove external fixator
3. Femoral distractor using calcaneal external fixator (± tibial pin)
4. Fluoroscopic adjustment of reduction with distractor
5. Anterior approach just off crest and adequate skin bridge
6. Work through anterior lateral fragment/medial malleolar piece; joint arthrotomy to attain reduction
7. Provisional fixation with K-wires; Anterior-posterior lag screws
8. Contour and insert plate percutaneously (9 hole scalloped)
9. Medial to lateral lag screws fixing medial cortical piece to anterolateral fragment
10. Proximal fixation
11. Place iliac crest bone graft into metaphyseal defect
12. Skin closure

Figure 3 Same patient as described in Figure 1. Preoperative plan for definitive open reduction and internal fixation of the pilon fracture including delta frame removal, fluoroscopic-aided reduction using a femoral distractor, and placement of a bone graft and scallop plate.

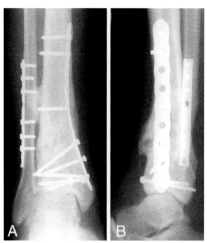

Figure 4 AP (**A**), and lateral (**B**) views of the patient as described in Figure 1, 1 year after percutaneous fixation with a scallop plate.

guide to proper restoration of length of the plafond. Anatomic landmarks are assessed intraoperatively with the use of fluoroscopy to prevent over-distraction through the external frame.

The affected limb is then maintained in a well-padded posterior splint and elevated on a Bohler-Braun frame until such time as the soft-tissue swelling allows further surgery. Definitive surgery is delayed until resolution of the acute phase of soft-tissue edema, typically 7 to 14 days after injury and evidenced by wrinkling of the skin over the medial and anterior aspects of the ankle. Open wounds are treated with serial irrigations and débridement and delayed soft-tissue closure or coverage is obtained within 5 to 7 days of the injury.

For minimally invasive plate osteosynthesis of a distal tibial frac-ture, the patient is placed supine on a radiolucent table, a roll is placed beneath the ipsilateral buttock, and a pneumatic tourniquet is applied to the proximal thigh. The ipsilateral iliac crest and entire lower extremity are made ready for surgery in the usual sterile fashion. After exsan-guination of the extremity, the tourniquet is inflated to 300 mm Hg.

Initial attention is paid to the fracture lines, which extend into the tibial plafond and are identified by careful evaluation of the CT scan (Figures 1 through 3). Articular fragments are anatomically reduced percutaneously, using fluoroscopy and pointed reduction forceps, or via direct open reduction using small incisions and arthrotomies. Once articular reduction is obtained, the articular fragments are stabilized with either 2.7-mm or 3.5-mm lag screws. An additional T

plate, one third or even smaller plates (Synthes) may be applied through limited approaches to buttress a large metaphyseal defect or act as washer in the face of significant comminution.

Once the articular fragments are stabilized, the metaphyseal fracture is addressed. The appropriate length of the semitubular plate, scallop plate (Synthes), or precontoured periarticular medial distal tibia plate (Synthes; Zimmer, Warsaw, IN) is determined by placing a plate along the anterior aspect of the leg and adjusting it so that under fluoroscopy the distal end of the plate is at the level of the tibial plafond and the proximal end extends at least three screw holes proximal to the proximal extent of the fracture. A 3-cm incision is made along the antero-medial aspect of the tibia and proximal to the fracture. A subcutaneous tunnel is created along the medial aspect of the tibia by blunt dissection using a large Kelly clamp. The plate can then be advanced directly beneath the soft tissues often with a suture to pull the leading edge

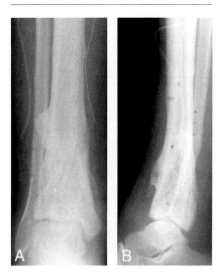

Figure 5 Same patient as described in Figure 1. AP (**A**) and lateral (**B**) views 2 years after hardware removal.

through the tunnel. The position of the plate is adjusted under fluoroscopy in both the coronal and sagittal planes to assure correct length and that it lies along the medial aspect of the tibia.

Cortical screws (3.5 or 4.0 mm) are placed through the plate via small percutaneous stab incisions to achieve an indirect reduction from distal to proximal or proximal to distal, depending on the fracture pattern. The distal metaphyseal articular fragment is indirectly reduced to the proximal fragment in this fashion. Percutaneous lag screws are placed across the fracture planes as needed to maintain the reduction, provide interfragmentary compression, and increase the stability of the construct (Figures 4 and 5). Radiographs are taken in the operating room to assess the overall alignment of the limb and ensure proper placement of the implants. The surgical incisions are irrigated and closed, sterile dressings are applied, and the limb is immobilized in a well-padded posterior and U splint, with

the ankle maintained in neutral position.

Clinical Results
The senior author recently reviewed retrospectively 17 patients treated between 1999 and 2001 for tibial plafond fractures, using a newly designed and minimally invasive ultra-slim scallop plate (Synthes). As per protocol, staged surgical treatment with open reduction and fixation of the fibular fracture and application of an external fixator was initially performed in 12 patients. As soon as the soft tissues and swelling allowed, (ie, skin wrinkling occurred), the articular surface was reconstructed and anatomically reduced through a small incision, and the articular block was fixed to the diaphysis using a medially placed, percutaneously introduced flat scallop plate (DL Helfet, MD, unpublished data, 2003).

Hemovac drains were removed when the drainage was less than 20 mL per 8 hours and generally within the first 24 to 48 hours. All patients received 48 hours of perioperative prophylactic antibiotic therapy. Postoperatively, the limb was elevated while the patient was in bed, and ambulation training was begun on postoperative day one with toe-touch weight bearing of 20 lb with crutches. On postoperative day two, gentle range-of-motion exercises of the ankle were begun, the patients were instructed on the use of a theraband, and a fracture boot was applied.

The patients were discharged when able to perform toe-touch weight bearing of 20 lb in their fracture boots. Sutures were removed at 10 to 14 days after surgery. Radiographs including an AP, lateral, and mortise views of the distal tibia and fibula were taken at 2 weeks, 6

weeks, and 3 months postoperatively to assess healing and alignment. Patients were progressed to partial weight bearing and then full weight bearing depending on the results of clinical and radiographic evaluation.

All patients achieved bony union at an average of 14.1 weeks. Eleven fractures (65%) were high-energy injuries. Two fractures were open. There were no plate failures or loss of fixation or reduction. Two superficial wound-healing problems resolved with local wound care. At an average follow-up of 17 months (range, 6 to 29 months), eight patients (47%) had excellent results, seven (41%) had fair results, and two (12%) had poor results. The average American Orthopaedic Foot and Ankle Society Ankle-Hindfoot Score was 86.1 (range, 61 to 100). Four patients subsequently required hardware removal, and one of these patients required ankle arthrodesis. Most importantly, there were no chronic or deep infections and no soft-tissue sloughs, flaps, etc. Based on initial results, a minimally invasive surgical technique using a new low-profile plate can decrease soft-tissue problems while leading to fracture healing and obtaining results that are comparable to those reported in other more recent series. The new scallop plate is appropriate for the treatment of pilon fractures and should be used in conjunction with a staged procedure in the acute trauma setting.

Summary
Open reduction and internal fixation of fractures of the distal tibia with articular involvement (ie, pilon fractures) has been plagued by complications. In keeping with modern trends for less invasive surgery, the protocol of (1) initial fibula fixation and spanning external fixation to

manage the soft-tissue injury; (2) limited open arthrotomies and fixation of the displaced distal tibial articular segment; and (3) percutaneous plate osteosynthesis of the articular segment to the tibial diaphysis has proved efficacious with an acceptably low rate of complications, especially to the soft-tissue envelope.

References

1. Destot EAJ (ed): *Traumatismes du pied et rayons x: Malleoles, Astragale, Calcaneum, Avant-pied.* Paris, France, Masson, 1911.

2. Helfet DL, Koval K, Pappas J, Sanders RW, DiPasquale T: Intra-articular "pilon" fracture of the tibia. *Clin Orthop* 1994;298:221-228.

3. Lambotte A: *Chirurgie operatoire des fractures.* Paris, France, Masson, 1913.

4. Muhr G, Breitfuss H: Complications after pilon fractures, in Tscherne H, Schatzker J (eds): *Major Fractures of the Pilon, the Talus, and the Calcaneus: Current Concepts of Treatment.* Berlin, Germany, Springer-Verlag, 1993, pp 65-67.

5. Ovadia DN, Beals RK: Fractures of the tibial plafond. *J Bone Joint Surg Am* 1986;68:543-551.

6. Ruedi TP, Allgower M: The operative treatment of intra-articular fractures of the lower end of the tibia. *Clin Orthop* 1979;138:105-110.

7. Sanders R, Pappas J, Mast J, Helfet D: The salvage of open grade IIIB ankle and talus fractures. *J Orthop Trauma* 1992;6:201-208.

8. Ruedi T, Allgower M: Fractures of the lower end of the tibia into the ankle-joint. *Injury* 1969;1:92-99.

9. Mast JW, Spiegel PG, Pappas JN: Fractures of the tibial pilon. *Clin Orthop* 1988;230:68-82.

10. Blauth M, Bastian L: Krettek C, Knop C, Evans S: Surgical options for the treatment of severe tibial pilon fractures: A study of three techniques. *J Orthop Trauma* 2001;15:153-160.

11. Borelli J Jr, Ellis E: Pilon fractures: Assessment and treatment. *Orthop Clin North Am* 2002;33:231-245.

12. Moller BN, Krebs B: Intra-articular fractures of the distal tibia. *Acta Orthop Scand* 1982;53:991-996.

13. Ruedi TP: Fractures of the lower end of the tibia into the ankle joint: Results 9 years after open reduction and internal fixation. *Injury* 1973;5:130-134.

14. Sirkin M, Sanders R: The treatment of pilon fractures. *Orthop Clin North Am* 2001;32:91-102.

15. Kellam JF, Waddell JP: Fractures of the distal tibial metaphysis with intra-articular extension: The distal tibial explosion fracture. *J Trauma* 1979;19:593-601.

16. Bone L, Stegemann P, McNamara K, Seibel R: External fixation of severely comminuted and open tibial pilon fractures. *Clin Orthop* 1993;292:101-107.

17. Bonnin JG (ed): *Injuries to the Ankle,* ed 1. London, England, Heinemann, 1950, pp 248-260.

18. Ruoff AC III, Snider RK: Explosion fractures of the distal tibia with major articular involvement. *J Trauma* 1971;11:866-873.

19. Heim U (ed): *The Pilon Tibial Fracture: Classification, Surgical Techniques, Results.* Philadelphia, PA, WB Saunders, 1995.

20. Helfet DL, Shonnard PY, Levine D, Borrelli J Jr: Minimally invasive plate osteosynthesis of distal fractures of the tibia. *Injury* 1997;28(suppl 1):A42-A48.

21. Beck E: Results of operative treatment of pilon fractures, in Tscherne H, Schatzker J (eds): *Major Fractures of the Pilon, the Talus, and the Calcaneus: Current Concepts of Treatment.* Berlin, Germany, Springer-Verlag, 1993, pp 49-51.

22. McFerran MA, Smith SW, Boulas HJ, Schwartz HS: Complications encountered in the treatment of pilon fractures. *J Orthop Trauma* 1992;6:195-200.

23. Bourne RB: Pylon fractures of the distal tibia. *Clin Orthop* 1989;240:42-46.

24. Maale G, Seligson D: Fractures through the distal weight-bearing surface of the tibia. *Orthopedics* 1980;3:517-521.

25. Fitzpatrick DC, Marsh JL, Brown TD: Articulated external fixation of pilon fractures: The effects on ankle joint kinematics. *J Orthop Trauma* 1995;9:76-82.

26. Pierce RO Jr, Heinrich JH: Comminuted intra-articular fractures of the distal tibia. *J Trauma* 1979;19:828-832.

27. Teeny SM, Wiss DA: Open reduction and internal fixation of tibial plafond fractures: Variables contributing to poor results and complications. *Clin Orthop* 1993;292:108-117.

28. Wyrsch B, McFerran MA, McAndrew M, et al: Operative treatment of fractures of the tibial plafond: A randomized prospective study. *J Bone Joint Surg Am* 1996;78:1646-1657.

29. Tornetta P III, Weiner L, Bergman M, et al: Pilon fractures: Treatment with combined internal and external fixation. *J Orthop Trauma* 1993;7:489-496.

30. Allgower M, Muller ME, Willenegger H: *Technik der operativen Frakturbehandlung.* New York, NY, Springer-Verlag, 1963.

31. Marsh JL, Bonar S, Nepola JV, Decoster TA, Hurwitz SR: Use of an articulated external fixator for fractures of the tibial plafond. *J Bone Joint Surg Am* 1995;77:1498-1509.

32. Manca M, Marchetti S, Restuccia G, Faldini A, Giannini S: Combined percutaneous internal and external fixation of type-C tibial plafond fractures: A review of twenty-two cases. *J Bone Joint Surg Am* 2002;84(suppl 2):109-115.

Fractures of the Tibial Plafond

J. Lawrence Marsh, MD
Joseph Borrelli, Jr, MD
Douglas R. Dirschl, MD
Michael S. Sirkin, MD

Abstract

Tibial plafond fractures comprise a diverse group of articular, metaphyseal, and occasionally diaphyseal injuries and have in common injury to the articular surface of the distal tibia and significant associated soft-tissue injury. Injury to the soft tissues combined with the complex fracture patterns has led to high complication rates from surgical attempts to reduce and stabilize these fractures. Currently, there is a wide range of treatment techniques available for a wide spectrum of injury severity, surgeon experience, and surgeon preferences. Patient outcomes vary widely. Because these injuries are relatively uncommon, the amount of clinical data available to guide treatment decisions is limited. Careful classification and assessment of the fracture pattern and associated soft-tissue injury and an understanding of the principles of modern concepts of treatment should allow the surgeon to choose from among several treatment protocols, all of which emphasize minimizing complications to optimize patient outcomes.

This chapter reviews the latest concepts in assessment, management, and expected outcomes for patients with fractures of the tibial plafond. The ongoing controversy between whether to treat these complex fractures with external fixation or plate fixation will be highlighted, and the factors that relate to outcome will be reviewed.

Classification and Assessment
Fracture Classification
The two most common classification systems used currently to assess fractures of the distal tibia are that of the AO/Orthopaedic Trauma Asso-

ciation (OTA) (Figure 1) and the system described by Ruedi and Allgöwer (Figure 2). Although both of these classification systems are commonly discussed in the literature, recent publications favor the AO/OTA classification.

The AO/OTA classification system is a complex fracture classification that assesses which bone is involved, the part of the bone that is involved, the number of fragments, the complexity of the fracture pattern, and in patients with articular injuries, the amount of joint involvement. For distal tibia fractures, the designation of bone involve-

ment is 43: 43-A fractures are extra-articular, 43-B fractures are partial articular, and 43-C fractures are complete articular. Although further subclassifications are based on these criteria, it has been shown that beyond the most rudimentary divisions of A, B, and C, the classification is not reliable; therefore, any usefulness beyond this level may be limited,[1-3] especially when comparing results of treatment.

The classification system of Ruedi and Allgöwer is based on the amount of comminution of the articular surface[4] (Figure 2). Type I fractures are nondisplaced, type II fractures are displaced but not comminuted, and type III fractures are displaced and comminuted. Although this classification system is simple and easy to remember, it has been shown to have poor observer reliability and may not provide enough detail to meaningfully guide treatment.[2]

Soft-Tissue Assessment and Classification
Understanding the importance of the soft-tissue injury in tibial plafond fractures is paramount to successful treatment. Complications

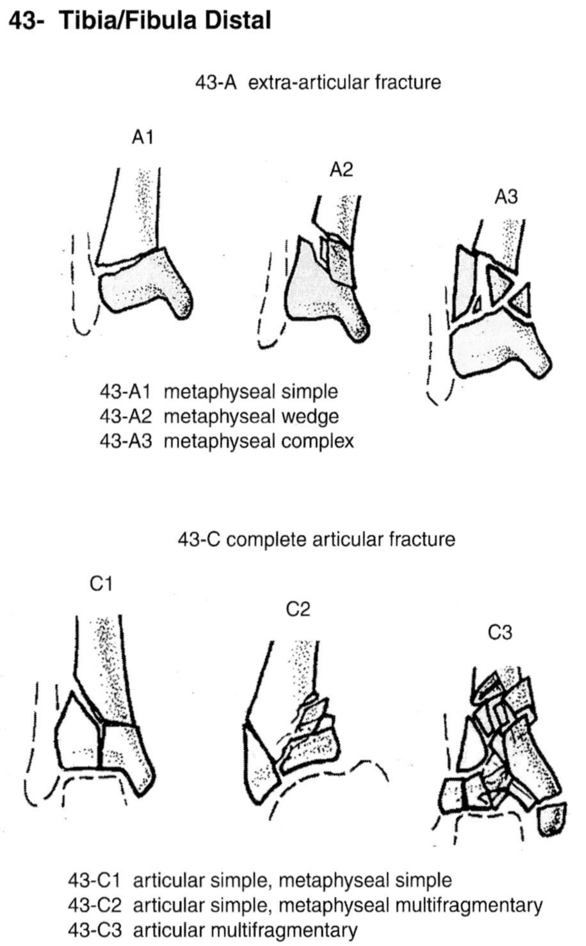

43- Tibia/Fibula Distal

43-A extra-articular fracture

A1

A2

A3

43-A1 metaphyseal simple
43-A2 metaphyseal wedge
43-A3 metaphyseal complex

43-B partial articular fracture

B1

B2

B3

43-B1 pure split
43-B2 split depression
43-B3 multifragmentary depression

43-C complete articular fracture

C1

C2

C3

43-C1 articular simple, metaphyseal simple
43-C2 articular simple, metaphyseal multifragmentary
43-C3 articular multifragmentary

Figure 1 The AO/OTA classification system for distal tibia fractures. (Reproduced with permission from Muller ME, Nazarian S, Koch P, Schatzker J (eds): *The Comprehensive Classification of Fractures of Long Bones.* New York, NY, Springer-Verlag, 1990, pp 172-173.)

related to the surrounding soft-tissue envelope may be the most difficult to treat and are responsible for devastating and long-term problems, such as chronic osteomyelitis or even amputation. The most commonly used system to classify soft-tissue injuries associated with fractures is that described by Tscherne[5] (Table 1).

The degree and amount of soft-tissue injury at times can be difficult to fully appreciate. Surgeons can assess the presence or absence of fracture blisters; if present, it can be determined whether they are clear or hemorrhagic. Blisters are one sign of severe soft-tissue injury. Visible bruising and contusion over the injured area as described in the Tscherne classification system are other signs of soft-tissue injury (Figure 3). However, even in the absence of blisters or visible bruising and contusion, swelling itself can represent a soft-tissue injury that should preclude aggressive surgery until it resolves. The presence of the wrinkle sign has been described as one measure of resolution of swelling, but to the authors' knowledge, the usefulness of this measure has not been systematically tested. If there is any concern for the status of the soft tissues, definitive treatment should be delayed, especially when considering formal open reduction of the articular component. Performing surgery through swollen, contused, and damaged tissue is unwise and will typically lead to disastrous complications.

Before surgeons had full understanding of the significance of the associated soft-tissue injury, treating high-energy pilon fractures was fraught with complications.[6-11] To prevent these severe soft-tissue–related problems, several strategies have been developed and tested, including definitive unilateral external fixation,[12-17] hybrid external fixation,[18-25] staged protocols with open reduction,[26-28] and most re-

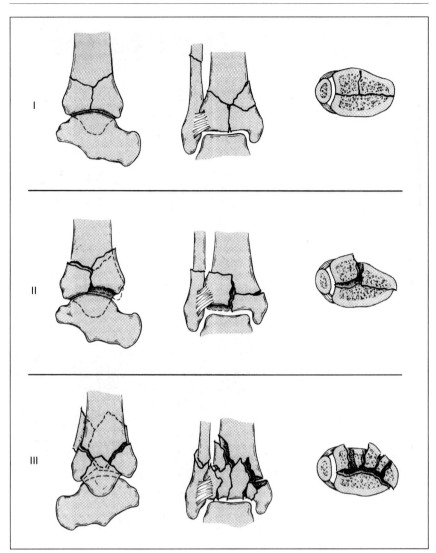

Figure 2 The classification system for fractures of the tibial plafond as described by Ruedi and Allgöwer is based on the amount of comminution of the articular surface. Type I fractures are nondisplaced, type II fractures are displaced but not comminuted, and type III fractures are displaced and comminuted. (Reproduced with permission from Ruedi TP, Allgöwer M: The operative treatment of intra-articular fractures of the lower end of the tibia. *Clin Orthop Relat Res* 1979;138:105-110.)

Table 1
Classification System for Soft-Tissue Injuries Associated With Fractures

Type 0	Minimal soft-tissue injury, torsion fractures
Type I	Superficial abrasion or contusion, mild to moderate fracture configuration
Type II	Deep, contaminated abrasion or muscle contusion, segmental fractures
Type III	Extensive soft-tissue injury, decompressed compartment syndromes

(Adapted with permission from Tscherne H, Oestern HJ: A new classification of soft-tissue damage in open and closed fractures (author's transl). *Unfallheilkunde* 1982;85:111-115.)

cently limited open reduction and percutaneous plating.[26,29-31] Soft-tissue complications from treatment have been reduced to a more acceptable level by using one or more of these techniques.

Temporizing Spanning External Fixation

Most modern treatment protocols recommend delaying definitive surgery to allow soft-tissue recovery. During this time, the use of a temporizing external fixator allows the patient to be mobilized while the length and alignment of the fracture is maintained. Use of these devices has become commonplace in the management of high-energy tibial plafond fractures.

Temporizing spanning external fixation uses the fixator to provide portable traction. Distraction and ligamentotaxis realign the limb; and although the fixator maintains length and rotation, it does not typically restore articular congruity. The ankle spanning external fixator can only facilitate the approximation of the articular fracture fragments (via ligamentotaxis); it cannot accurately reduce articular fragments.

Definitive articular reduction and bony stabilization is performed after swelling and edema have resolved, making surgical incisions safer. The spanning fixator provides some stability to the fractured area that minimizes additional soft-tissue injury and improves patient comfort, while the soft tissues recover. Once the surgeon determines that the soft tissues have recovered sufficiently, the fracture pattern has been thoroughly assessed, and a preoperative plan has been developed, additional surgical stabilization of the distal tibia, such as plate fixation and removal of the external fixator, can safely be performed.[27,28]

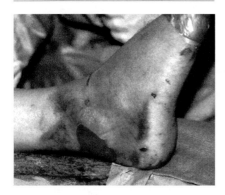

Figure 3 Photograph of a Tscherne type III soft-tissue injury in a patient with a tibial plafond fracture. (Reproduced with permission from Tscherne H, Oestern HJ: A new classification of soft-tissue damage in open and closed fractures (author's transl). *Unfallheilkunde* 1982;85:111-115.)

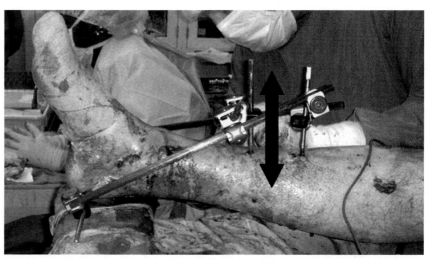

Figure 4 Photograph showing application of the temporizing transarticular fixator. The distal pin in the tibia controls the position of the foot in the sagittal plane. By sliding the frame up or down on this pin (*arrow*), the ankle can be translated anterior or posterior in relation to the tibial shaft. After locking this clamp, the alignment will be maintained even if an anteriorly directed force is placed on the distal segment by resting the foot on the bed.

Temporizing spanning external fixation uses half-pins in the tibia and a calcaneal transfixation pin. Two pins initially are placed into the tibia on the anteromedial portion of the tibial crest in the sagittal plane. These pins should be placed well proximal away from the zone of injury and away from the area where the future plate may be placed. It is best to avoid overlapping the pin sites with definitive implants to avoid contamination. A transcalcaneal pin is then placed. This centrally threaded pin is placed through the posterior calcaneus in the safe zone to avoid injury to the lateral plantar nerve, the most posterior plantar nerve, and the medial calcaneal nerve.[32] This pin should be placed parallel to the distal tibial articular surface and parallel to floor, with the patient's foot pointing straight up. Bars are then connected in a triangle from the most proximal tibial pin to the calcaneal pin, manual traction is applied, and a reduction is obtained. The distal tibial pin is then connected to the construct to maintain rigidity in the sagittal plane and allow for small adjustments to the

ankle reduction (Figure 4). If the foot lies in equinus after the frame is tightened, a supplemental 4-mm pin can be inserted into the base of the first metatarsal and attached to the medial rod of the frame to maintain the foot and ankle in a plantigrade position.

Radiographs should be obtained after reduction and carefully assessed for any residual shortening or ankle subluxation. Guides to correct length include the fibula or the Chaput fragment (anterolateral tibial fragment). Correct length of the tibia must be obtained with this initial fixator to avoid undue tension on the skin at the time of definitive fixation when tibial length must be restored (Figure 5). The talus must be reduced under the tibia, especially on a lateral radiograph; if not, anterior skin necrosis may occur from direct pressure of underlying bone. A poorly applied spanning frame that does not achieve length and overall alignment serves little purpose.

Although a large, multiplanar, one-piece external fixator typically used for definitive treatment can accomplish these same goals, it has two important disadvantages when used as a temporary spanning frame. First, one of the distal pins is placed within the talar neck, which therefore is close to the location of secondary incisions for internal fixation. Second, the cost of these external fixators is considerable compared with the cost of half-pins and bars. Simpler frames with transfixation pins placed through the tibia and the calcaneus can also be applied to accomplish the same goals, but offer no additional benefits and are associated with increased risk of neurovascular injury. The frames previously described are sometimes placed in the emergency department without bringing the patient to the operating room.

Rationale for Plate Fixation
Open reduction and internal fixation of intra-articular distal tibia

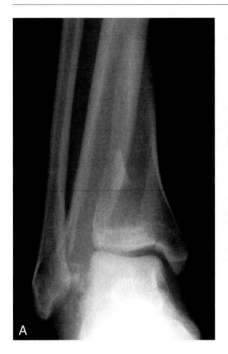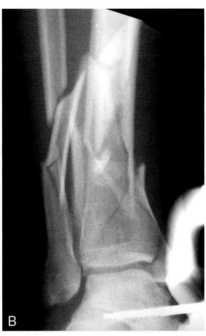

Figure 5 Radiographs of transarticular fixation in which the talus is left shortened and limb length is not realigned. Note the position of the intact fibula and lateral tibia as the guide to length (**A**) and the short fibula (**B**).

Table 2
Advantages of Open Reduction and Internal Fixation Over External Fixation in the Treatment of Pilon Fractures

Anatomic reduction of moderate to severely displaced articular fracture fragments is only possible with formal open reduction and internal fixation, particularly for fractures with centrally displaced fragments

With newer plating techniques and approaches, reduction and stabilization of the articular block to the tibial diaphysis can be performed with less soft-tissue stripping and smaller incisions; as a result, formal open reduction and internal fixation is safer, more soft-tissue friendly, and results in a considerably lower complication rate when combined with use of an initial spanning external fixator

Locking plate technology has allowed fixation of very distal fractures and in patients with osteoporosis, without having to span the ankle and subtalar joints, making early range of motion possible

Patients treated with open reduction and internal fixation do not require long-term pin site care and are therefore not subject to the morbidity commonly associated with the use of external fixators; additionally, if subsequent surgical procedures are necessary (bone graft of the metaphysis to treat delayed union or nonunion), contaminated pins and pin sites do not have to be prepped into the field

Although an external fixator can be used as effectively as a plate to buttress metaphyseal fractures, the longer the fracture takes to heal, the longer the frame has to remain in place, making pin tract complications even more likely

fractures was originally popularized in the 1970s.[4,33] Unfortunately, because of many unfavorable outcomes, including wound dehiscence, deep infection, and amputation, this technique fell out of favor for the treatment of these challenging injuries. Over the past 30 years, methods and implants have changed to make this technique safer and more beneficial to the patient. One such advance is the temporary ankle spanning external fixator, which helps delay surgery in patients with acute injury. Other advances have been made in the surgical approaches used to treat distal tibia fractures, which are often high-energy injuries.[27-29,34] The decrease in the rate of complications has allowed plate fixation to again be one of the more popular techniques of treatment of articular fractures of the distal tibia. Formal open reduction and internal fixation of pilon fractures also offers certain advan-

tages over the use of external fixation. These advantages are listed in Table 2 .

Treatment of high-energy displaced intra-articular distal tibia fractures is challenging. Although several treatment options are available, many surgeons continue to prefer formal open reduction and internal fixation to maximize the articular reduction and avoid the use of external fixators. The surgical approaches to the distal tibia allow direct visualization of fracture reduction, which optimizes the reconstruction of the damaged articular surface. Conversion of the temporary external fixator to internal fixation frees the ankle, allowing patients to perform range-of-motion exercises without encumbering the external fixation components.

There are several potential surgical approaches to the distal tibia through which plate fixation can be accomplished. Each of these ap-

proaches has relative indications and its own sets of advantages and disadvantages. The choice of approach should depend on the extent and location of the soft-tissue damage, the fracture pattern, and the surgeon's familiarity, training, and comfort with the approach.

Approaches and Techniques of Definitive Plate Fixation
Anteromedial Approach
The "workhorse" for the open treatment of distal intra-articular tibia fractures is the anteromedial ap-

proach, which is commonly used to treat fractures with involvement of the anterior, medial, and central plafond and with limited involvement of the lateral aspect. The anteromedial approach should only be undertaken once the soft tissues surrounding the distal leg have recovered from the trauma. Recovery of the skin, including reduction of swelling, is often evident by wrinkling of the skin at the base of the toes and the ankle and reepithelization of the blistered areas.[35] Care should be taken during the anteromedial approach, manipulation of the fracture fragments, and closure to minimize further soft-tissue trauma. Additional trauma to these areas can be avoided by not grasping the skin edges with forceps and by minimizing the use of self-retaining retractors and inattentive assistants.[36,37] If open reduction and internal fixation of the fibula is to be performed, the fibular incision should be placed slightly posterior to the midcoronal plane to ensure that at least a 7-cm skin bridge is present between the fibular and tibial incisions.

The anteromedial approach is started proximally at (or just above) the proximal extent of the fracture, one-half fingerbreadth lateral to the palpable tibial crest. The incision is extended distally, curving gently toward the talonavicular joint, paralleling the path of the anterior tibialis tendon. The incision should not be curved sharply around the medial malleolus because this will limit the exposure of the plafond. The extensor retinaculum is exposed medial to the anterior tibialis tendon and incised, leaving the tendon(s) undisturbed within the paratenon. The periosteum is left attached to the underlying fracture fragments, and the anterior tibialis, extensor hallu-

cis longus, and extensor digitorum communis tendons, along with the dorsalis pedis artery and venae and the superficial peroneal nerve, are retracted laterally. Previously, it was recommended that this approach be performed between the anterior tibialis and extensor hallucis longus tendons by retracting the anterior tibialis tendon medially and the extensor hallucis longus tendon laterally.[38] This technique, however, exposes the nearby neurovascular bundle and theoretically increases the risk of injury. Once the joint capsule is exposed, an arthrotomy is performed, and the articular surface and fragments are exposed. While gently retracting the skin, tendons, and dorsalis pedis arteries, the articular fragments of the distal tibia can be further displaced in a manner comparable to opening the pages of a book. Reconstruction of the joint should generally begin with the largest, least displaced fracture fragments and then proceed to the smaller, more displaced fragments. Occasionally, large articular fragments can first be reduced to the distal tibial diaphysis, and then the rest of the articular fragments reduced next. If this method is chosen, it is imperative that the articular fragments are anatomically reduced to the diaphysis because any malposition of these fragments will result in an even greater displacement at the articular surface. In either instance, image intensification in the AP, lateral, and oblique views will aid in assessing the reduction of the articular surface. If possible, the articular reduction can also be assessed via direct visualization by looking into the joint from below. It is important to keep in mind that if the metaphyseal aspect of the fibula has been plated, then the plate will obscure the articular surface when the

image intensifier is in the true lateral position. If recognized in advance, temporary stabilization of the fibula can be performed with small reduction forceps, and then definitive fixation can be performed after the tibial plafond has been reduced and stabilized. If the fibula has already been reduced and plated, oblique images of the distal tibia can be used to assess the adequacy of the reduction. Temporary stabilization of the reduced articular fragments is obtained with Kirschner wires (1.6 mm or 2.0 mm) and pointed reduction forceps, which are subsequently replaced with interfragmentary small-fragment lag screws or cannulated screws. Once the articular block is reconstructed, it is then reduced to the tibial shaft. It is held reduced with pointed reduction forceps and/or Kirschner wires (1.6 mm or 2.0 mm) while making sure that length, alignment, and rotation are restored. Definitive fixation of the distal tibia is then performed with small, low-profile implants. Generally, plates are placed along the medial aspect of the tibia to secure the articular block while resisting varus drift. Small plates are often needed anteriorly to buttress the anterior articular and metaphyseal fragments. Again, small, low-profile plates are best for this area. If the soft-tissue attachments are maintained during the surgery, these fragments will often heal relatively quickly; large fragment plates are not needed for strength and, because of their size, can become quite bothersome to the overlying soft tissues[29,39,40] (Figure 6).

Anterolateral Approach

An alternative approach to the tibial plafond that is gaining in popularity is the anterolateral approach. The relative indications for this approach

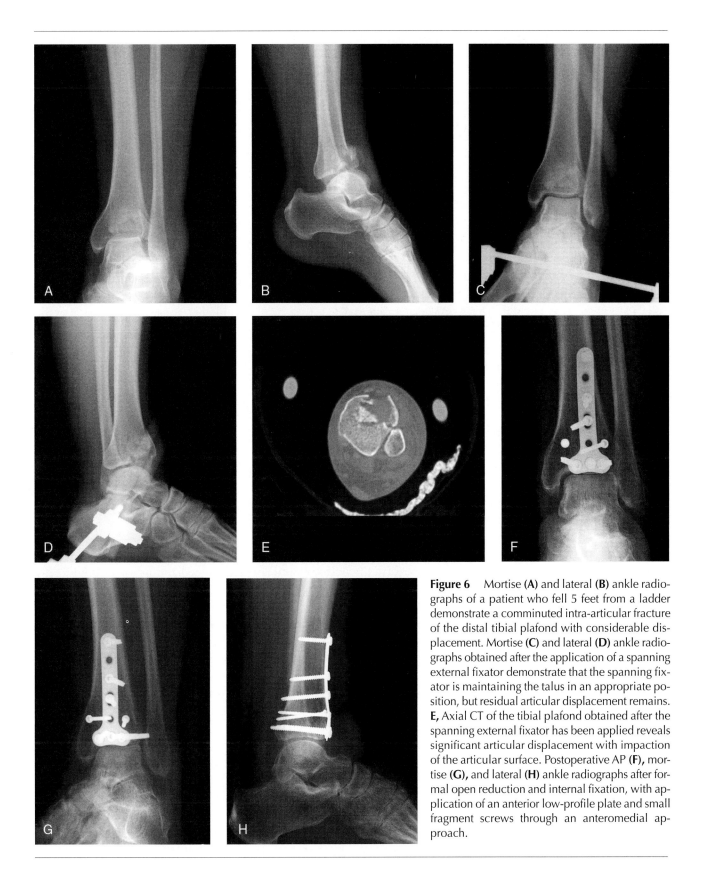

Figure 6 Mortise **(A)** and lateral **(B)** ankle radiographs of a patient who fell 5 feet from a ladder demonstrate a comminuted intra-articular fracture of the distal tibial plafond with considerable displacement. Mortise **(C)** and lateral **(D)** ankle radiographs obtained after the application of a spanning external fixator demonstrate that the spanning fixator is maintaining the talus in an appropriate position, but residual articular displacement remains. **E,** Axial CT of the tibial plafond obtained after the spanning external fixator has been applied reveals significant articular displacement with impaction of the articular surface. Postoperative AP **(F),** mortise **(G),** and lateral **(H)** ankle radiographs after formal open reduction and internal fixation, with application of an anterior low-profile plate and small fragment screws through an anteromedial approach.

over the anteromedial approach are the presence of an open or previously open medial wound, significant medial soft-tissue swelling and contusion, fractures with primarily lateral and anterolateral articular comminution, and fractures with widely displaced Chaput fragments. The primary advantages this approach has over the anteromedial approach are that on closure there is a thicker, more vascular coverage of the implants and fracture and, because the skin and soft tissues in this area are usually less severely injured than they are medially, both the fibula and the tibia can be stabilized through this single approach.[41] Although the dorsalis pedis artery can be injured from below, the superficial peroneal nerve is more at risk during this approach. Specially contoured plates are typically used when this approach is used to repair distal tibial fractures.

The approach is started along the anterolateral aspect of the distal leg parallel to and just anterior to the fibula. The incision is taken down through the skin and subcutaneous tissue, and the superficial peroneal nerve is identified, carefully mobilized, and retracted medially. The superior and inferior retinaculae are exposed and incised longitudinally for later repair. The interval between the extensor digitorum communis and the fibula is developed, the tendons and muscle bellies are elevated off of the interosseous membrane, and the distal tibia and ankle joint are exposed. In this approach, all of the tendons and dorsalis pedis and superficial peroneal nerves are retracted medially. The fibula is exposed and can be stabilized with an anterolateral or laterally placed plate; the articular fragments are reduced, and restoration of limb length, alignment, and rotation are achieved. Stabilization of the ar-

ticular fragments is typically performed with small fragment lag screws or cannulated screws, and specially designed distal tibial plates and other low-profile plates are used to restore continuity between the articular block and the diaphysis (Figure 7).

Posterolateral Approach
A posterolateral approach for the treatment of high-energy distal tibia fractures has been described, although the safety and indications for this approach have not been fully developed.[34] The rationale for the posterolateral approach, as with the anterolateral approach, is that the incision is made through skin that is less severely injured than with the anteromedial approach. Because of the robust nature of the posterior soft tissues, the implants and fracture will be well covered. In addition, because these tissues are more robust, they will be less likely to break down postoperatively. The disadvantages of this approach include limited access to the anterior articular fragments, patient positioning (prone), and the risk of injury to the sural nerve.

To perform the posterolateral approach to the distal tibia, the patient is positioned prone. The incision is made just medial, posterior, and parallel to the distal fibula and the peroneal tendons. The incision is carried down through the subcutaneous tissues, and the sural nerve is isolated and protected throughout. The interval between the peroneal brevis or peroneal longus and the flexor hallucis longus tendons is developed. The flexors are elevated off of the interosseous membrane and the posterior aspect of the distal tibia, and the fracture fragments are addressed in the usual manner. Plate fixation of the distal fibula and tibia are performed through the same incision,

with either specialty plates or straight plates contoured to the bone.

Medial Approach
A direct medial approach to the distal tibia for the treatment of intraarticular distal tibia fractures should be avoided for two reasons. First, the medial soft tissues are often compromised and cannot tolerate further surgical trauma and therefore are prone to develop wound dehiscence that can lead to deep infections. Second, even if these tissues are capable of tolerating a second insult, often, to close the incision over the implant and tibia, considerable tension of the skin is required. In this instance, wound dehiscence can occur and there is further loss of surrounding soft tissues, requiring a vascularized free-tissue transfer for secondary coverage.[10] If a wound problem occurs when using the other recommended approaches (anteromedial, anterolateral, and posterolateral), the wound, because of its location over muscle, retinaculum, and tendons, can be treated with local wound care and allowed to heal, thereby avoiding major soft-tissue reconstruction.

A medial approach should only be used for true percutaneous plating. With this technique, the articular surface is either not injured (AO/OTA type A fracture) or is reduced and fixed percutaneously. A precontoured plate is then placed medially to stabilize the articular segment to the tibial shaft using small percutaneous incisions.

Rationale for External Fixation for Definitive Treatment
Whether to treat high-energy tibial plafond fractures with open reduction and internal fixation or external fixation is a controversial issue among orthopaedic traumatologists.

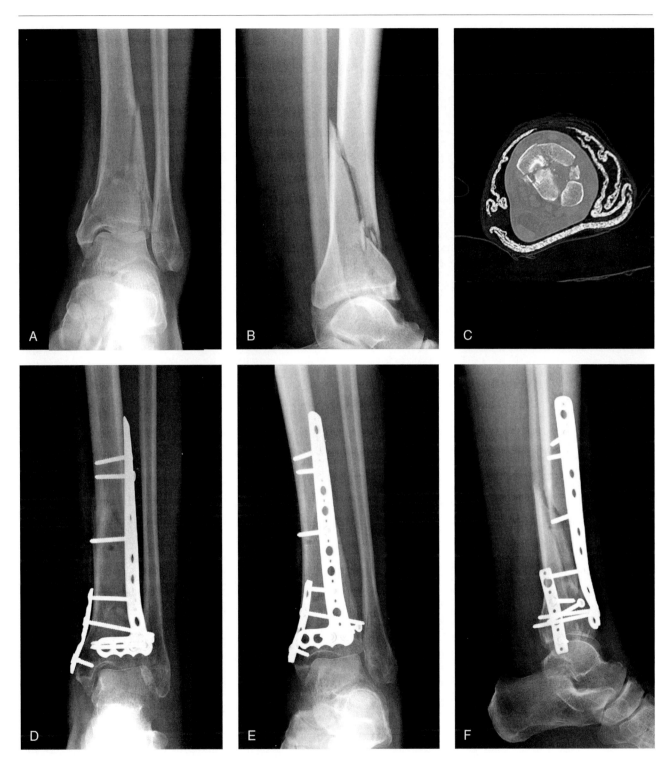

Figure 7 Mortise (**A**) and lateral (**B**) ankle radiographs of a patient who was involved in a high-speed vehicle crash demonstrate a comminuted, intra-articular fracture with shortening and a long posterolateral fragment. **C,** Axial CT scan demonstrates the intra-articular displaced fractures. Postoperative AP (**D**), mortise (**E**), and lateral (**F**) ankle radiographs after open reduction and internal fixation was performed via an anterolateral approach and supplemental stabilization was performed via a percutaneously placed medial plate.

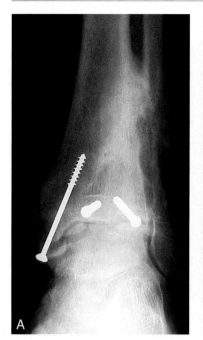
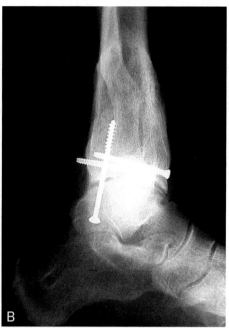
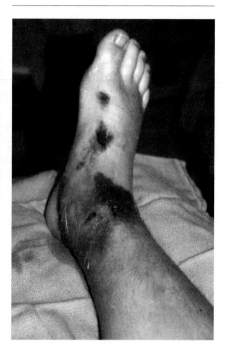

Figure 8 AP (**A**) and lateral (**B**) radiographs obtained 5 years after a highly comminuted tibial plafond fracture reveal nonanatomic reduction and severe osteoarthrosis. The patient had no pain and an excellent ankle score.

Figure 9 Photograph of a patient with a tibial plafond fracture shows massive soft-tissue swelling, fracture blisters, and deep contusion to the skin and muscle. Early open surgical treatment in this situation should be avoided.

It is not uncommon to hear dogmatic statements about the treatment of these injuries, with dichotomous terms such as "always/never" or "good/evil" used to describe treatment choices and their relative merits. In examining why this controversy exists, five factors come to mind. First, dogma and surgeon biases indicate that intra-articular fractures should undergo anatomic reduction; the literature, however, is divided on the preeminence of articular reduction.[42-48] Second, there is a strong legacy of using open reduction and internal fixation to treat these injuries, beginning in the 1970s with the work of Ruedi and Allgöwer.[33] Third, individual surgeon training and experience provide varying levels of expertise and comfort with the various reduction and stabilization techniques. Fourth, the functional outcomes of these injuries are unpredictable and do not correlate well at all with the ra-

diograph appearance.[49] Fifth, valid functional outcomes data indicating one technique is superior to another simply do not exist.

Tibial plafond fractures are devastating injuries to both the bone and soft tissues; consequently, the outcomes following treatment of these injuries are unpredictable. A patient with an anatomic reduction with a stable fixation and radiographic evidence of healing often will still have severe pain and a poor functional outcome. Conversely, a patient with a great deal of comminution and a nonanatomic reduction, who, after healing, has radiographic evidence of severe arthrosis, may have no pain and an excellent functional result (Figure 8). In trying to understand why this is so, surgeons must consider whether the extent of the soft-tissue and articular cartilage injury may have as much or more influence on the functional outcome as the bony injury.[47,48]

High-energy tibial plafond fractures are characterized by severe, early, soft-tissue swelling and the frequent occurrence of fracture blisters. These fractures often result in chronic soft-tissue changes such as swelling, extensive scar formation, tendon impingement, or complex regional pain syndrome. The extent and nature of soft-tissue injury are the factors that increase the risk of treatment complications in the management of these injuries.[36,50] The sequelae of such complications can be devastating and include amputation of the limb. Thus, the treatment undertaken for these injuries must ensure that devastating soft-tissue complications can be avoided (Figure 9).

External fixation as definitive treatment of high-energy tibial plafond fractures can help avoid

Table 3
Advantages of Using External Fixation to Treat High-Energy Tibial Plafond Fractures

External fixation completely spans the zone of injury and requires minimal or no soft-tissue dissection within the zone of injury; furthermore, it burns no bridges—it can always be converted later to internal fixation if the need arises

Surgery for articular reduction and stabilization (usually done on a delayed basis) can be performed with an external fixator in place; the fixator assists in maintaining length and alignment during surgery

External fixation is the easiest of the available techniques to apply and, once the spanning external fixator is in place, it allows a graded approach to the articular surface; fractures with minimal soft-tissue swelling are amenable to open reduction techniques, but those with massive soft-tissue swelling and scarring should have limited approaches to the articular surface

External fixation affords one technique for all fractures (there is no need to worry about whether to do a medial, lateral, or even a posterior approach); the technique for fixator application is the same in all fractures

An external fixator is as good a buttress as is a plate. This is a fact that is often ignored by those who prefer internal fixation; however, an external fixator, if appropriately applied, serves as an effective buttressing device in the same way as does a plate applied inside the body

It is not possible to achieve perfect anatomic reduction in all high-energy tibial plafond fractures because comminution of the central portion of the tibial plafond is present in almost all of these injuries and there is often loss of bone or articular cartilage from this central area of the plafond; therefore, restoration of the cortical rim of the plafond is nearly always possible with any technique, but restoration of the central bone and the lost articular cartilage is almost always impossible in the highest-energy fractures—external fixation acknowledges this fact because the goal of this technique is not to make the articular surface perfect in every patient

External fixation has good long-term (5- to 11-year) outcomes reported in the literature

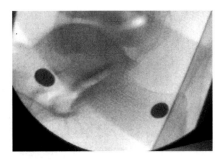

Figure 10 Lateral intraoperative fluoroscopic view of the foot illustrating the appropriate positions for half-pins in the talus and calcaneus. Care should be taken to ensure that the pins are parallel to the talar dome on the AP radiograph and that the subtalar joint is in neutral alignment when the second pin is inserted.

complications because it is the safest technique available for the treatment of these fractures.[49] External fixation offers several advantages, which are listed in Table 3.

It is clear that external fixation of high-energy distal tibia fractures began as a reaction to the high complication rates encountered with using open reduction and internal fixation to treat these fractures.[36,50] However, external fixation has now evolved and has been integrated into a philosophy of care for patients with high-energy periarticular fractures, a philosophy that involves spanning the zone of injury with the fixation device and making limited approaches to the fracture fragments with minimal dissection within the zone of injury.[12,49]

To apply the technique of definitive external fixation, the surgeon must understand that soft-tissue injuries are major contributors to poor outcomes. Therefore, further soft-tissue injury—particularly further surgical dissection within the zone of injury—should be limited. The surgeon must understand that reconstruction of a stable and functional ankle mortise is paramount, but that this does not necessarily mean reconstructing the entire tibia and fibula. The surgeon must understand that proper alignment of the mortise—both in an angular and rotational fashion—beneath the tibial shaft is important.

Spanning External Fixation as Definitive Treatment
The application of an external fixator for definitive care is similar to that used for temporary spanning external fixation. There is, however, one key difference: the external fixator used in this technique serves as

a buttressing device for at least 12 weeks after injury. Thus, the fixator pins used and the fixator construct attached to those pins must be strong and able to withstand physiologic forces for at least 12 weeks.[51] To achieve these goals, the following key points should be considered.

The pins inserted in the hindfoot should be large in diameter (the authors use 6-mm to 5-mm tapered pins), should be inserted in the coronal plane (directly from the medial side), and should have a cortical thread profile. The cortical thread profile maximizes the core diameter of the pin, which is important because these pins are loaded primarily in bending rather than in pullout.

One pin should be inserted in the talus and one in the calcaneus (Figure 10). The quality of the bone in the talar neck is superior to that in the calcaneus; this is an important factor to consider when using an external fixator frame that is to remain in place for 12 weeks. Because pins in this configuration will immobilize the subtalar joint, the surgeon must be careful to ensure that the joint is in neutral or slight valgus alignment at the time of fixator application.

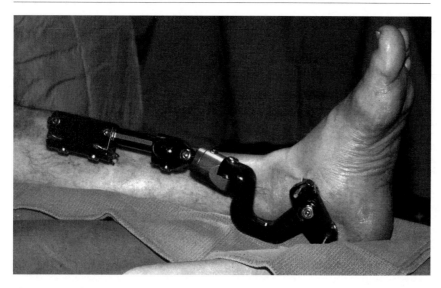

Figure 11 Photograph showing that pins should be inserted in the coronal plane in the tibial shaft to ensure that the tibial pins are in nearly the same plane as the pins in the foot and will allow for more potential for angular adjustment in the frame and a more cosmetic appearance of the device.

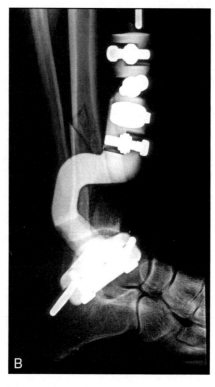

Figure 12 After application of the external fixator, the limb should be out to length and the talus centered under the tibial shaft on both AP (**A**) and lateral (**B**) radiographic views. Anterior translation of the talus relative to the tibial shaft should be avoided.

Varus alignment should be avoided.

Pins inserted into the tibial shaft must be outside (superior to) the zone of injury and in the coronal plane. It is important that the tibial pins remain outside the zone of injury as well as proximal to where any plate would lie on the tibia, should the surgeon choose at a later date to plate the fracture. Putting pins in the coronal plane, rather than perpendicular to the subcutaneous border of the tibia, allows for better alignment of the external fixator frame and easier adjustment of the position of the ankle and the limb within the frame.

The authors use a unified body type of external fixator frame (as opposed to a pin-to-bar construct) for this application (Figure 11). The unified body type of frame has been shown to provide excellent performance in static and fatigue testing,[51] is highly adjustable, and offers a lower profile and more cosmetic appearance than a pin-to-bar construct. Additionally, the unified body type of device is designed for use with the stronger 6-mm to 5-mm tapered external fixator pins.

Once the frame is applied, the limbs should be distracted with a frame to restore the limb to anatomic length and alignment. At the completion of the fixator application, the limb should be out to length and the talus should be centered beneath the tibial shaft on both AP and lateral fluoroscopic views. The surgeon should be particularly aware of (and should not accept) any anterior translation of the talus relative to the tibial shaft, a phenomenon that is common with highly comminuted fractures (Figure 12).

With the spanning fixator properly applied, limited internal fixation is then delayed until soft-tissue swelling has subsided and fracture blis-

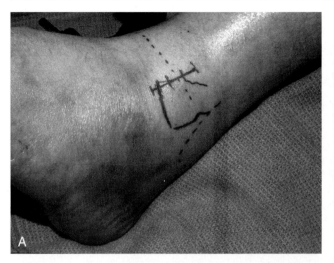

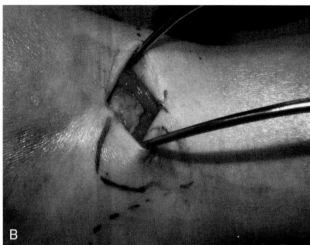

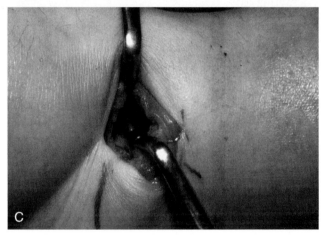

Figure 13 **A,** The incision should be centered on the ankle joint (*dotted line*) and made over the major anterolateral fracture fragment (*marked*). **B,** Dissection proceeds lateral to the peroneus tertius and the fracture fragment is exposed and retracted laterally. **C,** With the anterolateral fragment retracted laterally, the ankle joint is visualized, and the coronal split in the distal tibia can be identified and reduced.

ters have epithelialized. In many patients, this delay is 14 to 21 days before performing the secondary procedure. Several principles should be followed in performing limited internal fixation of the articular surface in these injuries.

The external fixator should be prepped into the surgical field—it cannot be removed because it is needed to obtain overall limb alignment. It is the authors' preference to wash the fixator thoroughly with chlorhexidine, cleanse it further with alcohol, and then paint it with povidone-iodine as part of the skin preparation.

The patient should be positioned supine in such a way that allows easy access to the limb for both surgery and obtaining the necessary AP and lateral fluoroscopic views. Using a narrow foot piece for the operating room table, with the opposite leg in a hemilithotomy position, is ideal; however, a regular operating room table with the surgical leg elevated on towels is also acceptable.

The surgeon should ensure that the limb is out to length and the talar dome is centered beneath the tibial shaft in both AP and lateral fluoroscopic views before proceeding with internal fixation. Appropriate length and rotational and angular alignment in the fixator should be ensured before an incision is made for limited open reduction and internal fixation. The external fixator serves to obtain and maintain length and overall alignment to make reduction and limited internal fixation of the articular fragments easier.

The surgical incisions should be centered on the joint line and positioned so as to use the major fracture lines as windows to see into the ankle joint (Figure 13). To facilitate this positioning, it is helpful to understand that there are some fracture fragments that are consistently present in most tibial plafond fractures. The anterolateral (Tillaux) fracture fragment is the most consis-

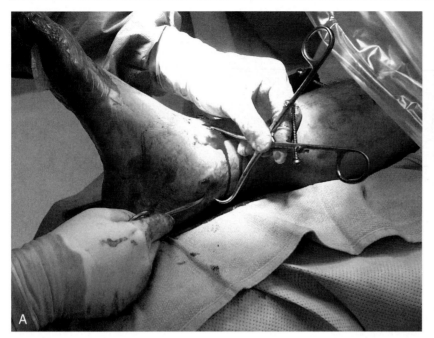

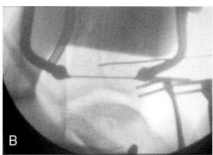

Figure 14 **A,** Intraoperative photograph showing reduction forceps and Kirschner wires used through stab incisions to reduce and stabilize the articular fragments. **B,** The reduction is assessed fluoroscopically.

tently present fragment in fractures of the distal tibia; as such, the anterolateral fracture line is the most frequent location in which the skin incision is made. A skin incision over this fracture line places the surgical approach lateral to the peroneus tertius tendon in a safe interval. Lateral retraction of this fracture fragment allows viewing of the ankle joint and also allows for visualization of the coronal split, which is also a typical finding in tibial plafond fractures. The comminuted central portion of the articular surface—another consistently present feature of these fractures—also can be visualized through this small window. The medial malleolar articular fragment, yet another consistently present fracture fragment in these injuries, is the only fracture fragment that cannot be visualized well through this small surgical approach centered at the level of the ankle joint.

Probes, dental picks, small elevators, tenacula, and pointed forceps are then used to "tease" the various articular fracture fragments into

place. These reduction tools are used through the small surgical incisions or through stab incisions made at various locations about the ankle to enable them to provide a bit of pressure on the articular fragments to gently rotate or translate them into proper position (Figure 14, *A*).

Once fracture fragments have been realigned (alignment is confirmed by visualization through the ankle joint and by fluoroscopy), they can then be stabilized with Kirschner wires or guide pins for cannulated screws. Screws are then inserted to compress the fracture fragments together and complete the reconstruction of the articular surface (Figure 14, *B*).

When using this methodology, care should be taken that surgical dissection does not extend proximally into the area of metaphyseal comminution because any dissection into this area will place it at risk for delayed union or nonunion. It is difficult at times to resist the temptation to expose this area for a lag screw or a small plate, but this

should be avoided. The external fixator will serve as an effective buttressing device such that additional fixation in the metaphysis or diaphysis is not necessary (Figure 15).

Final adjustments to the external fixator are made to ensure that the articular block of the tibial plafond is perfectly aligned beneath the tibial shaft with the appropriate angular and rotational alignment.

When the articular fragments have been stabilized with screws and the limb is aligned and stabilized by the external fixator, which now serves as a buttressing device, the surgical procedure is complete. Although this procedure will adequately stabilize the fracture against physiologic forces, it does not provide rigid stabilization. Rigid stability, however, is not necessary because the fixator will remain as the buttressing device during the entire treatment period. Essentially, the fixator serves as a buttress plate applied outside of the body.

Postoperatively, routine pin care is begun in 48 hours (at the time of

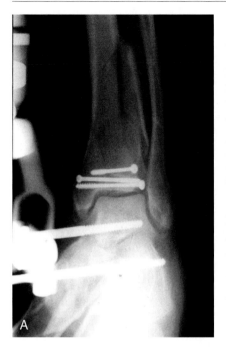
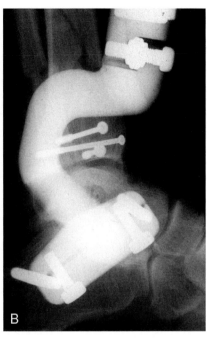

Figure 15   AP **(A)** and lateral **(B)** radiographs showing the articular fragments stabilized with screws. Final adjustments of the external fixator achieve proper alignment. No plate is required because the external fixator serves as a buttressing device. No dissection in the area of the tibial shaft is performed; this fracture will heal well without intervention (dissection in this area may lead to soft-tissue complications and will delay healing).

removal of the surgical dressing). Patients are also permitted at this time to bathe and shower the leg and fixator. The limb and fixator may be washed with regular soap and water in either the shower or the bath, but patients are encouraged not to enter swimming pools and/or hot tubs in which chemical additives are in the water. Patients should not bear weight (touch down only) on the limb for approximately 8 weeks after surgery. Following that period, patients are encouraged to bear weight as tolerated on the limb, with the fixator still in place, for 8 to 12 weeks following surgery. During the third postoperative month, the calcaneal pin typically will become inflamed and will be somewhat loose by 12 weeks after surgery. This is of no concern because the fixator will have done its job and will be re-

moved in the office at 12 weeks, provided the radiographs show healing of the metaphyseal portion of the fracture and the patient can bear weight without pain in the office with the frame removed and the pins still in place. After fixator removal, patients are usually placed in a short leg walking cast or removable orthotic device for an additional 4 weeks. Return to work almost never occurs before 6 months in patients who are laborers.

Hybrid External Fixation

When using hybrid external fixation to treat fractures of the distal tibia, there are no fixator elements distal to the ankle joint. Motion of the ankle joint is allowed and encouraged through most of the treatment course. Fixation is accomplished with diaphyseal half-pins connected

to metaphyseal or epiphyseal multiple thin tensioned wires through the use of rings, bars, and clamps. As this technique has evolved, it has become a staged protocol consisting of initial spanning fixation accompanied by definitive articular reconstruction and conversion to a non-bridging frame.[18,52] The articular reconstruction may occur at the time of initial external fixation or it may occur at conversion to a non-bridging construct. The timing will depend on the amount of articular displacement, the conditions of the soft tissue, and whether an open or a percutaneous technique of reduction will be used.

The technique of hybrid external fixation is initially similar to that of temporizing fixation. After soft-tissue stabilization has occurred, definitive fixation may be safely performed. If articular reduction has not been accomplished, this is performed first. Limited incisions, based on imaging, should be placed directly over articular fragments that need to be reduced. Percutaneously placed clamps and lag screws are then used to gain and hold reductions of the articular surface. Once articular congruity has been established, the reduction must be stabilized by way of the hybrid fixator.

Thin wires (usually 2 mm) are placed in the distal tibia. The first of these wires is typically placed from posterolateral, through the fibula, to anteromedial, and exiting the tibia medial to the tendon of the tibialis anterior. The second wire is placed from posteromedial on the tibia, beginning anterior to the neurovascular bundle and aimed to come out between the anterior and lateral compartments of the leg. The greater the angle that can be obtained between these two key wires, the more stable the fixation.[53] Even when us-

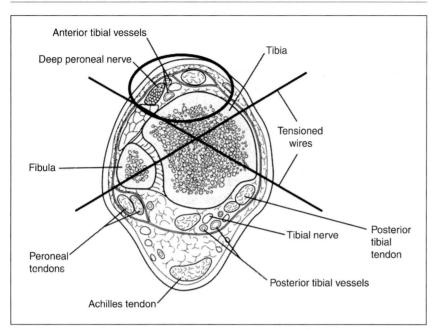

Figure 16 Illustration of the safe zone position for placement of thin wires in distal tibia; anterior compartments are the structures that are at risk (*circle*). (Reproduced with permission from Tornetta P III, Weiner L, Bergman M, et al: Pilon fractures: Treatment with combined internal and external fixation. *J Orthop Trauma* 1993;7:489-496.)

ing these "safe corridors," the thin wires across the distal tibia will impale a tendon in 55% of patients and a neurovascular structure in 38% of patients. Wires within 20 mm of the anterior joint line or 30 mm of the tip of the medial malleolus will be intracapsular and therefore may put patients at risk for septic arthritis[54] (Figure 16).

After these wires have been placed and tensioned to a ring, they are connected to the previously placed half-pins. The limb is manipulated and a reduction is obtained while the frame is tightened to maintain the fracture reduction.

Postoperatively, after the incision has healed, patients are allowed a 5-minute shower and are instructed to wash their legs and frames with soap and water. Weight bearing, except in patients with the most severe articular injuries, is begun quickly, with progression to full weight bear-

ing at approximately 6 to 8 weeks postoperatively. Frame removal occurs in the operating room after fracture healing has progressed, which is typically at 4 months after injury.

Factors Related to Outcome

To make informed choices on treatment decisions, a surgeon must have an understanding of the factors that affect patient outcome. Patient outcomes vary widely, and often the factors that surgeons believe are most important seem to have little bearing on the eventual function of the ankle and patient pain and impairment. Clinical data are either not available or are not robust enough to answer important questions. For all these reasons, assessing the most important factors for optimal outcome for a given patient is difficult and challenging.

Outcomes after rotational ankle

fractures are generally good, and the factors that affect good versus poor outcomes are well known. Patient factors such as advanced age, diabetes, and obesity have been shown to correlate with poor results. Factors associated with the injury are also important, including associated open wounds, osteochondral fractures, and the number of malleoli involved. The type and quality of treatment is clearly important because an accurate reduction of the talus in the mortise is critical to avoid early posttraumatic osteoarthritis. After high-energy axial loading plafond fractures, outcomes are less favorable and the important factors are less well understood. For instance, the relative effect of an anatomic articular reduction and the severity of injury are unknown.

It is important, therefore, that surgeons have an understanding of what can be expected at 1 year, 2 years, and at greater than 5 years after a tibial plafond fracture. To do so, surgeons must be familiar with available data on the interaction between the effect of the severity of injury and the quality of the articular reduction on outcome as well as the effects of other injury and patient demographic factors.

Complications

It is well known that complications during treatment such as infection, wound breakdown, nonunion, and malunion create grave situations that may lead to amputation and other unfortunate outcomes.[55] Data from studies performed in the 1990s indicate that complications during that period were frequent. For instance, Wyrsch and associates[11] reported that three of 18 closed fractures treated with plates resulted in amputation. In one study in which infections occurred in 37% of patients with high-energy fractures, more than 30 additional surgeries were required in 18 of 30 patients with Ruedi and Allgower type III fractures.[50]

Current techniques have substantially reduced but not eliminated complications. Table 4 details complication rates that have been reported in recent publications on the treatment of tibial plafond fractures using three contemporary techniques.

Changes in treatment techniques that have decreased complication rates include a long delay to definitive surgery, temporary spanning fixation, definitive external fixation, low-profile implants, indirect reduction techniques, and percutaneous techniques for reduction and placement of implants. Because complications have not been eliminated to the extent that there is always a risk of serious complications, surgeons must remember that when complications occur, they significantly influence patient outcome—often negatively. If a surgeon can minimize complications, the overall results for the patients will be positively influenced.

Typical Outcomes

Compared with other types of injury, other fracture problems, and specifically other articular fractures, patients with high-energy fractures of the tibial plafond have poorer outcomes and near-normal ankle function is rarely restored. For instance, compared with similar multiply injured patients without foot and ankle trauma, multiply injured patients with foot and ankle trauma have poorer outcomes, which demonstrates the negative effect of severe foot and ankle injuries.[56,58] As another example, patients with high-

Table 4
Complication Rates From Treatment With Current Techniques

Technique	Authors (year of study)	No. of Patients	Complication Rate (%)
Spanning external fixator	Marsh et al[16] (1995)	43	0
	Wyrsch et al[11] (1996)	20	5
	Mitkovic et al[17] (2002)	26	0
External fixation same side	Court-Brown et al[56] (1999)	24	4
	Tornetta et al[25] (1993)	26	7
Delayed plating	Patterson and Cole[27] (1999)	22	5
	Wyrsch et al[11] (1996)	20	5
	Mitkovic et al[17] (2002)	26	0

energy tibial plateau fractures have significantly better outcomes for the involved joint and better general health status than patients with tibial plafond fractures.[49,59] This point is illustrated by comparing two series of patients who were treated at the same institution. In a series of patients with high-energy tibial plateau fractures, all of whom were treated with external fixation, Weigel and Marsh[59] found that in the second 5-year period after injury the knee scores averaged 90 on a 100-point scale and that few knees had progressive osteoarthritis. In contrast, at a similar follow-up, patients with tibial plafond fractures had decreased general health status, marked ankle pain and disability, and a high percentage of severe posttraumatic osteoarthritis.[49] These two studies demonstrate that unlike the knee, which seems to tolerate high-energy articular fractures reasonably well, the ankle frequently develops posttraumatic osteoarthritis, secondary pain, and decreased function after high-energy articular fractures.

The measurable effect on the general health status of patients with tibial plafond fractures has been illustrated in studies in which the Medical Outcomes Study 36-Item Short-Form Health Survey (SF-36) was administered years after injury.

This long-lasting negative effect appears to be irrespective of treatment technique because it has been reported in separate series of patients who were treated with plates, external fixators, and both devices.[16,49,60,61] At 2 to 4 years after injury, most patients can expect to still have some pain that prevents full participation in normal recreational activities.[16,60] Most patients, however, will return to work, and arthrodesis is unusual. In the second 5-year period after injury, tibial plafond fractures have been shown to still affect the lives of patients. In one study, SF-36 scores showed that tibial plafond fractures had a significant effect on physical function, the role of physical function, and bodily pain compared with the scores of age-matched control subjects at 5 to 11 years after injury.[49] Not surprisingly, Ankle Osteoarthritis Scale scores were dramatically different in both groups as well; however, most patients were satisfied with the results and most had not required late arthrodesis (arthrodesis rate, 5.4%).

Most data indicate that recovery is slow and prolonged. In the first 2 years after injury, most patients can expect to still be recovering and improving by having gradually less pain and increasing function. In one study, patients reported that maximum medical improvement occurred at an average of 2.4 years after injury; in nine patients from whom sequential ankle scores were obtained (at 2 years and at < 5 years after injury), all reported improvement between these time points.[49] Because these data suggest a high likelihood of continued improvement, surgeons should delay reconstructive procedures in the first 12 to 18 months after injury.

Arthrosis is common and nearly universal after severe fractures. In one study, moderate or severe arthrosis was present in 30% of fractures by 2 to 4 years after injury; in another study, more than 70% of ankles were moderately or severely arthritic in the second 5-year period after injury.[16,49]

Factors Affecting Outcome

It is reasonable to conclude that high-energy, more comminuted fractures have poorer outcomes than low-energy, less comminuted fractures; these outcomes may be modified to a certain extent by the skill of the surgeon and the quality of the surgical repair. However, the limited data available indicate that patient outcome after these fractures is difficult to predict based on any criteria, including severity of injury and quality of articular reduction (Figures 17 and 18). In two studies using the same assessment of reduction, fair reductions were reported in 14% of patients and arthrodesis was required in 9%,[27] whereas another study reported fair or poor reductions in 30% of patients and arthrodesis was required in only 3%.[16] Two other studies that specifically assessed the quality of reduction and severity of injury found these variables were associated with arthrosis but not with clinical outcome.[62,63]

Severe injuries may result in an ankle that is as good as or better (in terms of function and pain) than ankles with less severe injuries because severe fractures develop peripheral buttressing osteophytes that cause ankylosis of the joint, thereby protecting the remaining articular surface from painful and damaging shear stresses. Less severe injuries preserve movement, and the loads on the damaged articular surfaces are not protected, leading to a higher risk of progressive cartilage loss. This concept is illustrated in a rotational ankle fracture in which a slightly wide mortise (a relatively nonsevere injury) left untreated can lead to rapidly progressive posttraumatic osteoarthritis.

Patient demographics have been shown to be an important predictor of outcome after calcaneal fractures to the extent that sex, age, and work status can be used to guide treatment. For fractures of the tibial plafond, the data are less robust; therefore, the effect of patient demographics on patient outcome is uncertain. In one study, females and white-collar workers had better outcomes at 2 to 4 years after injury.[16,62] These results were not seen in another study at 5 to 11 years after injury.[49] The effect of workers' compensation status on patient outcome, which has been shown to have a strong negative effect for other injuries, has not been studied for patients with fractures of the tibial plafond.

Important clinical implications arise from the inability to predict the outcome of a certain patient with a certain fracture pattern. First, based on the lack of a strong correlation of outcome with severity of injury, surgeons should not be quick to recommend arthrodesis for patients with severe injuries or for injuries with

poor articular reductions. Most patients improve over time, and most do not require arthrodesis. Because some of the worst fractures can actually have satisfactory outcomes, patience may be rewarded. Another important clinical consideration arises when making treatment decisions during the early treatment phases for patients with tibial plafond fractures. The risk versus benefit ratio of treatment choices must be considered. Complications always lead to bad outcomes, and the extent that outcome is improved with aggressive surgical approaches is at best unclear.

Summary

Tibial plafond fractures have a long-lasting adverse effect on patient general health status and a more significant adverse effect on ankle pain and function. Few patients with tibial plafond fractures experience restoration of normal ankle function. Many patients begin to show radiographic evidence of arthrosis by 2 years after injury, and most have significant posttraumatic arthrosis by the second 5-year period after injury. The effect of radiographic findings on clinical outcome is not clear, however, because most patients improve over time and most do not require arthrodesis. Patients may continue to experience some pain and decreased function, but they typically do not have enough symptoms to warrant reconstructive surgery. Complications must be avoided because they typically lead to repeat surgeries and poor patient outcomes. The factors that affect variations in outcome are uncertain. In particular, the severity of injury and the quality of articular reduction do not have as close an association with subsequent clinical outcome as has generally been believed.

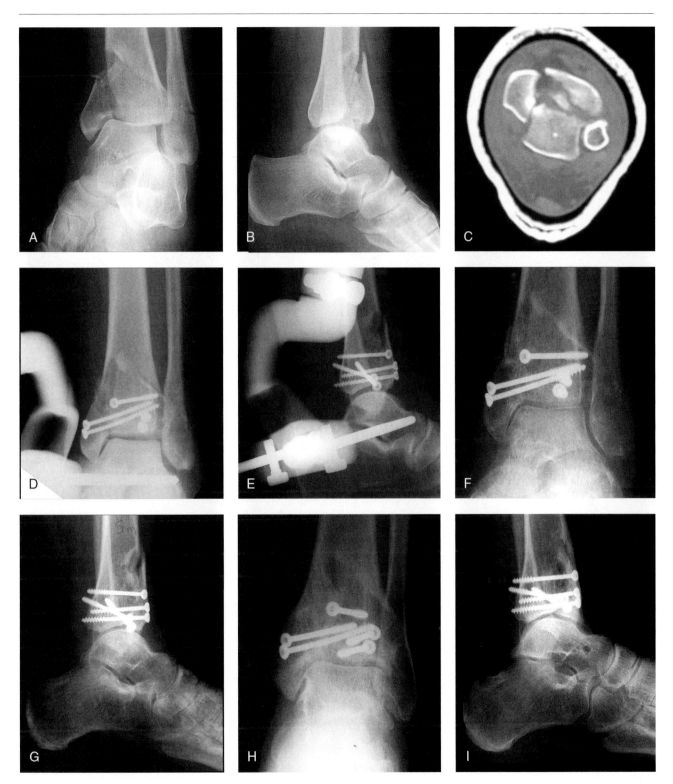

Figure 17 AP radiograph (**A**), postreduction lateral radiograph (**B**), and CT scan (**C**) of a B-3 fracture in a 38-year-old woman who fell from a horse show that only mild comminution is present. AP (**D**) and lateral (**E**) radiographs obtained after the application of a spanning fixator and fixation of the articular surface with screws show that articular reduction is excellent. AP (**F**) and lateral (**G**) radiographs obtained 6 months after injury show evidence of healing; however, the patient reported severe pain and inability to walk. At 4 years after injury, AP (**H**) and lateral (**I**) radiographs show an anterior osteophyte and anterior joint narrowing. The patient was fitted with a brace, reported moderate pain, and was able to return to work in a hospital kitchen; her ankle score was 72.

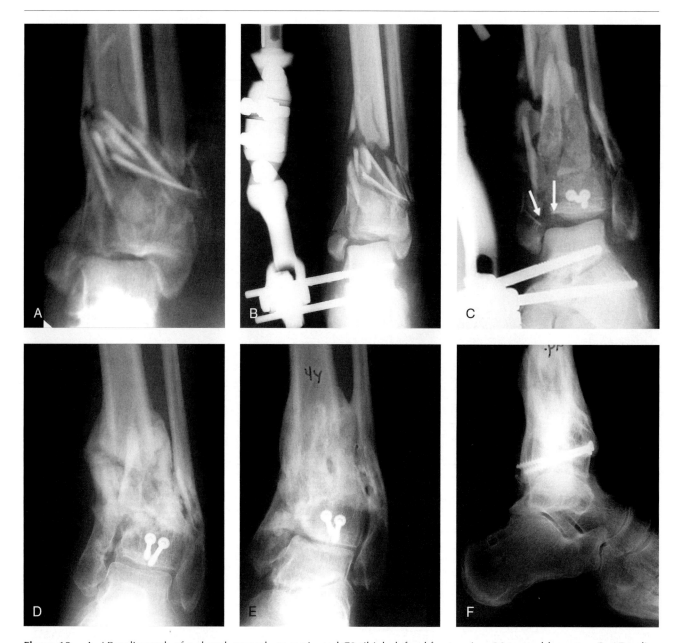

Figure 18 **A,** AP radiograph of a closed, severely comminuted C3 tibial plafond fracture in a 30-year-old woman. **B,** AP radiograph showing alignment in a spanning fixator. **C,** Radiograph of the fracture after fixation of the articular surface demonstrates residual articular incongruity (*arrows*). **D,** Radiograph obtained 1 year after injury shows a varus malunion. AP **(E)** and lateral **(F)** radiographs obtained 4 years after injury show maintained joint space. The patient, a teacher, was able to return to work and return to full participation in recreational activities; her ankle score was 95.

Because of the lack of clear data for preferred treatment techniques based on patient outcome, surgeons should choose treatment based both on characteristics of an injury and their own surgical skill and experience. Satisfactory results have been reported in series using predominantly plate fixation and in series using predominantly external fixation. With either technique, priority must be given to the soft-tissue injury to minimize complications. Techniques discussed in this chapter such as temporary spanning fixation, long delays to definitive surgery, the use of external fixation, low-profile plates, limited approaches, and avoiding the medial tibia have all had a role in decreasing complications and therefore improving outcomes.

References

1. Dirschl DR, Adams GL: A critical assessment of factors influencing reliability in the classification of fractures, using fractures of the tibial plafond as a model. *J Orthop Trauma* 1997;11:471-476.

2. Martin JS, Marsh JL, Bonar SK, DeCoster TA, Found EM, Brandser EA: Assessment of the AO/ASIF fracture classification for the distal tibia. *J Orthop Trauma* 1997;11:477-483.

3. Swiontkowski MF, Sands AK, Agel J, Diab M, Schwappach JR, Kreder HJ: Interobserver variation in the AO/OTA fracture classification system for pilon fractures: Is there a problem? *J Orthop Trauma* 1997;11:467-470.

4. Ruedi T: Fractures of the lower end of the tibia into the ankle joint: Results 9 years after open reduction and internal fixation. *Injury* 1973;5:130-134.

5. Tscherne H, Oestern HJ: [A new classification of soft-tissue damage in open and closed fractures (author's transl)]. *Unfallheilkunde* 1982;85:111-115.

6. Bourne RB, Rorabeck CH, Macnab J: Intra-articular fractures of the distal tibia: The pilon fracture. *J Trauma* 1983;23:591-596.

7. Ovadia DN, Beals RK: Fractures of the tibial plafond. *J Bone Joint Surg Am* 1986;68:543-551.

8. Helfet DL, Koval K, Pappas J, Sanders RW, DiPasquale T: Intraarticular "pilon" fracture of the tibia. *Clin Orthop Relat Res* 1994;298:221-228.

9. Mast JW, Spiegel PG, Pappas JN: Fractures of the tibial pilon. *Clin Orthop Relat Res* 1988;230:68-82.

10. Trumble TE, Benirschke SK, Vedder NB: Use of radial forearm flaps to treat complications of closed pilon fractures. *J Orthop Trauma* 1992;6:358-365.

11. Wyrsch B, McFerran MA, McAndrew M, et al: Operative treatment of fractures of the tibial plafond: A randomized, prospective study. *J Bone Joint Surg Am* 1996;78:1646-1657.

12. Bonar SK, Marsh JL: Unilateral external fixation for severe pilon fractures. *Foot Ankle* 1993;14:57-64.

13. Bonar SK, Marsh JL: Tibial plafond fractures: Changing principles of treatment. *J Am Acad Orthop Surg* 1994;2:297-305.

14. Bone L, Stegemann P, McNamara K, Seibel R: External fixation of severely comminuted and open tibial pilon fractures. *Clin Orthop Relat Res* 1993;292:101-107.

15. Marsh JL: External fixation is the treatment of choice for fractures of the tibial plafond. *J Orthop Trauma* 1999;13:583-585.

16. Marsh JL, Bonar S, Nepola JV, Decoster TA, Hurwitz SR: Use of an articulated external fixator for fractures of the tibial plafond. *J Bone Joint Surg Am* 1995;77:1498-1509.

17. Mitkovic MB, Bumbasirevic MZ, Lesic A, Golubovic Z: Dynamic external fixation of comminuted intra-articular fractures of the distal tibia (type C pilon fractures). *Acta Orthop Belg* 2002;68:508-514.

18. Anglen JO: Early outcome of hybrid external fixation for fracture of the distal tibia. *J Orthop Trauma* 1999;13:92-97.

19. Barbieri R, Schenk R, Koval K, Aurori K, Aurori B: Hybrid external fixation in the treatment of tibial plafond fractures. *Clin Orthop Relat Res* 1996;332:16-22.

20. French B, Tornetta P III: Hybrid external fixation of tibial pilon fractures. *Foot Ankle Clin* 2000;5:853-871.

21. Gaudinez RF, Mallik AR, Szporn M: Hybrid external fixation in tibial plafond fractures. *Clin Orthop Relat Res* 1996;329:223-232.

22. Griffiths GP, Thordarson DB: Tibial plafond fractures: Limited internal fixation and a hybrid external fixator. *Foot Ankle Int* 1996;17:444-448.

23. Manca M, Marchetti S, Restuccia G, Faldini A, Faldini C, Giannini S: Combined percutaneous internal and external fixation of type-C tibial plafond fractures: A review of twenty-two cases. *J Bone Joint Surg Am* 2002;84(Suppl 2): 109-115.

24. Pugh KJ, Wolinsky PR, McAndrew MP, Johnson KD: Tibial pilon fractures: A comparison of treatment methods. *J Trauma* 1999;47:937-941.

25. Tornetta P III, Weiner L, Bergman M, et al: Pilon fractures: Treatment with combined internal and external fixation. *J Orthop Trauma* 1993;7:489-496.

26. Blauth M, Bastian L, Krettek C, Knop C, Evans S: Surgical options for the treatment of severe tibial pilon fractures: A study of three techniques. *J Orthop Trauma* 2001;15:153-160.

27. Patterson MJ, Cole JD: Two-staged delayed open reduction and internal fixation of severe pilon fractures. *J Orthop Trauma* 1999;13:85-91.

28. Sirkin M, Sanders R, DiPasquale T, Herscovici D Jr: A staged protocol for soft tissue management in the treatment of complex pilon fractures. *J Orthop Trauma* 1999;13:78-84.

29. Helfet DL, Shonnard PY, Levine D, Borrelli J Jr: Minimally invasive plate osteosynthesis of distal fractures of the tibia. *Injury* 1997;28(Suppl 1):A42-A47.

30. Khoury A, Liebergall M, London E, Mosheiff R: Percutaneous plating of distal tibial fractures. *Foot Ankle Int* 2002;23:818-824.

31. Oh CW, Kyung HS, Park IH, Kim PT, Ihn JC: Distal tibia metaphyseal fractures treated by percutaneous plate osteosynthesis. *Clin Orthop Relat Res* 2003;408:286-291.

32. Casey D, McConnell T, Parekh S, Tornetta P III: Percutaneous pin placement in the medial calcaneus: Is anywhere safe? *J Orthop Trauma* 2002;16:26-29.

33. Ruedi TP, Allgöwer M: The operative treatment of intra-articular fractures of the lower end of the tibia. *Clin Orthop Relat Res* 1979;138:105-110.

34. Gobezie RG, Ponce BA, Vrahas MS: Pilon fractures: Use of the posterolateral approach for ORIF. *Operative Techniques in Orthopaedics* 2003;13:113.

35. Tull F, Borrelli J Jr: Soft-tissue injury associated with closed fractures: Evaluation and management. *J Am Acad Orthop Surg* 2003;11:431-438.

36. McFerran MA, Smith SW, Boulas HJ, Schwartz HS: Complications encountered in the treatment of pilon fractures. *J Orthop Trauma* 1992;6:195-200.

37. Thordarson DB: Complications after treatment of tibial pilon fractures: Prevention and management strategies. *J Am Acad Orthop Surg* 2000;8:253-265.

38. Hoppenfeld DP, Hutton R (eds): *Surgical Exposures in Orthopaedics: The Anatomic Approach*. Philadelphia, PA, Lippincott, 1994.

39. Borrelli J Jr, Catalano L: Open reduction and internal fixation of pilon fractures. *J Orthop Trauma* 1999;13:573-582.

40. Borrelli J Jr, Ellis E: Pilon fractures: Assessment and treatment. *Orthop Clin North Am* 2002;33:231-245.

41. Shantharam SS, Naeni F, Wilson EP: Single-incision technique for internal fixation of distal tibia and fibula fractures. *Orthopedics* 2000;23:429-431.

42. Wright V: Post-traumatic osteoarthritis: A

medico-legal minefield. *Br J Rheumatol* 1990;29:474-478.

43. Mitchell N, Shepard N: Healing of articular cartilage in intra-articular fractures in rabbits. *J Bone Joint Surg Am* 1980;62:628-634.

44. Llinas A, McKellop HA, Marshall GJ, Sharpe F, Kirchen M, Sarmiento A: Healing and remodeling of articular incongruities in a rabbit fracture model. *J Bone Joint Surg Am* 1993;75: 1508-1523.

45. Matta JM: Fractures of the acetabulum: Accuracy of reduction and clinical results in patients managed operatively within three weeks after the injury. *J Bone Joint Surg Am* 1996;78:1632-1645.

46. Honkonen SE: Degenerative arthritis after tibial plateau fractures. *J Orthop Trauma* 1995;9:273-277.

47. Marsh JL, Buckwalter J, Gelberman R, et al: Articular fractures: Does an anatomic reduction really change the result? *J Bone Joint Surg Am* 2002;84-A:1259-1271.

48. Dirschl DR, Marsh JL, Buckwalter JA, et al: Articular fractures. *J Am Acad Orthop Surg* 2004;12:416-423.

49. Marsh JL, Weigel DP, Dirschl DR: Tibial plafond fractures: How do these ankles function over time? *J Bone Joint Surg Am* 2003;85-A:287-295.

50. Teeny SM, Wiss DA: Open reduction and internal fixation of tibial plafond fractures: Variables contributing to poor results and complications. *Clin Orthop Relat Res* 1993;292:108-117.

51. Dirschl DR, Obremskey WT: Mechanical strength and wear of used EBI external fixators. *Orthopedics* 2002;25:1059-1062.

52. Watson JT, Moed BR, Karges DE, Cramer KE: Pilon fractures: Treatment protocol based on severity of soft tissue injury. *Clin Orthop Relat Res* 2000;375:78-90.

53. Geller J, Tornetta P III, Tiburzi D, Kummer F, Koval K: Tension wire position for hybrid external fixation of the proximal tibia. *J Orthop Trauma* 2000;14:502-504.

54. Vives MJ, Abidi NA, Ishikawa SN, Taliwal RV, Sharkey PF: Soft tissue injuries with the use of safe corridors for transfixion wire placement during external fixation of distal tibia fractures: An anatomic study. *J Orthop Trauma* 2001;15:555-559.

55. Dillin L, Slabaugh P: Delayed wound healing, infection, and nonunion following open reduction and internal fixation of tibial plafond fractures. *J Trauma* 1986;26:1116-1119.

56. Court-Brown CM, Walker C, Garg A, McQueen MM: Half-ring external fixation in the management of tibial plafond fractures. *J Orthop Trauma* 1999;13:200-206.

57. Turchin DC, Schemitsch EH, McKee MD, Waddell JP: Do foot injuries significantly affect the functional outcome of multiply injured patients? *J Orthop Trauma* 1999;13:1-4.

58. Tran T, Thordarson D: Functional outcome of multiply injured patients with associated foot injury. *Foot Ankle Int* 2002;23:340-343.

59. Weigel DP, Marsh JL: High-energy fractures of the tibial plateau: Knee function after longer follow-up. *J Bone Joint Surg Am* 2002;84-A:1541-1551.

60. Sands A, Grujic L, Byck DC, Agel J, Benirschke S, Swiontkowski MF: Clinical and functional outcomes of internal fixation of displaced pilon fractures. *Clin Orthop Relat Res* 1998;347:131-137.

61. Pollak AN, McCarthy ML, Bess RS, Agel J, Swiontkowski MF: Outcomes after treatment of high-energy tibial plafond fractures. *J Bone Joint Surg Am* 2003;85:1893-1900.

62. Williams TM, Nepola JV, DeCoster TA, Hurwitz SR, Dirschl DR, Marsh JL: Factors affecting outcome in tibial plafond fractures. *Clin Orthop Relat Res* 2004;423:93-98.

63. DeCoster TA, Willis MC, Marsh JL, et al: Rank order analysis of tibial plafond fractures: Does injury or reduction predict outcome? *Foot Ankle Int* 1999;20:44-49.

Avoiding Complications in the Treatment of Pronation-External Rotation Ankle Fractures, Syndesmotic Injuries, and Talar Neck Fractures

Dolfi Herscovici Jr, DO
*Jeffrey O. Anglen, MD
*Michael T. Archdeacon, MD, MSE
*Lisa K. Cannada, MD

Abstract

Fractures of the foot and ankle are common injuries that often are successfully treated nonsurgically; however, some injuries require surgical intervention. To restore anatomy and avoid the need for additional surgery, surgeons must pay attention to detail and understand common, avoidable complications. The surgeon should have an understanding of the pathologic characteristics of three common injuries of the foot and ankle as well as the potential complications and their prevention.

Almost 2% of the general population will sustain an ankle fracture during their lifetime.[1] These fractures are so common that their treatment seems routine, leading to a certain disregard for their seriousness and potential complications. In an effort to provide guidelines for treatment, investigators have developed classification schemes such as the Lauge-Hansen system,[2] a two-part system based on the mechanism of injury. In this scheme, the first word denotes the position of the foot at the time of injury and the second, the direction of the deforming force. There are four basic injury patterns in this system: supination-external rotation, seen in 40% to 75% of cases; supination-adduction, seen in 10% to 20%; pronation-abduction, seen in 5% to 21%; and pronation-external rotation, seen in 7% to 19%.

Pronation-External Rotation Ankle Fractures

Introduction and Pathologic Findings

The pronation-external rotation pattern, one of the least common injuries but arguably the one most likely to be treated poorly, occurs when an external rotation force is applied to a pronated foot. The injury begins medially and, depending on the amount of force exerted on the ankle, progresses toward the fibula and the tibiofibular ligaments. There are four described stages. Initially, stage 1 produces a rupture of the deltoid ligament or an avulsion of the medial malleolus. A disruption of the anterior-inferior tibiofibular ligament occurs in stage 2, and a diaphyseal fracture of the fibula occurs in stage 3. Stage 3 is identified on the basis of the pathognomonic fibular fracture patterns, described as a spiral or oblique fracture occurring

Jeffrey O. Anglen, MD, or the department with which he is affiliated has received research or institutional support from NIH and DePuy, has received royalties from EBI, and is a consultant for or an employee of Stryker. Michael T. Archdeacon, MD, or the department with which he is affiliated has received research or institutional support from Stryker and is a consultant for or an employee of Stryker. Lisa Cannada, MD, or the department with which she is affiliated has received research or institutional support from Zimmer and the Foundation for Orthopaedic Trauma and is a consultant for or an employee of Medtronic.

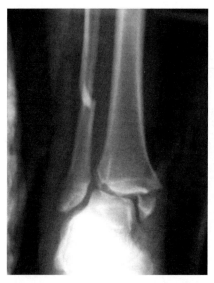

Figure 1 AP radiograph of a pronation-external rotation injury. Note the diaphyseal fibular fracture, the medial malleolar fracture, and widening of the syndesmosis.

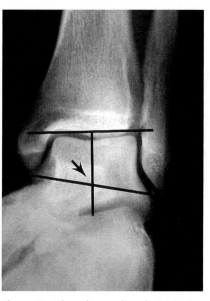

Figure 2 The talocrural angle (arrow) is determined by drawing a line perpendicular to the plafond, which intersects a line connecting the tips of the malleoli.

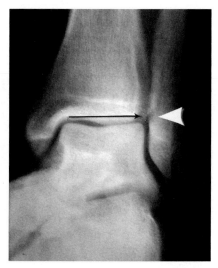

Figure 3 The Shenton line is drawn from the Wagstaffe tubercle (*white arrowhead*) on the fibula toward the medial malleolus. If the fibula is of adequate anatomic length, the line should pass through the tibial plafond (*black arrow*).

proximal to the plafond and continuing from anterior-proximal to posterior-distal. Continued force leads to stage 4, which is a failure of the posterior-inferior tibiofibular ligament or a fracture of the posterior malleolus.

The importance of this supra-articular fibular fracture is the potential for failure of the entire ligamentous connection between the tibia and fibula. In such a situation, radiographs frequently demonstrate, in addition to the fractures of the medial malleolus and the fibula, a diastasis or dislocation of the syndesmosis (Figure 1). Because as little as 1 mm of lateral talar displacement can decrease the contact area of the ankle joint by more than 40%, it is important to restore normal anatomy.[3,4] A combination of lateral talar displacement with persistent external rotation and fibular shortening ultimately contributes to early degenerative arthritis of the ankle.[5] Obtaining an anatomic reduction of

the ankle with nonsurgical techniques is difficult. To avoid these complications, open surgical reduction and fixation usually are required. The key to obtaining an anatomic reduction of the mortise is to first obtain an adequate reduction of the lateral malleolus,[6,7] then obtain a reduction of the medial malleolus, and finally repair any remaining osseous and soft-tissue injuries.

Radiographic Evaluation

Routine radiographic studies of the ankle, consisting of AP, mortise, and lateral plain radiographs, are the mainstay of imaging of ankle injuries. A critical analysis of these three plain radiographs should identify any shortening of the fibula, widening of the joint space, or malrotation of the fibula. A persistently widened medial clear space seen on radiographs often is an indication that fibular length has not been adequately restored. Three measurements are used to ascertain whether

the correct fibular length has been restored: the talocrural angle,[8] the tibiofibular (or Shenton) line,[9] and the circle sign.[10] The talocrural angle is created by a line drawn perpendicular to the tibial plafond intersecting a line drawn from the tips of the medial and lateral malleoli; the normal angle ranges from 79° to 87° (Figure 2). The tibiofibular line, which should intersect the distal (Wagstaffe) tubercle of the fibula, is drawn parallel to and through the subchondral bone of the tibial plafond (Figure 3). The circle sign is an unbroken curve between the lateral process of the talus and the recess in the distal tip of the lateral malleolus (Figure 4). Radiographs to evaluate syndesmotic widening are discussed in the next section.

Factors Producing Malreduction of Pronation-External Rotation Injuries

Three of the most common causes of persistent malreduction of pronation-

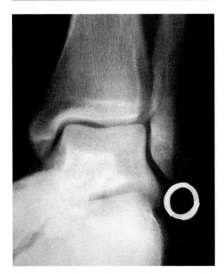

Figure 4   The circle sign is seen on the mortise radiograph and should be an unbroken curve connecting the recess in the distal tip of the fibula and the lateral process of the talus when the fibula is of adequate anatomic length.

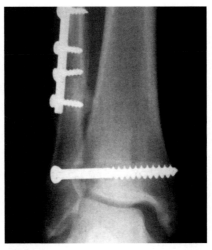

Figure 5   Radiograph of an inadequately reduced pronation-external rotation injury, demonstrating a shortened fibula with widening of the medial clear space. A syndesmotic screw was added in an attempt to "squeeze" the tibia and fibula together to reduce the mortise, which cannot be done until fibular length has been restored.

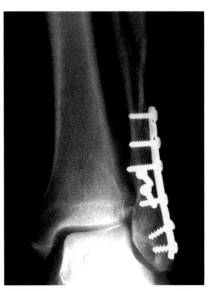

Figure 6   Postoperative radiograph demonstrating malreduction of the ankle mortise. The implant is too short and should be revised so that the fixation extends past the proximal fragments of the fibula.

external rotation injuries are inadequate restoration of fibular length, persistent external rotation of the fibula, and inadequate fixation of the fibula.

A widened medial clear space usually indicates continuing lateral talar subluxation. This often is due to a shortened fibula. To correct the lateral talar shift, the talus needs to be "pushed" toward the medial malleolus. This is achieved by lengthening the fibula. The most common mistake when trying to reduce the size of the medial clear space is to "squeeze" the tibia and fibula together with bone clamps or syndesmotic screws (Figure 5). This maneuver does not reduce the mortise, and a widened medial clear space persists. The anatomic length of the fibula needs to be restored with a distraction technique. When adequate fibular length is achieved, the mortise will be reduced, and the widening of the medial clear space will disappear.

Once adequate fibular length has been achieved, it is important to identify any persistent malrotation of the fibula. To correct malrotation, it is important to remember that the articular surface of the fibula articulates with the lateral border of the talus.[11] If there is any question regarding rotation, the dissection should be extended distally to expose the lateral malleolus and ensure that it articulates with the talus. Once proper length and rotation are verified, definitive fixation of the fibula can be applied.

The third common mistake is inadequate fixation. This is a mechanical problem caused by a plate that is either too short to provide adequate fixation or too malleable to hold the reduction of the fibula. Both situations can result in failure of the fixation (Figure 6). The fracture forces with this injury are unlike those seen with the more common supination-external rotation fracture. The fibular fracture of the pronation-external rotation injury is in the hard diaphyseal bone rather than the soft metaphyseal region, and the associated ligamentous injuries prevent neutralization of the forces across the fracture with a short malleable plate. The solution is the use of longer, stouter 3.5-mm plates (LCP Metaphyseal Plate; Synthes, Paoli, PA). The attraction of these plates is that they are available in lengths of up to 242 mm, allowing at least three screws to be placed proximal to the fracture; have a lower profile so they can be better contoured to the distal metaphyseal bone; and provide a sturdier proximal portion to stabilize the diaphyseal injury.

Syndesmotic Injuries of the Ankle
Introduction and Pathologic Findings
The syndesmosis complex is made up of an osseous component—the

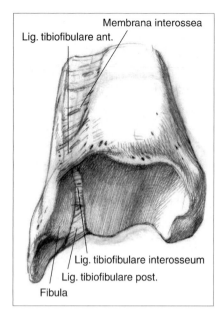

Figure 7 Drawing depicting the components of the syndesmotic complex. (Reproduced with permission from Grass R, Zwipp H: Syndesmosenplastik bei chronischer Insuffizienz des distalen tibiofibularen Syndesmosenkomplexes. *Operat Orthop Traumatol* 2003;15:208-225.)

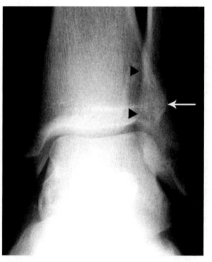

Figure 8 On an AP radiograph, tibiofibular overlap should be measured from the medial edge of the fibula (arrowheads) to the lateral border of the tibia (arrow), and it should exceed 6 mm.

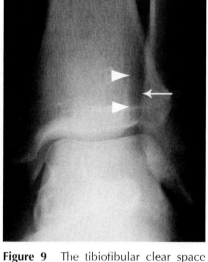

Figure 9 The tibiofibular clear space should be measured on the AP radiograph from the medial border of the fibula (arrow) to the lateral border of the tibial incisura (arrowheads).

fibular shaft (the lateral malleolus articulating with the recessed area of the tibia [the tibial incisura])—and four soft-tissue restraints, consisting of the anterior-inferior tibiofibular ligament, the posterior tibiofibular ligament, the interosseous ligament, and the interosseous membrane (Figure 7). These four ligaments stabilize the syndesmosis by preventing lateral displacement of the fibula. The anterior tibiofibular ligament provides 35% of the syndesmotic strength; the posterior ligament, 40%; and the interosseous ligament, 22%.[12] When the syndesmosis is disrupted, it alters the normal gliding and rotational motion between the talar dome and the distal part of the tibia. In a study quantifying the amount of diastasis produced by sectioning of these ligaments, a complete disruption of all four ligaments produced an average of 7.3 mm of tibiofibular diastasis.[12] When the soft-tissue restraints were individually divided, a loss of the anterior tibiofibular ligament produced 2.3 mm of diastasis, a loss of the posterior tibiofibular ligament produced 2.8 mm, and every 2 cm of sectioned interosseous ligament produced an additional 0.5 mm of diastasis.[12]

Radiographic Evaluation

Plain radiographs are used as the initial means of screening for a syndesmotic injury. The radiographs are either static or dynamic studies. Static radiographs are made without any stress applied to the ankle, whereas dynamic radiographs are made with an applied stress. Three measurements used to evaluate the syndesmosis are the tibiofibular overlap, the tibiofibular clear space, and the medial clear space.[13-15] Tibiofibular overlap is best measured 1 cm proximal to the joint on an AP radiograph. There should be more than 6 mm of overlap between the medial border of the fibula and the lateral border of the tibia (the anterior tubercle of the incisura; Figure 8). The tibiofibular clear space is one of the most sensitive indicators of syndesmotic injuries and is measured on the AP view. At 1 cm proximal to the ankle joint, widening is demonstrated by a distance of more than 6 mm between the medial border of the fibula and the medial cortical density of the tibia (the posterior tubercle of the incisura; Figure 9). Finally, the medial clear space should measure less than 4 mm; however, to detect subtle changes, this measurement may need to be compared with that in the contralateral extremity. If, after the performance of these studies, there is still a question about whether there is a syndesmotic injury, comparison radiographs of the contralateral extremity or CT can help to detect a subtle diastasis.

The two dynamic evaluations used to evaluate the integrity of the syndesmosis are the Cotton test and the modified Cotton test.[16,17] The

Cotton test, which has been attributed to F.J. Cotton, often is performed intraoperatively. It is done by grasping the distal part of the fibula and pulling it laterally. When the syndesmosis is compromised, the syndesmosis or the mortise or both are widened. The modified Cotton test also is intraoperatively done by obtaining a lateral radiograph of the ankle while pushing or pulling the fibula in the sagittal plane. Again, evaluation of the contralateral extremity may be necessary to identify subtle differences. Because the fibula often displaces posteriorly and laterally, the modified Cotton test may be more valuable than the Cotton test, but both should be done.

Factors Producing Malreduction of the Syndesmosis

Three common reasons why the syndesmosis cannot be anatomically reduced are malreduction of one or both malleoli, osseous or soft-tissue interposition, and malreduction of the fibula within the tibial incisura.

Malreduction of the malleoli will affect the syndesmosis, especially if substantial external rotation and shortening of the fibula remain (Figure 10). This occurs more often in association with comminuted fractures of the fibula because correct alignment of the fibula is difficult to achieve. Persistent external rotation does not allow the fibula to lie within the boundaries of the incisura. It is a mistake to accept a malreduction just because it is within the "acceptable" range for treatment of these injuries. Such malrotation ultimately affects the rotation and gliding motion of the ankle. The solution is to revise the fixation of the fibula to correct both malrotation and shortening.

Both osseous or soft-tissue interposition and malreduction of the

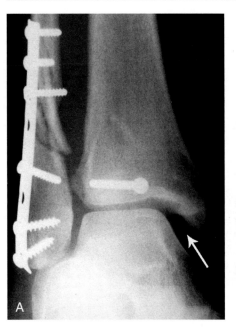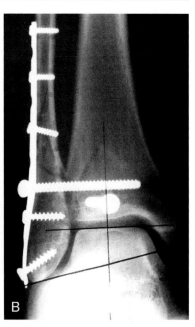

Figure 10   A, Mortise radiograph demonstrating malreduction of the ankle. The fibula is shortened, producing widening of the medial clear space (*arrow*) and widening of the syndesmosis. **B,** Following revision of the fixation, the fibula is now of adequate anatomic length. Use of a longer plate resulted in a reduction of the mortise and syndesmosis.

fibula within the incisura are strictly mechanical issues. After fixation of the malleoli, dynamic and static radiographs often demonstrate persistent widening of the syndesmosis. As is the case with pronation-external rotation injuries, the mistake is trying to "squeeze" the tibia and fibula together with a bone clamp. Too often, a closed reduction is done, and the tibiofibular relationship is deemed adequate on the basis of intraoperative static radiographs, even when the reduction is not anatomic. This is often a result of an inadequate radiographic assessment of the syndesmosis. When a closed manipulation does not produce an anatomic reduction, the solution is open reduction of the syndesmosis (Figure 11). The approach uses the fibular incision, with the dissection directed anterior to the fibula and onto the tibia. A lamina spreader can be used to separate the tibia and fibula and allow removal of

debris from the incisura. The incisura should be carefully examined to confirm that all blocks to reduction have been removed, allowing reduction of the fibula into its correct anatomic position. When this is confirmed radiographically, the fibula is securely fixed to the tibia.

Fractures of the Talar Neck
Introduction and Pathologic Findings

The talus contributes to the motion of the subtalar, tibiotalar, and transverse tarsal joints and plays a major role in the entire function of the foot and ankle. Approximately 50% of all talar fractures occur through the neck, the portion of the talus that is weakest and has the smallest cross-sectional area. These fractures are produced by hyperdorsiflexion of the foot, an axial load on the plantar surface of the fixed talus, or a direct blow.[18] The most common clas-

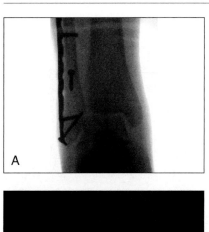
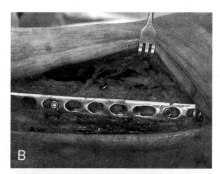
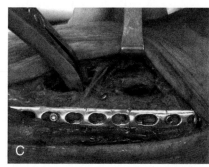
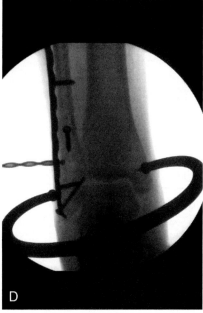
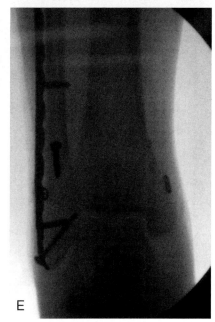

Figure 11 **A,** Intraoperative radiograph demonstrating some persistent widening of the syndesmosis after fixation of the fibula. **B,** Intraoperative photograph demonstrating how the syndesmosis is approached by dissecting anterior to the fibula. **C,** When the syndesmosis has been identified, a lamina spreader is placed between the tibia and fibula to facilitate removal of any loose osseous or soft-tissue structures within the incisura. **D,** Once the loose fragments have been removed, a bone clamp is used to reduce the fibula back into the incisura. An attempt should be made to place the bone clamp along the intermalleolar line and parallel to the line of syndesmosis fixation. **E,** The reduction is completed with suture (TightRope, Arthrex, Naples, FL) fixation. The radiograph demonstrates reduction of the syndesmosis.

sification system for fractures of the talar neck is that of Hawkins,[19] who described four distinct fracture patterns. The type I pattern is a nondisplaced fracture. Type II is a displaced fracture with a dislocation or subluxation of the subtalar joint. Type III is a fracture in which the talar body is displaced from both the subtalar and the tibiotalar joint. Type IV, originally described by Canale, is a fracture associated with subluxation or dislocation of the talonavicular joint.[20]

The problems associated with fractures of the neck of the talus are necrosis of the talar body, posttraumatic arthritis, and malunions and nonunions, resulting in the loss of ankle and subtalar motion. The causes of these complications are an interruption of the blood supply to the talar body, direct chondral damage produced at the time of the injury, malalignment of the fracture, excessive motion at the fracture site, and prolonged immobilization of the injured foot and ankle. As a general rule, as the severity of the injury increases, so do the complication rates. However, the two complications over which surgeons have the least control are necrosis of the bone and the development of posttraumatic arthritis. Current studies[21] have demonstrated that historical rates of necrosis are inaccurate. The incidence of posttraumatic arthritis is higher than that of osteonecrosis, and the timing of fixation does not seem to affect either of these two complications. However, even when an anatomic reduction has been achieved, osteonecrosis is still seen with 40% of type II fractures and 40% to 65% of type III fractures.[21]

Malunions and nonunions are usually caused by surgeon error. Although union rates are between 88% and 94%,[21] most malreductions occur as a result of inadequate reduction or insufficient methods of fixation. Malunion often produces varus malalignment of the hindfoot and shortening and deformity of the medial column (adduction of the midfoot and forefoot), with or without a cavus foot deformity. This deformity limits motion of the subtalar joint and decreases ankle dorsiflexion.[22,23]

Radiographic Evaluation

Plain AP, oblique, and lateral radiographs of the ankle and foot are used to identify fractures and displacement of the talar neck. In addition, the Canale view provides a direct AP view of the talar neck (Figure 12). This radiograph is made by placing the ankle into equinus and rotating the foot into 15° of pronation while the x-ray tube is angled 75° from the horizontal plane.[20] CT scans can also be extremely helpful for assessing comminution and displacement of the fracture as well as providing images of the ankle, subtalar, and transverse tarsal joints.

Factors Producing Malreduction of the Talar Neck

Four common reasons for malreduction of talar neck fractures are poor visualization of the fracture during reduction, medial compression of comminuted fractures, inadequate fixation, and early weight bearing by the patient.

Inadequate visualization of the fracture is an avoidable surgical error. Using percutaneous screws to stabilize the fracture because some or all of the displacement appears to have been corrected with a closed reduction technique is an error that should be avoided (Figure 13). Too often, there is residual malreduction that has not been corrected with the closed reduction and is not fully appreciated on fluoroscopic images. Inadequate preoperative planning (usually because preoperative CT scans were not ordered or were inadequately reviewed) or acceptance of "very little step-off" will result in a less-than-anatomic reduction of

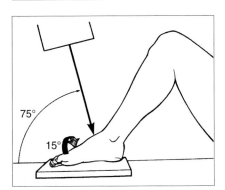

Figure 12 The position of the foot and the angle of the x-ray beam needed to produce a Canale radiograph of the talus. (Reproduced with permission from Heckman JD: Fractures of the talus, in Bucholz RW, Heckman JD (eds): *Rockwood and Green's Fractures in Adults*, ed 5. Philadelphia, PA, Lippincott Williams & Wilkins, 2001, vol 2, p 2097.)

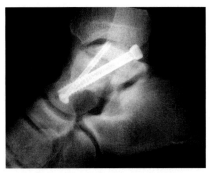

Figure 13 Percutaneous fixation resulting in malreduction of a talar fracture.

the fracture. The solution is an open reduction, with a two-incision approach, to verify an anatomic reduction of both the neck and the subtalar joint.[24] This two-incision approach consists of a medial incision that begins at the anterior border of the medial malleolus and extends toward the navicular tuberosity, just dorsal to the posterior tibial tendon, and an anterolateral incision that begins at the Chaput tubercle on the tibia and extends toward the bases of the third and fourth metatarsals.[25]

Another cause of malreduction is medial compression of a comminuted fracture. Comminution of the talar neck makes it difficult to judge the proper length of the neck, especially the medial column. Although descriptions of standard techniques include a recommendation for the use of a lag screw, this compresses the medial side of the neck, leading to a malreduction. The solutions are to obtain adequate visualization, use a bone graft when there is loss of bone, use a transfix-

ion (noncompression) screw technique to avoid compression, and consider adding a small plate and screw fixation to prevent medial collapse[26] (Figure 14).

Weight bearing before the fracture is healed and inadequate fixation are two of the prime reasons for failures. Often, a closed reduction improves the alignment of the fragments. The surgeon then wants to "hold" this position by stabilizing the fracture with pins. The mistake is that pins alone cannot maintain an adequate reduction of the fracture. This type of fixation allows gaps and motion to persist, increasing the risk of nonunion and osteonecrosis (Figure 15). The solution, after a formal open reduction technique, is to use screw and screw-plate combinations to maintain the reduction until healing has occurred.

Postoperative Care

Early weight bearing is avoided following all three of these injuries by applying a short leg, non–weight-bearing cast, which is worn until the sutures are removed (at 2 to 3 weeks). The patient then wears a cam-walker boot, begins range-of-motion and strengthening exercises, and maintains no weight bearing for the first 3 months after surgery.

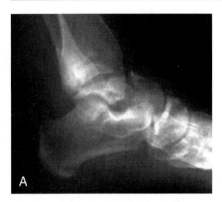
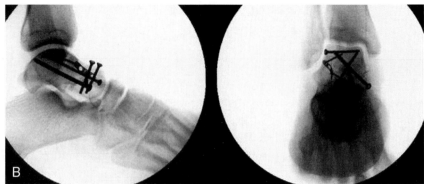

Figure 14 **A,** Lateral radiograph of a comminuted fracture of the talar neck. Compression of this fracture will result in malreduction of the hindfoot. **B,** Postoperative radiographs demonstrating the use of a transfixion screw technique augmented with a small plate to maintain the correct length of the talus.

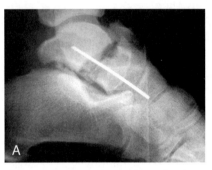
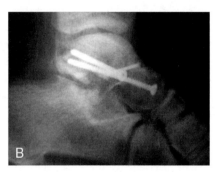

Figure 15 **A,** Radiograph made after pin fixation of a talar neck fracture, demonstrating shortening and angular malalignment of the neck. **B,** Revision with the use of screw fixation allowed the length of the talus to be restored.

Summary

Pronation-external rotation ankle fractures, syndesmotic injuries, and talar neck fractures are common conditions seen by most orthopaedic surgeons. Adequate preoperative evaluations, sufficient visualization of the pathological characteristics, and good surgical techniques should decrease the rates of complications associated with the management of these injuries.

References

1. Daly PJ, Fitzgerald RH Jr, Melton LJ, Ilstrup DM: Epidemiology of ankle fractures in Rochester, Minnesota. *Acta Orthop Scand* 1987;58:539-544.

2. Lauge-Hansen N: Fractures of the ankle: II. Combined experimental-surgical and experimental-roentgenologic investigations. *Arch Surg* 1950; 60:957-985.

3. Ramsey PL, Hamilton W: Changes in the tibiotalar area of contact caused by lateral talar shift. *J Bone Joint Surg Am* 1976;58:356-357.

4. Curtis MJ, Michelson JD, Urquhart MW, Byank RP, Jinnah RH: Tibiotalar contact and fibular malunion in ankle fractures: A cadaver study. *Acta Orthop Scand* 1992;63:326-329.

5. Thordarson DB, Motamed S, Hedman T, Ebramzadeh E, Bakshian S: The effect of fibular malreduction on contact pressures in an ankle fracture malunion model. *J Bone Joint Surg Am* 1997;79:1809-1815.

6. Yablon IG, Heller FG, Shouse L: The key role of the lateral malleolus in displaced fractures of the ankle. *J Bone Joint Surg Am* 1977;59:169-173.

7. Joy G, Patzakis MJ, Harvey JP Jr: Precise evaluation of the reduction of severe ankle fractures: Technique and correlation with end results. *J Bone Joint Surg Am* 1974;56:979-993.

8. Sarkisian JS, Cody GW: Closed treatment of ankle fractures: A new criterion for evaluation. A review of 250 cases. *J Trauma* 1976;16:323-326.

9. Morris M, Chandler RW: Fractures of the ankle. *Tech Orthop* 1987;2: 10-19.

10. Weber BG, Simpson LA: Corrective lengthening osteotomy of the fibula. *Clin Orthop Relat Res* 1985;199:61-67.

11. Sarrafian SK: Osteology, in *Anatomy of the Foot and Ankle: Descriptive, Topographic, Functional*, ed 2. Philadelphia, PA, Lippincott, 1993, pp 37-112.

12. Ogilvie-Harris DJ, Reed SC, Hedman TP: Disruption of the ankle syndesmosis: Biomechanical study of the ligamentous restraints. *Arthroscopy* 1994;10:558-560.

13. Xenos JS, Hopkinson WJ, Mulligan ME, Olson EJ, Popovic NA: The tibiofibular syndesmosis: Evaluation of the ligamentous structures, methods of fixation, and radiographic assessment. *J Bone Joint Surg Am* 1995;77: 847-856.

14. Ebraheim NA, Lu J, Yang H, Mekhail AO, Yeasting RA: Radiographic and CT evaluation of tibiofibular syndesmotic diastasis: A cadaver study. *Foot Ankle Int* 1997;18:693-698.

15. Daffner RH: Ankle trauma. *Radiol Clin North Am* 1990;28:395-421.

16. Cotton FJ: *Dislocations and Joint-Fractures*. Philadelphia, PA, WB Saunders, 1910, pp 615-616.

17. Candal-Couto JJ, Burrow D, Bromage S, Briggs PJ: Instability of the tibio-fibular syndesmosis: Have we been pulling in the wrong direction? *Injury* 2004;35:814-818.

18. Daniels TR, Smith JW: Talar neck fractures. *Foot Ankle* 1993;14:225-234.

19. Hawkins LG: Fractures of the neck of the talus. *J Bone Joint Surg Am* 1970;52:991-1002.

20. Canale ST, Kelly FB Jr: Fractures of the neck of the talus: Long-term evaluation of seventy-one cases. *J Bone Joint Surg Am* 1978;60:143-156.

21. Lindvall E, Haidukewych G, DiPasquale T, Herscovici D Jr, Sanders R: Open reduction and stable fixation of isolated, displaced talar neck and body fractures. *J Bone Joint Surg Am* 2004;86:2229-2234.

22. Daniels TR, Smith JW, Ross TI: Varus malalignment of the talar neck: Its effect on the position of the foot and on subtalar motion. *J Bone Joint Surg Am* 1996;78:1559-1567.

23. Sangeorzan BJ, Wagner UA, Harrington RM, Tencer AF: Contact characteristics of the subtalar joint: The effect of talar neck misalignment. *J Orthop Res* 1992;10:544-551.

24. Sangeorzan BJ, Mayo KA, Hansen ST: Intraarticular fractures of the foot: Talus and lesser tarsals. *Clin Orthop Relat Res* 1993;292:135-141.

25. Herscovici D Jr, Sanders RW, Infante A, DiPasquale T: Bohler incision: An extensile anterolateral approach to the foot and ankle. *J Orthop Trauma* 2000;14:429-432.

26. Fleuriau Chateau PB, Brokaw DS, Jelen BA, Scheid DK, Weber TG: Plate fixation of talar neck fractures: Preliminary review of a new technique in twenty-three patients. *J Orthop Trauma* 2002;16:213-219.

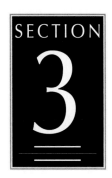

SECTION 3

Sports Medicine

Sports Medicine

The six chapters in this section are timely and provide valuable information about sports-related disorders of the foot and ankle, including diagnostic evaluation, nonsurgical management, and surgical treatments. There is controversy concerning the management of many sports-related foot and ankle conditions; therefore, these chapters are important because they provide the reader with a sound base of knowledge and may also stimulate further research that may help resolve some of the disagreements regarding the appropriate treatment for these conditions.

The chapter by Jones reviews Achilles tendon disorders and other causes of posterior and plantar heel pain such as retrocalcaneal bursitis, insertional Achilles tendinitis, pump bump, plantar fasciitis, and tarsal tunnel syndrome. Achilles tendon disorders are common in professional and recreational athletes. The Puddu classification of noninsertional Achilles disorders is reviewed, including peritendinitis, peritendinitis with tendinosis, and tendinosis. MRI may be useful in diagnosing tendinosis, which may be associated with prolonged recovery or failure of nonsurgical treatment.

Insertional Achilles tendon disorders can be recalcitrant and difficult to treat. Retrocalcaneal bursitis and a posterosuperior bony prominence are often associated with insertional tendinosis. A recent study of patients with insertional Achilles tendinosis showed that MRI could be useful in treatment decisions; more advanced tendon abnormalities noted on MRI may be associated with failure of nonsurgical treatment.[1] Jones reviews surgical approaches including the two-incision and central incision approaches; a more recently described S-shaped incision may decrease wound tension and dehiscence.[2]

Acute and chronic Achilles tendon ruptures are reviewed in chapter 13 by Myerson. Controversy remains concerning the nonsurgical or surgical treatment of acute Achilles tendon ruptures. A recent study has shown that ultrasonography may confirm apposition of ruptured tendon ends, allowing the possibility of good or excellent results with nonsurgical treatment with functional bracing and rehabilitation.[3] In addition, newer methods of minimally invasive surgery have been developed and evaluated, with satisfactory results reported.[4] Early postoperative weight bearing after surgical repair of acute Achilles tendon rupture may improve the patient's health-related quality of life and function in performing activities of daily living during the early postoperative period; however, at 6 months after surgery, there are only minimal differences between patients treated with early postoperative weight-bearing or non–weight-bearing regimens.[5]

As discussed in the chapter by Myerson, the surgical treatment of chronic Achilles tendon ruptures depends on the size of the gap between the tendon ends and may include V-Y tendon advancement, a turndown flap, or augmentation with peroneus brevis, flexor digitorum longus, or flexor hallucis longus (FHL) tendon. Recently, additional options have been reviewed, including augmentation with gracilis tendon, fascia lata, allograft, synthetic graft, or interposed scar tissue.[6] A study using isokinetic testing and MRI after Achilles tendon reconstruction with FHL transfer has demonstrated residual weakness despite satisfactory integration of the FHL tendon into the Achilles tendon and hypertrophy of the FHL muscle.[7]

Athletic injuries of the ankle syndesmosis are discussed in the up-to-date review by Porter, including evaluation, surgical treatment, and postoperative rehabilitation of unstable injuries. These injuries can be challenging to diagnose and may be associated with prolonged healing or residual symptoms. Syndesmosis screw fixation has been a reliable treatment for unstable syndesmosis injuries. However, attention to detail is required because malreduction of the syndesmosis may occur during open treatment of fractures and dislocations.[8] Recently, the successful use of bioabsorbable syndesmosis screw fixation has been reported for patients with ankle fractures or dislocations.[9] Preliminary success with suture-button fixation of the syndesmosis also has been reported[10] despite the significantly smaller failure torque with suture-button compared with screw fixation.[11]

The chapter by Frey provides a practical guide to the evaluation and treatment of ankle sprains, the most frequent sports injury of the foot and ankle. Acute ankle sprains frequently cause residual sequelae including chronic instability or symptoms associated with chondral damage.[12] A recent multicenter randomized trial of patients with acute ankle sprain showed that immobilization in a short leg cast for 10 days resulted in faster recovery than the use of a tubular compression bandage.[13] Although acute ankle sprains are usually treated nonsurgically, surgical repair may be considered for complete ligaments tears (grade III injuries) in competitive athletes or other patients. A recent review of 20 clinical trials, however, was inconclusive regarding the relative benefits of nonsurgical and surgical treatment for acute ankle sprain.[14]

In a patient with an ankle sprain, it is important to assess for associated injuries and predisposing disorders. The so-called ankle sprain is actually a twisting injury of the foot and ankle; further evaluation may reveal an osteochondral talar dome fracture, a lateral talar process fracture, an anterior process fracture of the calcaneus, a fifth metatarsal fracture, a subtalar joint injury, a peroneal tendon injury, or a tarsometatarsal fracture-dislocation.

Newer methods for treating chronic ankle instability are being evaluated, including arthroscopic ankle capsular shrinkage[15] and arthroscopic stabilization with a fibular anchor.[16] Risk factors for chronic instability include posterior position of the fibula,[17] varus alignment of the tibial plafond and hindfoot,[18] and sensorimotor factors such as static balance and neuromuscular function.[19] Comprehensive rehabilitation programs may improve functional limitations in patients with chronic ankle instability.[20]

The differential diagnosis, evaluation, and treatment of plantar heel pain are reviewed in the chapter by Pfeffer. The patient history and physical examination are of primary importance. A recent study on plantar fasciitis has confirmed previous findings that a prefabricated orthosis may be equally effective as a custom orthosis in relieving pain.[21] Additional research on plantar fasciitis has shown that a plantar fascia-specific stretching protocol may improve pain relief and function in patients with chronic plantar fasciitis.[22] A randomized, multicenter, placebo-controlled trial showed that extracorporeal shock wave therapy may significantly improve pain relief, function, and quality of life in patients with chronic plantar fasciitis.[23]

Other conditions causing plantar heel pain have recently received further study. Plantar fascia rupture in athletes has been treated with immobilization using a boot, with reported return to sports activity within 6 months.[24] Plantar midfoot pain may occur in dancers and those participating in kicking sports (such as soccer) because of overuse of the FHL and peroneus longus tendons, which dynamically stabilize the subtalar joint and midfoot arch when the foot and toes are actively plantar flexed.[25] Posterior tibial nerve entrapment

in the tarsal tunnel may be more aggravated by the decreased volume and increased pressure in the tarsal tunnel when the foot and ankle are in eversion or inversion compared with the neutral position; immobilization in the neutral position may be helpful.[26] Surgical decompression of the tarsal tunnel may be effective in relieving nerve entrapment symptoms.[27]

This section concludes with a current review of tarsometatarsal joint injuries in athletes by Myerson and Cerrato, including anatomy, mechanism of injury, classification, diagnosis, and treatment. These injuries may involve the intercuneiform and naviculocuneiform joints. Diagnosis may be difficult, prolonged time for healing may be required, and residual symptoms are common.

J. Chris Coetzee, MD
Orthopedic Foot and Ankle Surgeon
Minnesota Sports Medicine
Twin Cities Orthopedics
Minneapolis, Minnesota

Lowell D. Lutter, MD
Adjunct Professor of Orthopaedic
    Surgery
University of Minnesota
Minneapolis, Minnesota

References

1. Nicholson CW, Berlet GC, Lee TH: Prediction of the success of nonoperative treatment of insertional Achilles tendinosis based on MRI. *Foot Ankle Int* 2007;28:472-477.

2. Ong BC, Trepman E: Achilles tendon surgery: S-shaped surgical approach and postoperative positioning to minimize wound tension and external pressure. *Am J Orthop* 2001;30: 433-434.

3. Hufner TM, Brandes DB, Thermann H, Richter M, Knobloch K, Krettek C: Long-term results after functional nonoperative treatment

of Achilles tendon rupture. *Foot Ankle Int* 2006;27:167-171.

4. Aktas S, Kocaoglu B: Open versus minimal invasive repair with Achillon device. *Foot Ankle Int* 2009;30:391-397.

5. Suchak AA, Bostick GP, Beaupré LA, Durand DC, Jomha NM: The influence of early weight-bearing compared with non-weight-bearing after surgical repair of the Achilles tendon. *J Bone Joint Surg Am* 2008;90:1876-1883.

6. Maffulli N, Ajis A: Management of chronic ruptures of the Achilles tendon. *J Bone Joint Surg Am* 2008;90:1348-1360.

7. Hahn F, Meyer P, Maiwald C, Zanetti M, Vienne P: Treatment of chronic Achilles tendinopathy and ruptures with flexor hallucis tendon transfer: Clinical outcome and MRI findings. *Foot Ankle Int* 2008;29:794-802.

8. Miller AN, Carroll EA, Parker RJ, Boraiah S, Helfet DL, Lorich DG: Direct visualization for syndesmotic stabilization of ankle fractures. *Foot Ankle Int* 2009;30:419-426.

9. Ahmad J, Raikin SM, Pour AE, Haytmanek C: Bioabsorbable screw fixation of the syndesmosis in unstable ankle injuries. *Foot Ankle Int* 2009;30:99-105.

10. Cottom JM, Hyer CF, Philbin TM, Berlet GC: Treatment of syndesmotic disruptions with the Arthrex Tightrope: A report of 25 cases. *Foot Ankle Int* 2008;29:773-780.

11. Soin SP, Knight TA, Dinah AF, Mears SC, Swierstra BA, Belkoff SM: Suture-button versus screw fixation in a syndesmosis rupture model: A biomechanical comparison. *Foot Ankle Int* 2009;30:346-352.

12. Sugimoto K, Takakura Y, Okahashi K, Samoto N, Kawate K, Iwai M: Chondral injuries of the ankle with recurrent lateral instability: An arthroscopic study. *J Bone Joint Surg Am* 2009;91:99-106.

13. Lamb SE, Marsh JL, Hutton JL, Nakash R, Cooke MW, Collaborative Ankle Support Trial (CAST Group): Mechanical supports for acute, severe ankle sprain: A pragmatic, multicentre, randomised controlled trial. *Lancet* 2009;373:575-581.

14. Kerkhoffs GM, Handoll HH, de Bie R, Rowe BH, Struijs PA: Surgical versus conservative treatment for acute injuries of the lateral ligament complex of the ankle in adults. *Cochrane Database Syst Rev* 2007;2:CD000380.

15. de Vries JS, Krips R, Blankevoort L, Fievez AW, van Dijk CN: Arthroscopic capsular shrinkage for chronic ankle instability with thermal radiofrequency: Prospective multicenter trial. *Orthopedics* 2008;31:655.

16. Corte-Real NM, Moreira RM: Arthroscopic repair of chronic lateral ankle instability. *Foot Ankle Int* 2009;30:213-217.

17. McDermott JE, Scranton PE Jr, Rogers JV: Variations in fibular position, talar length, and anterior talofibular ligament length. *Foot Ankle Int* 2004;25:625-629.

18. Sugimoto K, Samoto N, Takakura Y, Tamai S: Varus tilt of the tibial plafond as a factor in chronic ligament instability of the ankle. *Foot Ankle Int* 1997;18:402-405.

19. Sefton JM, Hicks-Little CA, Hubbard TJ, et al: Sensorimotor function as a predictor of chronic ankle instability. *Clin Biomech (Bristol, Avon)* 2009;24:451-458.

20. Hale SA, Hertel J, Olmsted-Kramer LC: The effect of a 4-week comprehensive rehabilitation program on postural control and lower extremity function in individuals with chronic ankle instability. *J Orthop Sports Phys Ther* 2007;37:303-311.

21. Baldassin V, Gomes CR, Beraldo PS: Effectiveness of prefabricated and customized foot orthoses made from low-cost foam for noncomplicated plantar fasciitis: A randomized controlled trial. *Arch Phys Med Rehabil* 2009;90:701-706.

22. DiGiovanni BF, Nawoczenski DA, Malay DP, et al: Plantar fascia-specific stretching exercise improves outcomes in patients with chronic plantar fasciitis: A prospective clinical trial with two-year follow-up. *J Bone Joint Surg Am* 2006;88:1775-1781.

23. Gerdesmeyer L, Frey C, Vester J, et al: Radial extracorporeal shock wave therapy is safe and effective in the treatment of chronic recalcitrant plantar fasciitis: Results of a confirmatory randomized placebo-controlled multicenter study. *Am J Sports Med* 2008;36:2100-2109.

24. Saxena A, Fullem B: Plantar fascia ruptures in athletes. *Am J Sports Med* 2004;32:662-665.

25. Femino JE, Trepman E, Chisholm K, Razzano L: The role of the flexor hallucis longus and peroneus longus in the stabilization of the ballet foot. *J Dance Med Sci* 2000;4:86-89.

26. Bracilovic A, Nihal A, Houston VL, Beattie AC, Rosenberg ZS, Trepman E: Effect of foot and ankle position on tarsal tunnel compartment volume. *Foot Ankle Int* 2006;27:431-437.

27. Gondring WH, Shields B, Wenger S: An outcomes analysis of surgical treatment of tarsal tunnel syndrome. *Foot Ankle Int* 2003;24: 545-550.

J. Chris Coetzee, MD or a member of his immediate family has received royalties from Arthrex, Inc, and DePuy; has made paid presentations on behalf of Arthrex, Inc, and DePuy; serves as a paid consultant to or is an employee of Arthrex, Inc, and DePuy; and has received research or institutional support from DePuy. Neither Lowell D. Lutter, MD, nor a member of his immediate family has received anything of value from or owns stock in a commercial company or institution related directly or indirectly to the subject of this commentary.

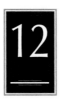

Achilles Tendon Problems in Runners

Donald C. Jones, MD

Incidence

Disorders of the Achilles tendon are very common in the running athlete, with a reported incidence ranging from 6.5% to 18.7%.[1-3] Welsh and Clodman[4] found that, of competitive track athletes with chronic Achilles tendinitis, 16% were forced to abandon their sports prematurely, while 54% continued to compete despite significant discomfort.

Achilles tendon injuries also occur in other sports, such as basketball, racquetball, soccer, football, and badminton. The mean age of patients with these injuries is between 24 and 30 years of age.[1,5,6]

Terms used to describe inflammation about the Achilles tendon and paratenon vary, which has led to considerable confusion when reviewing the literature. The classification used by Puddu and associates[7] provides a simple, but functional, arrangement. Peritendinitis refers to inflammation of the paratenon without an associated inflammatory response within the tendon. Peritendinitis with tendinosis describes a second stage of inflammation, in which both the Achilles tendon and paratenon are involved. The third stage, tendinosis, refers to asymptomatic degenerative lesions within the Achilles tendon, but without alteration of the paratenon. These changes may consist of mucoid or fatty change and/or fibroid degeneration, cartilage metaplasia, calcification, or bone metaplasia. Arner and associates[8] described these changes in biopsies taken at the time of repair of acute ruptures in asymptomatic patients.

Anatomy

The gastrocnemius and soleus muscles form the common Achilles. The gastrocnemius muscle originates from both the lateral and medial femoral condyles, and the soleus muscle originates from the posterior surface of the tibia and the fibula.

The soleus and gastrocnemius muscles contribute separately to the formation of the Achilles tendon. The gastrocnemius muscle segment ranges from 11 to 26 cm in length, and the soleus muscle portion measures 3 to 11 cm. The narrowest part of the tendon is 4 cm proximal to its insertion.

The tendinous portion of the triceps surae complex has a relatively poor blood supply, consisting primarily of longitudinal arteries that course the length of the tendon complex. These arteries are supplemented by vessels from the mesotenon. Studies have shown the least vascular area to be 2 to 6 cm above the insertion of the Achilles tendon into the calcaneus. As a result, this area of poor vascularity is susceptible to chronic inflammation and rupture.[1,9-11]

The Achilles tendon fibers rotate laterally as they descend. Cummins and associates[12] describe three patterns of rotation. In the most common pattern, the gastrocnemius muscle contributes two thirds of the fibers posteriorly and the soleus muscle contributes the remaining one third. In the second most common pattern, the gastrocnemius and the soleus muscle each contribute half of the fibers. In the least frequent pattern, the soleus muscle makes up the posterior two thirds and the gastrocnemius muscle the remaining one third. This rotation of the Achilles tendon plays an important part in the development of pathologic conditions.

Contributing Factors

The etiology of Achilles tendon disorders can be singular or multifactorial. According to Clement and associates,[1] the primary etiologic factors include training errors, such as an increase in training mileage, a single severe competitive session (10 km or a marathon), a sudden increase in training intensity, repetitive hill running, recommencement of training after an extended period of inactivity, and running on uneven or slippery terrain.

However, biomechanical variations, such as miserable malalignment, genu varum, and cavus foot, can also contribute to increased stress on the Achilles tendon and resultant bursitis. Excessive pronation of the forefoot has been implicated as the major biomechanical factor in running-induced injuries.[1,13,14]

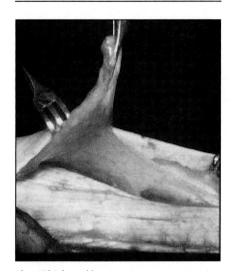

Fig. 1 Thickened hyperemic paratenon (peritendinitis).

An understanding of the biomechanics of the foot and ankle can help clarify the causal relationship between hyperpronation of the foot and Achilles tendon problems. In the initial phase of gait, the foot contacts the ground in supination. This supinated position results in a locked subtalar and midfoot joint, producing a very rigid structure. The rigidity of the foot provides the sturdy platform needed to absorb the tremendous amount of force transferred across the hindfoot at impact. Immediately after heel strike, the runner's body weight progresses over the center of the foot, and passive pronation is initiated. The calcaneus moves laterally, the talus drops off medially, and the forefoot begins to abduct. At this point, the foot becomes more flexible. As the body weight reaches the midline, maximum pronation is achieved and the hindfoot and forefoot are very flexible. Described as a "bag of bones," the foot is now capable of adapting to most unlevel running surfaces. As the weight transfer continues toward the toe-off position, the foot supinates and once again becomes a rigid lever for the function of push-off.

During this cycle, total range of motion of the subtalar joint, according to

James and associates,[15] is 31°, with 23° of inversion and 8° of eversion. This subtalar motion creates a "whipping" action of the tendon and the resultant shear forces across the Achilles tendon can result in chronic inflammation about the Achilles tendon complex.

Realizing that excessive hindfoot motion is not desirable in patients with Achilles problems, a decrease in subtalar motion is desirable in symptomatic patients. A number of studies have demonstrated that use of an orthosis can decrease this extreme motion.[16-18] The reduction of maximum eversion with an orthosis ranges from 6% to 12%. It is therefore assumed that the reduction of this extreme subtalar joint motion and the resultant "Achilles whip" can benefit patients with Achilles discomfort.

Achilles Tendon Disorders
Musculotendinous Junction Injury
Injuries to the musculotendinous junction are quite infrequent. These injuries usually occur in younger individuals with tight heel cords. Because of the excellent blood supply to this area, these injuries usually heal quite quickly.[15] Frequently, a decrease in vigorous activities for a short period of time is adequate treatment. However, on rare occasion, short-term immobilization is necessary. Total time from injury to recovery varies from 2 to 4 weeks.

Peritendinitis
The Achilles tendon is surrounded by the paratenon, not a synovial sheath. This paratenon is a loose, fatty, areolar tissue, which plays an important role in vascularization of the Achilles tendon.

Peritendinitis may result from abnormal biomechanics as previously described, or it may be caused by friction between the Achilles tendon and the adjacent tendon sheath. This friction may result from either intrinsic or extrinsic pressure. Examples of extrinsic causes of friction are ill-fitting shoes or poorly

applied tape about the ankle, which crimps the Achilles tendon. Intrinsic irritation may result from direct compression by a distal posterior tibial exostosis.

Symptoms of Achilles peritendinitis consist primarily of pain in the Achilles tendon area that is aggravated by activity and relieved by rest. The involved area may be only several centimeters in length or it can involve the entire tendon from its insertion to the musculotendinous junction.

Initial treatment of Achilles peritendinitis should consist of ice massage, contrast baths, and anti-inflammatory medication. If there is an alignment problem, orthoses that place the hindfoot in subtalar neutral are appropriate. With adequate conservative treatment, the athlete is usually asymptomatic in a relatively short period of time.

In more advanced or chronic cases, the paratenon becomes fibrotic and stenosed. An attempt may be made to dissect the adhered surrounding paratenon from the Achilles tendon. This is accomplished by placing a needle between the paratenon and Achilles tendon and rapidly injecting 15 ml of local anesthetic into the subparatenon space, creating a mechanical lysis of the adhesions. However, if this treatment fails, surgical decompression may be required.

The involved tendon is exposed through a medial peripatellar incision. Usually the involved paratenon is hyperemic, thickened, and somewhat adherent to the underlying tendon (Fig. 1). However, the paratenon may not be thickened and may only demonstrate a slight brownish blush over the tender area. Completely excise the involved paratenon medially, laterally, and posteriorly. Leave the anterior paratenon and fatty tissue intact, as this is a major area of blood supply to the tendon. Histology of the excised paratenon will frequently show only a relatively minimal acute inflammatory reaction, but a significant amount of hypervascularity.

Rehabilitation following open lysis of adhesions consists of immediate active and passive range of motion of the ankle along with protected weightbearing for 10 to 14 days. Two weeks postoperatively, full weightbearing is allowed and a vigorous rehabilitation program, consisting of range of motion, strengthening, and proprioception education, is initiated. The patient is allowed to return to a gradual running program at 6 to 8 weeks after surgery.

Peritendinitis and Tendinosis

As mentioned earlier, in some cases both the paratenon and Achilles tendon exhibit inflammation. Involvement of the Achilles tendon can be secondary to interstitial microscopic failure or obvious central necrosis with mucoid degeneration. As opposed to isolated peritendinitis, which frequently involves tenderness along the entire Achilles tendon, the combination of peritendinitis and tendinosis usually presents with a localized area of tenderness 2 to 6 cm above the insertion.[5,13,19] Swelling and nodular deformity may also be present (Fig. 2).

In the acute stage, pain is present with prolonged running and high impact-type activities, while lesser activities are asymptomatic. However, in chronic cases, pain may be present during both training and daily activities.

In the absence of nodular deformity, it may be difficult to differentiate between pure peritendinitis and peritendinitis with tendinosis. It is extremely important that this distinction be made. In peritendinitis alone, there is no need to violate the tendon at the time of surgical intervention. On the other hand, if peritendinitis and tendinosis exist together, the tendon must be opened and debrided. Evaluation by magnetic resonance imaging (MRI) is extremely helpful preoperatively in determining whether or not tendinosis is a component of the Achilles disorder (Fig. 3).

The conservative measures men-

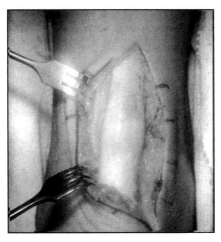

Fig. 2 Nodular deformity of the Achilles tendon (tendinosis).

tioned above are usually effective in resolving the problem. If not, a 1- to 2-week period of immobilization in a walking cast may be of benefit. If conservative treatment is unsuccessful after 6 months, surgery is an option for those athletes unable to train at the desired or needed level.

Expose the Achilles tendon through a posteromedial incision. Excise the paratenon and palpate the Achilles tendon for nodular deformities. In a tendon that is quite normal looking, but symptomatic, a preoperative MRI is helpful in locating the area of tendinosis.

A longitudinal incision is made through the tendon for a twofold purpose: (1) to see if there is an area of central necrosis or inflamed tissue that should be excised, and (2) to stimulate the healing reaction. After excising the involved area, the tendon is closed with absorbable sutures. If the defect is large, the tendon may require augmentation. Options include a plantaris weave,[20] a turn-down flap, or a flexor hallucis longus transfer.

Postoperatively, the period of immobilization depends on the amount of tissue excised. If a small defect is present, the patient is rigidly immobilized for 2 weeks, followed by mobilization in a

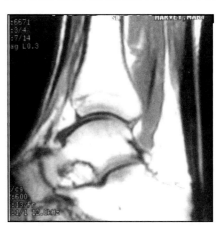

Fig 3 Magnetic resonance imaging reveals change in the Achilles tendon consistent with tendinosis.

removable boot for an additional 2 to 4 weeks. With a larger defect, 4 to 6 weeks of rigid immobilization may be necessary.

Athletes who undergo this type of surgery must exercise great patience. It is not uncommon for the recovery process to require 4 to 6 months for total rehabilitation and the ability to return to vigorous training.

Posterior Heel Pain

Pain along the posterior wall of the calcaneus is not uncommon in runners. Although not seen as frequently as pain in the Achilles tendon, posterior heel pain can be extremely limiting to the athlete. Conditions that cause posterior heel pain include retrocalcaneal bursitis and tendinosis, pre-insertional Achilles tendinitis, and pre-tendinous Achilles bursitis.

Anatomic Considerations

Familiarity with the anatomy of the hindfoot is important in understanding the etiology and treatment of hindfoot discomfort. The posterior calcaneus has three surfaces—posterior, middle posterior, and superior. The posterior surface is a continuation of the tuberosity of the calcaneus with the plantar aponeurosis, the flexor retinaculum, and the flexor digitorum brevis muscle. The middle posterior surface is where the Achilles tendon has its most proximal insertion, with the tendon fanning out into both medial and lateral expansions. It is important to understand that the insertion of the Achilles tendon extends much further inferiorly than is frequently appreciated. The fact that this insertion extends onto the plantar aspect of the calcaneus is a very important consideration when performing a partial retrocalcaneal ostectomy. The superior surface of the calcaneus extends from the talar articulation to the posterior border. Just above this border is the pre-Achilles fat pad, which occupies a portion of Kaeger's triangle.

The nerve supply of the posterior calcaneal area originates from the medial surocutaneous nerve, a combined branch from the tibial nerve, and the communicating branch of the common peroneal nerve. Vascularity of the posterior aspect of the calcaneus consists of both the medial calcaneal branches of the posterior tibial artery and the peroneal artery.

Numerous variations of posterior calcaneal morphology have been described. It is important to recognize the three most common variations in the shape of the superior tuberosity of the calcaneus: (1) hyperconcave, (2) normal, and (3) hypoconcave.

Two separate bursa reside along the posterior calcaneal wall. The adventitious superficial pre-Achilles tendinous bursa separates the Achilles tendon from the overlying skin and is present in about 50% of individuals. It becomes inflamed secondary to chronic irritation from external compression of shoe wear. The second bursa, the retrocalcaneal bursa, is present at birth and lies between the posterosuperior aspect of the calcaneus and the overlying Achilles tendon. This bursa is horseshoe shaped, with medial and lateral arms that extend distally along the medial and lateral edge of the Achilles tendon. With average measurements of 2 mm in length by 4 mm in width by 8 mm

in depth, it is a significant structure. The synovial lining in the proximal portion abuts against the Achilles fat pad. The anterior bursa wall is composed of fibrocartilage, while the posterior wall is indistinguishable from the epitenon of the Achilles tendon. Interestingly, the retrocalcaneal bursa has a consistently characteristic bursal fluid. Canoso and associates[21] demonstrated that the normal retrocalcaneal bursal fluid has a low cellular content, with predominantly mononuclear cells and a good mucin clot. The hyaluronic acid content of the fluid is noted to be higher than that of the fluid found in the olecranon and prepatellar subcutaneous bursa. The average volume of fluid in a normal retrocalcaneal bursa is 1.22 ml.

Retrocalcaneal Bursitis

Retrocalcaneal bursitis is inflammation of the retrocalcaneal bursa. I have biopsied multiple Achilles tendons distal to the inflamed retrocalcaneal bursa and have consistently found chronic inflammation. Therefore, the entity referred to as "retrocalcaneal bursitis" is actually retrocalcaneal bursitis and distal Achilles tendinitis. This condition can develop as the result of a systemic inflammatory disease process, direct pressure from shoe wear, or altered mechanics of the foot and ankle.

When treating a running athlete with recalcitrant retrocalcaneal bursitis, always exclude the possibility of a systemic inflammatory disease as the cause of the symptoms before considering surgical intervention. This is especially important if the process is bilateral. The overall instance of retrocalcaneal bursitis with rheumatoid arthritis is estimated to be between 2% and 10%.[22]

As previously stated, biomechanical abnormalities can also potentiate the development of retrocalcaneal bursitis. The most common associated abnormalities are rigid plantarflexed first ray, rearfoot varus, and hyperrotation. The

abnormal motion created by these deformities can lead to increased shear stress at the osseous soft tissue interface along the posterosuperior aspect of the calcaneus, resulting in traumatic inflammation of the retrocalcaneal bursa and the adjacent Achilles tendon.

Although a heel prominence may be contributory, it is not uncommon to see retrocalcaneal bursitis develop in runners without an associated calcaneal deformity. The bursa may become inflamed as the result of heel counter compression or secondary to a "nutcracker" effect of the Achilles and the calcaneus on the bursa during repeated episodes of forced ankle dorsiflexion. It is for this reason that many long distance runners who use uphill running (as a training method) develop retrocalcaneal bursitis-type symptoms. A deadly combination for a long distance runner is abnormal biomechanics of the hindfoot in tandem with maltraining.

Diagnosis

Signs of retrocalcaneal bursitis include swelling and erythema over the posterosuperior calcaneal tuberosity. Palpation of this area reveals tenderness both medial and lateral to the Achilles tendon along the extended arms of the retrocalcaneal bursa. Fluid within the bursa is occasionally ballotable. Infrequently, there is tenderness along the Achilles tendon above the bursa; however, most frequently there is tenderness distal to the retrocalcaneal bursa. The pain is aggravated by dorsiflexion of the ankle beyond the neutral position and is relieved by plantarflexion.

Clinical examination usually confirms the diagnosis of retrocalcaneal bursitis; however, when difficulty in diagnosis arises, an MRI and bone scan may be helpful. An MRI will show an enlarged, inflamed bursa (Fig. 4), while a bone scan (Fig. 5) will demonstrate marked increased uptake along the superior wall of the posterior calcaneus.

Treatment

The heel counter must first be inspected. If there is any evidence of extrinsic compression, the foot wear must be modified. Once the extrinsic pressure has been relieved, ice, nonsteroidal anti-inflammatory medication, and a 3/8- to 1-in temporary heel lift may help to relieve the symptoms. Because lower extremity malalignment may be a factor, mechanical problems, such as tibial vara, functional equinus, tight hamstrings or calf muscles, and cavus foot, must be excluded as an aggravating factor. Training mileage should be decreased and the use of a soft, stable running surface encouraged. If the symptoms are not relieved at this point, the ankle and the retrocalcaneal bursa may require immobilization in a short leg cast for 3 to 4 weeks. However, once the cast is removed, the treating physician must be very careful not to incorporate dorsiflexion exercises too rapidly into the physical therapy.

An injection of steroid solution into the retrocalcaneal bursa has been advocated. However, Kennedy and Willis,[23] who reported on the effects of local steroid injection into tendons, found the most significant effect of such an injection to be collagen necrosis, with the return of normal tensile strength not occurring in the tendon for 14 days after the injection. This effect puts the tendon at risk for rupture for a period of 2 weeks postinjection. Even though the injection is into the bursa, not the Achilles tendon, there is always the concern that some of the steroid solution may come in contact with the Achilles tendon. I, personally, avoid this form of treatment.

Historically, three procedures have been advocated for this condition. Ippolito and Ricciardi-Pollini[24] described three patients with this condition. They removed the retrocalcaneal bursa and reported complete clinical relief of symptoms. Keck and Kelley[25] also reported on a series of patients who gained complete relief from simple bursal excision.

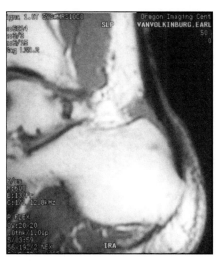

Fig. 4 Inflamed, enlarged retrocalcaneal bursa.

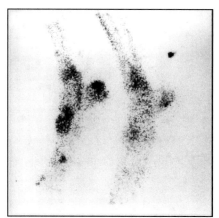

Fig. 5 Increased uptake along superior aspect of calcaneus consistent with retrocalcaneal bursitis.

Zadek[26] advocated a wedge osteotomy of the calcaneus. A dorsally based wedge of calcaneus is removed from the proximal half posteriorly, and the dorsal osteotomy site is closed, thereby foreshortening the calcaneus and theoretically decreasing the pressure across the calcaneal Achilles interface.

Stanley James and I have found that a partial retrocalcaneal ostectomy is a reliable procedure when dealing with this problem.[27] The objective of this procedure is to relieve pain by removing the underlying intrinsic source of irritation and pressure. Because of the associated Achilles tendinitis, bony decompression of the bursal area and distal Achilles tendon is mandatory. For this reason, we do not feel that simple excision of the bursa is adequate.

When surgically treating retrocalcaneal bursitis and Achilles tendinitis, controversy remains relating to the ideal incision. Numerous surgical approaches have been advocated. The most common incision used for this approach is a longitudinal incision parallel to the Achilles tendon. However, a lazy-L, reverse J-shape, and transverse incision also have been suggested. I recommend using two incisions, a parallel medial incision and a

lateral longitudinal incision (Fig. 6). Of a large number of failed retrocalcaneal ostectomies seen in my office, most occurred following the use of a single incision, which in many instances does not allow adequate visualization of the calcaneus and the Achilles tendon.

The technique for partial ostectomy using two incisions is as follows. The patient is placed in a prone position with a bolster placed under the distal leg. Longitudinal incisions are made from the insertion of the Achilles tendon to 7 to 10 cm proximal on either side of the Achilles tendon. Carry the incision distal to the superior portion of the plantar heel skin. Great care is taken to avoid damage to the sural nerve, which lies approximately 1 to 2 cm anterior to the lateral border of the Achilles tendon. The retrocalcaneal area and the superior aspects of the calcaneus are then exposed by a combination of blunt and sharp dissection. Once the tendon has been adequately exposed to the insertion site, which is much more distal than is generally appreciated, an oblique partial ostectomy of the superior angle of the calcaneus is carried out. The ostectomy begins approximately 1 cm anterior to the superior angle and then angles well downward past the point of tenderness.

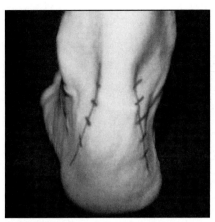

Fig. 6 Double incision technique used for partial retrocalcaneal ostectomy.

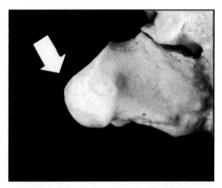

Fig. 7 Ostectomy must be perpendicular to the longitudinal axis of the calcaneus.

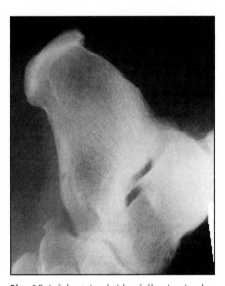

Fig. 8 Painful retained ridge following inadequate partial retrocalcaneal ostectomy.

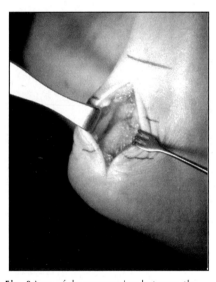

Fig. 9 Area of decompression between the posterior calcaneus and Achilles tendon.

Occasionally, a fairly large piece of posterior calcaneus must be resected in order to decompress the individual area of tendon. Kodziej and Nunley presented a study in which they showed that up to 75% of the length of insertion site may be resected without fear of tendon failure (Kolodziej P, Nunley JA, personal communication).

The reciprocating saw blade must be observed through both incisions so that the cut does not angle to one side or the other, but remains perpendicular to the longitudinal axis of the calcaneus (Fig. 7).

The inflamed bursa is removed in tandem with the bony fragment.

Often a ridge of bone is left at the distal insertion site (Fig. 8). This must be carefully removed with a small curette or rongeur so that no irritating prominence remains below the distal Achilles tendon. Next, the medial and lateral margins of the calcaneus are chamfered with small osteotomes and rasped smooth. The posterior calcaneus is repeatedly palpated through the overlying skin to make certain that all bony ridges and bony prominences are removed. With dorsiflexion of

the ankle, a visible space between the calcaneus and the adjacent Achilles insures adequate decompression (Fig. 9). Prior to closure, the Achilles tendon is inspected for inflamed or necrotic areas that require resection. The wound is closed in a routine fashion over a hemovac. A postoperative film should be taken (Fig. 10).

Insertional Achilles Tendinitis

It is not uncommon in the Masters age group runner to encounter insertional Achilles tendinitis associated with a calcific projection.[22] This projection, frequently referred to as a "fish hook" osteophyte (Fig. 11), is related to an inward angulation of the lower half of the posterior calcaneal tuberosity, which causes the Achilles tendon to begin its insertion at an anatomically low point. The resultant abnormal traction in the lower half of the posterior tuberosity produces a reactive osteosclerosis and formation of a prominent spur. This calcification may become very painful as a result of local pressure and associated Achilles inflammation. At the time of surgery, it is not uncommon to note erosion of the central portion of the Achilles tendon at the site of the fish hook osteophyte. Therefore, the pain in this condition is caused not only by extrinsic pressure on a prominent calcaneal spur, but also by the associated Achilles tendinitis and erosion.

A long period of conservative care is essential before considering surgery. We have found the previously mentioned conservative forms of care to be beneficial. In addition, in recalcitrant cases, I find that immobilizing the foot and ankle in a short leg walking cast is frequently beneficial.

If surgery is necessary, great care must be taken with skin retraction, because this condition usually occurs in older individuals and skin necrosis and wound breakdown are serious threats. If adequate circulation is present, two incisions may be used for the purpose of debridement, as in the cases of retrocalcaneal bursa treat-

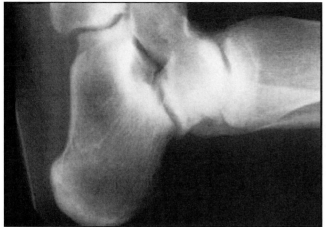

Fig. 10 Pre- and postoperative film.

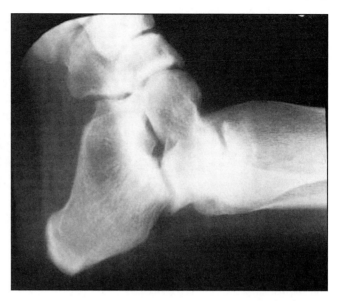

ment. Baxter and Thigpen,[28] who use a single longitudinal central incision for debridement, have found the results satisfactory.

Superficial Peritendinous Achilles Bursitis (pump bumps)

Superficial peritendinous Achilles bursitis develops secondary to chronic inflammation caused by direct compression from shoes or blunt trauma. As mentioned in the discussion on anatomy, this bursa is present only 50% of the time. The location of the bursa corresponds to the upper edge of the offending shoe heel counter. It is not uncommon to see associated thickened and inflamed skin overlying the irritated superficial bursa. Clinically, it is important to realize that this pump bump may exist with or without underlying intrinsic pressure from a hyperconvex retrocalcaneal tuberosity. A bony prominence of this sort is best evaluated radiographically.

Conservative measures are almost always effective. A 3/16-in heel lift and modification of the shoe heel counter will usually suffice. The heel counter may be raised, lowered, or softened in an attempt to decrease the direct pressure and irritation.

If surgery is warranted, the offending prominent superior portion of the calcaneus can usually be removed through a single incision.

Heel Pain

The most common causes of heel pain in the runner are plantar fasciitis, nerve entrapment about the heel, and fat pad trauma/atrophy. These disabling entities are most frequently seen in distance runners, because most distance runners are midfoot strikers, while most sprinters are forefoot strikers.

Plantar Fasciitis

Plantar fasciitis is a term used to describe a painful condition located about the posterior medial surface of the foot just distal to the attachment of the plantar fascia to the calcaneus. It is caused by microtears and chronic inflammation where the plantar fascia attaches to the medial tubercle of the calcaneus.

During the early phase of plantar fasciitis, the symptoms occur gradually and are of relatively low intensity. However, as the patient continues to train, the pain becomes more noticeable and can cause serious disability for the athlete. The patient gives a history of

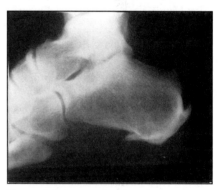

Fig. 11 Calcific insertional tendinosis, the "fish hook" osteophyte.

severe pain in the morning upon rising. The pain decreases with initial walking activities; however, it quickly returns with activities such as walking on hard surfaces, prolonged running, or climbing. If the athlete continues to run despite the pain, the gait pattern is usually altered. In order to decrease the stress on the plantar fascia, the foot assumes a fixed supinated and inverted posture from foot strike to toe-off. Because of overloading of the lateral column of the foot in this supinated position, the runner may also develop lateral foot pain.

Physical examination usually reveals maximum tenderness over the medial edge of the plantar fascia just distal to its insertion into the calcaneus. Interestingly, considerable pressure may be required to locate the exact area of tenderness.

Tightness of the Achilles tendon is frequently noted in this condition. Leg-length inequality may also be a precipitating factor. If one leg is longer than the other, heel pain is more frequently seen in the shorter leg.

Conservative Treatment As with most running injuries, the cornerstone of nonsurgical treatment is alteration of training. Cycling and deep water running activities are effective in maintaining the cardiovascular fitness of the athlete and produce very little stress across the inflamed plantar fascia. In addition to these low impact cardiovascular workouts, abbreviated running workouts may also be continued. A stretching program, ice massage, and nonsteroidal anti-inflammatory medication are also recommended. The use of a night splint that holds the foot in 5° of dorsiflexion has also been helpful. Because the night splint prevents the foot from lying in the equinus position during sleep, the plantar fascia is not allowed to contract. Therefore, the hindfoot is much less painful in the morning. In recalcitrant cases, short-term full immobilization in a short leg walking cast is recommended. If a biomechanical abnormality such as hyperpronation, miserable malalignment, or a rigid cavus deformity is identified, orthoses are recommended.

In patients with continuing refractory symptoms, a steroid injection may be beneficial. However, great care must be taken when injecting this area with steroid solution. Multiple steroid injections may predispose the runner to plantar fascia rupture, which is not a benign complication. Disruption of the plantar fascia attachment from the calcaneus may have a detrimental effect on function. Daly and associates[29] demonstrated a change in both arch height and the ratio of arch height to arch length following complete plantar fascia release. With complete fascial rupture, increased compressive forces are transmitted to the dorsal aspect of the midfoot, while decreased flexion forces occur across the metatarsal phalangeal joint complex. Midfoot pain and metatarsalgia can result.

Surgical Treatment If the patient has 10 to 12 months of pain recalcitrant to conservative treatment, surgery is an option. An oblique incision 3 to 4 cm in length is made just distal and medial to the heel pad, near the junction of the thicker plantar heel pad skin. This incision must be anterior to the medial calcaneal branch of the posterior tibial nerve. Inadvertent injury to this branch of the posterior tibial nerve will result in a postoperative neuroma. Dissection proceeds through subcutaneous tissue. The medial and lateral borders of the proximal plantar fascia are identified. The medial 50% of the plantar fascia is incised 1 to 2 cm distal to its origin from the calcaneus. If a large heel spur is present, it may be removed. If a smaller heel spur is present, the more extensive dissection required for its excision is not indicated. Surgical removal of this heel spur is controversial, because numerous studies have indicated that such spurs play very little role in pain associated with plantar fasciitis.[29,30]

The tourniquet is released and hemostasis established. The wound is closed with interrupted sutures. Postoperatively, the patient is kept nonweightbearing for 1 week. Progressive weightbearing in a postoperative shoe is allowed as tolerated 1 week postoperatively. The sutures are removed in 10 to 14 days. No repetitive impact loading activities are allowed for a total of 6 weeks. It is not unusual for the rehabilitation process to take up to 3 months before the patient is able to carry out high-impact loading activities.

Nerve Entrapments About the Heel

Heel pain can also result from nerve entrapment syndromes. Perhaps the best known nerve entrapment syndrome in this area is tarsal tunnel syndrome. Tarsal tunnel syndrome is characterized by neurogenic pain described as burning in nature. In differentiating tarsal tunnel syndrome from plantar fasciitis, there is no tenderness over the medial tubercle in tarsal tunnel syndrome, but there is a positive Tinel sign over the posterior tibial nerve as it passes under the laciniate ligament. Nerve conduction studies are also quite helpful in making the diagnosis.

The most frequent nerve entrapment syndrome causing heel pain in the runner is entrapment of the first branch of the lateral plantar nerve.[31,32] Entrapment of this nerve occurs as the nerve changes from a vertical to a horizontal direction and passes under the heavy deep fascia of the abductor hallucis muscle. The abductor hallucis muscle is frequently hypertrophied in runners, which contributes to the entrapment process. The pathognomonic sign of entrapment of the first branch of the lateral plantar nerve is tenderness along its course, in association with burning, shooting pain from the ankle to the heel. No numbness is present with this entrapment process. Unlike plantar fasciitis, there is no early morning pain and no increase in symptoms when the patient arises after a prolonged period of sitting. Although no cutaneous sensory deficit occurs, motor weakness of the abductor digiti quinti may occasionally be detected. However, electrodiagnostic studies, electromyography, and nerve conduction studies are not helpful in making a diagnosis of entrapment of the first branch of the lateral nerve.[28,33-35]

Conservative Treatment Conservative treatment for athletes with this problem consists of modification of running activities, contrast baths, nonsteroidal anti-inflammatory medication, and ice massage. As with plantar fasciitis, if excessive pronation is present, a semi-rigid orthosis may decrease the stresses across the compressed nerve.

Baxter and Thigpen[28] have shown an 82% success rate in patients with this condition treated surgically. Baxter and Pfeffer[34] published a series that included 59 heels in 53 patients, with 89% excellent or good results following surgery.

Surgical Treatment A 4- to 5-cm oblique incision is made over the proximal abductor hallucis muscle, with the incision centered along the course of the first branch of the lateral plantar nerve. As with all incisions in this area, care must be taken to avoid damage to the medial calcaneal sensory nerve branches, which course posterior to this incision. The superficial fascia of the abductor hallucis muscle is exposed. This fascia is then divided. The abductor muscle belly is retracted superiorly with a right-angle retractor. The deep fascia of the abductor hallucis is exposed. The inferior edge of the deep fascia is incised, exposing the area where the nerve is compressed between this tight fascia and the medial border of the quadratus plantae muscle. Care should be taken to completely divide the fascia from inferior to superior. If the heel spur is felt to add additional compression to the nerve, it is removed as well. Leave the abductor hallucis muscle belly intact. At this point, the nerve should be thoroughly decompressed and a small hemostat should fit easily along the course of the nerve without impingement dorsally or plantarward. The plantar fascia is not incised unless there are associated symptoms of plantar fasciitis or the medial edge of the plantar fascia is compressing the nerve. Return to activities varies between 4 to 12 weeks.

Heel Pad Pain

Fat pad atrophy in the athlete can result from multiple steroid injections or repeated trauma. The pain is usually quite diffuse. There is no morning pain as seen in plantar fasciitis, and there is no neurogenic pain as seen in nerve entrapment syndromes.

On clinical examination, the heel paid is usually quite flat and relatively thin. Unfortunately, there is no surgical treatment for this entity. Treatment consists of cushioned heel cups and shock-absorbent sneakers or inserts. In some cases, a plastic heel cup may be helpful.

References

1. Clement DB, Taunton JE, Smart GW: Achilles tendinitis and peritendinitis: Etiology and treatment. *Am J Sports Med* 1984;12:179–184.

2. Krissoff WB, Ferris WD: Runners' injuries. *Phys Sports Med* 1979;7:55–64.

3. Jones DC, James SL: Overuse injuries of the lower extremity: Shin splints, iliotibial band friction syndrome, and exertional compartment syndromes. *Clin Sports Med* 1987;6:273–290.

4. Welsh RP, Clodman J: Clinical survey of Achilles tendinitis in athletes. *Can Med Assoc J* 1980;122:193–195.

5. Denstad TF, Roaas A: Surgical treatment of partial Achilles tendon rupture. *Am J Sports Med* 1979;7:15–17.

6. Nelen G, Martens M, Burssens A: Surgical treatment of chronic Achilles tendinitis. *Am J Sports Med* 1989;17:754–759.

7. Puddu G, Ippolito E, Postacchini F: A classification of Achilles tendon disease. *Am J Sports Med* 1976;4:145–150.

8. Arner O, Lindholm A, Lindvall N: Roentgen changes in subcutaneous rupture of the Achilles tendon. *Acta Chir Scand* 1959;116:496–500.

9. Gillies H, Chalmers J: The management of fresh ruptures of the tendo Achillis. *J Bone Joint Surg* 1970;52A:337–343.

10. Inglis AE, Sculco TP: Surgical repair of ruptures of the tendo Achillis. *Clin Orthop* 1981;156:160–169.

11. Lotke PA: Ossification of the Achilles tendon: Report of seven cases. *J Bone Joint Surg* 1970;52A:157–160.

12. Cummins EJ, Anson BJ, Carr BW, et al: The structure of the calcaneal tendon (of Achilles) in relation to orthopedic surgery: With additional observations on the plantaris muscle. *Surg Gynecol Obstet* 1946;83:107–116.

13. Clancy WG Jr, Neidhart D, Brand RL: Achilles tendonitis in runners: A report of five cases. *Am J Sports Med* 1976;4:46–57.

14. Buchbinder MR, Napora NJ, Biggs EW: The relationship of abnormal pronation to chondromalacia of the patella in distance runners. *J Am Podiatry Assoc* 1979;69:159–162.

15. James SL, Bates BT, Osternig LR: Injuries to runners. *Am J Sports Med* 1978;6:40–50.

16. Bates BT, Osternig LR, Mason MS, et al: Foot orthotic devices to modify selected aspects of

17. Cavanagh PR (ed): *The Running Shoe Book*. Mountain View, CA, Anderson World, 1980.

18. Clarke TE, Frederick EC, Cooper LB: Biomechanical measurement of running shoe cushioning properties, in Nigg BM, Kerr BA (eds): *Biomechanical Aspects of Sports Shoes and Playing Surfaces*. Calgary, Canada, University of Calgary, 1983, pp 25–34.

19. Fox JM, Blazina ME, Jobe FW, et al: Degeneration and rupture of the Achilles tendon. *Clin Orthop* 1975;107:221–224.

20. Lynn TA: Repair of the torn Achilles tendon, using the plantaris tendon as a reinforcing membrane. *J Bone Joint Surg* 1966;48A:268–272.

21. Canoso JJ, Wohlgethan JR, Newberg AH, et al: Aspiration of the retrocalcaneal bursa. *Ann Rheum Dis* 1984;43:308–312.

22. Turlik MA: Seronegative arthritis as a cause of heel pain. *Clin Podiatr Med Surg* 1990;7:369–375.

23. Kennedy JC, Willis RB: The effects of local steroid injections on tendons: A biomechanical and microscopic correlative study. *Am J Sports Med* 1976;4:11–21.

24. Ippolito E, Ricciardi-Pollini PT: Invasive retrocalcaneal bursitis: A report of three cases. *Foot Ankle* 1984;4:204–208.

25. Keck SW, Kelly PJ: Bursitis of the posterior part of the heel: Evaluation of surgical treatment of eighteen patients. *J Bone Joint Surg* 1965;47A:267–273.

26. Zadek I: An operation for the cure of achillobursitis. *Am J Surg* 1939;43:542–546.

27. Jones DC, James SL: Partial calcaneal ostectomy for retrocalcaneal bursitis. *Am J Sports Med* 1984;12:72–73.

28. Baxter DE, Thigpen CM: Heel pain: Operative results. *Foot Ankle* 1984;5:16–25.

29. Daly PJ, Kitaoka HB, Chao EY: Plantar fasciotomy for intractable plantar fasciitis: Clinical results and biomechanical evaluation. *Foot Ankle* 1992;13:188–195.

30. Sarrafian SK: Functional characteristics of the foot and plantar aponeurosis under tibiotalar loading. *Foot Ankle* 1987;8:4–18.

31. Rubin G, Witten M: Plantar calcaneal spurs. *Am J Orthop* 1963;5:38–41;53–55.

32. Lapidus PW, Guidotti FP: Painful heel: Report of 323 patients with 364 painful heels. *Clin Orthop* 1965;39:178–186.

33. Kenzora JE: The painful heel syndrome: An entrapment neuropathy. *Bull Hosp Jt Dis Orthop Inst* 1987;47:178–189.

34. Baxter DE, Pfeffer GB: Treatment of chronic heel pain by surgical release of the first branch of the lateral plantar nerve. *Clin Orthop* 1992;279:229–236.

35. Schon LC, Glennon TP, Baxter DE: Heel pain syndrome: Electrodiagnostic support for nerve entrapment. *Foot Ankle* 1993;14:129–135.

lower extremity mechanics. *Am J Sports Med* 1979;7:338.

Achilles Tendon Ruptures

Mark S. Myerson, MD

Acute Ruptures

Etiology and Epidemiology

Why do the majority of acute ruptures of the Achilles tendon occur in males? On evaluation of our institutional experience, the male-to-female ratio is 30:1, somewhat higher than that previously reported[1] where the ratio was noted to range between 2:1 and 19:1. This may reflect a difference in the sporting activity of our patient population, because it has been repeatedly documented that more than 75% of Achilles tendon ruptures occur during sports activity in patients between the ages of 30 and 40 years.[2] These statistics contrast with a more recent study from Copenhagen of 209 patients with Achilles tendon rupture over an 18-year period. In these patients there were ruptures in 55 women and 158 men, with a median age of 41 years.[3] Yet it should not be assumed that because ruptures occur predominantly during athletic activity that it is the latter which precipitates the rupture, because the incidence of Achilles tendon ruptures is much more common in industrialized countries, where lifestyles are generally sedentary and where the interest in recreational athletics has suddenly increased.[2,4] There appears to have been a dramatic change in the incidence of Achilles tendon ruptures over the past 40 years, but this increase has occurred predominantly

in developed countries. Interestingly, Achilles tendon ruptures are a rarity in developing countries, especially in Africa and East Asia. In Hungary, the number of patients with an Achilles tendon rupture increased 285% in men and 500% in women between two successive 7-year periods.[5] The stereotypical Achilles rupture therefore seems to occur in the adult male who is not well conditioned and does not participate regularly in sports, although rupture usually occurs during some athletic activity.

In addition to this epidemiologic data, there are likely biologic and mechanical events that precede rupture. Clearly, tendon degeneration occurs as a result of a combination of hypovascularity and repetitive microtrauma, resulting in diffuse tendon degeneration and ultimately rupture.[6,7] Regeneration with tendon healing cannot occur due to the recurrent microtrauma, and this condition is worsened by underlying hypovascularity, substantiated by the fact that the vast majority of ruptures occur 4 to 6 cm proximal to the insertion of the tendon, where the blood supply to the tendon is poor.[8] In addition to these underlying problems, a critical load must be applied to the tendon, resulting in rupture. This is well identified clinically, because the majority of ruptures occur during a sudden push-off during some sporting activity. Different stresses may precipitate

rupture, including pushing off with the weightbearing forefoot while extending the knee joint, as in sprinting, running, and jumping. Unexpected dorsiflexion of the ankle (which occurs, for example, when slipping is associated with a sudden deceleration when falling forward as well as more abrupt dorsiflexion on a plantarflexed foot when jumping from a height) will cause a rupture. The critical threshold for rupture, however, is not clear, although in addition to the factors identified above, genetics, the neuroendocrine environment, and growth factors also play a role. In addition, there are histopathologic changes, including hypoxic degeneration, mucoid degeneration, and calcifying tendinopathy, that occur in association with rupture. These factors may have some relevance for patients who sustain a rupture, because there is an increased likelihood of contralateral rupture when compared with the general population, and antecedent Achilles tendinitis occurs in 15% of patients who sustain a rupture.[9]

The use of corticosteroids, orally or injectable, has been associated with collagen necrosis and an increased incidence of rupture.[10] Despite this latter well-known fact, patients with various forms of Achilles tendinitis continue to receive steroid injection. In addition to corticosteroids, anabolic steroids and fluoroquinolone antibiotics have been shown to cause collagen dysplasia and reduced tensile strength of the Achilles tendon.[11] Other reported causes of tendon rupture include gout,[12] hyperthyroidism and renal insufficiency,[13] and arteriosclerosis.[14] It would be of some benefit to identify patients at risk for Achilles rupture, particularly those who experience chronic pain as a result of tendinitis. This pain is often a sign of progressive degeneration of the tendon, which can lead to its rupture. The clinical course and sonograms were studied prospectively in 36 patients with chronic degenerative tendinosis to find a prognostic parameter predictive of rupture. Analysis of the tendons that subsequently ruptured exhibited high-grade thickening, and these patients with sonographic findings had a worse clinical outcome after nonsurgical treatment. In this study, 28% of patients with thickening of the tendon associated with chronic pain had a spontaneous rupture.[15]

In summary, the Achilles tendon ruptures as a result of a sequence of events that is based on an underlying hypovascularity, resulting in localized degeneration and weakening of the tendon, which somehow lowers the tendon threshold for rupture. The precise position and load that causes the injury remains obscure, but it is probably a complex equation of neuromuscular control and external factors, including the applied load to the foot.

Diagnosis

Most patients present with a typical history, and describe an audible snap as if someone hit them in the back of the ankle. Although push-off strength is markedly compromised, the diagnosis of the acute rupture is surprisingly not always made, due in part to the strength of the remaining muscles

of plantarflexion. The combination of the use of all of the plantarflexor muscles, including the flexor hallucis longus (FHL) and flexor digitorum longus (FDL), and the posterior tibial and peroneal muscles, provides some strength for walking. Yet while patients are able to walk, and perhaps even function with respect to some activities of daily living, push-off strength is markedly compromised. Individuals are unable to perform a single or, even less likely, a repetitive heel rise, and activities that require greater amounts of push-off strength (including ascending and descending stairs, running, and jumping) are generally not possible. In addition to the acute pain and swelling, a limp and plantarflexion weakness are present on examination. The rupture commonly occurs approximately 4 cm proximal to the insertion of the tendon, and although avulsion of the calcaneus may occur, it is relatively uncommon unless antecedent insertional tendinitis has been present. A defect or indentation of the posterior tendon is either visible or palpable if there is not too much swelling of the limb present, and the diagnosis is always confirmed by a positive Thompson test.[16] In this test, the affected calf is squeezed, and a positive test indicates discontinuity of the muscle with the heel because loss of passive plantarflexion of the foot is present.

Imaging studies are not necessary as part of the diagnostic work-up for rupture. If one suspects an avulsion of the tendon off the insertion, a lateral radiograph may show a small fracture, and therefore may be helpful with respect to preoperative planning. Magnetic resonance imaging (MRI) is not necessary to make the diagnosis and does not seem to have a role in planning treatment. Ultrasonography has been used as a technique for defi-

nition of Achilles tendon pathology and rupture,[17] and although I have not found that this test is necessary to make the diagnosis, it may be useful when nonsurgical treatment is contemplated. Ultrasound can accurately determine the gap between tendon ends. The test is performed with the foot held in passive plantarflexion, noting whether the tendon ends approximate. If there is adequate apposition between the tendon ends, nonsurgical treatment may have a greater likelihood of success, and for the appropriately selected individual this remains a useful test. Richter and associates[18] demonstrated that functional treatment of the rupture in a brace without surgery is possible through careful sonographic analysis of the patients with Achilles rupture.

Treatment Alternatives

As part of the decision-making process for treatment, one should define the various functional goals and activities of daily living for each individual. While it may be argued that maximum and expeditious resumption of athletic activity may only reasonably be accomplished with surgical treatment, accurate parameters must be used to evaluate the success of treatment. To provide a valid means of comparison, all clinical parameters including pain, stiffness, muscle weakness, footwear restrictions, as well as range of motion of the ankle and isokinetic calf muscle strength, should be included as part of the patient evaluation process. The majority of these injuries occur in the setting of some athletic activity, and a prompt return to their sport may be important to the successful outcome of treatment. In 1993, Cetti and associates[19] showed that there were significantly fewer complaints 1 year after the injury in patients treated surgically. In a prospective randomized study of 111 patients with acute rupture, they found that those treated surgically had significantly higher rates of resuming sports activities at the same level, a lesser degree of calf atrophy, better ankle movement, and fewer complaints. Mandelbaum and associates[9] demonstrated a 92% return to sports by 6 months with a 2.6% deficit on isokinetic testing. Neumann and associates[20] demonstrated permanent kinematic and neuromuscular changes of the gait pattern after Achilles tendon rupture that was treated surgically but that included immobilization in a cast after surgery. Although these studies provide some insight into the outcome of treatment, a general lack of a standardized method for subjective and objective assessment of these injuries limits interpretation of the data reported in the literature. For the future, prospectively designed studies using standard and accepted tools will become most important to further assess patient selection for treatment protocols.

Nonsurgical Versus Surgical Management

The pendulum towards surgical or nonsurgical management of Achilles tendon ruptures has shifted repeatedly this century, and these swings are likely to continue.[21-24] Although there have been attempts to compare the results of patients treated surgically with those managed nonsurgically, the methods of patient evaluation have not been adequate, and, although many reports found that better results occurred in the surgical groups, the majority of studies were not randomized or carefully controlled.[25,26] Helgeland and associates[27] prospectively evaluated 38 patients with Achilles rupture whose treatment was randomized to surgical and nonsurgical treatment. They identified a markedly increased incidence

of complications after nonsurgical treatment. In particular, they noted that for these patients the plantarflexion range was markedly reduced in the injured foot when compared with the opposite foot, and there were also reduced muscle strength and an increased rate of rerupture in those treated without surgery.[27]

The methods of immobilization and rehabilitation used after surgery or nonsurgical treatment generally involved the use of prolonged casting with limited bearing of weight. After long immobilization periods in equinus after surgical treatment of Achilles tendon rupture, long-lasting motor patterns in functional movement have been identified. Thermann and associates[28] identified, in a experimental biomechanical model in rabbits, the results of surgical compared with functional nonsurgical treatment in a specially designed orthosis taped to the limb of the rabbit. They found that there were no significant biomechanical differences after 3 months, and when compared with the results reported in the literature for cast immobilization, their functional treatment resulted in a significantly faster course of healing. Neumann and associates[20] documented alterations in gait pattern, noting kinematic and neuromuscular changes 1 year after surgery and neuromuscular deficits. As a result of the noted complications after surgery, various studies began to support nonsurgical management of Achilles ruptures,[25,26] culminating in an editorial in 1973 that stated, ". . . in view of the excellent results obtainable by conservative treatment, it is doubtful whether surgical repair in closed rupture of the Achilles tendon can be justified."[29] However, over the past decade, numerous advances have been made with respect to both sur-

gical techniques and rehabilitation modalities in the entire field of sports-related injury. As a result of these technical and therapeutic improvements, studies began to demonstrate superior results with surgical repair.[19,30,31] During the last 20 years, as patient expectations and functional goals have increased, surgical options have gained acceptance and popularity. In keeping with these patient goals, the recent emphasis has focused on aggressive postoperative protocols after surgical treatment, with early weightbearing and controlled range-of-motion exercises. These latter postoperative treatment programs avoid cast immobilization and were found to be well tolerated, safe, and effective. Although these studies reported superior outcomes and demonstrated particular value for well-motivated patients and athletes, it is still unclear whether or not the results of these treatment protocols apply to all patients, or are limited to those who especially desire the highest functional outcome. Perhaps as improved methods of patient evaluation and the results of randomized prospective studies emerge, the pendulum will swing back toward nonsurgical methods of treatment. At the present time, however, it is our practice to limit nonsurgical treatment to the sick patient, the sedentary individual, or those with very limited functional and athletic goals.

The controversy regarding surgical and nonsurgical treatment alternatives does not end here, because, once a decision is made to perform surgery, it is necessary to choose from a plethora of technical alternatives for this repair. Any method of repair should perfectly restore continuity of the ruptured tendon ends, have them heal in a physiologic position, and restore normal dynamic muscle function. This goal is not always easy to accomplish, given the multiple strands of the tendon after the acute rupture, and this problem becomes more marked with percutaneous methods of repair. Perhaps the most important aspect of surgical repair, regardless of the method of suture used, is the accurate tensioning of the repair and establishing the exact dynamic resting length of the tendon. A repair may not be considered successful if the tendon-muscle-tendon unit is too short, and the foot is positioned in equinus. From a functional standpoint however, over-lengthening of the Achilles is worse, and severely compromises push-off strength. It is for this reason that one must view the results of percutaneous methods of repair with some scepticism, because the tendon ends can never be accurately apposed.

Bunnell[32] and Kessler[33] were the first to popularize the end-to-end suture technique for ruptured tendons. In 1977, Ma and Griffith[34] described a percutaneous repair, and although this method remains popular, there is an unacceptable incidence of sural nerve injury, a less than anatomic positioning of the tendon, and a higher incidence of rerupture. Various other methods of suture have been advocated, including a 3-bundle suture technique,[12] a suture weave,[35] a 6-strand-suture technique,[36] and the use of external fixation techniques.[22]

In addition to direct repair of the tendon, various augmentation techniques have been described to supplement the strength of the repair using part of the gastrocnemius fascia or the plantaris tendon, if the latter is present. The gastrocnemius may be used as an aponeurosis flap, performed as a slide of the superficial fascia overlying the muscle,[21] or rotation of 1 or 2 central flaps of fascia.[37] The use of the plantaris makes sense

when considering augmentation of a primary repair, because the direct repair may be followed by a weave of the plantaris through the Achilles tendon. Alternatively, the plantaris tendon may be used to prevent adhesion formation between the skin and the repaired tendon by fanning it out to use as a thin fascial membrane covering the repair.[37] All these methods aim to improve the continuity and strength of the repair construct, but in practice, the need for these augmentation procedures is not necessary to treat the acute rupture, because apposition of the tendon ends is always possible, and with appropriate suture techniques, reinforcement should not be required.

In addition to these methods of repair, more extensive techniques of reconstruction have been described using the fascia lata,[38] peroneus brevis,[39] FDL,[40] or FHL.[41] These reconstructive procedures are not necessary for treatment of the acute rupture, and they are discussed in more detail below with respect to management of chronic neglected ruptures. The use of various exogenous materials to reinforce the primary repair of the Achilles tendon have been reported, including carbon fiber,[42] marlex mesh,[14] dacron grafts,[43] and polypropylene braids,[44] but these are of historical interest only.

Surgical Technique

Regardless of the method of surgery selected, the surgeon should select a safe and effective procedure, one that will allow the patient to accomplish realistic goals in a timely manner. I prefer to delay surgery for approximately 1 week after rupture. The reduction of swelling prior to commencement of surgery is important in order to minimize the potential for problems with wound closure and infection. Not only does the swelling

decrease by this time, but the apposition of the tendon ends becomes easier, because some consolidation of the tendon ends occurs during this time, making the repair technically easier. Before this time, although surgery may be performed and accomplished satisfactorily, the tendon ends are very frayed, and establishing the correct tension on the tendon ends may be difficult. Surgery is performed with the patient in the prone position, and although any anesthesia may be used, my preference is to administer local anesthesia. In most cases, both feet are prepared as part of the operative field to permit accurate side-to-side comparison of the resting dynamic tension of the repaired tendon. An anteromedial incision is made along the length of the paratenon and the Achilles tendon, extending to the musculotendinous junction. Each end of the tear is sutured with 1 or 2 strands of a #2 nonabsorbable material using a modified whip-suture technique. It is important not to include too much tendon in each pass of the suture, so as to avoid potential tendon compression and necrosis.

The most important aspect of surgical repair, regardless of the method of suture used, is to correctly tension the tendon, and this can be facilitated by carefully commencing the suture at the correct position on the tendon. Insertion of the suture should not begin at the end of the frayed portion of the tendon ends. The tendon should be laid down with the frayed ends apposed to get a sense of the correct position of the repair, and then the suture strands should be inserted. Before tying the sutures, each strand is pulled to obtain a sense of the correct tension, and then this position is compared with the opposite limb. It is for this reason that I find that it is useful to include the opposite limb in the operative field to allow adequate comparison of the resting tension on both tendons while in the prone position. The sutures are then tied, with the knots passed to the anterior aspect of the tendon and secured. Wound closure after Achilles repair is generally difficult, and it is worsened by the swelling and bulk of the repaired tendon in the subcutaneous position, which creates tension on the skin edges and increases the likelihood of wound complications. To minimize this tension, I perform a fasciotomy of the posterior compartment of the leg, which increases the horizontal or cross-sectional diameter of the subcutaneous tissues and facilitates skin closure. If the plantaris tendon is present, it is used to cover the tendon repair. I have not found that it is necessary to augment the repair; however, the plantaris can be unravelled and used to create a thin layer over the repair to prevent adhesion formation between the tendon and the skin. The paratenon should be closed with 4-0 absorbable suture, and the ankle is taken through a complete range of motion to evaluate the stability of the repair. The wound is closed with interrupted nylon mattress sutures, and a posterior splint is applied with the foot positioned in neutral dorsiflexion.

Rehabilitation After Surgery

Historically, prolonged cast immobilization was used to treat ruptures when either surgical or nonsurgical methods were used. However, the use of a cast increases the likelihood of muscle atrophy, joint stiffness, cartilage atrophy, degenerative arthritis, adhesion formation, and deep venous thrombosis. In contrast, limb and joint mobilization limits muscle atrophy,[45] promotes fiber polymerization to collagen,[46] fosters an increased

organization of collagen in the repair site that leads to increased strength,[47] and increases tendon and muscle strength.[48] In addition to the biologic effects of immobilization, there are permanent deficits of the Achilles tendon, which can be demonstrated with isokinetic testing.[26,49–51] More recent work has emphasized early range of motion of the foot after surgery without the use of a cast. Mandelbaum and associates[9] reported on 29 athletes who were started early range-of-motion and conditioning programs postoperatively. By 6 weeks, 90% of the patients had full range of motion, and by 6 months, 92% returned to sports participation, and on isokinetic testing at 6 months these patients had no more than an average of 2.9% deficit in plantarflexion strength. Functional rehabilitation, which includes early motion and weightbearing, therefore appears to be safe and highly effective at returning athletes and other patients to activities of daily life and sport with the highest level of function. Other authors have since documented similar successes with immediate movement of the ankle and foot after surgical treatment, with no increase in wound complications, and a marked decrease in the formation of skin adhesions to the tendon scar. Motta and associates[52] reported on 78 physically active patients who were treated after surgery with early assisted movement of the ankle and foot with excellent results.

I therefore advocate initiation of weightbearing and range of motion once the sutures are removed, between 10 and 14 days after surgery, in a hinged range-of-motion walker boot that permits motion of the ankle. The hinge is set to permit full plantarflexion, but with a stop to dorsiflexion at the neutral position, and the boot is worn for 8 weeks. The

therapy program begins almost immediately, permitting range of motion and progressive exercise with accelerated weightbearing. During the early phases of rehabilitation, patients are encouraged to increase weightbearing. Riding a bicycle is permitted at 3 weeks, exercise in a pool by 4 weeks, and by 8 weeks, push-off strengthening is started with a stair-climbing device. By the beginning of the third month, the patient begins single-toe heel rises, jogging, and a general increase in push-off strengthening activities. Because overuse and fatigue can occur at any time, attention to symptoms of overuse during the retraining phase is essential.

The technique described above applies to ruptures that occur proximal to the insertion, with a sufficient stump distally for suture. In those cases in which the tendon is avulsed from the calcaneus, the tendon is reattached to the bone with a suture anchor. There is generally sufficient tendon on the medial and lateral margins of the posterior calcaneus for additional insertion of sutures, but this should not be relied upon. The postoperative routine is similar after this method of repair, although it is necessary to be aware of the increased potential for failure of the suture construct.

Complications

The reported incidence of complications after Achilles tendon repair varies considerably, although the largest review included 775 ruptures treated surgically with an incidence of 20% of complications, many of which were quite minor.[24] Complications include skin necrosis, wound infection, sural neuroma, and adhesion of the skin to the repaired tendon. Although the reported incidence of rerupture of the tendon is considerably higher after nonsurgical treatment, in my experience, the incomplete return of function and performance is more common and problematic. Perhaps the single largest problem of nonsurgical treatment is the inability to establish functional continuity of the tendon with a normal dynamic resting length of the tendon maintained. Theoretically, many of the complications of cast immobilization may be eliminated by commencing early weightbearing in a functional boot, allowing some active and passive plantarflexion of the foot. The potential for failure of nonsurgical treatment must be weighed against the increased possibility of infection, anesthetic problems, and wound dehiscence after surgery.

Infection can be a disastrous complication because the options for soft-tissue coverage over the Achilles tendon are very limited.[53] The problem is that large skin and soft-tissue defects over the Achilles tendon are difficult to treat because of the relative avascularity of the adjacent tissue and the likelihood of exposed tendon. Split-thickness skin grafts rarely are suitable, because the take over the exposed tendon is unlikely. Although local flaps are described and possible, the donor site is often unsightly and associated with unacceptable scarring. If a wound problem is encountered, weightbearing should be limited, and the limb should be elevated to reduce tissue swelling. Oral antibiotics are invariably sufficient, and wound debridements should be kept to a minimum to avoid inadvertent exposure of the Achilles. I use Silvadene ointment applied liberally over the incision until granulation tissue is present, at which time wet-to-dry dressings with saline may be used. The patient may get the wound wet in a shower, but not soak the limb in a tub, and after cleansing with soap and water, Silvadene is applied to cover the entire exposed tissue. Fortunately, this complication occurs relatively infrequently, yet even with exposed tendon, this method of wound care is effective, and rarely are local or free flaps necessary to solve the problem. When the defect is larger, a free microvascular flap will lead to acceptable coverage and function.[53] If a deep infection occurs, all the sutures must be removed, and hopefully some revascularization of the tendon will occur with healing, albeit in a compromised position. Other problems, such as scarring of the skin to the incision, have been minimized by the ambulatory program outlined above, but if problematic, various physical therapy modalities are used to decrease scarring and adhesion formation to the skin. If rerupture occurs, it is usually within the first 4 to 6 months after initiation of treatment. I have never encountered this problem with the surgical treatment and rehabilitation program outlined above, but the potential for complications exists and each requires special treatment, as described earlier.

Chronic Ruptures

Patients who sustain a rupture of the Achilles tendon are ideally treated expeditiously after injury, whether the treatment chosen is functional brace treatment or surgery.[25,30,31] Various terms, including the neglected or the missed rupture, have been applied to delayed diagnosis and treatment. As described above, I prefer to delay treatment for 1 or 2 weeks, when some fibrous reorganization of the tendon ends occur and there is less swelling present, before performing surgery. Certainly, if the rupture is diagnosed within the first few weeks of injury, this is not a neglected rupture, nor is it likely that any functional deficit will be experienced by this minimal delay. Boyden and associates[54] compared the results of early and later repair of Achilles rupture in 21 patients, but did not find significant differences between the 2 groups, who were treated before or after 6 weeks following injury. However, substantial losses of function were noted in both groups on isokinetic and isometric testing, which were notably worse than those recently reported. It is difficult to draw a conclusion regarding the timing of surgery with respect to these patients because a functional method of recovery with early weightbearing and rehabilitation was not used for any of these patients.[54]

It is likely that if treatment is delayed for 6 weeks after rupture, the expected outcome cannot parallel the results had the repair been performed more expeditiously, although this depends on the extent of the gap between the tendon ends and the potential for muscle recovery. Two weeks after rupture, the gap between the torn tendon ends begins to fill with fibrous scar tissue, which does not have the same contractile strength as the normal tendon. The fibroblasts are disorganized and not longitudinally oriented, and this scar will gradually stretch and elongate because it is unable to withstand the tensile forces applied by the gastrocnemius-soleus complex. Although the tendon may occasionally heal in continuity, albeit in an elongated position, a long-standing rupture more commonly results in a gap, the length of which is determined by the amount of retraction of the proximal stump. The extent to which the patient perceives this as a problem depends on his or her activities of daily living, because some patients are able to ambulate without any functioning Achilles tendon. It is of interest that the clinical presentation of the neglected rupture is quite similar to that in patients who were treated with or without surgery but with subsequent elongation of the muscle-tendon unit.

Patient Evaluation

The strength of the gastrocnemius-soleus complex is established by observing ambulation, which should include the ability to walk on tiptoe or on the heels. The patient should be evaluated in the prone and seated positions, while testing maximum passive dorsiflexion. The prone dorsiflexion test is reliable, and although the extent of passive dorsiflexion varies for each individual, it is generally symmetrical for both extremities, which makes it possible to assess the extent of excessive dorsiflexion. Plantarflexion strength is further determined manually, and then with a double and single heel-rise test. Some patients can perform a single heel rise with no functional Achilles, but a repetitive heel-rise test is generally not possible. If a more accurate measure of strength is necessary, manual muscle testing is not sufficient, and isokinetic strength and power should be determined using machines, such as a dynamometer, that adequately document power and strength. This testing is performed through motions of dorsiflexion and plantarflexion and is analyzed as a percentage deficit relative to the opposite limb normalized for body weight. At 60 degree-seconds, these correlate with strength, and at 120 degree-seconds, they correlate with power parameters.

The size of the gap between the tendon ends must be carefully assessed, and although this can at times be assessed by palpation, if surgery is planned the method of reconstruction does depend on the extent of this gap, which should

therefore be more accurately determined by MRI or ultrasound.

Management Options

Brace management is indicated for those patients who are not experiencing functional deficits as a result of the loss of push-off strength and who are not disabled in their activities of daily living. To this group should be added those who have potential problems with wound healing. Due to the magnitude of the dissection for correction of neglected ruptures, one must ensure that all potential for wound compromise is eliminated, including cigarette smoking, chronic dermatologic problems or chronic swelling of the limb, venous stasis, and arteriosclerosis causing lower limb ischemia. The brace options include a molded polypropylene ankle-foot orthosis (AFO), with or without a hinge at the ankle. A molded AFO is made, and the posterior ankle of the brace is transversely cut and reinforced by attaching a short piece of dense rubber to the medial and lateral margins of the brace. This AFO permits passive dorsiflexion with mild passive resistance, and the reinforced rubber contracts at the end point of dorsiflexion to forcibly plantarflex the foot. Some patients tolerate the brace well and find that it improves both stability and push-off strength such that surgery is not required.

Reconstruction of the Chronic Rupture

The ideal function of the gastrocnemius-soleus muscle can be regained only if the muscle is healthy, and without atrophy, both of which are unlikely if considerable time has elapsed since injury. Ideally, end-to-end tendon apposition of the tendon ends should be attempted, but this should be accomplished without

placing the foot in marked equinus, which may not be possible if the gap between the tendon ends is great. For these reasons, many techniques for repair, reconstruction, or augmentation of the chronic Achilles tendon rupture have been proposed.[38,39,43,55–58] Many of these methods of reconstruction depend on harvesting avascular autologous tissue, such as multiple strips of fascia lata,[38] proximal Achilles turn-down flaps,[59] and the plantaris tendon.[56] The V-Y tendon advancement of the more proximal gastrocnemius muscle-tendon complex, as described initially, is generally avascular, but this depends on the method of muscle detachment and how it is advanced. These tendinous flaps are revascularized from the surrounding tissue or paratenon. However, it is possible to perform a substantial V-Y advancement while maintaining muscle integrity and continuity posteriorly, and this procedure has the potential of being vascularized.

The tendon transfers that are used to augment a deficient Achilles, ie, the peroneus brevis, FHL, or FDL, similarly are able to function despite a markedly compromised blood supply, although the muscle remains viable. When selecting either of these tendons, one must consider the donor morbidity and the strength of the transfer itself. Each of the described tendons used for transfer, ie, the peroneus brevis, the FHL, and the FDL, create some deficit that must be anticipated. For example, the peroneus brevis transfer as originally described by Turco and Spinella[58] is able to augment the Achilles, but this will inevitably compromise eversion strength. The balance of the muscles of eversion (the peroneus longus and brevis) and inversion (the posterior tibial, and to a lesser extent, the anterior tibial muscle) is therefore affected. One may anticipate the muscle deficit created by tendon transfer based on the percentages of total muscle force acting on the ankle.[60] The total strength of the peroneus longus and brevis (as a percentage of force on the ankle) is 7.1%, with the peroneus brevis accounting for 2.6%. The remaining available eversion force of 4.5% is insufficient to counteract the strength of the posterior tibial muscle, which accounts for 6.4% of the force across the ankle. The anterior tibial muscle may further add to some dynamic inversion, and the inversion/eversion balance is theoretically markedly compromised. This dynamic disruption of inversion and eversion does not occur with the use of either the FDL or the FHL, although these too have their drawbacks.[40,41,61,62]

I base the decision as to which technique to use for the neglected Achilles rupture on the distance between the tendon ends, the presence of gastrocnemius-soleus muscle atrophy, and the age and athletic activities of the patient. Generally, the reconstruction is planned according to the size of the defect between the tendon ends, and it is helpful to plan the extent of the surgery preoperatively. As with repair of an acute rupture, it is essential to obtain an anatomic end result, and this requires correct tensioning of the repair. A tourniquet is optional for all procedures. If used, it should be applied to the thigh and not the calf, to avoid tethering the gastrocnemius-soleus complex. If a more distal or calf tourniquet is used, tethering will prevent the proximal stump from being pulled distally. Wound closure after any of the procedures described below must be performed carefully to avoid subsequent skin necrosis. The paratenon should be repaired when possible to help maintain the blood supply to the tendon, followed by

wound closure in layers. After surgery, the lower leg is immobilized in a bulky dressing, incorporating splints to hold the ankle in a neutral position. A neutral position is preferred after all reconstructive procedures unless the ankle is intentionally placed in equinus to facilitate end-to-end repair of smaller gaps between the tendon ends. The postoperative course is the same for all the different procedures, because the need for functional rehabilitation with early mobilization and strengthening is identical to that after repair of an acute rupture. Postoperatively, patients are allowed to commence range-of-motion exercises once the sutures are removed, and weightbearing commences at about 2 weeks in a removable hinged range-of-motion walker boot that allows complete flexion of the ankle but has a dorsiflexion block that can be adjusted during the recovery process.

Defects of 1 to 2 cm

End-to-end anastomosis of the tendon ends is clearly optimum but may not be possible after neglected ruptures, although for this minimal defect, it is usually possible to accomplish the repair without any augmentation or reconstruction. The muscle can usually be mobilized and the repair performed with the foot held in mild equinus, and the foot gradually assumes a plantigrade position during rehabilitation. Exact end-to-end apposition of the tendon is important, and the repair is no different from that described above for management of the acute rupture. The success of this repair depends on an adequate suture fixation followed by aggressive rehabilitation to maximize isokinetic function. This procedure is easily accomplished if the gap is 1 cm or less. If the gap is greater, it is necessary to rely on the tensile properties of the muscle-tendon unit

to achieve end-to-end tendon apposition. The exposure and method of suture is identical to that described above, but, prior to tying the sutures, tension is applied for approximately 10 minutes to "stress relax" the myotendinous junction. This technique will gain up to 2 cm in length, depending on the extent of atrophy and the elastic properties of the tissue. The ankle is then placed in the desired amount of plantarflexion to achieve end-to-end repair, and after posterior compartment fasciotomy and skin closure, the lower limb is immobilized in a neutral position. Postoperative management is similar to that described above.

Defects of 2 to 5 cm

For these larger defects, I use a V-Y myotendinous lengthening, although this can occasionally be augmented with the FHL transfer described below. As originally described, this procedure reportedly corrected strength deficit when performed without the addition of the FHL transfer, and it relies on remaining muscle function, regardless of the length of time elapsed since injury. Theoretically, if the muscle is scarred this is not likely to work; however, this has not been my experience and that of others because, despite muscle atrophy, after tendon advancement, muscle strength and function seem to return. However, this procedure cannot be used if the muscle is severely atrophied and scarred as, for example, after infection. Although the FHL may be used as a sole transfer for these defects, this unnecessarily sacrifices a healthy functioning muscle, and if any function can be anticipated from the gastrocnemius, the V-Y advancement is preferable.

The procedure is performed with the patient in the prone position. A long incision is made, beginning proximal to the myotendinous junction in the midline, and gently curving immediately posteromedial to the Achilles tendon distally. After debridement of the tendon ends, an additional 1 cm of tendon length is further lost, necessitating careful planning of the length required of the proximal tendon flap. An inverted V incision is made in the fascia of the gastrocnemius, taking care to leave the underlying muscle attached to the anterior paratenon. The length of the arms of the inverted V should be twice as long as the defect, usually about 12 to 18 cm long. The planning of the flap is important in order to preserve the muscle attachment to the fascia and tendon posteriorly. Leave a margin of at least 1 cm on each side of the tendon flap proximally, although this is not possible distally where the incision is made into the tendon itself. The flap is then gently advanced by separating the muscle edges bluntly so as to preserve the posterior muscle tissue attached. For defects of up to 5 cm it is not difficult to advance the entire flap and preserve the muscle in continuity posteriorly. However, if the defect is larger, then the muscle posteriorly may become detached as the flap is advanced. An end-to-end repair is performed using a whip suture as described above. The Y is then closed with 2-0 nonabsorbable suture. Routine closure is performed and a bulky splint is applied in 10° to 20° of plantarflexion. Postoperative rehabilitation is performed as described above.

The results of the V-Y advancement for treatment of neglected Achilles tendon ruptures were reported recently by Us and associates.[63] These authors examined their patients with isokinetic testing and found a deficiency in peak torque ranging from 2% to 22% when compared to the unaffected limb. However, they noted that all patients were able to return to their preinjury activities, including sports. Other authors have reported similar success using the V-Y advancement procedure, with a 25% deficit in peak torque testing on Cybex postoperatively.[64]

Defects > 5 cm

For defects of this magnitude, rely on a tendon transfer either alone or in combination with a V-Y advancement of the gastrocnemius muscle and tendon. A turn-down flap of tendon may be used, but this is not my preferred method of reconstruction because of the bulk of the tendon at the point at which it is passed inferiorly. Although the peroneus brevis has been successfully used in these circumstances,[58] because this tendon is a weaker flexor, its use will compromise eversion, and I do not recommend it. The alternatives are to use either the FDL[40] or the FHL[62] as previously described. The use of either of these tendons retains its function as a plantarflexor of the foot, although neither approximates the strength of the gastrocnemius-soleus. Each of these procedures has its theoretical advantages and, of course, its proponents; however, due to the greater strength and the proximity of the muscle to the Achilles, I prefer to use the FHL. Although weak in comparison, the FHL is the second strongest plantarflexor next to the gastrocnemius-soleus complex, although it is less than one-tenth the power and strength of the latter muscle.[60]

The patient is positioned slightly laterally with the affected side down and the ipsilateral hip and knee flexed, or, if preferred, the prone position may be used. The skin marking for the incision on the foot corresponds to the talonavicular joint proximally and the mid-portion of the first metatarsal distally. The plane of the dissection is superficial to the abductor hallucis and flexor hallucis brevis, which are reflected dorsally or away from the first metatarsal. The FHL and FDL are identified, with the FHL being the more medial structure. The medial plantar branch of the medial plantar nerve can be damaged by this dissection, and it must be identified and retracted. To prevent proximal and distal retraction of the FHL tendon ends, two sutures are inserted into the FHL tendon, 1 cm apart, at the level at which the FHL is to be cut. The FHL is sutured by tenodesis of its distal stump to the FDL, while the ankle and toes are held in a neutral position. There are invariably cross-connections between the FHL and the FDL, and suture of the two tendons distally may not be necessary if the FHL is harvested proximal to these cross-connections. The range of motion of the hallux is assessed and, unless full dorsiflexion of the hallux is possible after the tenodesis, the sutures must be changed to adjust the tension on the stump of the FHL. More proximally, at the level of the foot where the FHL and FDL tendons cross each other (the Knot of Henry), there are multiple fibrous cross-connections between these tendons, and these usually need to be released for the FHL to be pulled into the proximal wound. A second incision is made along the medial border of the Achilles tendon from the myotendinous junction to 2 cm distal to the Achilles insertion. The deep posterior compartment of the leg is then opened longitudinally. The FHL muscle is identified, and its tendon is pulled into the proximal wound. At times, it is necessary to open the flexor retinaculum as far distal as the sustentaculum tali to permit the tendon to pass into the proximal wound. A 4.5-mm drill hole is made

1 cm distal to the Achilles tendon insertion and 1.5 cm anterior to the posterior margin of the calcaneal cortex from medial to lateral. A 1-cm incision is made on the lateral posterior margin of the heel posterior to the sural nerve and immediately over the drill hole. The tendon is then passed from medial to lateral, and then back medially through a subcutaneous tunnel over the dorsal cortex of the calcaneus. In the past, I have tried drilling 2 holes, made at 90° to each other, but this construct seems too tenuous, because fracture of the calcaneus may occur. A suture passer may be used to pull the tendon of the FHL from proximal to distal through the drill hole. Alternatively, the end of a small metallic suction tip is passed from lateral to medial, and the suture on the FHL is sucked into the tip, facilitating passage of the tendon from medial to lateral. If the harvested FHL tendon is long, the FHL may be woven through the distal stump of the Achilles, although this does not appear to be necessary to obtain full function. The FHL is sutured in a side-to-side tenodesis manner to the Achilles with 2-0 nonabsorbable monofilament, and the muscle is sutured to the Achilles with 4-0 absorbable suture. The Achilles should be used in the final repair wherever possible, regardless of the length of time since rupture, in the hope that the gastrocnemius-soleus muscle strength will augment the transfer. The FHL, although strong, is markedly weaker than the gastrocnemius-soleus, and alone cannot be expected to return the patient to full activity. One must recognize, however, that the FHL is used here as a tendon transfer, and the strength and integrity of this transfer should not be compromised by a dead, atrophic, and nonyielding Achilles. If the proximal gastrocne-mius-soleus muscle has no contractility, a tenodesis of the FHL to the remaining Achilles may impair the ability of the FHL to function, and a tenodesis effect will occur.

The construct is tensioned with the ankle in neutral flexion. At the completion of the repair, the foot is taken through a full range of motion, and the ability of the construct to withstand dorsiflexion beyond neutral is carefully checked. The postoperative routine is identical to that described above for chronic rupture repair techniques.

Complications

The main complications associated with delayed repair of the Achilles tendon are wound necrosis, rerupture, infection, and inability to gain dorsiflexion. Wound-edge necrosis can best be avoided by using meticulous soft-tissue handling techniques, full-thickness flaps, and routine posterior fasciotomy. In addition, a bulky, cotton dressing with a posterior splint should be used to minimize initial motion pressure on the wound. Infection can be devastating if full-thickness necrosis occurs, exposing the tendon. In this case, the tendon must be kept constantly moist, to avoid desiccation, by using regular wet-dressing changes with oral antibiotics and permitting healing by secondary intention. An alternative method of wound management uses the application of Silvadene dressings followed by split-thickness skin grafting over the granulating surface.

Ankle stiffness can best be avoided by a regimented postoperative rehabilitation course and by ensuring that the repair does not require the ankle to be placed in excessive plantarflexion. Perhaps a more clinically significant complication is the lack either of free motion or of the ability to regain adequate push-off strength. Either of these may be caused by incorrect tensioning of the repair or by elongation of the repair construct postoperatively. Ankle stiffness results from insufficient length because the repair must be made with the foot held in equinus. This position is far less compromising than repairs performed in a functionally elongated position. A patient with the latter repair never fully regains push-off strength.

The chronic or neglected Achilles tendon rupture poses a difficult problem for the orthopaedic surgeon. Most patients will complain of an inability to perform a single toe-stance or heel-rise, weakness at push-off of the gait cycle, and the inability to participate in recreational sports due to lack of strength. Bracing with a spring-loaded, hinged AFO can improve function and power at push-off, but will not permit the patient to perform toe rises.

The etiology of the chronic rupture can be multifactorial, including missed initial diagnoses, inappropriate treatment of an acute rupture, chronic Achilles tendinosis leading to microtears with subsequent lengthening, and ruptures associated with inflammatory disorders, such as rheumatoid arthritis and systemic lupus erythematosus. Ruptures in patients with inflammatory disorders can be very difficult to diagnose and treat. Such patients frequently have involvement of multiple joints (causing a decreased range of motion and weakness), are on multidrug regimens (often including steroids that can increase the risk of postoperative complications), and can sustain spontaneous ruptures that may be undetected for years. There does not seem to be a time limit beyond which a repair of a chronic rupture will not improve function. Regardless of the etiology, the size of the defect, and the time since rupture, the decision-making algorithm and repair techniques outlined above provide patients with improved strength, function, and power, and freedom from a brace. However, it must be remembered that the patient must be motivated toward an aggressive rehabilitation course and be compliant with such a regimen.

References

1. Carden DG, Noble J, Chalmers J, Lunn P, Ellis J: Rupture of the calcaneal tendon: The early and late management. *J Bone Joint Surg* 1987; 69B:416–420.

2. Jozsa L, Kvist M, Balint BJ, et al: The role of recreational sport activity in Achilles tendon rupture: A clinical, pathoanatomical, and sociological study of 292 cases. *Am J Sports Med* 1989;17:338–343.

3. Levi N: The incidence of Achilles tendon rupture in Copenhagen. *Injury* 1997;28:311–313.

4. Sun Y-S, Yen T-F, Chie LH: Ruptured Achilles tendon: Report of 40 cases. *Zhonghua Yixue Zazhi* 1977;57:94–96.

5. Jozsa L, Kannus P: Histopathological findings in spontaneous tendon ruptures. *Scand J Med Sci Sports* 1997;7:113–118.

6. Fox JM, Blazina ME, Jobe FW, et al: Degeneration and rupture of the Achilles tendon. *Clin Orthop* 1975;107:221–224.

7. Lagergren C, Lindholm A: Vascular distribution in the Achilles tendon: An angiographic and microangiographic study. *Acta Chir Scand* 1959;116:491–495.

8. Arner O, Lindholm A: Avulsion fracture of the os calcaneus. *Acta Chir Scand* 1949;117:258–260.

9. Mandelbaum BR, Myerson MS, Forster R: Achilles tendon ruptures: A new method of repair, early range of motion, and functional rehabilitation. *Am J Sports Med* 1995;23:392–395.

10. Mahler F, Fritschy D: Partial and complete ruptures of the Achilles tendon and local corticosteroid injections. *Br J Sports Med* 1992;26: 7–14.

11. Laseter JT, Russell JA: Anabolic steroid-induced tendon pathology: A review of the literature. *Med Sci Sports Exerc* 1991;23:1–3.

12. Beskin JL, Sanders RA, Hunter SC, Hughston JC: Surgical repair of Achilles tendon ruptures. *Am J Sports Med* 1987;15:1–8.

13. Cirincione RJ, Baker BE: Tendon ruptures with secondary hyperparathyroidism: A case report. *J Bone Joint Surg* 1975;57A:852–853.

14. Hosey G, Kowalchick E, Tesoro D, et al: Comparison of the mechanical and histologic properties of Achilles tendons in New Zealand white rabbits secondarily repaired with Marlex mesh. *J Foot Surg* 1991;30:214–233.

15. Nehrer S, Breitenseher M, Brodner W, et al: Clinical and sonographic evaluation of the risk of rupture in the Achilles tendon. *Arch Orthop Trauma Surg* 1997;116:14–18.

16. Thompson TC, Doherty JH: Spontaneous rupture of tendon of Achilles: A new clinical diagnostic test. *J Trauma* 1962;2:126–129.

17. Harcke HT, Grissom LE, Finkelstein MS: Evaluation of the musculoskeletal system with sonography. *Am J Roentgenol* 1988;150: 1253–1261.

18. Richter J, Josten C, David A, Clasbrummel B, Muhr G: Sports fitness after functional conservative versus surgical treatment of acute Achilles tendon ruptures. *Zentralbl Chir* 1994;119:538–544.

19. Cetti R, Christensen SE, Ejsted R, Jensen NM, Jorgensen U: Operative versus nonoperative treatment of Achilles tendon rupture: A prospective randomized study and review of the literature. *Am J Sports Med* 1993;21:791–799.

20. Neumann D, Vogt L, Banzer W, Schreiber U: Kinematic and neuromuscular changes of the gait pattern after Achilles tendon rupture. *Foot Ankle Int* 1997;18:339–341.

21. Christensen I: Rupture of the Achilles tendon: Analysis of 57 cases. *Acta Chir Scand* 1953;106: 50–60.

22. Nada A: Rupture of the calcaneal tendon: Treatment by external fixation. *J Bone Joint Surg* 1985;67B:449–453.

23. Quenu J, Stoianovitch: Les ruptures du tendon d'Achille. *Rev Chir (Paris)* 1929;67:647–678.

24. Wills CA, Washburn S, Caiozzo V, Prietto CA: Achilles tendon rupture: A review of the literature comparing surgical versus nonsurgical treatment. *Clin Orthop* 1986;207:156–163.

25. Lea RB, Smith L: Non-surgical treatment of tendo achillis rupture. *J Bone Joint Surg* 1972; 54A:1398–1407.

26. Nistor L: Surgical and non-surgical treatment of Achilles tendon rupture: A prospective randomized study. *J Bone Joint Surg* 1981;63A: 394–399.

27. Helgeland J, Odland P, Hove LM: Achilles tendon rupture: Surgical or non-surgical treatment. *Tidsskr Nor Laegeforen* 1997;117:1763–1766.

28. Thermann H, Frerichs O, Biewener A, Krettek C, Schandelmeier P: Functional treatment of acute rupture of the Achilles tendon: An experimental biomechanical study. *Unfallchirurg* 1995;98:507–513.

29. Achilles tendon rupture. *Lancet* 1973;1: 189–190.

30. Inglis AE, Scott WN, Sculco TP, Patterson AH: Ruptures of the tendo Achillis: An objective assessment of surgical and non-surgical treatment. *J Bone Joint Surg* 1976;58A:990–993.

31. Jacobs D, Martens M, Van Audekercke R, Mulier JC, Mulier F: Comparison of conservative and operative treatment of Achilles tendon rupture. *Am J Sports Med* 1978;6:107–111.

32. Bunnell S: Primary repair of severed tendons: The use of stainless steel wire. *Am J Surg* 1940; 47:502–516.

33. Kessler I: The "grasping" technique for tendon repair. *Hand* 1973;5:253–255.

34. Ma GW, Griffith TG: Percutaneous repair of acute closed ruptured Achilles tendon: A new technique. *Clin Orthop* 1977;128:247–255.

35. Cetti R: Ruptured Achilles tendon: Preliminary results of a new treatment. *Br J Sports Med* 1988;22:6–8.

36. Mortensen NH, Saether J: Achilles tendon repair: A new method of Achilles tendon repair tested on cadaverous materials. *J Trauma* 1991; 31:381–384.

37. Kirschenbaum SE, Kelman C: Modification of the Lindholm procedure for plastic repair of ruptured Achilles tendon: A case report. *J Foot Surg* 1980;19:4–11.

38. Bugg EI Jr, Boyd BM: Repair of neglected rupture or laceration of the Achilles tendon. *Clin Orthop* 1968;56:73–75.

39. Perez Teuffer A: Traumatic rupture of the Achilles tendon: Reconstruction by transplant and graft using the lateral peroneus brevis. *Orthop Clin North Am* 1974;5:89–93.

40. Mann RA, Holmes GB, Jr, Seale KS, Collins DN: Chronic rupture of the Achilles tendon: A new technique of repair. *J Bone Joint Surg* 1991;73A:214–219.

41. Wapner KL, Hecht PJ, Mills RH Jr: Reconstruction of neglected Achilles tendon injury. *Orthop Clin North Am* 1995;26:249–263.

42. Jenkins DH, Forster IW, McKibbin B, Ralis ZA: Induction of tendon and ligament formation by carbon implants. *J Bone Joint Surg* 1977;59B:53–57.

43. Levy M, Velkes S, Goldstein J, Rosner M: A method of repair for Achilles tendon ruptures without cast immobilization: Preliminary report. *Clin Orthop* 1984;187:199–204.

44. Giannini S, Girolami M, Ceccarelli F, Catani F, Stea S: Surgical repair of Achilles tendon ruptures using polypropylene braid augmentation. *Foot Ankle Int* 1994;15:372–375.

45. Booth FW: Physiologic and biochemical effects of immobilization on muscle. *Clin Orthop* 1987;219:15–20.

46. Pepels WRJ, Plasmans CMT, Sloof TJJH: Abstract: The course of healing of tendons and ligaments. *Acta Orthop Scand* 1983;54:952.

47. Gelberman RH, Manske PR, Vande Berg JS, Lesker PA, Akeson WH: Flexor tendon repair in vitro: A comparative histologic study of the rabbit, chicken, dog, and monkey. *J Orthop Res* 1984;2:39–48.

48. Enwemeka CS, Spielholz NI, Nelson AJ: The effect of early functional activities on experimentally tenotomized Achilles tendons in rats. *Am J Phys Med Rehabil* 1988;67:264–269.

49. Bradley JP, Tibone JE: Percutaneous and open surgical repairs of Achilles tendon ruptures: A comparative study. *Am J Sports Med* 1990;18: 188–195.

50. Inglis AE, Sculco TP: Surgical repair of ruptures of the tendo Achillis. *Clin Orthop* 1981; 156:160–169.

51. Shields CL Jr, Kerlan RK, Jobe FW, Carter VS, Lombardo SJ: The Cybex II evaluation of sur-

gically repaired Achilles tendon ruptures. *Am J Sports Med* 1978;6:369–372.

52. Motta P, Errichiello C, Pontini I: Achilles tendon rupture: A new technique for easy surgical repair and immediate movement of the ankle and foot. *Am J Sports Med* 1997;25:172–176.

53. Leppilahti J, Kaarela O, Teerikangas H, Raatikainen T, Orava S, Waris T: Free tissue coverage of wound complications following Achilles tendon rupture surgery. *Clin Orthop* 1996;328:171–176.

54. Boyden EM, Kitaoka HB, Cahalan TD, An KN: Late versus early repair of Achilles tendon rupture: Clinical and biomechanical evaluation. *Clin Orthop* 1995;317:150–158.

55. Howard CB, Winston I, Bell W, Mackie I, Jenkins DH: Late repair of the calcaneal tendon with carbon fibre. *J Bone Joint Surg* 1984;66B:206–208.

56. Lynn TA: Repair of the torn Achilles tendon, using the plantaris tendon as a reinforcing membrane. *J Bone Joint Surg* 1966;48A:268–272.

57. Schedl R, Fasol P: Achilles tendon repair with the plantaris tendon compared with repair using polyglycol threads. *J Trauma* 1979;19:189–194.

58. Turco VJ, Spinella AJ: Achilles tendon ruptures: Peroneus brevis transfer. *Foot Ankle* 1987;7:253–259.

59. Bosworth DM: Repair of defects in the tendo Achillis. *J Bone Joint Surg* 1956;38A:111–114.

60. Silver RL, de la Garza J, Rang M: The myth of muscle balance: A study of relative strengths and excursions of normal muscles about the foot and ankle. *J Bone Joint Surg* 1985;67B:432–437.

61. Wapner KL, Hecht PJ: Repair of chronic Achilles tendon rupture with flexor hallucis longus tendon transfer. *Op Tech Orthop* 1994;4:132–137.

62. Wapner KL, Pavlock GS, Hecht PJ, Naselli F, Walther R: Repair of chronic Achilles tendon rupture with flexor hallucis longus tendon transfer. *Foot Ankle* 1993;14:443–449.

63. Us AK, Bilgin SS, Aydin T, Mergen E: Repair of neglected Achilles tendon ruptures: Procedures and functional results. *Arch Orthop Trauma Surg* 1997;116:408–411.

64. Kissel CG, Blacklidge DK, Crowley DL: Repair of neglected Achilles tendon ruptures: Procedure and functional results. *J Foot Ankle Surg* 1994;33:46–52.

14

Evaluation and Treatment of Ankle Syndesmosis Injuries

David A. Porter, MD, PhD

Abstract

Athletes sustain ankle syndesmosis injuries far less frequently than they do lateral ankle sprains; however, syndesmosis injuries are more challenging to detect and treat. Grade II injuries, which are occultly unstable, may be overlooked or treated too conservatively (nonsurgically), leading to latent diastasis, chronic instability, further injury, arthritic changes, chronic pain, osteochondral lesions, and other sequelae. Surgical intervention for chronic syndesmosis injuries produces mixed results and creates an uncertain future for athletes who desire to return to their sport. Optimal treatment starts with a comprehensive evaluation that includes a thorough physical examination as well as imaging studies to evaluate for instability (medial clear space widening and syndesmosis disruption). All acute unstable syndesmosis injuries (grades II and III) should be treated with surgery, which can include repair of the deltoid ligament with open reduction and internal fixation of the syndesmosis. Isolated deltoid sprains also are often repaired surgically in athletes. This more aggressive treatment helps avoid the chronic pain and instability and osteochondral abnormalities associated with chronic injury.

The annual incidence of ankle syndesmosis injuries is approximately 15 cases per 100,000 individuals in the general population.[1] The incidence is higher in athletes, whose susceptibility to this injury is increased because of their participation in activities that involve planting the foot and then cutting motions as well as direct blows to the lateral ankle. Exact figures are elusive because differences in injury reporting do not capture all cases, but estimates indicate 1% to 18% of all ankle sprains are syndesmosis injuries.[2,3]

Although this type of injury is seen less frequently than lateral ankle injuries, syndesmosis injuries can be more challenging to diagnose

and treat. Although a complete syndesmotic disruption is easy to detect, more subtle injuries often go unnoticed. One survey of physicians and trainers who care for professional athletes identified syndesmosis injuries as the foot and ankle injury that is most difficult to treat.[2]

Although significant morbidity is associated with such injuries,[4] syndesmotic disruption can cause persistent disability in competitive athletes. Patients with syndesmosis injuries frequently require almost twice as much time to return to sport compared with patients who have lateral ankle sprains.[3]

Early diagnosis with appropriate treatment is preferable to late diagnosis because a chronic injury can

be problematic, often leading to suboptimal and sometimes uncorrectable outcomes.[5]

Syndesmosis Anatomy and Physiology

The syndesmosis (also called the interosseous membrane) allows the tibia and fibula to work together as a single unit, providing stability to the lower leg and actions of the foot and ankle complex. At the distal ends of these two bones, the anterior-inferior tibiofibular ligament (AITFL), the posterior-inferior tibiofibular ligament, and the interosseous ligament lend stability to the ankle mortise and maintain the fibula in the incisura fibularis tibiae. The deltoid ligament helps maintain the syndesmosis indirectly by stabilizing the medial ankle mortise. Under normal circumstances, this configuration is so stable that the syndesmosis and the ankle mortise widen only approximately 1 mm during gait.[3] A syndesmosis sprain results from sustained forceful external rotation with abduction and dorsiflexion.

Classification of Injury

Syndesmosis injuries involve disruption of the ligamentous structures between the distal fibula and tibia as well as a disruption of the deltoid ligament medially. Forceful external rotation and abduction of the ankle widens the ankle mortise

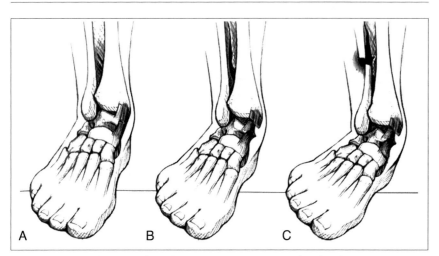

Figure 1 Classification of syndesmosis injury. See text for details. **A,** Grade I. **B,** Grade II. **C,** Grade III. (Reproduced with permission from Porter DA: Ligamentous injuries of the foot and ankle, in Fitzgerald RH, Kaufer H, Malkani AL (eds): *Orthopaedics.* St Louis, MO, Mosby, 2002, pp 1607-1621.)

as the talus pushes the distal fibula laterally away from its articulation with the distal tibia. Stretching or tearing of the syndesmosis, deltoid, and associated ligamentous structures results in diastasis. A proximal fibular fracture can be involved in more severe injuries.

A grade I injury involves injury to the anterior deltoid ligament and the distal interosseous ligament but without tearing of the more proximal syndesmosis or the deep deltoid ligament.[6] The AITFL often is very tender to palpation and may have a higher grade injury; because no diastasis is present, the injury is, by definition, stable.

A grade II injury involves disruption of the anterior and deep deltoid ligaments as well as a tear in a significant portion of the syndesmosis, resulting in an unstable ankle that is still normally aligned on nonstress radiographs. A grade II injury poses particular diagnostic challenges because the extent of the injury and its occult instability are often more difficult to recognize. Underestimating the injury or using a nonstabiliz-ing treatment can have devastating consequences for the patient. A chronic, unstable syndesmosis can predispose the patient to further injury, arthritic changes, chronic pain, osteochondral lesions, and other sequelae.[5]

A grade III injury involves severe external rotation and abduction, with complete disruption of the medial ligaments and extensive disruption of the syndesmosis, frequently accompanied by fracture of the proximal fibula (Maisonneuve). Such injuries are overtly unstable on initial examination and standard radiographs. The classification of injury is shown in Figure 1.

Understanding Why Syndesmosis Injuries Often Lead to Complications and Chronic Injury

The deltoid is twice as strong as the ankle's lateral ligaments.[1] Thus, a tear of the deltoid leads to collapse of the hindfoot into valgus (because of the tensile stresses). In contrast, severe plantar flexion with inversion can lead to a complete tear of the lat-

eral ligaments (anterior talofibular and calcaneofibular ligaments)—but because less tension is placed on them with walking (compressive forces laterally in a valgus-aligned hindfoot), healing often is unremarkable.

A grade II syndesmosis injury can lead to complications if not diagnosed and treated properly. Insight gained from observation of the varus-valgus resistance seen in the knee and mirrored in the ankle sheds light on potential pitfalls in assessing and treating occult syndesmosis instabilities. Current opinion is divided regarding surgical intervention of grade II injuries;[7] however, some authors agree that all acute unstable syndesmosis injuries (grades II and III) should be treated surgically.[8] Aggressive stabilization (open reduction and internal fixation) of the syndesmosis as well as surgical repair of the deltoid ligament is considered a more conservative approach to a grade II injury than nonsurgical treatment because repair of a chronic syndesmosis insufficiency yields poor results.

Although nonsurgical treatment of a grade II injury can be successful, a suboptimal result makes it difficult for the athlete to return to sports activity. The challenge is to uncover occult instabilities before they become chronic and debilitating.

Physical Examination

Palpation of the ankle produces tenderness along the anterior deltoid (in all grades) and the deep deltoid (particularly in grades II and III). Tenderness also is noted along the length of the syndesmosis in all grades of injury. With grade II and III injuries, the tenderness often extends at least one third to one half the length of the leg. The anterior talofibular ligament often is not tender, but significant tenderness is found in the AITFL, deltoid, and syndesmosis. Palpating the full length of the fibula can reveal evidence of a Maisonneuve fracture.

It is also helpful to examine areas of swelling. In particular, swelling medially over the deltoid is highly suggestive of deltoid injury and, thus, a syndesmosis injury also is likely. Fites and associates[5] recommended that "if swelling above the joint line between the tibia and fibula occurs less than 24 hours after injury, consider it a syndesmosis injury until proven otherwise." Although sometimes difficult to identify, it is important to attempt to determine if tenderness exists along the medial neck of the talus rather than along the deep deltoid. A high-grade lateral ankle sprain can result in medial impingement and medial talar neck pain (as opposed to soft-tissue tenderness of the deep deltoid).

Another important clinical finding is that patients have difficulty bearing weight with an unstable syndesmosis injury. This denotes a more significant injury than a lateral ankle sprain. Numerous biomechanical tests have been used to determine if diastasis is present in a syndesmosis injury. The most reliable test is an external rotation test (Figure 2). A positive test will produce pain at the ankle or the syndesmosis. However, the external rotation test is not always helpful in determining the stability or instability of the syndesmosis.

Imaging Studies

Much has been written about measuring the tibia-fibula interval and overlap on standard radiographs as a way to assess diastasis.[2,9] However, Gardner and associates[10] maintain that "no optimal radiographic mea-

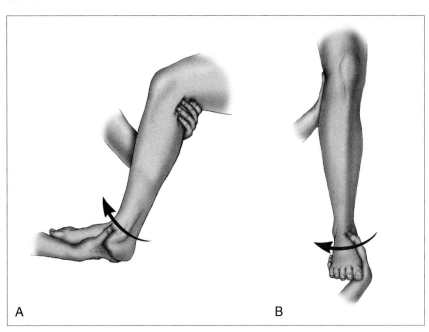

Figure 2 External rotation test. The foot and ankle are held with one hand and the upper leg stabilized with the other hand. The foot and ankle are externally rotated to check for pain in the ankle or leg. **A,** Medial view. **B,** Frontal view. (Reproduced with permission from Porter DA, Schon LC: Ankle sprains, ankle instability and syndesmosis injuries, in Porter DA, Schon LC (eds): *Baxter's The Foot and Ankle in Sport*, ed 2. Philadelphia, PA, Mosby, 2008, pp 273-290.)

surement exists for assessing syndesmotic integrity." Measurements of the tibia-fibula interval and overlap can be unreliable indicators of the stability of a diastasis because the measurements are highly dependent on the rotation of the ankle during positioning for radiographs. Also, the depth of the fibular notch varies because of size differences in the tibial tubercles that bind the lateral surface of the tibia anteriorly and posteriorly, thus making the measurements too variable to draw consistent conclusions.

The medial clear space is a reliable indicator of instability. Generally, the determination is made by assessing the cartilage interval between the dorsal talus and the distal tibia (the tibial-talar interval). The interval between the medial malleolus and medial talus should be the same as this or within 1 to 2 mm (Figure 3). With

the ankle in neutral dorsiflexion, any widening at the medial clear space of more than 2 mm larger than that of the tibial-talar interval is highly suggestive of deltoid rupture and instability. These measurements must be taken in the context of the patient's history and clinical findings (external rotation injury, significant swelling, tenderness over the deltoid and syndesmosis, positive external rotation stress test).

Routine radiographs are obtained on all patients with significant injuries, especially those in whom syndesmosis sprain is suspected. If possible, weight-bearing radiographs are obtained in the AP, lateral, and mortise views. If a proximal fibular fracture is suspected, weight-bearing radiographs of the entire tibia and fibula are obtained. External rotation stress radiographs of the ankle are obtained if the patient his-

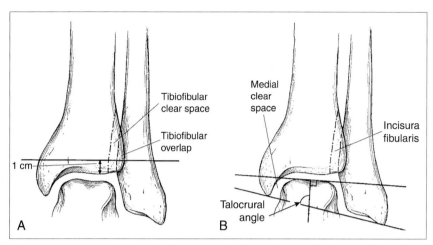

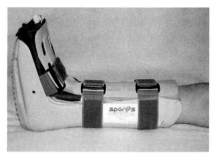

Figure 4 Removable walking boot with built-in cold compression.

Figure 3 Measurement of the tibiotalar interval compared with medial clear space. **A,** AP view. **B,** Mortise view. (Reproduced from Wuest TK: Injuries to the distal lower extremity syndesmosis. *J Am Acad Orthop Surg* 1997;5:172-181.)

tory, physical examination, and standard radiographs do not clearly delineate stability or instability. A local ankle block can be used, if necessary, to obtain these stress images. If stability is still in doubt after these assessments, the patient can return in 1 week for reevaluation and repeat imaging studies or an MRI can be obtained.

In some situations, MRI may be indicated to define the degree of anatomic injury. MRI also is helpful when the mechanism of injury is unknown or if stability is still in doubt. MRI and CT can provide images in the frontal, axial, and sagittal planes. Some believe that axial plane CT better shows small diastases (2 to 3 mm). Another advantage of MRI and CT is that three-dimensional reconstructions can be made of the distal tibia-fibula complex.[2,9]

Because the degree of injury can be difficult to determine, repeat examinations and radiographs of grade I injuries are recommended 1, 2, 4, and 6 weeks after injury. If the ankle is unstable, surgery is planned. A good reduction is the only significant predictor for func-

tional outcome in this type of injury.[8-10]

Treatment Overview

Grade I syndesmosis injuries are treated nonsurgically. Boot immobilization and cold therapy are used for comfort and assisting in rehabilitation (Figure 4).

To ensure that the syndesmosis is stable, the examination and radiographs are repeated every 1 or 2 weeks until long-term stability is ensured. Patients use crutches only 1 to 2 weeks for comfort; then the athlete gradually is weaned out of the boot between 3 and 6 weeks, into either an off-the-shelf stirrup brace or a custom short articulating ankle-foot orthosis. During this time, exercises are initiated, gradually moving from range of motion and stretching exercises to a bike program and balancing exercises. The average time to return to sport after this injury is between 4 and 8 weeks.

Grade II and III injuries, by definition, are unstable. There is a consensus that surgical intervention is always needed for grade III injuries. Although opinion is divided regard-

ing surgical treatment of grade II injuries,[7] some authors advocate surgical treatment for all unstable tears (grades II and III), believing that it is preferable to err on the side of surgical treatment with open reduction and internal fixation of grade II injuries than to risk the sequelae of chronic instability.[11]

Acute Versus Chronic Syndesmosis

An acute syndesmosis injury is one that has been present less than 4 weeks. The goal is to reestablish stability and prevent it from becoming a chronic injury. Patients with acute injuries can have a good outcome if anatomic alignment is restored. Various authors have documented that a good reduction is the only predictor of outcome with syndesmosis injuries.[8-10] A recent retrospective study found that 98% of surgically treated patients were still pain free after 2 years, and their overall functional scores on the AAOS Foot and Ankle Module Assessment averaged 96.5.[12]

A chronic injury is one that has been present at least 3 months. During the time it takes for an acute injury to develop into a chronic injury, outcome is uncertain. A chronic injury may be the result of many causes, including misdiagnosis, late diastasis, and subtle fibular malreduction.[10] Pain is the complaint that causes many patients to seek medical evaluation. The key goal of treatment of this difficult condition is to reestablish anatomic alignment with long-term stability. However, detailed evaluation is required to uncover the source of the patient's symptoms. MRI and CT can uncover distal adhesions, malreductions, and other conditions that plain radiographs might miss. Gardner and associates[10] reported that the prevalence of malreduction of the fibula may be three times higher than previously published. If previous screw fixation has failed, the syndesmosis must be reconstructed.

A preoperative injection of local anesthesia into the area of pain can be both diagnostic and therapeutic in uncovering heterotopic ossification as a source of pain;[2,8] such ossification can be excised surgically. Debris that was not detected or removed previously may be a source of malreduction; this can be excised and the syndesmosis fixed with screws. The medial side of the ankle must be examined and any scar tissue or debris removed to allow anatomic reduction.

Treatment may involve excision of medial soft-tissue debris, open reduction with long-term use of screws, reconstruction of lateral ankle ligaments (AITFL and distal syndesmosis), or other interventions.

A modified Broström-like procedure can be used to reconstruct the medial deltoid ligament. If insufficient tissue remains for repair, an autologous graft can be taken from the plantaris, the second or third toe extensor, the semitendinosus, or the gracilis.[2] These autografts also can be used to reconstruct the syndesmosis ligament itself, if needed. An autogenous gracilis graft is the author's tissue of choice.

A synostosis fusion may be a last resort to maintain stability of the tibia-fibula joint; it may be required if the patient is not an athlete and has a very large body mass (more than 250 lb) or has evidence of early significant arthritic changes in the ankle. Complete ankle fusion is a salvage procedure for extensive tibiotalar arthrosis after failed treatment or chronic injury that has progressed with cartilage destruction.

Open Reduction and Internal Fixation for Syndesmosis

Reestablishing the correct tibia-fibula relationship through anatomic reduction is crucial in unstable syndesmosis injuries. The correct tibia-fibula interval, fibula length, and proper alignment of the fibula in the incisura must be established and maintained.

Consideration should be given to repairing the deltoid ligament to allow evaluation of the talar dome and distal tibial cartilage surfaces, including the posterolateral tibia where bone contusions and cartilage injury are most common, and to allow early motion and early weight bearing, which promote cartilage health and collagen repair.[13] In addition, poor surgical and functional outcomes have occurred with chronic deltoid insufficiency. The talar dome bears more weight per unit area than any other joint surface.[1] If the deltoid injury causes even a 1-mm lateral talar shift, the joint contact area decreases by 42%.[7] A lateral talar displacement of more than 2 mm results in a more than 90% chance of degenerative changes unless it is properly realigned.[1]

There is no clear scientific evidence for the number of screws or cortices needed to maintain anatomic alignment.[14] Options include two

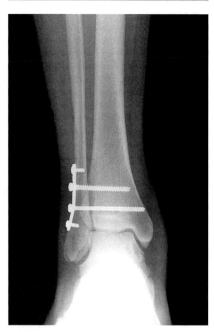

Figure 5   Positioning of syndesmosis screws.

screws and four cortices, although three cortices may be used.

A four-hole, one third tubular plate with 3.5-mm unicortical screws in the proximal and distal holes for positioning of the plate is used for fixation. With the ankle in neutral dorsiflexion, the reduction is held with a large forceps reduction clamp. Under fluoroscopic guidance, a partially threaded 4.5-mm screw is placed transsyndesmotically 1 cm above the distal tibial plafond. This first screw achieves adequate reduction of the fibula to the tibia. The second, more proximal 4.5-mm screw is a fully threaded neutralization screw that is used for added stability (Figure 5).

If an associated Weber C fibular fracture is present, the fibula is fixed anatomically. Sometimes the same plate is used for the syndesmosis screws and the screws to fix the fibular fracture; at other times, two separate plates are used. If the fibular fracture is more than halfway up

Table 1
Postoperative Rehabilitation Protocol

Postoperative	Crutches; no weight bearing; elevate leg Walking boot and cold therapy Start home exercise program for stretching
1 week	Home exercises (stretches and range-of-motion exercises) Protected weight bearing as tolerated Wean to one crutch
2 weeks	Assess range of motion Start home exercises with resistance bands Start weaning out of boot over next 2 weeks to stirrup brace
3 weeks	Normal gait in walking boot

1 month	Increase in weight-bearing exercises
	Proprioception (for example, biomechanical ankle platform system or
	  BAPS board) and gait training with brace and athletic shoe are
	  initiated; includes resistance band exercises, stationary bike

6 weeks	Start progression from bike to elliptical trainer to stair climbing
8 to 10 weeks	Running
2 months	Strengthen entire lower extremity; work on sport-specific agility drills
3 months	Remove screws
4 to 6 months	Return to sport

the shaft, fibular fixation is not performed. Reduction is confirmed with an intraoperative stress test. After documented reduction, sutures are tied medially in the deep deltoid and augmented with sutures in the anterior deltoid.

The syndesmosis screws (as well as the lateral plate) can be removed from 2 to 4 months after placement. The author's recommendation is that this hardware be removed at 3 months or later, depending on the athlete's choice. Although some sources might argue that this technique causes changes in ankle mechanics and limits range of motion over the short term, this limitation is not as crucial as obtaining and maintaining correct reduction of the syndesmosis and the mortise.[11]

Lingering diastasis is a concern with syndesmosis injuries, but with this surgical approach persistent diastasis has not occurred. This surgical technique also allows early weight bearing, prevents disuse atrophy, promotes proprioception training, and hastens return to normal activities.

Complications

Complications of chronic syndesmosis instability may include deltoid insufficiency, a significant cause of instability, and no good solution currently exists for repair of chronic deltoid injuries.

Arthritic changes may develop within 1 year of surgery because of significant impaction injury at the time of the syndesmosis sprain, a fracture that occurred during the injury, or the presence of osteochondral lesions on the tibia or talus. If such lesions occur on the tibia, surgical interventions produce mixed results at best. Tibial osteochondral lesions that are located far posteriorly have better outcomes because they can be resected without significantly affecting the weight-bearing surface. Treatment of other tibial osteochondral lesions is not as successful.

Osteochondral changes can occur on the posterolateral area of the ankle because of plantar flexion and slight eversion that occurs with many syndesmosis injuries. However, osteochondral lesions on the ta-

lus usually can be treated successfully. The difference in treatment outcomes of osteochondral lesions of the tibia and talus may be because the tibia always is weight bearing, whereas the weight-bearing surface of the talus moves with plantar flexion and dorsiflexion so that an area containing an osteochondral lesion on the talus is only intermittently weight bearing.

Screws may break. If this occurs late in the course of treatment and the deltoid ligament is stable, the screws can be removed without compromising stability. However, screw extraction may pose a challenge. Broken cannulated 4.5-mm screws used for syndesmosis fixation can be removed rather easily using the broken-screw removal set with reverse thread extractor. Also, if four cortices are used, the distal broken portion of the screw can be removed from the medial side with less difficulty.

Postoperative Rehabilitation

The rehabilitation protocol after open reduction and internal fixation of the syndesmosis begins with early protected weight bearing, followed by stretching, proprioception, and weight-bearing exercises, then progression to a bike and stair or elliptical program. Running and sport-specific exercises are incorporated (Table 1).

A short articulating ankle-foot orthosis is recommended for protection and to facilitate training.

New Treatment Technique: Tightrope Fixation

Some surgeons are using a tightrope fixation for syndesmosis injuries. Scientific studies are emerging regarding the effectiveness of this permanent suture and washer approach for such a significant ligament injury.[15] If the fixation is adequate, it will have the advantage of not requiring a second surgical procedure to remove the hardware.

Summary

The key to treating syndesmosis injuries is to make the correct initial diagnosis and initiate treatment that will produce optimal stability and outcomes with the least chance for complications or chronicity. Tibiafibula diastasis often is overlooked or misdiagnosed. If a diastasis is undetected or inadequately treated, chronic ankle syndesmosis instability, pain, arthritic changes, and other problems will occur.[16] All acute unstable syndesmosis injuries (grades II and III) need surgical intervention. Appropriate treatment of the acute injury is the best solution for avoiding the adverse conditions associated with chronic injury.

References

1. van den Bekerom MPJ, Lamme B, Hogervorst M, Bolhuis HW: Which ankle fractures require syndesmotic stabilization? *J Foot Ankle Surg* 2007; 46:456-463.

2. Clanton TO, Paulos P: Syndesmosis injuries in athletes. *Foot Ankle Clin North Am* 2002;7:529-549.

3. Lin CF, Gross MT, Weinhold P: Ankle syndesmosis injuries: Anatomy, biomechanics, mechanism of injury, and clinical guidelines for diagnosis and intervention. *J Orthop Sports Phys Ther* 2006;36:372-384.

4. Nonfatal Occupational Injuries and Illnesses Requiring Days Away from Work. *United States Department of Labor News.* Washington, DC, Bureau of Labor Statistics, USDL 07-1741. November 2007.

5. Fites B, Kunes J, Madaleno J, Silvestri P, Johnson DL: Latent syndesmosis injuries in athletes. *Orthopedics* 2006; 29:124-127.

6. Porter DA: Ligamentous injuries of the foot and ankle, in Fitzgerald RH, Kaufer H, Malkani AL (eds): *Orthopaedics.* St. Louis, MO, Mosby, 2002, pp 1607-1621.

7. Jenkinson RJ, Sanders DW, Macleod MD, Domonkos A, Lydestadt J: Intraoperative diagnosis of syndesmosis injuries in external rotation ankle fractures. *J Orthop Trauma* 2005;19: 604-609.

8. Nicholson CW, Anderson RB: Operative treatment of syndesmotic injuries in the competitive athlete. *Tech Foot Ankle Surg* 2006;5:38-44.

9. Zalavras C, Thordarson D: Ankle syndesmotic injury. *J Am Acad Orthop Surg* 2007;15:330-339.

10. Gardner MJ, Demetrakopoulos D, Briggs SM, Helfet DL, Lorich DG: Malreduction of the tibiofibular syndesmosis in ankle fractures. *Foot Ankle Int* 2006;27:788-792.

11. Ebraheim NA, Elgafy H, Padanilam T: Syndesmotic disruption in low fibular fractures associated with deltoid ligament injury. *Clin Orthop Relat Res* 2003;409:260-278.

12. Porter DA, May BD, Berney T: Functional outcome after operative treatment for ankle fractures in young athletes: A retrospective case series. *Foot Ankle Int* 2008;29:887-894.

13. Porter DA, Schon LC: Ankle sprains, ankle instability and syndesmosis injuries, in *Baxter's The Foot and Ankle in Sport*; ed 2. Philadelphia, PA, Mosby, 2007, pp. 273-390.

14. Moore JA, Shank JR, Morgan SJ, Smith WR: Syndesmosis fixation: A comparison of three or four cortices of screw fixation without hardware removal. *Foot Ankle Int* 2006;27: 567-572.

15. Thornes B, McCartan D: Ankle syndesmosis injuries treated with the TightRope suture-button kit. *Tech Foot Ankle Surg* 2006;5:45-53.

16. Ebraheim NA, Taser F, Shafiq Q, Yeasting RA: Anatomical evaluation and clinical importance of the tibiofibular syndesmosis ligaments. *Surg Radiol Anat* 2006;28:142-149.

Ankle Sprains

Carol Frey, MD

Introduction

Inversion injuries to the ankle are one of the most common injuries seen in sports.[1] The incidence has been reported as high as one injury per 10,000 persons per day. The most common injury is to the anterior talofibular ligament followed by a combined injury to the anterior talofibular ligament and the calcaneofibular ligament. Although it has been noted that an isolated injury to the calcaneofibular ligament can exist, it is rarely seen. It is important for the orthopaedic surgeon to recognize that with a twisting injury to the foot and ankle, many structures are at risk for injury, including the peroneal tendons, syndesmosis, base of the fifth metatarsal, subtalar joint, lateral and anterior processes of the talus, Stieda process or the os trigonum, superficial peroneal and sural nerves, and the calcaneal-cuboid and Lisfranc joints. The complete differential diagnosis should be considered when evaluating the patient with an ankle sprain because a significant injury can be missed. Recent studies indicate that the subtalar joint may also be injured in the majority of grade II and III ankle sprains. In the case of an associated subtalar injury, the evaluating surgeon may note ecchymosis along the medial aspect of the heel, also known as the battle sign.

Lateral Collateral Ligament Injuries
Mechanism of Injury

Most injuries to the lateral collateral ligaments occur with a plantar flexion inversion injury to the ankle.[2-4] The lateral collateral ligaments are comprised of the anterior talofibular ligament, calcaneofibular ligament, and the posterior talofibular ligament. The anterior and posterior talofibular ligaments are capsular ligaments that represent discrete thickenings of the ankle joint capsule; the extracapsular calcaneofibular ligament is a distinct structure that is closely approximated to the inferior sheath of the peroneal tendons and is independent of the joint capsule. The anterior talofibular ligament is under maximum tension with the ankle in plantar flexion; in contrast, the calcaneofibular ligament is under most tension with the ankle in dorsiflexion.

Dynamic stabilization of the ankle is achieved with the help of the peroneal tendons, which protect the joint from the strong plantar flexion and inversion forces placed on it by the posterior tibial tendon. The nerves of proprioception that exist in the ankle joint and ligaments signal the peroneal tendons to contract when needed in order to stabilize the ankle joint.

Other biomechanical factors such as tight Achilles tendons, a varus hindfoot, or limited motion in the subtalar joint (for example, tarsal coalition) will cause excessive forces to fall to the lateral side of the foot and ankle and can place the ankle at an increased risk for inversion sprains.

Classification and Evaluation

Ankle sprains are classified as grades I, II, or III. The differences between these grades are outlined in Table 1. Physical examination with stress tests, radiographic stress tests, MRI, arthrograms, and tenograms have been recommended to help grade or assess the severity of the injury.[5-7]

Arthrograms and tenograms are rarely used because their results are difficult to obtain and interpret. The tests lack specificity and must be performed within the first 72 hours of an injury before fibrous clots develop.

MRI is a valuable tool in the evaluation of the patient with chronic ankle pain but does not provide information about ligamentous laxity and is not recommended in the workup of a patient with an acute ankle sprain.

Radiographic stress tests can sometimes provide objective data as to the extent of ligament damage.[8-10] The radiographic anterior drawer test (Fig. 1) is an evaluation of anterior talofibular damage and should be performed in approximately 10° of plantar flexion, the position that places most stress on the anterior talofibular ligament. The tibia is stabilized and the talus is pushed anteriorly, noting any subluxation of the talus with respect to the tibia. Any anterior displacement greater than approximately 4 mm has been considered abnormal, but a comparison should always be made to the opposite ankle.

The radiographic talar tilt test (Fig. 2) is performed by placing the ankle in neutral position (the position that places more stress on the calcaneofibular ligament) or in slight plantar flexion. A comparison is

Table 1
Classification of Ankle Sprains

	Anatomic Injury*	Physical Examination	Radiographic Findings
Grade I	Partial Tear ATF or CF	Negative or 1+ Drawer	– Drawer – Talar tilt
Grade II	Torn ATF Intact CF	2+ Drawer	+ Drawer – Talar tilt
Grade III	Torn ATF Torn CF	3+ Drawer	+ Drawer + Talar tilt

*ATF=anterior talofibular ligament; CF=calcaneofibular ligament

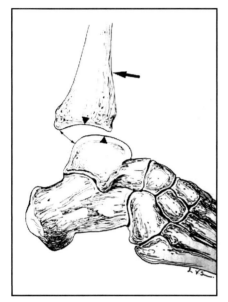

Fig. 1 Anterior instability demonstrated in a stress view. An anterior translation of more than 4.0 mm is usually considered abnormal. (Reproduced with permission from Pfeffer G, Frey C: Ankle instability, in *Current Practice in Foot and Ankle Surgery*. New York, NY, McGraw-Hill, 1993, pp 112-128.)

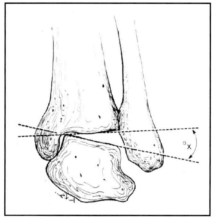

Fig. 2 Lateral instability demonstrated on an inversion stress view. Using this measurement technique varies tilt. A value of 10° or a difference of more than 6° from the uninjured ankle is considered abnormal. (Reproduced with permission from Pfeffer G, Frey C: Ankle instability, in *Current Practice in Foot and Ankle Surgery*. New York, NY, McGraw-Hill, 1993, pp 112-128.)

always made to the opposite ankle. The tibia and the hindfoot are stabilized, and a varus stress is applied. The talar tilt is measured by drawing a line tangential to the distal aspect of the tibia and a line tangential to the proximal aspect of the talus. The angle where these two lines meet is the talar tilt angle. On average, a difference between the injured and the uninjured ankle of greater than 6° denotes a positive test.

Radiographic stress tests are considered by many to be unreliable because the results may vary depending on whether a machine or manual testing was performed; the position of the ankle; amount of relaxation, pain, or swelling; and amount or duration of load applied. Furthermore, normal values have been reported to range from 5° to 23° for the talar tilt test and 2 mm to 9 mm for the anterior drawer test. Although useful in evaluating chronic ankle instability, radiographic stress tests are not indicated in the workup of a

patient with an acute lateral collateral ligament sprain.

The physical examination of the acute lateral ankle sprain should include an assessment of ligamentous laxity. If the patient's level of pain prevents a thorough evaluation, a local anesthetic may be used to block the injured ligaments. The anterior drawer test is performed as described for the radiographic stress tests.

The varus stress test is performed on both ankles for comparison. The ankle should be placed in neutral position to place more stress on the calcaneofibular ligament. The tibia is stabilized in one hand and the hindfoot in the other, making sure that varus stress is being applied through the ankle joint alone. The differences in the two ankles should be noted.

Treatment
Most authors agree that grade I and II ankle sprains should be treated conservatively. Phase 1 of treatment includes rest, ice, compression, elevation, and anti-inflammatory medications. Phase 2 includes range-of-motion stretching, particularly of the Achilles tendon, and strengthening, particularly of the peroneal tendons. Plantar flexion is deemphasized during this phase because this is the position that allows the most stress on the anterior talofibular ligament. Once the patient has full range of motion and has regained strength in the peroneal tendons, Phase 3 of treatment is instituted, which includes assessment of proprioception and agility, and a return to sports participation. A brace is recommended for grade II sprains through all phases of treatment and for sports participation until the end of the season or for a 3-month period, whichever is longer. It usually takes ankles with grade II sprains 2 to 4 weeks to regain full function.

There is some controversy with respect to the appropriate treatment of grade III ankle sprains.[11,12] Primary surgical treatment, cast immobilization, and early mobilization have been advocated.

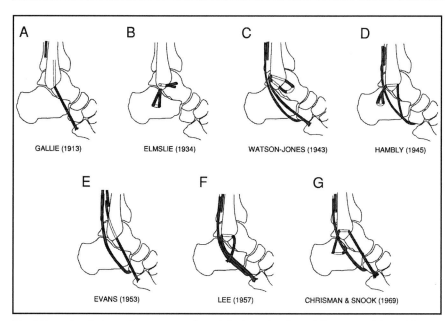

Fig. 3 Several techniques for reconstruction of the lateral collateral ligaments of the ankle are shown. (Reproduced with permission from Pfeffer G, Frey C: Ankle instability, in *Current Practice in Foot and Ankle Surgery*. New York, NY, McGraw-Hill, 1993, pp 112-128.)

damage to the proprioception fibers in the ankle ligaments and capsule or by peroneal weakness. Studies have indicated that balance exercises and a peroneal muscle strengthening program can restore functional stability to even a mechanically unstable ankle.[13,14] Exercise can increase the dynamic reaction time and ankle protection provided by the peroneal muscles. Failure to properly rehabilitate the peroneal muscles and proprioceptors is a major cause of chronic ankle instability.

Chronic Ankle Instability

A significant percentage of athletes will develop chronic instability of the ankle that will require further treatment. Chronic ankle instability may be documented by physical findings and radiographic stress tests. Prior to surgical intervention, the patient should complete an ankle rehabilitation program that includes peroneal muscle strengthening, proprioception training, and Achilles tendon stretching. If functional instability still exists after completion of this program, reconstruction of the ligaments is indicated. More than 50 procedures have been described to reconstruct the lateral collateral ligaments of the ankle. Many of these procedures use a portion or all of the peroneus brevis tendon to reconstruct the lateral ligaments. The most common are the Chrisman-Snook and the Evans procedures (Fig. 3). Most of these procedures have resulted in good outcomes.[15]

Anatomic repair of the ligaments, such as a direct ligament repair, will help preserve maximum ankle function[16] (Fig. 4). In some cases this repair has been augmented with the inferior extensor retinaculum. Because the inferior extensor retinaculum has deep fibers that insert on the floor of the sinus tarsi, augmentation with the inferior extensor retinaculum is indicated in patients who have combined subtalar and ankle instability. The direct ligament repair has the advantages of preserving the peroneal tendons, creating minimal complications, and

In a review of all randomized prospective studies that compare primary surgical treatment versus the nonsurgical treatment of grade III ankle sprains, not one study shows the surgically treated patients to have better outcomes. Exceptions may be ballet dancers and other elite-level performers and athletes, although no randomized prospective study exists to support surgery in this group, either. Furthermore, even though acute repair may result in less talar tilt, patients may take a longer time to become symptom-free and at 1 year, a greater number of patients treated surgically have residual symptoms. In addition, there are more complications reported with acute surgical repair.

Generally, the same treatment protocol is used with grade III injuries as for grade I and II injuries. Grade III injuries progress more slowly through the phases of treatment. During phase 1 of treatment, grade III injuries require an ankle brace with a hindfoot lock or a short leg walking cast.

If a cast is elected, it should be a dorsiflexion walking cast that should not be used for more than 2 weeks. At 2 weeks,

the repair process has commenced with the anterior talofibular ligament in apposition, and significant contracture formation has not begun. After this period, the patient progresses through phases 2 and 3 of treatment.

The patient with the grade III injury should wear a brace and/or have the injury taped for 3 months or until the end of the season, whichever is longer. A strength and balance program should continue through this period, especially for athletes and dancers. Bracing and tape can be used to stabilize the ankle by increasing mechanical stability and decreasing the range of ankle motion (particularly plantar flexion), and by amplifying and transferring the proprioception signals from the ankle. However, it should be kept in mind that tape is expensive to apply and can loosen after 20 to 30 minutes of play.

Proprioception

Freeman[13] introduced the concept of functional instability to describe the patient's subjective complaints of giving way. Functional ankle instability may be caused by

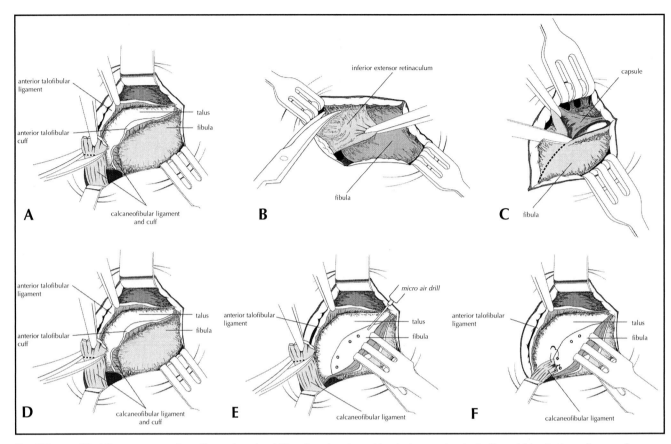

Fig. 4 The modified Brostrum procedure. The patient should be placed supine with a bolster under the ipsilateral hip. **A,** A small, curved incision at the tip of the lateral malleolus can be used. The inferior extensor retinaculum, peroneal tendons, and the lateral collateral ligaments are identified. **B,** The inferior extensor retinaculum is identified and freed to be used later for reinforcing the direct ligament repair. **C,** The capsule is opened in the region of the anterior talofibular ligament. **D,** The lax ligaments are transected, retaining approximately one third of the ligament attached to the distal fibula. **E,** The fibula is roughened with a burr inferior to the original ligaments' attachment. **F,** The distal stump of the anterior talofibular ligament and the calcaneofibular ligament is reattached to the fibula through drill holes, using a nonabsorbable braided suture. The ankle is placed in slight dorsiflexion and maximal eversion, and the sutures are tied. (Reproduced with permission from Pfeffer G, Frey C: Ankle instability, in *Current Practice in Foot and Ankle Surgery.* New York, NY, McGraw-Hill, 1993, pp 112-128.)

allowing retention of greater ankle and subtalar range of motion. Good long-term results have been reported using the direct ligament repair in high-performance athletes.

Exogenous ligament substitutes such as carbon fibers and bovine xenografts have been used more recently, but long-term results have not been reported.

Arthroscopic repair of the lateral collateral ligaments has been reported using suture anchors, staples, and capsular shrinkage (Figs. 5 through 8). Functional stability has been reported following these procedures but no long-term results have been reported.

Whatever the surgical technique selected, the athlete with a varus hindfoot places an added stress on the surgical repair and is at greater risk for reinjury. When extreme varus of the heel is present, a calcaneal osteotomy may be indicated.

Syndesmosis Injuries
Anatomy and Mechanism of Injury
The three ligaments that unite the distal fibula with the distal tibia are the anterior tibiofibular ligament, posterior tibiofibu-

lar ligament, and interosseous ligament. The lower aspect of the interosseous membrane also participates in stabilizing the distal fibula. When the ankle moves from full plantar flexion to full dorsiflexion, the fibula moves laterally 1.5 mm and takes a 2.5° lateral turn on its long axis.

Biomechanical tests have indicated that the anterior inferior tibiofibular ligament provides 35% of the strength of the syndesmosis, the interosseous ligament, 22%, and the posterior inferior tibiofibular ligament, 33%. The interosseous membrane does not add to the resistance to diastasis.

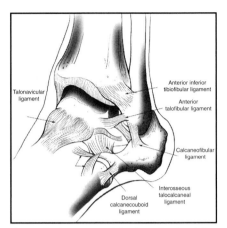

Fig. 5 The ligaments of the lateral side of the ankle.

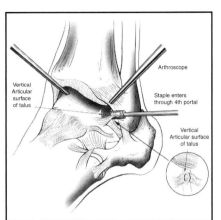

Fig. 7 A staple technique to stabilize the ankle is shown.

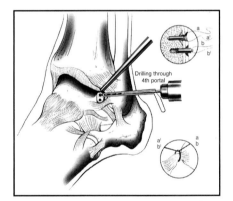

Fig. 6 A suture anchor technique to stabilize the ankle is shown.

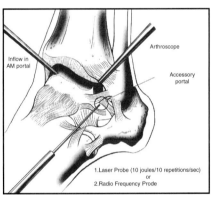

Fig. 8 Laser capsular shrinkage technique to stabilize the ankle.

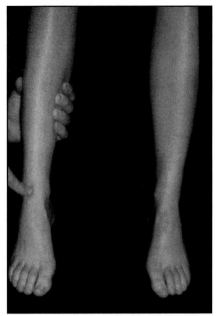

Fig. 9 The squeeze test demonstrates injury to the syndesmosis.

Injuries and sprains to the syndesmosis occur with much less frequency than do those to the lateral collateral ligament. They have been reported to represent approximately 11% of all ankle sprains. Disruption of the syndesmosis has been well described as occurring with or without fractures of the fibula. The mechanism of injury to the syndesmosis is primarily through external rotation or hyperdorsiflexion. This injury is commonly seen in skiers and football players.

Diagnosis

The patient's ankle is typically tender over the anterior syndesmosis, on the anterior lateral aspect of the ankle joint just proximal to the joint line. This may or may not be associated with swelling or tenderness over the deltoid ligament. The squeeze test may be performed by squeezing the fibula and the tibia at the midcalf area (Fig. 9). If the test is positive, it will elicit pain over the anterior syndesmosis. If there is an associated Maisonneuve fracture, the maximum tenderness will be felt in the area of the fracture. The syndesmosis may also be tested by performing the external rotation stress test. When performing this test, the foot is externally rotated on a stabilized leg with the knee flexed at a right angle. The external rotation stress test will create pain at the site of the syn-

desmosis if it is injured. These two tests should be included in any evaluation of an injured athlete after an ankle sprain. Syndesmosis injuries often have a longer rehabilitation time, requiring more long-term disability than injuries to the lateral collateral ligaments of the ankle.

Radiographs of the ankle are required in the evaluation of the athlete with a possible syndesmosis injury. In up to 50% of these cases, there may be a bone avulsion fracture from the anterior or posterior tubercle of the tibia. It is also important to evaluate the syndesmotic space. The tibiofibular clear space, measured 1 cm up from the joint line on the anteroposterior (AP) and mortise views, should be less than 6 mm. This is considered to be the most reliable criteria for detecting widening of the syndesmosis. The tibiofibular overlap on the AP view should be greater than 6 mm. The tibiofibular overlap on the mortise view should be greater than 1 mm. If there is any question as to widening of the syndesmosis, comparison views can be made of the opposite, uninjured ankle or external rotation stress views can be taken. Stress tests have been reported as difficult to obtain in many cases and occasionally other tests such as bone scans, CT, MRI, and arthrograms have been recommended. A positive bone scan will show increased uptake at the talofibular joint.

Treatment

There is universal agreement that sprains of the syndesmosis take considerably longer to heal than sprains to the lateral collateral ligaments of the ankle. It has also been noted that approximately one third of patients with syndesmotic ankle sprains have chronic mild to moderate pain with activity after recovery.

A partial injury to the syndesmosis should be treated in a walking cast for 2 to 4 weeks followed by an ankle rehabilitation program and tape/brace for 3 months or until the end of the season, whichever is longer. If syndesmosis widening is noted on plain or stress radiographs, then surgical repair is recommended. Surgery should include direct surgical repair of the torn anterior tibiofibular ligaments or repair of an avulsion fracture if present. Furthermore, the distal tibiofibular syndesmosis should be transfixed with a syndesmosis screw placed 1 to 2 cm proximal to the distal tibiofibular articulation, with the ankle held in maximum dorsiflexion. Postoperatively, the patient is treated in a non–weight-bearing short leg cast for 4 weeks, followed by 4 more weeks in a weight-bearing cast. The syndesmosis screw should be removed in approximately 12 weeks. It is not uncommon for heterotopic bone to form in the area of the syndesmosis injury, regardless of the treatment program. Unless there is frank synostosis that affects the normal motion of rotation and distal migration of the fibula with respect to the tibia, the results are not affected by heterotopic bone formation.

If a synostosis does occur, the athlete will particularly note pain during push-off and forced dorsiflexion. Dorsiflexion is limited. If symptoms cannot be managed with conservative treatment, including physical therapy, anti-inflammatory agents, and a cushioned heel lift, surgery to remove the synostosis is indicated when the heterotopic bone has matured. The recurrence rate is high with this type of surgery.

References

1. Holmer P, Sondergaard L, Konradsen L, Nielsen PT, Jorgensen LN: Epidemiology of sprains in the lateral ankle and foot. *Foot Ankle Int* 1994;15:72-74.

2. Kannus P, Renstrom P: Treatment for acute tears of the lateral ligaments of the ankle: Operation, cast, or early controlled mobilization. *J Bone Joint Surg Am* 1991; 73: 305-312.

3. Burks RT, Morgan J: Anatomy of the lateral ankle ligaments. *Am J Sports Med* 1994;22:72-77.

4. Colville MR, Marder RA, Zarins B: Reconstruction of the lateral ankle ligaments: A biomechanical analysis. *Am J Sports Med* 1992;20:594-600.

5. Johnson EE, Markolf KL: The contribution of the anterior talofibular ligament to ankle laxity. *J Bone Joint Surg Am* 1983;65:81-88.

6. Colville MR, Marder RA, Boyle JJ, Zarins B: Strain measurement in lateral ankle ligaments. *Am J Sports Med* 1990;18:196-200.

7. Rasmussen O: Stability of the ankle joint: Analysis of the function and traumatology of the ankle ligaments. *Acta Orthop Scand* 1985;211(suppl):1-75.

8. Ahovuo J, Kaartinen E, Slatis P: Diagnostic value of stress radiography in lesions of the lateral ligaments of the ankle. *Acta Radiol* 1988;29:711-714.

9. Louwerens JW, Ginai AZ, van Linge B, Snijders CJ: Stress radiography of the talocrural and subtalar joints. *Foot Ankle Int* 1995;16: 148-155.

10. Ishii T, Miyagawa S, Fukubayashi T, Hayashi K: Subtalar stress radiography using forced dorsiflexion and supination. *J Bone Joint Surg Br* 1996;78:56-60.

11. Thermann H, Zwipp H, Tscherne H: Treatment algorithm of chronic ankle and subtalar instability. *Foot Ankle Int* 1997;18:163-169.

12. Black HM, Brand RL, Eichelberger MR: An improved technique for the evaluation of ligamentous injury in severe ankle sprains. *Am J Sports Med* 1978;6:276-282.

13. Freeman MAR: Instability of the foot after injuries to the lateral ligaments of the ankle. *J Bone Joint Surg Br* 1965;47:669-677.

14. Mascaro TB, Swanson LE: Rehabilitation of the foot and ankle. *Orthop Clin North Am* 1994;25:147-160.

15. Colville MR, Grondel RJ: Anatomic reconstruction of the lateral ankle ligaments using a split peroneus brevis tendon graft. *Am J Sports Med* 1995;23:210-213.

16. Gould N, Seligson D, Gassman J: Early and late repair of lateral ligaments of the ankle. *Foot Ankle* 1980;1:84-89.

Plantar Heel Pain

Glenn B. Pfeffer, MD

Introduction

Plantar heel pain is one of the most common problems treated in orthopaedic practice.[1] Despite its frequency, little is known about the pathophysiology of this condition. Patients and physicians are often frustrated by symptoms refractory to varied and prolonged treatment modalities. The ability to effect a cure correlates with the precision of the diagnosis and is dependent on an understanding of both the complex anatomy of the heel and the multiple causes of plantar heel pain.

Diagnosis

The differential diagnosis of plantar heel pain includes atrophy of the fat pad; stress fracture of the calcaneus; rupture of the plantar fascia; proximal (and distal) plantar fasciitis; plantar fibromatosis; tendinitis of the flexor hallucis longus; tumor of the calcaneus; and nerve injury such as that to the first branch of the lateral plantar nerve, tarsal tunnel syndrome, and postoperative neuroma of the medial calcaneal sensory nerve.

In differentiating these varied diagnoses, a comprehensive medical history is essential. The history should include the patient's general medical condition, any substantial change in weight, the exact location and duration of pain and whether it radiates, and the relationship of pain to athletic activities, particularly those requiring running and jumping. The time of day that maximal pain occurs should be noted. Patients with proximal plantar fasciitis will frequently complain of disabling pain with the first few steps

out of bed in the morning. Chronic pain at rest may be caused by a tumor of the calcaneus. Radiculopathy in the L5-S1 distribution should be considered in the patient with low back pain and, particularly when the heel pain is bilateral, a systemic process should be excluded. Pain at the sites of tendinous insertions (enthesiopathy) is often a prominent feature in patients with a seronegative spondyloarthropathy.[2,3] Ankylosing spondylitis, psoriatic arthritis, Reiter's syndrome, intestinal arthropathies, and Behçet's syndrome must be excluded in the patient with heel pain that occurs in conjunction with skin lesions, conjunctivitis, arthritis, back pain, or abdominal complaints. An HLA/B27 test and erythrocyte sedimentation rate are useful screening methods for these diagnoses. Gout, Paget's disease, or sarcoidosis are rare with isolated painful inflammation in the plantar heel. The ischemic changes of peripheral vascular disease are also an unusual cause of plantar heel pain.

The key to the examination of plantar heel pain is to determine the specific focal area of maximal tenderness (Fig. 1). Each diagnosis has a maximally tender spot. The medial calcaneal tuberosity, lateral calcaneal tuberosity, proximal plantar fascia, distal plantar fascia, proximal abductor (overlying the first branch of the lateral plantar nerve), tarsal tunnel, flexor hallucis longus at the knot of Henry, the fat pad, and any scar from a previous surgery should be percussed and compressed to determine tenderness and the reproduction of a patient's

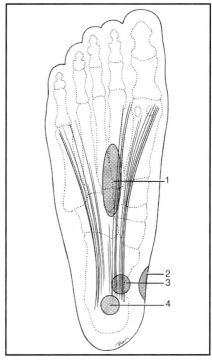

Fig. 1 Areas of maximal focal tenderness: 1 = midfoot plantar fasciitis, 2 = compression of first branch lateral plantar nerve, 3 = proximal plantar fasciitis, 4 = fat pat atrophy. (Reproduced with permission from Pfeffer GB, Baxter DE: Surgery of the adult heel, in Jahss MH (ed): *Disorders of the Foot and Ankle*, ed 2. Philadelphia, PA, WB Saunders, 1991, pp 1396-1416.)

symptoms. Deep pressure may often have to be applied. The windlass mechanism puts tension on the plantar fascia and may cause an increase in the patient's pain[4,5] (Fig. 2). When the fascia is taut, the plantar fascia should be palpated for defects proximally (rupture) or masses distally (plantar fibromatosis).

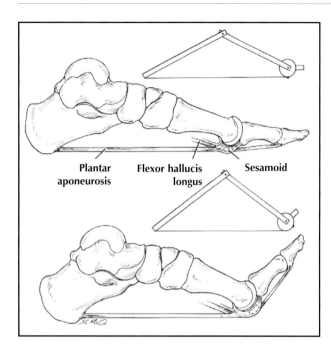

Fig. 2 The windlass mechanism. (Reproduced with permission from Richardson EG: The foot in adolescents and adults, in Crenshaw AH (ed): *Campbell's Operative Orthopaedics,* ed 7. St. Louis, MO, CV Mosby, 1987.)

Plantar aponeurosis   Flexor hallucis longus   Sesamoid

The presence of a neuroma in a previous surgical scar will have a positive percussion sign directly over the cut nerve. Achilles tendon tightness is often associated with various causes of plantar heel pain (proximal plantar fasciitis and distal plantar fasciitis) and is tested by holding the foot in a neutral position and passive dorsiflexion of the ankle.

A patient's weight should also be documented on the physical examination. Increased body weight is associated with proximal plantar fasciitis.[6] It is often impossible, however, for a patient to achieve weight loss while a painful heel causes limitation of activity.

Anatomy of the Fat Pad
The fat pad cushions the foot with each heel strike.[7] A healthy middle-aged man has a gait velocity of approximately 82 m/min and a cadence of 116. This rate results in 58 heel strikes/min with a force of 110% of body weight. A middle- or long-distance runner generates a force of 200% of body weight. Considering timing, impact forces, and an average heel area of 23 cm², the loading pressure

of a 70-kg man is approximately 9.3 kg/cm² when running.

Anatomic studies of the human heel pad have identified structural specialization that is capable of meeting these high impacts.[8,9] The anatomy of the heel pad was first described by Teitze in 1921. He emphasized the specialized anatomy of the heel pad, with elastic adipose tissue organized as spiral fibrous tissue septa anchored to one another, the calcaneus, and the skin. Designed to resist compressive loads, the tissue septa are U-shaped or comma-shaped, fat-filled columns.[10] The septa are reinforced internally with elastic transverse and diagonal fibers that connect the thicker walls and separate the fat into compartments.[11] The thickness of the heel pad is the most important factor in determining the stresses seen in the tissue beneath it. After age 40 years, the adipose tissue begins to deteriorate, with the insidious loss of collagen, elastic tissue, water, and overall thickness of the heel pad. These changes result in softening and thinning in the heel pad, loss of shock absorbency, and

decreased protection of the underlying calcaneal tuberosity.

Causes of Chronic Heel Pain
The Fat Pad
Advanced atrophy of the plantar heel is an unusual problem and almost always occurs in the elderly patient. Heel pad atrophy can also occur in patients with rheumatoid arthritis.[12] A patient with calcaneodynia secondary to fat pad atrophy complains of plantar heel pain aggravated by hard-soled shoes and walking on non-resilient surfaces.[10,13] By clinical examination, the patient has soft, flattened heel pads, with prominence of the underlying calcaneal tubercles. Compression of this area by the examiner duplicates the symptoms, with pain maximal over the central weight-bearing portion of the heel pad. There is no radiation of the pain and the plantar fascia is not tender distally. The overlying plantar skin almost always demonstrates inflammation, from underlying bony irritation. This is not seen in any other cause of plantar heel pain. There is no reliable surgical treatment for this problem. A steroid solution should never be injected into the fat pad because it will promote further atrophy. The patient's symptoms are best treated with soft-soled shoes and a heel cup. A plastic heel cup that elevates the painful area and centralizes the fat pad under the prominent tuberosity is often the treatment of choice. A shock-absorbing insert, such as a cellular rubber gel or silicone pad, may also be beneficial. In addition, a slight heel elevation can be useful by shifting some of the weight bearing more anteriorly.

A rare cause of heel pain related to the fat pad is piezogenic ("piezo" meaning pressure) papules.[11] The normal fat chambers coalesce with degenerative changes in the dermis, creating piezogenic papules on the heel that appear with weight bearing. Multiple small papules are a common occurrence. Large, painful papules can form occasionally. It is not well understood why these larger papules are painful. Herniation of subcutaneous fat through defects in the dermis with subsequent local ischemia may be the cause. Heel cups may be sufficient treatment, but a custom orthosis molded to take pressure off of the painful papules is often required. In the absence of any papules, pinpoint tenderness on the heel can be caused by a glomus tumor, which is exquisitely tender to local pressure and changes in temperature. Surgical excision of the glomus tumor is curative.[14]

Another unusual cause of fat pad pain is separation of the fat pad from its anchor on the plantar aspect of the calcaneus. The heel pad becomes painful and freely mobile. The likely etiology for this separation is the presence of a fluid-filled cyst between the calcaneus and the fat pad, usually following direct trauma to the heel. MRI of the heel can confirm the diagnosis. Aspiration of the cyst and immobilization in a non-weight-bearing cast may permanently close the dead space. Surgical treatment consists of excision of the cyst through either a medial or lateral incision and removal of several millimeters of the plantar calcaneus. A compression dressing and adequate closed drainage should be used. The goal is for the heel pad to re-adhere to the underlying calcaneus.

Stress Fracture of the Calcaneus

Diffuse pain over the fat pad can occasionally be caused by an underlying stress fracture of the calcaneus.[15] Stress fractures of the calcaneus are uncommon and only occur in patients who place a significant stress on their heels. Military recruits who trained for more than 16 hours per day were found to be at particular risk for a calcaneal stress fracture. The stress fracture appears on the lateral radiographs as a vertical sclerotic band running from the posterior superior plateau into the cancellous region of the calcaneus. The trabecular pattern of bone is perpendicular to the line of the stress fracture. Often the stress fracture does

not appear on initial radiographs and a technetium-99m bone scan may be required to detect early cases. The bone scan will demonstrate significant increased uptake on delayed images of the calcaneus. Although rare, a tumor of the calcaneus should be considered in the differential diagnosis of an abnormal bone scan.[16,17] Careful examination of the radiographs is essential. The sclerotic band of the stress fracture usually becomes evident on radiographs by 3 to 4 weeks after the onset of symptoms. On occasion, MRI may be required to evaluate the problem. Patients with proximal plantar fasciitis or heel pain syndrome will often have a hot bone scan directly over the medial calcaneal tuberosity related to inflammation of the periosteum. This finding is in clear distinction from a true stress fracture of the body of the calcaneus.

Clinically, a stress fracture of the calcaneus presents with diffuse pain about the entire heel. The patient has a history of progressive calcaneal pain almost always associated with a period of prolonged, intense activity. Mild erythema and swelling may be present. The hallmark of this condition is significant tenderness with simultaneous medial and lateral compression of the calcaneus. The pain is not localized to the plantar aspect of the heel alone. Casting is not required and symptoms usually resolve over 6 to 8 weeks. Weight bearing is allowed as tolerated with crutches. A removable cast may facilitate ambulation. Nonsteroidal anti-inflammatory agents, contrast baths, and a shock-absorbent heel insert may all be beneficial. Activity modification is essential to avoid recurrent injury.

Acute Rupture of the Plantar Fascia

If an active patient experiences the acute onset of proximal heel pain, rupture of the plantar fascia should be considered. Rupture is much less common than chronic proximal plantar fasciitis and can be easily differentiated on the basis of

physical examination and history. A palpable defect in the proximal plantar fascia is present just distal to the medial calcaneal tuberosity. Ecchymosis and local hemorrhage occur with significant tenderness over the proximal plantar fascia. An athletic patient will often relate acute hyperextension of the midfoot that occurred while jamming the foot into a small pothole during running. There is often a history of proximal plantar fasciitis that has been treated with a steroid injection.[18-20] A short leg cast is helpful in a patient who needs to bear weight. Otherwise, crutches with weight bearing as tolerated is an appropriate treatment. Exercises directed at stretching the plantar fascia should be started when the acute inflammation lessens after several weeks.

Patients with a history of plantar fasciitis who rupture their plantar fascia often experience relief of their chronic plantar pain. However, they often develop a variety of new foot problems, including dorsal and lateral midfoot pain, midfoot swelling, metatarsalgia, and decreased toe-off strength.[21] These symptoms are best treated with supportive shoes, a medial longitudinal arch support, and, in refractory cases, prolonged casting for 8 weeks.

Proximal Plantar Fasciitis

Proximal plantar fasciitis is the most common cause of plantar heel pain, accounting for approximately 80% of patients with plantar symptoms. The average age of a patient with proximal plantar fasciitis is 45 years. The condition is twice as common in women as in men. There may be a history of increased stress on the foot from prolonged standing or athletic activity. There may be a history of recent weight gain. Symptoms are usually insidious in onset and often worse with the first few steps upon awakening. During sleep, the foot is in a plantar-flexed position, which allows the proximal plantar fascia to contract. The stretch placed on the plantar fascia by standing produces significant symptoms. The pain often resolves during the day, exacerbated by prolonged standing or athletic activity.[1,22-29]

Patients with proximal plantar fasciitis experience pain where the plantar fascia arises from the medial calcaneal tuberosity. A patient presents with maximal tenderness over the medial calcaneal tuberosity that may be associated with discomfort over the plantar fascia distally for 1 to 2 cm. The examiner frequently has to apply a considerable amount of pressure to localize this painful area. Radiation of pain is unusual. Contrary to many reports, the patient almost never has increased pain or duplication of symptoms with passive dorsiflexion of the toes, which causes traction on the plantar fascia by the windlass mechanism. Patients with proximal plantar fasciitis often have tightness of the Achilles tendon.[30,31] Achilles tendon tightness should be evaluated with the foot held in neutral position. In addition, there is a possible loss of dorsiflexion when compared to the contralateral, asymptomatic leg. A correlation has been postulated between proximal plantar fasciitis, pes planus, and pes cavus, although this relationship has never been clearly documented.

The diagnosis of proximal plantar fasciitis should be differentiated from other sources of plantar heel pain, especially distal plantar fasciitis and entrapment of the first branch of the lateral plantar nerve. Conservative and surgical treatments of these diagnoses are different. Proximal plantar fasciitis is a condition of chronic tears and inflammation in the origin of the plantar fascia where it arises from the medial calcaneal tuberosity. During gait, the plantar fascia places a repetitive traction stress on this area. The mechanism for this probably lies in the particular anatomic relationship of the plantar fascia to the calcaneus.[32]

The plantar fascia is a multilayered fibrous aponeurosis.[8] It arises predominantly from the medial calcaneal tuberosity and inserts distally through several slips into the plantar plates of the metatarsophalangeal joints, the flexor tendon sheaths, and the bases of the proximal phalanges of the digits. When the metatarsophalangeal joints are dorsiflexed during gait, the windlass of the plantar fascia tightens and raises the longitudinal arch.[5] A secondary effect is traction on the calcaneus by the inelastic plantar fascia fibers.[4]

Over time with repetitive stress, microtears can occur in the origin of the plantar fascia. Along with continued traumatic fatigue in the fascia, a reparative inflammatory response develops. As documented by MRI, the inflamed proximal plantar fascia becomes thickened, increasing from a mean thickness of 3 mm in a normal heel to a mean thickness of 7.4 mm in patients with chronic heel pain.[10] Surgical biopsy specimens of the origins of the plantar fascia in patients with proximal plantar fasciitis reveal collagen necrosis, angiofibroblastic hyperplasia, chondroid metaplasia, and matrix calcification. A similar process in all likelihood develops in the flexor brevis muscle directly deep to the plantar fascia, which accounts for the plantar spur that develops in the origin of that muscle in approximately 50% of patients with proximal plantar fasciitis. Nirschl and Pettrone[33] describe similar pathologic changes to the proximal planter fascia occurring in the extensor carpi radialis brevis origin in patients with tennis elbow. The striking similarity of these two conditions has in the past led clinicians to refer to chronic proximal plantar fasciitis as "tennis heel."

The diagnosis of proximal plantar fasciitis is largely a subjective one, based on tenderness and a reproduction of a patient's symptoms with pressure over the medial calcaneal tuberosity and proximal plantar fascia. Multiple tests have been suggested for the evaluation of this condition, including three-phase bone scan, ultrasound, CT scan, MRI, and sonography.[34-36]

It has also been suggested that oblique radiographs of the heel can reveal a fatigue fracture in the area of the medial calcaneal tuberosity. Ultrasound, sonography, and MRI are all able to demonstrate a thickening of the proximal plantar fascia consistent with chronic inflammatory changes.[37-39] All of these studies rarely contribute to the diagnosis and treatment of proximal plantar fasciitis, however, and should be reserved for the patient who presents a diagnostic challenge. Even the commonly obtained standing lateral radiograph of the painful heel is not required for the initial evaluation and treatment of a patient who presents with a classic history and examination for proximal plantar fasciitis.

A periosteitis of the medial calcaneal tuberosity frequently occurs in conjunction with the degenerative changes of the proximal plantar fascia. The majority of painful heels, in fact, have a positive delayed technetium-99m bone scan. The focal uptake in the medial calcaneal tuberosity is in clear distinction to the intense diffuse uptake on bone scan of a calcaneal stress fracture.

Conservative Treatment More than 90% of patients with proximal plantar fasciitis are cured with conservative care.[1,24,25,40,41] Nonsurgical treatment modalities include activity modification, shoe alteration, prefabricated inserts, custom-fabricated orthoses, stretching exercises, physical therapy, nonsteroidal anti-inflammatory agents, ultrasound, cortisone injections, night splints, casting, and recently, shock wave therapy.[42] The appropriate sequence of these treatments or which are most efficacious and cost-effective is not known. A large, prospective, randomized study of 236 patients demonstrated that an 8-week treatment course of Achilles tendon and plantar fascia stretching improved 72% of patients with proximal plantar fasciitis.[27] Stretching in addition to the use of a silicone or rubber heel cup yielded improvement in 95% and 88% of patients, respectively. The addition of a custom-made polypropylene orthotic device added no benefit to stretching alone. A reasonable conclusion, therefore, is that an 8-week program of stretching and the use of a prefabricated cushioned heel cup is a reasonable cost-effective first line of treatment for proximal plantar fasciitis.[43] Contrast baths, ice, massage, and anti-inflammatory agents may be of some additional benefit. Achilles tendon and plantar fascia stretching should be performed frequently during the day. If a patient is unable to master these techniques through a home program, a short formal consultation with a physical therapist may be helpful.

In the athletic patient, modification in training is essential. Mileage reduction, alternating activities, work reduction, and shortened workouts should be considered. Low-resistance cycling and running in the swimming pool are effective cardiovascular activities that are usually not stressful to the heel. A motion-control running shoe in the patient with pes planus or a cushioned shoe in the patient with pes cavus should also be prescribed.

If significant symptoms persist after 8 weeks of initial conservative care, a steroid injection is often beneficial. If a radiograph has not already been taken, it should be obtained prior to injecting the steroid. Care should be taken to inject deep to the plantar fascia so as not to cause atrophy of the fat pad.[21] A medial approach is easy to use and allows the steroid to spread along the broad origin of the plantar fascia[44] (Fig. 3). The needle is walked across the anterior border of the calcaneus just deep to the plantar fascia, thereby avoiding the plantar nerves. Multiple steroid injections may predispose a patient to plantar fascia rupture. Ninety-five percent of patients should expect improvement in their symptoms within the first few days after the injection. The maximum benefit of the injection, however, generally only lasts 6 to 8 weeks, with significant long-term benefits in less than 50% of patients.[21]

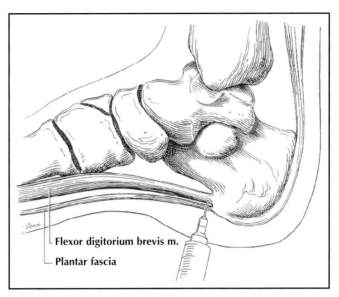

Flexor digitorium brevis m.

Plantar fascia

Fig. 3 Injection for proximal plantar fasciitis. (Reproduced with permission from Pfeffer GB, Baxter DE: Surgery of the adult heel, in Jahss MH (ed): *Disorders of the Foot and Ankle,* ed 2. Philadelphia, PA, WB Saunders, 1991, pp 1396-1416.)

Iontophoresis of dexamethasone is another popular treatment for a patient with persistent symptoms. A recent randomized double-blind placebo-controlled study, however, demonstrated that the iontophoresis provided no long-lasting benefit at only 1 month after treatment.[45] Patients who underwent iontophoresis did experience greater immediate relief of symptoms than those treated with traditional modalities alone. In the rare patient who requires immediate reduction of symptoms, such as the elite athlete, the modality of iontophoresis should be considered.

In patients who remain refractory to these initial conservative measures, other options include a custom orthotic device, a short-leg walking cast for 6 weeks, shoe modification with a rocker bottom and steel shank, and a dorsiflexion night splint.[46-48] The night splint has recently gained widespread acceptance with significant improvement in symptoms demonstrated in multiple studies.[49] A commercially available night splint provides a dorsiflexion stretch to the plantar fascia and metatarsophalangeal joints. Using this technique, a recent study by Powell and associates,[47] demonstrated that 88% of patients with refractory symptoms

improved after only 1 month of treatment. Given the success of this device in patients with refractory symptoms, it should be considered as an addition to the initial treatment protocol.

Historically, the presence of a calcaneal spur was of great importance in the treatment of proximal plantar fasciitis.[50] In 1963, however, Tanz[51] demonstrated that only 50% of patients with plantar heel pain had a heel spur and that 16% with nonpainful heels also had a heel spur. Rubin and Witton[52] determined that same year that only 10% of patients with heel spurs were symptomatic. Multiple authors have since demonstrated that the successful treatment of proximal plantar fasciitis is not contingent on the surgical removal of a heel spur. This is not surprising, given that the spur arises deep to the plantar fascia in the non-weight-bearing substance of the flexor brevis muscle.

Surgical Treatment The majority of patients with proximal plantar fasciitis can be treated conservatively. A few patients will have symptoms that extend beyond several months. For patients with significant disability and more than 6 months of persistent pain, surgical intervention should be considered.[6,18,24,53,54] There are several options for the surgical treatment

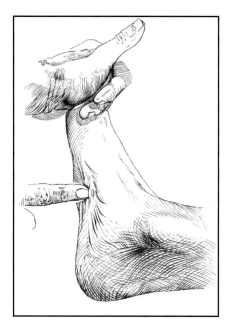

Fig. 4 Maximal tenderness exacerbated by the windlass mechanism in patient with midfoot plantar fasciitis. (Reproduced with permission from Campbell JW, Inman VT: Treatment of plantar fasciitis and calcaneal spurs with the UCBL shoe insert. *Clin Orthop* 1974;103:57.)

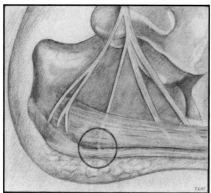

Fig. 5 Entrapment of the first branch of the lateral plantar nerve. (Reproduced with permission from Pfeffer GB, Baxter DE: Surgery of the adult heel, in Jahss MH (ed): *Disorders of the Foot and Ankle*, ed 2. Philadelphia, PA, WB Saunders, 1991, pp 1396-1416.)

of a patient with refractory proximal plantar fasciitis. All surgical treatments, however, have in common a partial, not complete, release of the plantar fascia where it arises from the medial calcaneal tubercle.

The plantar fascia plays a critical role in the static and dynamic stabilization of the longitudinal arch.[55] Nonsurgical, spontaneous rupture of the plantar fascia leads to some degree of a flatfoot deformity in patients and a complete surgical release produces a similar result. Several recent studies demonstrate the deleterious effect of a complete surgical plantar fascia release in that patients walk less energetically on the side treated surgically, place less force on the heel, and demonstrate a decrease in arch stability by 25%, creating a less rigid and more deformable arch.[56-59] Even a partial plantar fasciotomy decreases the arch-

supporting function of the plantar fascia, but to a less significant degree than a complete release.[60] The average width of the entire plantar fascia, including the medial, central, and lateral bands, is approximately 3 cm. When the medial plantar fascial fibers are divided at surgery, an attempt should be made to preserve at least 50% of the lateral fibers.

The two most common surgical options for proximal plantar fasciitis are open and endoscopic partial plantar fascia release. An open release provides direct visualization of the plantar fascia, allowing the surgeon to divide only the thickened portion that is involved in the inflammatory process.[61-66] The endoscopic approach provides less morbidity and a more rapid return to function postoperatively.[67] Partial plantar fascia release is usually performed under regional anesthesia with intravenous sedation and standby general anesthesia. An ankle block is very useful, using a 1:1 solution of 0.25% bupivacaine hydrochloride (Marcaine) and 1% lidocaine, both without epinephrine. A well-padded ankle tourniquet set at 250 mm Hg is beneficial, although not required.

Distal Plantar Fasciitis and Tendinitis of the Flexor Hallucis Longus

An unusual but quite disabling cause of chronic heel pain is distal plantar fasciitis. The patient has tenderness over the midportion of the plantar fascia. As opposed to proximal plantar fasciitis, dorsiflexion of the toes almost always exacerbates the patient's symptoms by the windlass mechanism stretching the midfascial fibers. There is usually only minimal tenderness over the most proximal fascial fibers (Fig. 4). Distal plantar fasciitis is most frequently seen in sprinters and middle-distance runners who run on their toes. Significant pes cavus or pes planus may also predispose to this condition by placing increased stress on the midportion of the plantar fascia.

Tendinitis of the flexor hallucis longus tendon can be characterized by pain in the plantar medial midfoot. This condition can easily be distinguished from distal plantar fasciitis. Passive dorsiflexion of the great toe aggravates both plantar fasciitis and flexor hallucis longus tendinitis, but resisted flexion of the toe is painful only with involvement of the tendon. Careful palpation with motion of the tendon is usually sufficient to confirm the diagnosis. A painful plantar fibromatosis involving the midplantar fascia can also be detected by careful examination.

A medial longitudinal arch support is often not tolerated in a patient with distal plantar fasciitis because it pushes up on the inflamed plantar fascia and increases tension on its fibers. Circumferential taping of the foot with 1-in adhesive tape applied over a nonadhesive elastic wrap is usually most beneficial. Rest, alteration of training, nonsteroidal anti-inflammatory agents, ice, massage, contrast baths, and stretching exercises that emphasize plantar fascia and Achilles tendon stretching are also helpful. A 1/8-in medial heel wedge may take tension off the plantar fascia. If these modalities fail, a successful treatment option is the University of California Biomechanical Laboratory (UCBL) orthosis.[68] The theory of the UCBL orthosis is to hold the foot in supination and thereby decrease tension on the plantar fascia. The UCBL insert is usually not helpful in patients with proximal plantar fasciitis, as the rigid material used in construction of the insert often aggravates the inflamed heel. It is extremely unusual to operate on a patient for distal plantar fasciitis. If prolonged conservative treatment of more than 6 months fails, however, a partial plantar fascia release may help reduce symptoms.

Nerve Injury

Entrapment of the First Branch of the Lateral Plantar Nerve One of the most commonly overlooked causes of chronic plantar heel pain is entrapment of the first branch of the lateral plantar nerve.[69] Entrapment of the nerve accounts for approximately 15% of chronic plantar heel pain.[70] The first branch innervates the periosteum of the medial calcaneal tuberosity, the long plantar ligament, the abductor digiti quinti, and flexor brevis muscles. Entrapment occurs as the nerve changes from a vertical to a horizontal direction around the medial plantar aspect of the heel.[71-73] The exact site of compression is between the heavy deep fascia of the abductor hallucis muscle and the medial caudal margin of the medial head of the quadratus plantae muscle (Fig. 5). Athletes who spend a significant amount of time on their toes, such as sprinters, ballet dancers, and figure skaters, are prone to entrapment of the first branch of the lateral plantar nerve by the well-developed abductor hallucis. The medial calcaneal branches that innervate the plantar and medial aspects of the heel pass superficial to the abductor hallucis muscle and are not involved with the entrapment of the first branch.

Another potential site of entrapment of the first branch is where the nerve passes just distal to the medial calcaneal tuberosity. Inflammation and spur formation in the origin of the flexor brevis muscle can produce sufficient swelling to cause compression of the nerve against the long plantar ligament. The inflammatory changes of proximal plantar fasciitis can therefore predispose to chronic entrapment of the nerve, with both conditions often occurring simultaneously.

The diagnosis of entrapment of the first branch of the lateral plantar nerve is a clinical one. It is therefore incumbent on the examiner to differentiate entrapment of the first branch from other more common causes of heel pain. Early morning pain is not common with isolated nerve entrapment, which tends to cause more pain at the end of the day or after prolonged activity. The pathognomonic sign of entrapment of the first branch of the lateral plantar nerve is maximal tenderness where the nerve is compressed between the deep, taut fascia of the abductor hallucis muscle and the medial caudal margin of the quadratus plantae muscle. If simultaneous inflammation of the fascia occurs, the patient may have associated tenderness over the proximal plantar fascia and medial calcaneal tuberosity. Without maximal tenderness over the course of the nerve on the plantar medial aspect of the foot, the diagnosis of entrapment should not be made. Some patients may have paresthesias elicited with pressure over the nerve at the entrapment site, although this is not a common occurence. Entrapment of the isolated medial plantar nerve ("jogger's foot") occurs more distally at the level of the navicular tuberosity and should not be confused with entrapment of the first branch of the lateral plantar nerve more proximally.[74]

Motor weakness in the abductor digiti quinti may be detected, although no cutaneous sensory deficit occurs. Electromyography and nerve conduction studies are not consistent in the diagnosis entrapment of the first branch of the lateral plantar nerve.[75] Measurement of nerve conduction slowing across the site of entrapment is technically demanding, and denervation potentials in the intrinsic foot muscles may only rarely occur because of the possible dynamic nature of this particular compression neuropathy. A comparison may be drawn to the diagnosis of a posterior interosseous nerve entrapment in the upper extremity.

Treatment for athletes with entrapment of the first branch of the lateral plantar nerve is similar to that for proximal plantar fasciitis. Conservative care consists of rest, activity modification, nonsteroidal anti-inflammatory agents, contrast baths, ice, massage, stretching exercises, and the injection of a cortisone preparation. The addition of a prefabricated shock-absorbent heel insert will also help decrease inflammation in the area. In athletes with excessive pronation, especially long-distance runners, a nonrigid medial longitudinal arch support can decrease compression of the nerve.

The vast majority of patients can be cured with conservative care. As with the treatment of proximal plantar fasciitis, in a patient with persistent disabling symptoms of more than 6 months, surgical intervention should be considered. Eighty-five percent of patients can be expected to have a good or excellent result from surgical decompression of the nerve. Decompression of the first branch of the lateral plantar nerve requires an open procedure.[69] Adequate decompression of the nerve cannot be performed endoscopically. The endoscope is reserved for patients who have isolated proximal plantar fasciitis without evidence of nerve entrapment. The mean recovery time to resumption of everyday activity is 3 months.

Tarsal Tunnel Syndrome In making the diagnosis of entrapment of the first branch of the lateral plantar nerve, it is important not to miss a more extensive nerve entrapment consistent with a tarsal tunnel syndrome.[76] Posttraumatic adhesions, bony spurs from the medial

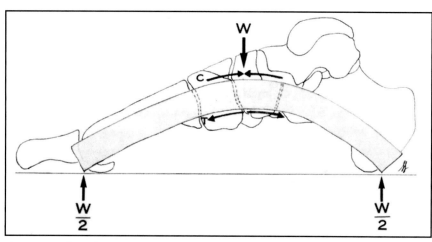

Fig. 6 Truss effect of plantar aponeurosis. (Reproduced with permission from Sarrafian FK: Functional characteristics of the foot and plantar aponeurosis under tibiotalar loading. *Foot Ankle* 1987;8:4-18.)

calcaneus or talus, chronic inflammation, benign tumors, and varicosities can all cause compression of the posterior tibial nerve within the tarsal tunnel. Excessive pronation has been postulated, but has never proven, to predispose to tarsal tunnel syndrome by placing repeated stress on the structures within the tarsal tunnel.

In general, the plantar heel pain produced by tarsal tunnel syndrome is more diffuse and less focal than that of either proximal plantar fasciitis or entrapment of the first branch of the lateral plantar nerve. A careful clinical examination should easily distinguish among these three entities. The salient clinical feature of tarsal tunnel syndrome is direct focal tenderness over the nerve as it passes beneath the flexor retinaculum. Percussion of the nerve in this area will reproduce the patient's symptoms, which can include pain, burning, or tingling on the plantar aspect of the foot. Subjective numbness of the toes may occur, although objective decreased sensibility is rarely demonstrated. Some patients may complain of proximal radiation of their symptoms. Electromyography and nerve conduction studies can be helpful in making a diagnosis. A nor-

mal study, however, does not exclude the diagnosis of tarsal tunnel syndrome. Entrapment of the first branch of the lateral plantar nerve with an associated chronic proximal plantar fasciitis may occur rarely in conjunction with a tarsal tunnel syndrome.

A medial heel wedge can decrease tension on the posterior tibial nerve and its branches. A steroid injection into the tarsal tunnel can also be beneficial, but usually produces only transient relief of symptoms. Surgical release of the flexor retinaculum and exploration of the tarsal tunnel can be expected to provide relief in a majority of patients, especially when the symptoms are unilateral and easily reproducible on preoperative examination. Internal neurolysis of the nerve is rarely indicated.

Complications of Heel Surgery
The most common problem encountered after plantar heel surgery is persistent pain. It is essential to determine if the pain is similar to or different from the patient's preoperative symptoms. Causes of similar continued heel pain include incorrect preoperative diagnosis, insufficient release of the plantar fascia, inadequate release of a nerve entrapment, and

inadequate recovery time. The most common causes for postoperative pain that is different from preoperative symptoms are: incisional neuromas and biomechanical imbalance of the foot.

In the patient with persistent postoperative heel pain that has not changed in nature, it is essential to make sure that the initial diagnosis was correct. The plantar fascia may have been adequately treated, but the source of persistent symptoms may be tarsal tunnel sundrome that was overlooked. A partial release of the plantar fascia may have been performed for the diagnosis of proximal plantar fasciitis, without addressing the simultaneous occurrence of an entrapment of the first branch of the lateral plantar nerve. Careful postoperative examination of the patient to document areas of maximal tenderness can distinguish these diagnoses.

Persistent pain consistent with proximal plantar fasciitis is often a result of inadequate release of the plantar fascia. This problem most commonly occurs after minimal-incision heel surgery. Performed through a 1-cm incision, an attempt is made to divide the plantar fascia blindly just distal to the medial calcaneal tuberosity. Using this approach, it is possible to completely miss the plantar fascia, performing no release at all. A similar inadequate release can occur with endoscopic plantar fascia release. There is a clear learning curve using endoscopic technique and, unless the plantar fascia fibers are clearly visualized, it is easy to miss them entirely.

If the correct diagnosis has been made and the appropriate treatment carried out, a patient may have persistent heel pain simply on the basis of inadequate recovery time. The mean time to recovery after release of the first branch of the lateral plantar nerve is approximately 3.5 months, with some patients requiring up to 9 months. There is a similar range of recovery time after a partial release of the plantar fascia for proximal plantar fasciitis. In order to reduce the recovery period, an attempt should be made to minimize edema and decrease inflammation in the immediate postoperative period. Full weight bearing should be discouraged for at least 2 weeks after surgery, and the use of non-steroidal anti-inflammatory agents and contrast baths can be helpful during the first 6 weeks of recovery. An injection of a steroid preparation may also be considered if some symptoms persist 4 months postoperatively. Continued plantar fascia stretching exercises can also be beneficial, especially in the patient recovering from a partial division of the plantar fascia.

Postoperative pain that is dissimilar to the patient's preoperative symptoms is most likely iatrogenic. An incisional neuroma is the most common significant complication of this type. Once a painful neuroma develops postoperatively, the results can be disastrous. Anything that touches the medial or lateral scar causes extreme pain and shoe wear is often impossible. A positive percussion/Tinel sign is present over the incision line, causing dysesthesias in the nerve distribution. Distal to the incision, there is a decrease in sensibility. While division of the superficial medial calcaneal sensory nerve is possible in an open procedure, nerve injury has increased because of the popularity of the endoscopic technique and inadequate visualization of the superficial sensory nerves.

Initial treatment should include a course of systematic desensitization performed by an experienced therapist. One injection of a steroid preparation into the painful area is also reasonable. More than one injection over a short period of time is unlikely to be beneficial and causes atrophy of the subcutaneous tissue. A transcutaneous electrical nerve stimulator may be helpful in some patients, as may modalities to decrease local edema and inflammation. A postoperative neuroma may serve as a trigger for a complex regional pain syndrome that may require sympathetic blocks and medical management.

If a patient is unable to tolerate the neuroma symptoms, surgical intervention should be considered. Repair of the nerve is usually impossible at this level because of the small size of the distal fibers and the difficulty in mobilizing the nerve. Excision of the neuroma with resection of the proximal nerve to a level within the tarsal tunnel above the shoe line is recommended. Rather than resecting the entire superficial medial or lateral sensory nerve, which would leave a significant area of numbness on the heel, only the branch involving the neuroma should be resected. This can be accomplished by intrafascicular dissection of the nerve branch under loupe magnification. The tourniquet should be deflated before closing the wound to obtain hemostasis and to prevent a hematoma postoperatively. No subcutaneous sutures should be used and a 3-0 nonabsorbable nylon skin suture will help minimize postoperative inflammation.

The first branch of the lateral plantar nerve can be cut inadvertently during surgery or significant postoperative adhesions can develop. Because this nerve runs deep to the abductor fascia, however, if a neuroma forms it is often asymptomatic. If chronic pain is present, the proximal fibers of the first branch of the lateral plantar nerve should be resected back to within the tarsal tunnel. If the patient complains of any symptoms referable to the posterior tibial nerve or its branches, a wide tarsal tunnel release should be performed simultaneously.

In some cases of persistent postoperative heel pain, a specific etiology cannot be determined. Previous surgery may obscure a definitive diagnosis. In these patients, there is often diffuse tenderness over the tarsal tunnel, the first branch of the lateral nerve, and the proximal plantar fascia. Salvage surgery consists of a release of the tarsal tunnel, decompression of entrapment of the first branch of the lateral plantar nerve, and complete division of the plantar fascia from its insertion on the calcaneal tuberosity. If at the original surgery the posterior tibial nerve and its branches have already been released in an adequate manner (proximal to the medial malleolus and distal beneath the abductor hallucis muscle), there is unlikely to be a benefit reexploration and neurolysis of the posterior tibial nerve is unlikely to be beneficial.

Perhaps the most difficult complication that can develop following surgery for proximal plantar fasciitis is a biomechanical imbalance of the foot. Patients have surgery to treat plantar heel pain, only to develop metatarsalgia or pain in the dorsal midfoot or calcaneocuboid joints. This clinical condition is referred to as lateral column syndrome. A truss mechanism exists in the foot through the plantar fascia as demonstrated by the windlass mechanism (Fig. 6). If the plantar fascia is divided surgically, either partially or completely, there are increased compressive forces transmitted to the dorsal and lateral aspect of the midfoot, and decreased flexion forces on the metatarsophalangeal joint complex.[31,58] These changes often produce pain with weight bearing.

As originally described, the endoscopic technique often involved complete release of the plantar fascia, and many patients developed lateral column symptoms. Complete plantar fascia release by either endoscopic or open techniques is no longer recommended, although inadvertent complete division of the plantar fascia may still cause similar symptoms. Treatment consists of either a custom-fabricated orthotic device or a short-leg walking cast. Metatarsalgia can often be treated with a custom-made orthotic device. Dorsal and lateral foot symptoms usually require a short-leg walking cast. Up to 12 weeks of casting may be needed before symptoms begin to abate. The lateral plantar heel pain that occasionally occurs following a partial plantar fascia release results from increased stress on the lateral calcaneal tuberosity from the remaining plantar fascia fibers. This condition usually resolves spontaneously without the need for an orthotic device or cast.

References

1. Gill LH: Plantar fasciitis: Diagnosis and conservative management. *J Am Acad Orthop Surg* 1997;5:109-117.

2. Gerster JC: Plantar fasciitis and Achilles tendinitis among 150 cases of seronegative spondarthritis. *Rheumatol Rehabil* 1980;19:218-222.

3. Gerster JC, Piccinin P: Enthesopathy of the heels in juvenile onset seronegative B-27 positive spondyloarthropathy. *J Rheumatol* 1985;12:310-314.

4. Hedrick MR: The plantar aponeurosis. *Foot Ankle Int* 1996;17:646-649.

5. Hicks JH: The mechanics of the foot. Part II: The plantar aponeurosis and the arch. *J Anat* 1954;88:25-30.

6. Hill JJ Jr, Cutting PJ: Heel pain and body weight. *Foot Ankle* 1989;9:254-256.

7. Miller WE: The heel pad. *Am J Sports Med* 1982;10:19-21.

8. Sarrafian SK (ed): *Anatomy of the Foot and Ankle: Descriptive, Topographic, Functional*, ed 2. Philadelphia, PA, JB Lippincott, 1993.

9. Jahss MH, Michelson JD, Desai P, et al: Investigations into the fat pads of the sole of the foot: Anatomy and histology. *Foot Ankle* 1992;13:233-242.

10. Prichasuk S: The heel pad in plantar heel pain. *J Bone Joint Surg Br* 1994;76:140-142.

11. Lin E, Ronen M, Stampler D, Suster S: Painful piezogenic heel papules: A case report. *J Bone Joint Surg Am* 1985;67:640-641.

12. Resnick RB, Hudgins LC, Buschmann WR, Kummer FJ, Jahss MH: Analysis of the heel pad fat in rheumatoid arthritis. *Foot Ankle Int* 1999;20:481-484.

13. Jorgensen U: Achillodynia and loss of heel pad shock absorbency. *Am J Sports Med* 1985;13:128-132.

14. Quigley JT: A glomus tumor of the heel pad: A case report. *J Bone Joint Surg Am* 1979;61: 443-444.

15. Protzman RR, Griffis CG: Stress fractures in men and women undergoing military training. *J Bone Joint Surg Am* 1977;59:825.

16. Hertzanu Y, Mendelsohn DB, Gottschalk F: Aneurysmal bone cyst of the calcaneus. *Radiology* 1984;151:51-52.

17. Khermosh O, Schujman E: Benign osteoblastoma of the calcaneous. *Clin Orthop* 1977;127:197-199.

18. Anderson RB, Foster MD: Operative treatment of subcalcaneal pain. *Foot Ankle* 1989;9:317-323.

19. Leach R, Jones R, Silva T: Rupture of the plantar fascia in athletes. *J Bone Joint Surg Am* 1978;60:537-539.

20. Sellman JR: Plantar fascia rupture associated with corticosteroid injection. *Foot Ankle Int* 1994;15:376-381.

21. Bordelon RL: Subcalcaneal pain: A method of evaluation and plan for treatment. *Clin Orthop* 1983;177:49-53.

22. Karr SD: Subcalcaneal heel pain. *Orthop Clin North Am* 1994; 25:161-175.

23. Furey JG: Plantar fasciitis: The painful heel syndrome. *J Bone Joint Surg Am* 1975;57: 672-673.

24. Gill LH, Kiebzak GM: Outcome of nonsurgical treatment for plantar fasciitis. *Foot Ankle Int* 1996;17:527-532.

25. Lapidus PW, Guidotti FP: Painful heel: Report of 323 patients with 364 painful heels. *Clin Orthop* 1965;39:178-186.

26. Pfeffer G, Bacchetti P, Deland J, et al: Comparison of custom and prefabricated orthoses in the initial treatment of proximal plantar fasciitis. *Foot Ankle Int* 1999;20:214-221.

27. Snook GA, Chrisman OD: The management of subcalcaneal pain. *Clin Orthop* 1972;82: 163-168.

28. Wolgin M, Cook C, Graham C; Mauldin D: Conservative treatment of plantar heel pain: Long-term follow-up. *Foot Ankle Int* 1994; 15:97-102.

29. Kibler WB, Goldberg C, Chandler TJ: Functional biomechanical deficits in running athletes with plantar fasciitis. *Am J Sports Med* 1991;19:66-71.

30. Carlson RE, Fleming LL, Hutton WC: The biomechanical relationship between the tendoachilles, plantar fascia, and metatarsophalangeal joint dorsiflexion angle. *Foot Ankle Int* 2000;21:18-25.

31. Sarrafian SK: Functional characteristics of the foot and plantar aponeurosis under tibiotalar loading. *Foot Ankle* 1987;8:4-18.

32. Cardinal E, Chhem RK, Beauregard CG, Aubin B, Pelletier M: Plantar fasciitis: Sonographic evaluation. *Radiology* 1996;201: 257-259.

33. Nirschl RP, Pettrone FA: Tennis elbow. *J Bone Joint Surg Am* 1979;61:832-839.

34. Wall JR, Harkness MA, Crawford A: Ultrasound diagnosis of plantar fasciitis. *Foot Ankle* 1993;14:465-470.

35. Williams PL, Smibert JG, Cox R, Mitchell R, Klenerman L: Imaging study of the painful heel syndrome. *Foot Ankle* 1987;7:345-349.

36. Berkowitz JF, Kier R, Rudicel S: Plantar fasciitis: MR imaging. *Radiology* 1991;179:665-667.

37. Sewell JR, Black CM, Chapman AH, Statham J, Hughes GR, Lavender JP: Quantitative scintigraphy in diagnosis and management of plantar fasciitis (calcaneal periostitis): Concise communication. *J Nucl Med* 1980;21:633-636.

38. Vasavada PJ, DeVries DF, Nishiyama H: Plantar fasciitis: Early blood pool images in diagnosis of inflammatory process. *Foot Ankle* 1984;5:74-76.

39. Davis PF, Severud E, Baxter DE: Painful heel syndrome: Results of nonoperative treatment. *Foot Ankle Int* 1994;15:531-535.

40. Lutter LD: Surgical decisions in athletes' subcalcaneal pain. *Am J Sports Med* 1986;14: 481-485.

41. Spiegl PV, Johnson KA: Heel pain syndrome: Which treatments to choose? *J Musculoskel Med* 1984;66-71.

42. Knuttgen HG: Ossatron: New treatment for sports injuries? *Georgia Tech Sports Medicine and Performance Newsletter* 1999;1:1.

43. Miller RA, Torres J, McGuire M: Efficacy of first-time steroid injection for painful heel syndrome. *Foot Ankle Int* 1995;16:610-612.

44. Dasgupta B, Bowles J: Scintigraphic localisation of steroid injection site in plantar fasciitis. *Lancet* 1995;346:1400-1401.

45. Gudeman SD, Eisele SA, Heidt RS, et al: Treatment of plantar fasciitis by iontophoresis of 0.4% dexamethasone: A randomized, double-blind, placebo-controlled study. *Am J Sports Med* 1997;25:312-316.

46. Mizel MS, Marymont JV, Trepman E: Treatment of plantar fasciitis with a night splint and shoe modification consisting of a steel shank and anterior rocker bottom. *Foot Ankle Int* 1996;17:732-735.

47. Powell M, Post WR, Keener J, Wearden S: Effective treatment of chronic plantar fasciitis with dorsiflexion night splints: A crossover prospective randomized outcome study. *Foot Ankle Int* 1998;19:10-18.

48. Tisdel CL, Harper MC: Chronic plantar heel pain: Treatment with a short leg walking cast. *Foot Ankle Int* 1996;17:41-42.

49. Wapner KL, Sharkey PF: The use of night splints for treatment of recalcitrant plantar fasciitis. *Foot Ankle Int* 1991;12:135-137.

50. DuVries HL: Heel spur (calcaneal spur). *Arch Surg* 1957;74:536-542.

51. Tanz SS: Heel pain. *Clin Orthop* 1963;28: 169-177.

52. Rubin G, Witten M: Plantar calcaneal spurs. *Am J Orthop* 1963;5:38-41; 53-55.

53. Lester DK, Buchanan JR: Surgical treatment of plantar fasciitis. *Clin Orthop* 1984;186:202-204.

54. Davies MS, Weiss GA, Saxby TS: Plantar fasciitis: How successful is surgical intervention? *Foot Ankle Int* 1999;20:803-807.

55. Daly PJ, Kitaoka HB, Chao EY: Plantar fasciotomy for intractable plantar fasciitis: Clinical results and biomechanical evaluation. *Foot Ankle* 1992;13:188-195.

56. Arangio GA, Chen C, Kim W: Effect of cutting the plantar fascia on mechanical properties of the foot. *Clin Orthop* 1997;339:227-231.

57. Huang CK, Kitaoka HB, An KN, Chao EY: Biomechanical evaluation of longitudinal arch stability. *Foot Ankle* 1993;14:353-357.

58. Katoh Y, Chao EY, Laughman RK Schneider E Morrey BF: Biomechanical analysis of foot function during gait and clinical applications. *Clin Orthop* 1983;177:23-33.

59. Kitaoka HB, Luo ZP, An KN: Mechanical behavior of the foot and ankle after plantar fascia release in the unstable foot. *Foot Ankle Int* 1997;18:8-15.

60. Thordarson DB, Kumar PJ, Hedman TP, Ebramzadeh E: The effect of partial versus complete plantar fasciotomy on the windlass mechanism. *Foot Ankle Int* 1997;18:16-20.

61. Kahn C, Bishop JO, Tullos HS: Plantar fascia release and heel spur excision via plantar route. *Orthop Rev* 1985;14:222-225.

62. Kinley S, Frascone S, Calderone D, Wertheimer SJ, Squire MA, Wiseman FA: Endoscopic plantar fasciotomy versus traditional heel spur surgery: A prospective study. *J Foot Ankle Surg* 1993;32:595-603.

63. Ward WG, Clippinger FW: Proximal medial longitudinal arch incision for plantar fascia release. *Foot Ankle* 1987;8:152-155.

64. Sammarco GJ, Helfrey RB: Surgical treatment of recalcitrant plantar fasciitis. *Foot Ankle Int* 1996;17:520-526.

65. Barrett SL, Day SV: Endoscopic plantar fasciotomy for chronic plantar fasciitis/heel spur syndrome: Surgical technique: Early clinical results. *J Foot Surg* 1991;30:568-570.

66. Barrett SL, Day SV, Pignetti TT, Robinson LB: Endoscopic plantar fasciotomy: A multi-surgeon prospective analysis of 652 cases. *J Foot Ankle Surg* 1995;34:400-406.

67. Palumbo R, Kudros SA, Baxter DE: Endoscopic plantar fasciotomy: Indications, techniques, and complications. *Sports Med Arthrosc Rev* 1994;2:317-322.

68. Baxter DE, Pfeffer GB: Treatment of chronic heel pain by surgical release of the first branch of the lateral plantar nerve. *Clin Orthop* 1992;279:229-236.

69. Baxter DE, Thigpen CM: Heel pain: Operative results. *Foot Ankle* 1984;5:16-25.

70. Przylucki H, Jones CL: Entrapment neuropathy of muscle branch of lateral plantar nerve: A cause of heel pain. *J Am Podiatry Assoc* 1981; 71:119-124.

71. Rondhuis JJ, Huson A: The first branch of the lateral plantar nerve and heel pain. *Acta Morphol Neerl Scand* 1986;24:269-279.

72. Rask MR: Medial plantar neurapraxia (jogger's foot): Report of 3 cases. *Clin Orthop* 1978;134:193-195.

73. Schon LC, Glennon TP, Baxter DE: Heel pain syndrome: Electrodiagnostic support for nerve entrapment. *Foot Ankle* 1993;14:129-135.

74. Radin EL: Tarsal tunnel syndrome. *Clin Orthop* 1983;181:167-170.

75. Clancy WG: Tendinitis and plantar fasciitis in runners. *Orthopedics* 1983;6:217-233.

76. Campbell JW, Inman VT: Treatment of plantar fasciitis and calcaneal spurs with the UC-BL shoe insert. *Clin Orthop* 1974;103:57-62.

Current Management of Tarsometatarsal Injuries in the Athlete

Mark S. Myerson, MD

Rebecca Cerrato, MD

Abstract

The frequency of foot injuries is increasing in certain athletes, particularly injuries to the tarsometatarsal joint complex. A high index of suspicion for this injury is required to make the diagnosis because the clinical signs often are subtle. A comprehensive examination along with bilateral weight-bearing plain radiographs of the foot should be obtained in any suspected midfoot injury. Further imaging studies and stress radiographs may assist in the diagnosis and direct management. Nonsurgical treatment can be considered in a stable sprain with less than 2 mm of diastasis between the first and second metatarsal bases on a weight-bearing AP foot radiograph. Any tarsometatarsal injury with displacement of more than 2 mm or instability requires surgical treatment. Various techniques and approaches have been described, depending on the injury pattern, including primary arthrodesis and ligament reconstruction. Anatomic reduction is the most critical goal in the treatment of these injuries.

The current management of injuries to the tarsometatarsal complex depends on the type and mechanism of the injury, the forces involved, whether the injury is high or low energy, and whether it occurred in an athlete. Foot and ankle injuries are some of the more common injuries in athletes, with foot injuries accounting for 16% of all sports-related injuries.[1] Some athletes are at higher risk. Midfoot sprains occur in 4% of football players per year, with offensive linemen incurring 29.2% of these injuries.[2] Tarsometatarsal injuries in athletes are distinctly different from those caused by high-energy trauma. Athletes tend to have subtle clinical and radiographic findings, and a high index of suspicion is necessary to recognize and diagnose these injuries appropriately. A wide spectrum of injuries to the tarsometatarsal and associated interrelated joints is now recognized. Treatment concepts have evolved over the past decade, with the use of more rigid forms of fixation and, most importantly for the athlete, intensive rehabilitation.

Anatomy

The tarsometatarsal joint complex includes the three cuneiforms, the cuboid, and the bases of the five metatarsals. From a functional perspective, this complex can be divided into three columns.[3] The medial column includes the first metatarsal-medial cuneiform joint, the middle column includes the second and third tarsometatarsal joints as well as the articulations between the middle and lateral cuneiforms, and the lateral column consists of the articulations between the fourth and fifth metatarsals and the cuboid. The distal articulation of the middle cuneiform (and the corresponding second metatarsal) is recessed 8 mm proximally relative to the medial cuneiform and 4 mm relative to the lateral cuneiform.[4] This "keystone" configuration allows the base of the second metatarsal to articulate with five adjacent bones, creating a tight mortise that provides substantial stability to the entire tarsometatarsal complex. Additionally, the anatomic shape of the transverse arch provides inherent osseous stability. In cross section, the trapezoidal shape of the middle three metatarsal bases and the corresponding shape of the cuneiforms create a Roman arch, which also adds stability to the midfoot. Although the columns of the tarsometatarsal joint complex function interdependently, the motion of each is quite different, which has implications for both diagnosis and treatment. The medial column allows approximately 3.5 mm of dorsoplantar movement. The middle column permits only approximately 0.6 mm of sagittal plane motion, whereas the lateral column allows an average of 13 mm of movement in this plane.[5] It is therefore interesting to note that most injuries to the tarsometatarsal joint complex involve the second metatarsocuneiform joint (or the middle column). There is almost no sagittal movement of the second metatarsal and, despite the inherent anatomic rigidity conferred by the recessed position of the base of the metatarsal and despite the strength of the oblique Lisfranc ligament, fracture and/or dislocation (isolated or in combination with additional joint instability) is most common in this articulation.

Additional stability is conferred on the entire articulation by strong ligamentous attachments, which are classified by topography (dorsal, interosseous, and plantar) and by course (longitudinal, oblique, and transverse).[6] There is a certain symmetry to all of these ligaments, with the exception of those at the second metatarsal, where no intermetatarsal ligament is present. The longitudinal and oblique fibers connect the cuneiforms and cuboid to the metatarsals, and the transverse ligaments connect the metatarsal bases. The plantar ligaments are stronger and stiffer than the dorsal ligaments. Between the first and second metatarsals, there is no intermetatarsal ligament; rather, the Lisfranc ligament runs obliquely from the medial cuneiform to the plantar base of the second metatarsal. Biomechanical studies have shown that, of all ligaments in the tarsometatarsal complex, the Lisfranc ligament has the most strength and highest load to failure.[7]

Mechanism of Injury

It is important to understand the different mechanisms of injuries to the tarsometatarsal joint complex. Obviously, a high-energy injury as-

sociated with a motor-vehicle crash, a fall from a height, or a crushing injury is vastly different from an injury caused by low-velocity indirect forces, which are responsible for the injuries in athletes. Over the past decade, there has been a greater frequency of low-energy twisting injuries in athletes. To a large extent, this is caused by changes in the interface between the athletic shoe and the playing surface, particularly when the athlete is playing on artificial turf. Injuries of the tarsometatarsal joints that take place on regular turf in American football are influenced by the type of shoe and cleat worn and by the forces on the foot when another athlete falls on it while it is in a compromised or fixed position. These athletic injuries to the tarsometatarsal complex can be divided broadly into plantar flexion injuries and abduction injuries, although this is an oversimplification because there are probably varying patterns of each force. Plantar flexion injuries occur when an axial force is applied along the longitudinal axis of a foot that is in slight equinus with the metatarsals firmly planted on the ground distally, resulting in failure under tension dorsally.[8,9] As the body moves forward over the forefoot, twisting with rotation and abduction of the forefoot occurs, causing the various patterns of dislocation. The classic example is in an American football lineman who, during a block, has his foot plantar flexed and the metatarsophalangeal joints maximally dorsiflexed. He sustains the injury when a force, such as a tackle, is directed onto the heel or when someone falls onto the firmly planted foot. Abduction injuries occur when the forefoot is forcefully abducted with the hindfoot fixed. As the abduction force increases, the recessed base of the

second metatarsal dislocates, and the remaining metatarsals displace laterally. These injuries also can occur in sports in which a stirrup creates a fulcrum effect on the forefoot, such as equestrian sports and windsurfing.[8,10] This is an oversimplification because many patterns of injury can occur, either as fractures of the metatarsals or as subluxation of the tarsometatarsal and intercuneiform joints.

Classification

Several classification schemes have been applied to injuries of the tarsometatarsal joints. In 1909, Quénu and Küss[11] described different patterns of tarsometatarsal injuries. They organized these patterns into three groups: homolateral, isolated, and divergent. In 1982, Hardcastle and associates[12] discussed their experience with treating 119 tarsometatarsal injuries, reporting that the prognosis depended more on articular incongruity than on the mechanism of injury. They modified the classification system of Quénu and Küss by dividing the injuries into types A, B, and C. Type A indicates complete displacement of all of the metatarsals or complete incongruity of the tarsometatarsal joint complex, type B reflects partial incongruity, and type C is a divergent pattern. Myerson and associates[13] refined this classification system after reviewing 76 fracture-dislocations of the tarsometatarsal joint complex. Type B injuries were divided into medial dislocations (type B1) and lateral dislocations (type B2). Type C injuries were divided into those with partial incongruity (type C1) and those with total incongruity (type C2). Later, Chiodo and Myerson[3] described the three-column theory to classify these injuries, emphasizing the separate motion segments of the midfoot. That classification system helps with treatment planning because the metatarsals within a column often work as a functional unit. The system also highlights the importance of movement of various parts of the midfoot, which in turn is important with respect to the outcome. Subtle incongruity is less well tolerated in the middle than in the medial or lateral column. It was demonstrated that symptomatic posttraumatic arthritis is most common at the base of the second metatarsal.[14] The lateral column, which has the greatest sagittal plane motion, is the least likely to be involved in posttraumatic arthritis. This is an interesting concept because the movement of these joints must somehow be correlated with the functional outcome of treatment.

It should not be assumed that an injury to the tarsometatarsal joints includes only the base of the metatarsals and the corresponding cuneiform and cuboid. Frequently, there is involvement of the intercuneiform space or the naviculocuneiform joints. This involvement was first reported in 1986. Since that time, this pattern of injury has been observed far more frequently in athletes and particularly in American football players in the United States.[13] The instability, and therefore the potential for posttraumatic arthritis, is greater with this pattern of tarsometatarsal as well as intertarsal injury, and treatment of these injury patterns differs from that of the more common isolated middle-column subluxation. The use of the eponym Lisfranc injuries as well as the term tarsometatarsal joint should be avoided; the broader term tarsometatarsal joint complex should be used to refer to all types of injuries in the midfoot.

Classification systems are useful for comparing one study with another, and they can help to guide treatment and describe the radiographic appearance of traumatic high-energy injuries. They are less helpful in the diagnosis and management of the more isolated and subtle injuries in athletes. Regardless, they still provide a good framework for the concept of three functional columns. Ligamentous injuries in athletes are routinely classified with the American Medical Association's Standardized Nomenclature of Athletic Injuries.[15] First- and second-degree sprains are defined as partial tears, and a third-degree sprain is a complete rupture of the ligamentous support. Nunley and Vertullo[16] reported on the management of midfoot sprains in 15 athletes and created a new classification system to address subtle tarsometatarsal injuries with minimal or no displacement seen on weight-bearing radiographs. They classified the injury on the basis of clinical findings, radiographs, and bone scintigrams. With stage I injuries, patients were able to bear weight but could not return to playing sports; less than 2 mm of diastasis between the first and second metatarsals was seen on the weight-bearing AP radiographs. The physical findings associated with stage II injuries were similar to those seen in stage I, but there were 2 to 5 mm of diastasis between the first and second metatarsals. Despite the instability of the first-second tarsometatarsal joint seen on AP radiographs, lateral radiographs showed no collapse of arch height (Figure 1). Stage III included injuries to both the first and the second intermetatarsal space, with diastasis, but there was loss of arch height, defined by a decreased distance between the fifth metatarsal

and the medial cuneiform as seen on lateral weight-bearing radiographs. When using this classification system, the patient should be able to fully bear weight because weight-bearing and/or stress radiographs are an important tool in the diagnosis and planning of treatment.

Diagnosis

A midfoot sprain is often subtle, and, when examining an athlete, there should be a high index of suspicion for a tarsometatarsal injury because it is not as easily diagnosed as a high-velocity injury. Often, the athlete describes a "pop" in the foot occurring at the time of injury and has pain that is aggravated by bearing weight.[9] The foot should be examined for asymmetry between the first and second toes, subtle swelling, and point tenderness over the midfoot.[17] Plantar ecchymosis confined to the midfoot is a clinical finding that is highly suggestive of a midfoot injury in an athlete.[18] Gentle manipulation of the midfoot by passively pronating and abducting the forefoot can be used to assess the stability of the tarsometatarsal complex (Figure 2). Passive dorsiflexion and abduction of the forefoot place a strain across the medial column, and pain will serve as an apprehension sign.[17,19] Shapiro and associates[9] described two provocative maneuvers that they found to produce pain in some athletes with a tarsometatarsal injury: (1) compression of the midfoot and (2) dorsal and plantar deviation of the first metatarsal head while the examiner stabilizes the second metatarsal head. It should not be assumed that simple manipulation of the first metatarsal in the sagittal plane is diagnostic because the medial column is frequently not involved in the injury and the first metatarsocuneiform joint may be

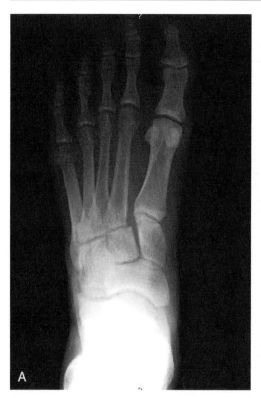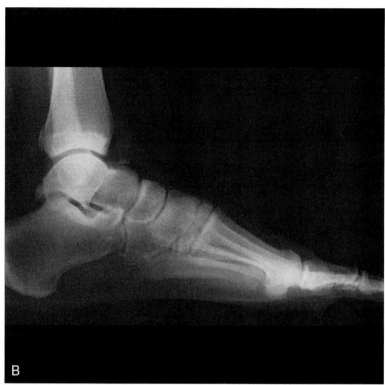

Figure 1　The AP **(A)** and lateral **(B)** radiographs demonstrate diastasis between the medial and middle columns; however, no loss of arch height is seen on the lateral weight-bearing radiograph. This is a stage II injury.

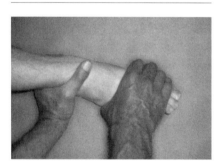

Figure 2　Manipulation of the midfoot with the passive pronation-abduction maneuver.

asymptomatic. Another clinical stress test consists of squeezing the first-second interspace in the coronal place to stress the base of the middle and the medial column in an attempt to elicit pain or a palpable click (Figure 3). This test is more specific for the diagnosis of injury. There can be a diastasis between the first and second metatarsals or a diastasis between the medial and middle cuneiforms combined with a diastasis between the first and second metatarsals. In the latter situation, compression of the interspace under fluoroscopy will confirm the extent of the instability.

When an injury to the tarsometatarsal joint complex is suspected, standard radiographs of the foot (preferably made while the patient is bearing weight), including AP, 30° internal oblique, and lateral views, should be made. The goal of diagnosis is to determine if there is displacement or instability of the joints because this indicates whether surgical treatment is needed. Normally, the medial border of the second metatarsal lines up with the medial border of the middle cuneiform on the AP radiograph, and the medial border of the fourth metatarsal lines up with the medial border of the cuboid on the oblique radiograph. Displacement of more than 2 mm between the first and second metatarsal bases should raise the suspicion of a tarsometatarsal injury and must be compared with the first-second intermetatarsal space in the contralateral foot. The fleck sign, which is a small avulsion fragment arising from either the lateral edge of the medial cuneiform or the medial aspect of the second metatarsal base, has been described.[13] These fragments are the points of attachment of the tarsometatarsal (Lisfranc) ligament. A lateral radiograph should show normal continuity from the dorsal cortex of the first metatarsal to the medial cuneiform. Faciszewski and associates[20] emphasized that the lateral weight-bearing

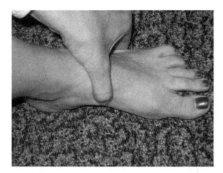

Figure 3 Stressing the bases of the middle and medial columns can be performed by squeezing the first-second interspace.

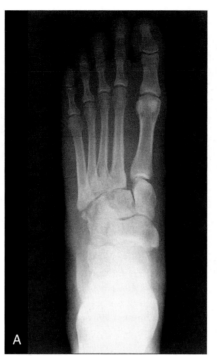
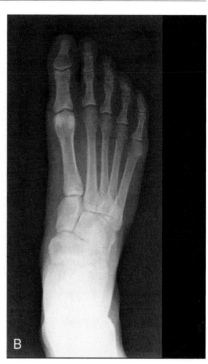

Figure 4 The bilateral weight-bearing radiographs of this patient show asymmetric widening between the first and second metatarsal bases when the left foot **(A)** is compared with the right foot **(B)**.

radiograph helps to differentiate a simple sprain from a complex ligamentous disruption. They calculated the distance from the plantar base of the fifth metatarsal to the base of the medial cuneiform and compared it with the distance in the uninjured foot. Patients with a negative value (the medial cuneiform was plantar to the base of the fifth metatarsal) had collapse of the longitudinal arch and poor outcomes.

If a patient presents with pain in the midfoot following an injury and radiographs demonstrate normal findings, the next step should be to evaluate the stability of the midfoot. A tarsometatarsal injury and its stability are documented with bilateral radiographs made with the patient bearing as much weight as tolerated on the injured foot (Figure 4). Because of pain, weight bearing on the injured foot may not be easy for the patient, but weight bearing will often demonstrate subtle shifts of the midfoot that are otherwise not apparent. It has been estimated that 20% of tarsometatarsal joint injuries are missed on the initial radiographs.[21] Stress radiographs, CT, and MRI are indicated if initial radiographs show normal or equivocal findings when a tarsometatarsal injury is suspected.

Stress radiographs are very important if a diagnosis of midfoot injury is suspected because of tenderness over the tarsometatarsal joint complex and the radiographic findings are either normal or equivocal. Stress radiographs should be performed with the patient under appropriate anesthesia and with fluoroscopy. Curtis and associates[17] recommended manipulation of the midfoot with passive pronation and simultaneous abduction. They believed that the pronation-abduction stress test was sensitive and assisted in determining patterns of instability, and they found it to be particularly useful for distinguishing unstable third-degree sprains from stable first- and second-degree sprains in athletes. There can be variation between the instability in the medial column and that in the middle column, and the instability can extend

between the cuneiforms. This pattern of injury is not easy to demonstrate with a standard passive pronation-abduction test; therefore, another stress test, consisting of squeezing between the medial and middle columns and looking for radiographic evidence of instability can be used.[22] Nunley and Vertullo[16] disputed the use of stress radiographs because the investigator can exert only limited force (compared with weight bearing) on the tarsometatarsal complex manually, and there is lack of standardized criteria for defining the result. This has not been the authors' experience because stress radiographs are always obtained with the patient under anesthesia and are believed to be a reliable indicator of the pattern of instability that is present. When a patient has a suspected midfoot injury and the weight-bearing radiographs do

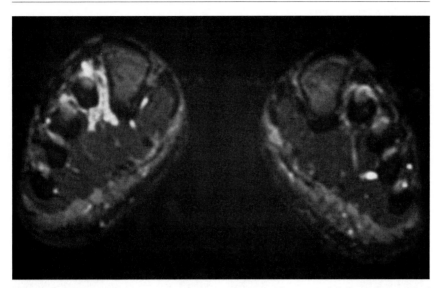

Figure 5 T2-weighted coronal MRI scan comparing the injured (left) and uninjured (right) feet of a patient who had normal radiographs but pain in the left midfoot that worsened with manipulation. There is increased signal intensity between the first and second metatarsal bases of the left foot, consistent with soft-tissue edema at the midfoot.

not demonstrate instability, stress radiographs with the patient under anesthesia are routinely obtained to guide treatment. The most frequent unexpected pattern of displacement or instability that the authors have seen on stress radiographs is displacement at the first metatarsocuneiform joint or the intercuneiform joints.

CT can detect subtle injuries of the tarsometatarsal joint complex. In a cadaver study, Lu and associates[23] compared the sensitivity of CT scans and plain radiographs in detecting subtle injuries at the tarsometatarsal region. Displacements of less than 2 mm were seen on the CT scans of all 12 specimens but were appreciated on the plain radiographs of only 2. However, CT can be too sensitive, often demonstrating fractures that do not require treatment if the foot is stable. Furthermore, CT imaging is a static test that cannot be used to assess stability. The most appropriate indication

for performing a CT scan for a patient with a tarsometatarsal injury is a complex midfoot injury with comminution because the choice of surgical management may be affected by the findings.

MRI is another sensitive study that can be used to diagnose subtle and purely ligamentous midfoot injuries in the absence of subluxation or dislocation[24,25] (Figure 5). MRI scanning is not necessary in the presence of obvious diastasis. Rather, it should be used to confirm the diagnosis and guide the treatment of a stable tarsometatarsal sprain as determined by stress radiographs.

Bone scintigraphy is another imaging tool that can be used to help diagnose subtle midfoot injuries or those for which the diagnosis was delayed.[2] Nunley and Vertullo[16] reported that 15 athletes with a midfoot sprain all had positive bone scans. They argued that bone scans are widely available, easy to interpret, inexpensive, and can remain

positive for more than 1 year after a midfoot injury.

Nonsurgical Treatment

Nonsurgical treatment is rarely indicated for unstable injuries of the tarsometatarsal joint complex. The extent of displacement correlates with the outcome.[8,12,17,26] Residual displacement of as little as 2 mm decreases the articular contact area, and surgery is probably indicated for even minimally displaced fracture-dislocations of the tarsometatarsal joints.[13,27] Left untreated, most displaced midfoot sprains lead to arthritis.[12,13] Surgical treatment is recommended for all obviously displaced injuries. However, the role of nonsurgical treatment of stable and minimally displaced injuries, particularly in an athlete, has been less clearly delineated in the literature. Curtis and associates[17] performed a retrospective study of 19 athletes with a tarsometatarsal joint injury. Seven of nine patients with no diastasis had a good-to-excellent result with nonsurgical treatment. Two of three patients with a third-degree sprain were treated with open reduction and internal fixation and had a good or excellent result, whereas the third patient, treated with cast immobilization, was unable to return to sports. It was concluded that poor functional results were commonly correlated with a delay in diagnosis and inadequate treatment of unstable injuries with nonsurgical immobilization.[17] Faciszewski and associates[20] reviewed the cases of 15 patients with a subtle tarsometatarsal injury, defined as a diastasis between the first and second metatarsal bases of between 2 and 5 mm. They recognized that some patients with residual displacement had a good result and tried to identify factors that might be associated with good or poor functional outcomes. They found no correlation between the extent of the diastasis and the patient's functional outcome. They proposed that maintenance of the longitudinal arch is the critical factor necessary to achieve a good outcome. Shapiro and associates[9] reported on nine athletes with an isolated rupture of the tarsometatarsal ligament. Eight were treated with a removable splint for 4 to 6 weeks followed by progressive weight bearing. One patient, with the widest diastasis (5 mm), chose surgical treatment. All patients were able to return to sports activities; however, the average time until they returned was 14.5 weeks. On the basis of a review of the results in 15 athletes with a tarsometatarsal injury, Nunley and Vertullo[16] recommended that stage I (nondisplaced) injuries be treated conservatively with a non–weight-bearing cast for 6 weeks, followed by the use of a custom orthosis, and that stage II injuries (those with diastasis) and stage III injuries (those with diastasis combined with loss of arch height) should be treated with anatomic reduction and internal fixation.

If the midfoot is injured but no instability is noted on weight-bearing or stress radiographs, the injury is a stable sprain and can be treated with immobilization in a boot. If the foot remains stable on repeat weight-bearing radiographs made 2 weeks later, weight-bearing is permitted as tolerated. A firm, off-the-shelf, padded orthotic arch support inside the boot is typically added and is used until there is no midfoot pain on firm palpation and on stress examination with forced (but gentle) passive pronation and abduction of the midfoot. At 6 to 8 weeks, the midfoot is examined

for tenderness. Weight bearing out of the boot may commence once there is no pain on stress, but the return to activities must be closely monitored. The athlete is permitted to resume training and exercise but may not engage in any activity that involves pronation, torque, or twisting of the midfoot. It is recommended that a stiff-soled shoe with a rigid orthotic support inside it be worn for 6 months. These modifications are for both daily shoe wear as well as athletic shoes. An alternative to the stiff orthotic device is a steel shank added to the sole of the shoe to inhibit midfoot motion and minimize midfoot torque. The athlete is allowed to return to exercises but initially performs them in a swimming pool and on stationary machines, including running on a treadmill. Running on an uneven surface and twisting or cutting activities are not permitted for 4 months. Many athletes return to activities including running, football, and other ball sports by 3 months after a nondisplaced sprain, but it is not realistic to expect a full recovery before this time. The timing of the return to full athletic activities by these patients depends on the severity of the sprain and the type of treatment. The protocol for rehabilitation is the same as that after surgical treatment, but the return to full athletic activity can be as long as 8 to 9 months after severe sprains.

Surgical Management
Surgery is indicated for displaced fractures and dislocations as well as unstable ligamentous injuries. Once it is decided to proceed with surgery, several questions should be asked. When should the surgery be performed? If there has been a delay in diagnosis, is it too late for surgery? Should the procedure be performed

percutaneously or open? Which type of fixation is better: Kirschner wires, screws, or a ligament reconstruction? When should a primary arthrodesis be performed? How should the patient be managed postoperatively? When should the hardware be removed? When can the athlete expect to return to functional and sports activities?

Timing of Surgery
As a general rule, the sooner that surgery can be performed, the quicker the rehabilitation. It is ideal, however, to perform the surgery when the swelling has decreased, unless a percutaneous approach to fixation is to be used. The most important factor influencing the decision regarding the timing of surgery is the associated injury to the soft tissues, particularly when there has been a direct crushing type of injury to the foot. In the absence of a compartment syndrome, the use of an intermittent-compression foot-pump device can facilitate reduction of the soft-tissue edema.[28] If the diagnosis is missed, delayed surgery without arthrodesis may still be performed successfully, but preferably the surgery should be done within 6 weeks after the injury.[29] Displaced fractures and dislocations are difficult to reduce after 2 months, and a satisfactory outcome is less likely if deformity persists. However, successful open reductions of tarsometatarsal joint subluxations, associated with neither a fracture nor arthritis, have been performed up to 1 year after the injury. The success of such a late reduction depends on the extent of articular incongruity, and it cannot be accomplished in the presence of a malunited fracture. Generally, in these cases of late reduction, it is preferable to do an open reduction and perhaps even a

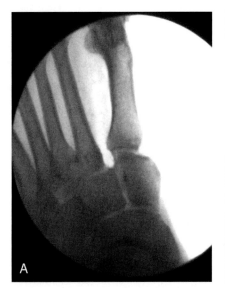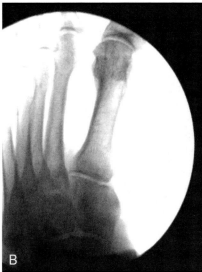

Figure 6   Reduction of the first tarsometatarsal joint is performed by pulling the hallux into varus (**A**), while pushing laterally against the base of the first metatarsal (**B**).

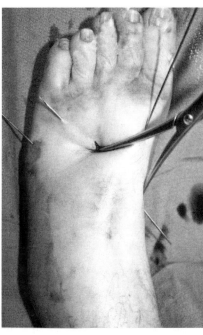

Figure 7   The middle column is reduced to the stabilized medial column with a bone-reduction clamp.

delayed primary arthrodesis rather than the percutaneous method of treatment because the thick scar in the first web space must be resected to reduce the joints.

Percutaneous Compared With Open Fixation

An anatomic reduction is the most important goal of treating injuries of the tarsometatarsal joint complex, and the quality of the reduction has been shown to correlate with the outcome.[12,13,26,30,31]   Dislocations are easy to reduce closed, and closed reduction should be attempted for all patients regardless of the type of fixation that is to be used. Under fluoroscopic visualization, first gentle axial traction is applied by pulling on the hallux and lesser toes while the hindfoot is pulled posteriorly. Then, slight pressure is applied at the midfoot, and the forefoot is pulled medially. Once the articulation is noted to be in reasonable alignment, the reduction is maintained with a large bone-reduction clamp, applied between the base of

the second metatarsal and the medial cuneiform. When the clamp is carefully squeezed, the base of the second metatarsal is gradually reduced into its anatomic position.

Once the dislocation has been reduced, the type of internal fixation can be chosen. Cannulated screws placed over a guide pin are generally used. The sequence of fixation is important.[32] Although the middle column is the point around which the rest of the midfoot gains stability, the medial column is fixed first. Assessment of instability of the first tarsometatarsal joint is therefore important, and this is where stress evaluation of the joint helps. Although subluxation of the second tarsometatarsal joint is usually obvious, manipulation of the foot with passive pronation and abduction will identify subluxation of the first tarsometatarsal joint. The fixation of the first tarsometatarsal joint is performed by pulling the hallux into varus and simultaneously pushing laterally on the base of the first metatarsal with the thumb, which

forces the first metatarsal into alignment with the medial cuneiform (Figure 6). Once the first metatarsal is fixed with a guide pin, the middle column is reduced with the bone-reduction clamp, and a partially threaded screw is inserted obliquely from the medial cuneiform into the second metatarsal, compressing the base of the second metatarsal into the mortise, which locks it into place (Figure 7).

If closed reduction does not succeed, the failure is usually caused by a bone fragment or soft tissue interposed at the base of the second metatarsal. Soft-tissue interposition (for example, a torn tarsometatarsal ligament) does not typically block reduction because the ligament falls to the plantar surface of the foot. If, however, it is not possible to reduce the injury by closed means, open reduction and internal fixation are indicated. One longitudinal incision

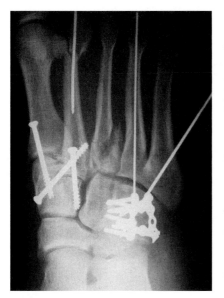

Figure 8 Plate fixation of the cuboid was used to establish lateral column length.

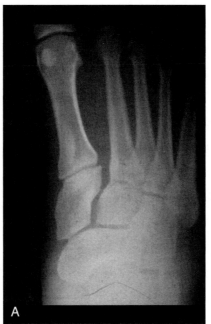

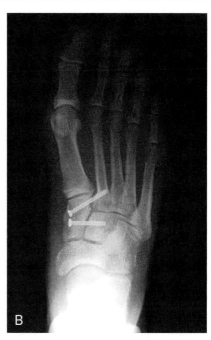

Figure 9 **A,** This patient presented with a typical longitudinal instability pattern, with diastasis between the medial cuneiform and the second metatarsal base as well as between the medial and middle cuneiforms. **B,** Fixation was obtained with 3.5-mm transarticular screws.

placed over the dorsum of the involved tarsometatarsal joints is preferred. If more than one incision is used, then it is important to maintain as wide a skin bridge as possible.

One exception to the order of reduction is in the presence of a Lisfranc injury with a fracture and a shortened cuboid. The length of the cuboid and the lateral column of the foot must be restored to normal to avoid a permanent abduction deformity of the forefoot. Although fractures of the cuboid are infrequently associated with low-energy athletic injuries, if the cuboid is fractured, the first step should be a lateral reduction. This restores the length of the cuboid, which in turn helps to align and reduce the middle and medial columns. If the cuboid cannot be reduced manually, an indirect reduction technique with temporary external fixation to lengthen the lateral column of the foot can be used. Pins are placed into the fifth metatarsal and the calcaneus, and a distractor is applied between the pins.

The articular surfaces of the cuboid are inspected. Comminuted fragments should be elevated if that is necessary to restore the surface congruity. Fixation of the cuboid is frequently difficult. An H-plate can be used to maintain its length (Figure 8). Spanning the cuboid with the H-plate either to the bases of the fourth and fifth metatarsals or to the calcaneus may be necessary. The plate is removed once the cuboid fracture has healed.

Fixation
Early reports described pin fixation alone, and supporters of Kirschner-wire fixation can be found in the literature.[12,33] Kirschner wires have a limited role in the treatment of midfoot injuries, but they should rarely be used as the sole form of fixation. Kirschner wires are easy to insert and easy to pull out. Thus, if they are used, the reduction may be lost if

they become loose or back out. This leads to failure because the joints must be reduced and held reduced for at least 4 months. Kirschner wires can be used to stabilize the lateral column of the foot, where rigid fixation can result in functional loss of motion. They are inserted obliquely from the bases of the fourth and fifth metatarsals into the cuboid or more medially into the cuneiforms. Kirschner wires should be buried subcutaneously to decrease the risk of infection.

Current recommendations generally are for more rigid fixation than can be obtained with Kirschner wires. Lee and associates[34] found that screw fixation provided more stability to the medial and middle columns than did Kirschner-wire fixation in a cadaver model of the tarsometatarsal joint complex (Figure 9). Thordarson and Hurvitz[35] studied 14 patients treated with polylactide screws to fix tarsometatarsal injuries. At 20 months, there was no local soft-tissue reaction, osteolysis, or loss of reduction. Because screw fixation placed across articular surfaces clearly can damage the joint, application of a dorsal plate to the first and/or second tarsometatarsal articulation to avoid the use of crossing intra-articular screws has been studied. Alberta and associates[36] compared fixation with transarticular 3.5-mm screws with fixation with a dorsal one-third tubular plate in a tarsometatarsal cadaver model and found no difference in the resistance to tarsometatarsal joint displacement with a weight-bearing load. These plates can be removed at the same time that screws traditionally have been removed—once the articulation is stable, between 14 and 16 weeks.

Primary Arthrodesis

Primary arthrodesis has recently been advocated for some tarsometatarsal injuries.[37] This may be an alternative treatment of severely comminuted intra-articular fractures, but such fractures are not typical of the low-energy injuries encountered in athletes. There is minimal motion in the middle-column joints, and an arthrodesis may have the same outcome as reduction and internal fixation. However, when a primary arthrodesis is performed, more dissection is required, more bone is removed, small articular fragments are removed, larger defects may require bone grafting, and it is more difficult to achieve fixation. The authors rarely perform a primary arthrodesis in an athlete.

In a randomized prospective study, Ly and Coetzee[37] compared open reduction and internal fixation with primary arthrodesis in 41 patients who had an isolated ligamentous tar-

sometatarsal injury. They found that the group treated with the primary arthrodesis had more rapid recovery, a higher final foot function score, and a superior return to function. Furthermore, five patients in the open reduction and internal fixation group were ultimately treated with an arthrodesis. However, these five patients all had a high-energy injury, and none were high-performance athletes. Mulier and associates[38] studied a group of patients randomized to treatment by two surgeons, one who performed an arthrodesis and one who performed an open reduction and internal fixation, and found far more complications and reports of stiffness in the group treated with the arthrodesis. Although arthrodesis decreased the symptoms of posttraumatic arthritis, most of these patients had a preoperative deformity that required correction, and few underwent an isolated single-column arthrodesis. In summary, although primary arthrodesis has been advocated by a few authors, it is a difficult operation and the resulting stiffness may not be desirable when compared with the outcome in a patient who recovers well from open reduction and internal fixation or closed reduction and internal fixation. Primary arthrodesis is not recommended for athletes, regardless of the potential for a rapid return to activity. The maintenance of motion in the medial column as well as the limited motion in the middle column is necessary to restore full function in these patients.

Ligament Reconstruction

Ligament reconstruction is an option for the treatment of an acute midfoot subluxation. The procedure is particularly applicable to an isolated subluxation that is associated with diastasis between the mid-

dle and medial columns. In the ideal case, the tarsometatarsal ligament would be restored directly or indirectly, but it is not possible to directly repair this ligament. It passes from the base of the second metatarsal obliquely into the distal-lateral edge of the medial cuneiform. It is extremely strong and is situated on the plantar surface of the joint, making direct repair impossible. However, indirect reconstruction of the ligament was described with different tendon-graft substitutes, passed through drill holes placed to recreate the isometry and anatomy of the Lisfranc ligament (C Nery, MD, Seattle, WA, unpublished data presented at the American Orthopaedic Foot and Ankle Society annual meeting, 2004). Eighteen patients were followed for an average of 6 years after treatment of a tarsometatarsal injury with a "neoligamentplasty." Fifteen of the 18 patients had a good-to-excellent result according to their foot function score. No other studies evaluating this technique are available; therefore, ligamentous repair or reconstruction should be considered investigational.

Postoperative Management

In the postoperative period, several issues must be addressed, including the durations of immobilization and limited weight bearing, when activity and exercise can be resumed, and, most importantly, when to remove the internal fixation. Most athletes do not return to full athletic function until at least 8 months after an open reduction, and it may take up to 1 year before high-performance athletes are asymptomatic. Nunley and Vertullo[16] reported a 93% rate of excellent outcomes in athletes with a stage I or II injury who had been treated with open reduction, with the athletes returning to sports participation at an average of 14.4 weeks. This rapid return to sports activity has not been the experience of the authors. Rather, it has been rare that an athlete has been able to return to unrestricted sports activity, particularly those involving twisting and cutting movements, before 6 months.

Early active motion of the adjacent joints combined with protected weight bearing is ideal for patients treated with rigid screw fixation. No weight bearing is allowed for 2 weeks, but partial protected weight bearing in a walking boot is permitted once the incisions have healed. Athletes can begin activity in a swimming pool 3 weeks postoperatively, followed by exercise on a stationary bicycle with high repetitions and little resistance by 4 weeks. Progressive weight bearing in a boot is begun at 6 weeks, and use of the boot is discontinued between 8 and 10 weeks, as dictated by the symptoms. When the athlete begins walking without the boot, a shoe that has been stiffened as much as possible with the addition of a very rigid orthotic arch support is worn. Alternatively, a carbon-fiber or graphite orthotic plate can be placed inside the shoe. This rigid support is particularly important when the patient returns to athletic activity because most athletic shoes are quite flexible. As the athlete increases sports activity participation, monitoring for aching, soreness, and swelling of the midfoot is performed. Once the athlete is able to run in a swimming pool, more activity on a bicycle and an elliptical trainer is allowed, and ultimately, running on a treadmill is permitted. Running on grass or the beach with cutting activities is not permitted for approximately 6 months because of the torsion

that these activities place on the midfoot.

Removal of Hardware

Internal fixation is maintained for a minimum of 4 months to allow ligamentous healing. Compared with fractures of the forefoot, these dislocations take far longer to heal and far more time is needed to achieve joint stability. There are even times when the hardware is left in permanently if the patient is asymptomatic. Motion does occur between the medial and middle columns of the foot, and this will ultimately lead to fatigue failure of the fixation in some patients. In some patients, aching and pain start to develop in the midfoot at approximately 3 months following surgery. If there is any concern about the stability of the midfoot and healing of the ligaments, the patient should start wearing the boot again, and the rehabilitation intensity should be decreased until the symptoms fully resolve. Another alternative that has recently been discussed but not yet described in the published literature is to remove the screws and substitute a fixation suture (the so-called tightrope system) to stabilize the midfoot. This permits motion at the first-second articulation, is less rigid than screw fixation, and may facilitate rehabilitation with less risk of recurrent subluxation. If there is any uncertainty regarding the stability of the foot, it is prudent to maintain fixation for as long as possible.

References

1. Garrick JG, Requa RK: The epidemiology of foot and ankle injuries in sports. *Clin Sports Med* 1988;7:29-36.

2. Meyer SA, Callaghan JJ, Albright JP, Crowley ET, Powell JW: Midfoot sprains in collegiate football players. *Am J Sports Med* 1994;22:392-401.

3. Chiodo CP, Myerson MS: Developments and advances in the diagnosis and treatment of injuries to the tarsometatarsal joint. *Orthop Clin North Am* 2001;32:11-20.

4. Sarrafian S: Syndesmology, in Sarrafian SK (ed): *Anatomy of the Foot and Ankle: Descriptive, Topographic, Functional*, ed 2. Philadelphia, PA, Lippincott, 1993, pp 204-207.

5. Ouzounian TJ, Shereff MJ: In vitro determination of midfoot motion. *Foot Ankle* 1989;10:140-146.

6. de Palma L, Santucci A, Sabetta SP, Rapali S: Anatomy of the Lisfranc joint complex. *Foot Ankle Int* 1997;18:356-364.

7. Solan MC, Moorman CT III, Miyamoto RG, Jasper LE, Belkoff SM: Ligamentous restraints of the second tarsometatarsal joint: A biomechanical evaluation. *Foot Ankle Int* 2001;22:637-641.

8. Myerson M: The diagnosis and treatment of injuries to the Lisfranc joint complex. *Orthop Clin North Am* 1989;20:655-664.

9. Shapiro MS, Wascher DC, Finerman GA: Rupture of Lisfranc's ligament in athletes. *Am J Sports Med* 1994;22:687-691.

10. Ceroni D, De Rosa V, De Coulon G, Kaelin A: The importance of proper shoe gear and safety stirrups in the prevention of equestrian foot injuries. *J Foot Ankle Surg* 2007;46:32-39.

11. Quénu E, Küss GE: Étude sur les luxations du métatarse (Luxations métatarso-tarsiennes). Du diastasis entre le 1er et le 2e métatarsien. *Rev Chir* 1909;39:1-72.

12. Hardcastle PH, Reschauer R, Kutscha-Lissberg E, Schoffmann W: Injuries to the tarsometatarsal joint: Incidence, classification and treatment. *J Bone Joint Surg Br* 1982;64:349-356.

13. Myerson MS, Fisher RT, Burgess AR, Kenzora JE: Fracture dislocations of the tarsometatarsal joints: End results correlated with pathology and treatment. *Foot Ankle* 1986;6:225-242.

14. Komenda GA, Myerson MS, Biddinger KR: Results of arthrodesis of the tarsometatarsal joints after traumatic injury. *J Bone Joint Surg Am* 1996;78:1665-1676.

15. American Medical Association: *Standardized Nomenclature of Athletic Injuries.* Chicago, IL, American Medical Association, 1986.

16. Nunley JA, Vertullo CJ: Classification, investigation, and management of midfoot sprains: Lisfranc injuries in the athlete. *Am J Sports Med* 2002; 30:871-878.

17. Curtis MJ, Myerson M, Szura B: Tarsometatarsal joint injuries in the athlete. *Am J Sports Med* 1993;21: 497-502.

18. Ross G, Cronin R, Hauzenblas J, Juliano P: Plantar ecchymosis sign: A clinical aid to diagnosis of occult Lisfranc tarsometatarsal injuries. *J Orthop Trauma* 1996;10:119-122.

19. Lattermann C, Goldstein JL, Wukich DK, Lee S, Bach BR Jr: Practical management of Lisfranc injuries in athletes. *Clin J Sport Med* 2007;17: 311-315.

20. Faciszewski T, Burks RT, Manaster BJ: Subtle injuries of the Lisfranc joint. *J Bone Joint Surg Am* 1990;72: 1519-1522.

21. Mantas JP, Burks RT: Lisfranc injuries in the athlete. *Clin Sports Med* 1994;13:719-730.

22. Coss HS, Manos RE, Buoncristiani A, Mills WJ: Abduction stress and AP weightbearing radiography of purely ligamentous injury in the tarsometatarsal joint. *Foot Ankle Int* 1998; 19:537-541.

23. Lu J, Ebraheim NA, Skie M, Porshinsky B, Yeasting RA: Radiographic and computed tomographic evaluation of Lisfranc dislocation: A cadaver study. *Foot Ankle Int* 1997;18:351-355.

24. Potter HG, Deland JT, Gusmer PB, Carson E, Warren RF: Magnetic resonance imaging of the Lisfranc ligament of the foot. *Foot Ankle Int* 1998; 19:438-446.

25. Preidler KW, Brossmann J, Daenen B, Goodwin D, Schweitzer M, Resnick D: MR imaging of the tarsometatarsal joint: Analysis of injuries in 11 patients. *AJR Am J Roentgenol* 1996;167:1217-1222.

26. Arntz CT, Hansen ST Jr: Dislocations and fracture dislocations of the tarsometatarsal joints. *Orthop Clin North Am* 1987;18:105-114.

27. Ebraheim NA, Yang H, Lu J, Biyani A: Computer evaluation of second tarsometatarsal joint dislocation. *Foot Ankle Int* 1996;17:685-689.

28. Myerson MS, Henderson MR: Clinical applications of a pneumatic intermittent impulse compression device after trauma and major surgery to the foot and ankle. *Foot Ankle* 1993;14: 198-203.

29. Trevino SG, Kodros S: Controversies in tarsometatarsal injuries. *Orthop Clin North Am* 1995;26:229-238.

30. Kuo RS, Tejwani NC, Digiovanni CW, et al: Outcome after open reduction and internal fixation of Lisfranc joint injuries. *J Bone Joint Surg Am* 2000;82:1609-1618.

31. Teng AL, Pinzur MS, Lomasney L, Mahoney L, Havey R: Functional

outcome following anatomic restoration of tarsal-metatarsal fracture dislocation. *Foot Ankle Int* 2002;23: 922-926.

32. Thordarson DB: Fractures of the midfoot and forefoot, in Myerson MS (ed): *Foot and Ankle Disorders.* Philadelphia, PA, Saunders, 2000, pp 1272-1277.

33. Resch S, Stenström A: The treatment of tarsometatarsal injuries. *Foot Ankle* 1990;11:117-123.

34. Lee CA, Birkedal JP, Dickerson EA, Vieta PA Jr, Webb LX, Teasdall RD: Stabilization of Lisfranc joint injuries: A biomechanical study. *Foot Ankle Int* 2004;25:365-370.

35. Thordarson DB, Hurvitz G: PLA screw fixation of Lisfranc injuries. *Foot Ankle Int* 2002;23:1003-1007.

36. Alberta FG, Aronow MS, Barrero M, Diaz-Doran V, Sullivan RJ, Adams DJ: Ligamentous Lisfranc joint injuries: A biomechanical comparison of dorsal plate and transarticular screw fixation. *Foot Ankle Int* 2005;26:462-473.

37. Ly TV, Coetzee JC: Treatment of primarily ligamentous Lisfranc joint injuries: Primary arthrodesis compared with open reduction and internal fixation. A prospective, randomized study. *J Bone Joint Surg Am* 2006;88: 514-520.

38. Mulier T, Reynders P, Dereymaeker G, Broos P: Severe Lisfrancs injuries: Primary arthrodesis or ORIF? *Foot Ankle Int* 2002;23:902-905.

SECTION 4

Arthroscopy

Arthroscopy

This section provides a guide to advanced arthroscopic and extra-articular endoscopic techniques for treating foot and ankle conditions. Much progress has been made in using arthroscopy for foot and ankle disorders because of the development of small diameter endoscopes with excellent optical resolution along with improvements in precise small joint techniques. If nonsurgical management fails to relieve symptoms for select foot and ankle conditions, the surgeon may choose an arthroscopic or endoscopic treatment option. Arthrodesis, when indicated, can be accomplished with advanced arthroscopic techniques; however, as with arthroscopic procedures in other regions such as the knee, the surgeon may perform an open procedure if necessary.

"Arthroscopic Ankle Arthrodesis" by Tasto and associates provides a much broader overview of arthroscopic ankle and hindfoot surgery than implied by the title. The chapter also reviews arthroscopic treatment of osteochondral lesions of the talar dome, ankle instability, syndesmosis injuries, and subtalar joint pathology. The second chapter authored by Tasto, "Arthroscopy of the Subtalar Joint and Arthroscopic Subtalar Arthrodesis," provides an updated overview of subtalar joint arthroscopy using anterolateral and posterolateral portals.

Since the publication of these chapters, multiple studies have been published to document recent advances in the use of arthroscopy in evaluating and managing ankle and hindfoot conditions. A recent follow-up study of patients treated for osteochondral talar dome lesions with arthroscopic excision and abrasion or drilling showed that many patients had good clinical results, but more than one third of patients had deterioration of results by 5 years after the procedure.[1] Arthroscopic débridement with microfracture for osteochondral talar dome lesions is more successful for lesions smaller than 15 mm; outcomes are worse for older patients, those with a greater body mass index, those with a history of trauma, or when osteophytes are present.[2] Repeat débridements of an osteochondral talar dome lesion may be helpful in some patients.[3] Three-dimensional, computer-guided, retrograde drilling and bone grafting may enable more precise treatment of some osteochondral talar dome lesions without violating the intact talar dome cartilage.[4]

Arthroscopic methods are available for autologous chondrocyte implantation for treating osteochondral talar dome lesions, with average clinical improvement reported at 3 years after treatment.[5] Large, cystic-type talar dome lesions may be successfully treated with a cored osteochondral graft from the ipsilateral knee; however, the technique is demanding and medial malleolar osteotomy may be required in approximately 50% of the ankles.[6] A randomized, controlled trial for patients with osteochondral talar dome lesions showed no difference in results of treatment with chondroplasty, microfracture, or osteochondral autograft transplantation; however, the conclusions of this study may have been limited by the small sample size.[7]

Arthroscopic evaluation of ankles with chronic lateral ligament instability has shown that chondral damage is associated with older patients, greater talar tilt angle, and increased varus inclination of the tibial plafond.[8] Arthroscopic treatment of chronic lateral ankle instability with a suture anchor in the fibula can provide satisfactory results despite a high (29%) complication rate.[9] Treating chronic lateral ankle instability with thermal capsular shrinkage is controversial, but one recent study showed improvement of symptoms and functional ankle scores even though there was no demonstrable improvement of mechanical laxity.[10]

For latent ankle syndesmotic instability, arthroscopically assisted repair with percutaneous fixation may decrease pain and improve function and radiographic parameters of instability.[11] The diagnosis of chronic ankle syndesmotic instability (widening of the syndesmosis by more than 2 mm) with arthroscopy correlates well with MRI findings; arthroscopic débridement of the syndesmosis may result in clinical improvement of pain resulting from impingement.[12] Arthroscopy also may be useful for the reduction and fixation of acute syndesmotic disruption.[13]

Recent studies have confirmed that arthroscopically assisted ankle arthrodesis provides high rates of union with cost savings compared with open arthrodesis techniques.[14-16] Successful fusion can be achieved with arthroscopic methods even in the presence of marked deformity.[17]

Subtalar joint arthroscopy can clarify the anatomic cause and provide successful treatment of the clinical syndrome known as sinus tarsi syndrome, which may be a result of an interosseous talocalcaneal ligament tear, synovitis, a cervical ligament tear, arthrofibrosis, or soft-tissue impingement.[18] Subtalar joint arthroscopy may be indicated for persistent sinus tarsi pain, despite noncontributory MRI findings, because of the greater diagnostic sensitivity of arthroscopy.[19] In some patients, subtalar arthroscopic release can relieve pain and stiffness after an intra-articular calcaneal fracture.[20] Subtalar arthroscopy also has been used for lateral calcaneal ostectomy to decompress lateral calcaneofibular impingement after calcaneal fracture and excision of painful os trigonum.[21,22]

In the first two chapters in this section, the authors report that arthroscopic subtalar arthrodesis can be accomplished from the anterolateral and posterolateral subtalar arthroscopic portals, with the occasional addition of an accessory anterolateral portal. A recent study has confirmed that arthroscopic subtalar arthrodesis using the anterolateral and posterolateral portals appears to achieve a high rate of union and patient satisfaction.[23] Arthroscopic subtalar arthrodesis also may be done from three posterior portals with the patient in the prone position.[24]

The chapter by van Dijk reviews the posterior endoscopic approach for examining and treating the posterior ankle and subtalar joint; the os trigonum and posterior impingement; the posterior tibial, peroneal, flexor hallucis longus, and Achilles tendons; and the retrocalcaneal

space. Careful placement of portals and knowledge of ankle and hindfoot anatomy are necessary. Posterior ankle portals, including the combined use of the posterolateral and posteromedial portals, may improve the arthroscopic working area and expand treatment options.[25] A cadaver study showed that arthroscopic equipment can be placed posteriorly without gross injury to neurovascular structures; however, the distance between the arthroscopic cannula and neurovascular structures, such as the sural or tibial nerves, may be 0 mm in some instances.[26] A recent clinical study showed that temporary numbness at the posterior portal scars occurred in 5 of 15 patients (33%) treated with posterior ankle arthroscopy for os trigonum excision, prominent posterior talar process decompression, flexor hallucis longus tenolysis, removal of loose body, or osteochondritis dissecans débridement; however, all patients were satisfied with the procedure.[27]

Endoscopic visualization has facilitated percutaneous repair of acute Achilles tendon rupture and treatment of chronic Achilles tendinopathy with débridement or multiple tenotomies.[28-30] In addition, endoscopic retrocalcaneal bursectomy and

excision of Haglund deformity may provide satisfactory results in most patients.[31]

The chapter by Frey and van Dijk presents an overview of first metatarsophalangeal (MTP) joint arthroscopy. Indications for this treatment include first MTP joint osteophytes, arthritis (hallux rigidus), chondromalacia, osteochondral lesions, loose bodies, arthrofibrosis, posttraumatic synovitis, recurrent swelling, locking, persistent pain, and stiffness.[32-34] Recent reports of first MTP joint arthroscopy have expanded the potential indications for this procedure to include pigmented villonodular synovitis, first MTP joint arthrodesis, sesamoid disorders, ganglion cysts, intra-articular fractures, gouty arthritis, and hallux valgus deformities.[35-44] Small joint arthroscopy in the foot also has been described for first metatarsocuneiform arthrodesis and lesser MTP joint conditions.[45,46]

Carol C. Frey, MD
Assistant Clinical Professor
Department of Orthopaedic Surgery
University of California, Los Angeles
Co-Director and Chief, Foot and Ankle
  Surgery
West Coast Sports Medicine Foundation
Manhattan Beach, California

References

1. Ferkel RD, Zanotti RM, Komenda GA, et al: Arthroscopic treatment of chronic osteochondral lesions of the talus: Long-term results. *Am J Sports Med* 2008;36:1750-1762.

2. Chuckpaiwong B, Berkson EM, Theodore GH: Microfracture for osteochondral lesions of the ankle: Outcome analysis and outcome predictors of 105 cases. *Arthroscopy* 2008;24:106-112.

3. Savva N, Jabur M, Davies M, Saxby T: Osteochondral lesions of the talus: Results of repeat arthroscopic debridement. *Foot Ankle Int* 2007;28:669-673.

4. Geerling J, Zech S, Kendoff D, et al: Initial outcomes of 3-dimensional imaging-based computer-assisted retrograde drilling of talar osteochondral lesions. *Am J Sports Med* 2009;37:1351-1357.

5. Giannini S, Buda R, Vannini F, Di Caprio F, Grigolo B: Arthroscopic autologous chondrocyte implantation in osteochondral lesions of the talus: Surgical technique and results. *Am J Sports Med* 2008;36:873-880.

6. Scranton PE, Frey CC, Feder KS: Outcome of osteochondral autograft transplantation for type-V cystic osteochondral lesions of the talus. *J Bone Joint Surg Br* 2006;88:614-619.

7. Gobbi A, Francisco RA, Lubowitz JH, Allegra F, Canata G: Osteochondral lesions of the talus: Randomized controlled trial comparing chondroplasty, microfracture, and osteochondral autograft transplantation. *Arthroscopy* 2006;22:1085-1092.

8. Sugimoto K, Takakura Y, Okahashi K, Samoto N, Kawate K, Iwai M: Chondral injuries of the ankle with recurrent lateral instability: An arthroscopic study. *J Bone Joint Surg Am* 2009;91:99-106.

9. Corte-Real NM, Moreira RM: Arthroscopic repair of chronic lateral ankle instability. *Foot Ankle Int* 2009;30:213-217.

10. de Vries JS, Krips R, Blankevoort L, Fievez AW, van Dijk CN: Arthroscopic capsular shrinkage for chronic ankle instability with thermal radiofrequency: Prospective multicenter trial. *Orthopedics* 2008;31:655.

11. Schuberth JM, Jennings MM, Lau AC: Arthroscopy-assisted repair of latent syndesmotic instability of the ankle. *Arthroscopy* 2008;24:868-874.

12. Han SH, Lee JW, Kim S, Suh JS, Choi YR: Chronic tibiofibular syndesmosis injury: The diagnostic efficiency of magnetic resonance imaging and comparative analysis of operative treatment. *Foot Ankle Int* 2007;28:336-342.

13. Chan KB, Lui TH: Isolated anterior syndesmosis diastasis without fracture. *Arch Orthop Trauma Surg* 2007;127:321-324.

14. Ferkel RD, Hewitt M: Long-term results of arthroscopic ankle arthrodesis. *Foot Ankle Int* 2005;26:275-280.

15. Nielsen KK, Linde F, Jensen NC: The outcome of arthroscopic and open surgery ankle arthrodesis: A comparative retrospective study on 107 patients. *Foot Ankle Surg* 2008;14:153-157.

16. Winson IG, Robinson DE, Allen PE: Arthroscopic ankle arthrodesis. *J Bone Joint Surg Br* 2005;87:343-347.

17. Gougoulias NE, Agathangelidis FG, Parsons SW: Arthroscopic ankle arthrodesis. *Foot Ankle Int* 2007;28:695-706.

18. Lee KB, Bai LB, Song EK, Jung ST, Kong IK: Subtalar arthroscopy for sinus tarsi syndrome: Arthroscopic findings and clinical outcomes of 33 consecutive cases. *Arthroscopy* 2008;24:1130-1134.

19. Lee KB, Bai LB, Park JG, Song EK, Lee JJ: Efficacy of MRI versus arthroscopy for evaluation of sinus tarsi syndrome. *Foot Ankle Int* 2008;29:1111-1116.

20. Lee KB, Chung JY, Song EK, Seon JK, Bai LB: Arthroscopic release for painful subtalar stiffness after intra-articular fractures of the calcaneum. *J Bone Joint Surg Br* 2008;90:1457-1461.

21. Lui TH: Endoscopic lateral calcaneal ostectomy for calcaneofibular impingement. *Arch Orthop Trauma Surg* 2007;127:265-267.

22. Horibe S, Kita K, Natsu-ume T, Hamada M, Mae T, Shino K: A novel technique of arthroscopic excision of a symptomatic os trigonum. *Arthroscopy* 2008;24:121.

23. Glanzmann MC, Sanhueza-Hernandez R: Arthroscopic subtalar arthrodesis for symptomatic osteoarthritis of the hindfoot: A prospective study of 41 cases. *Foot Ankle Int* 2007;28:2-7.

24. Lee KB, Saltzman CL, Suh JS, Wasserman L, Amendola A: A posterior 3-portal arthroscopic approach for isolated subtalar arthrodesis. *Arthroscopy* 2008;24:1306-1310.

25. Phisitkul P, Tochigi Y, Saltzman CL, Amendola A: Arthroscopic visualization of the posterior subtalar joint in the prone position: A cadaver study. *Arthroscopy* 2006;22:511-515.

26. Sitler DF, Amendola A, Bailey CS, Thain LM, Spouge A: Posterior ankle arthroscopy: An anatomic study. *J Bone Joint Surg Am* 2002;84:763-769.

27. Willits K, Sonneveld H, Amendola A, Giffin JR, Griffin S, Fowler PJ: Outcome of posterior ankle arthroscopy for hindfoot impingement. *Arthroscopy* 2008;24:196-202.

28. Doral MN, Bozkurt M, Turhan E, et al: Percutaneous suturing of the ruptured Achilles tendon with endoscopic control. *Arch Orthop Trauma Surg* 2009;129:1093-1101.

29. Thermann H, Benetos IS, Panelli C, Gavriilidis I, Feil S: Endoscopic treatment of chronic midportion Achilles tendinopathy: Novel technique with short-term results [published online ahead of print March 14, 2009]. *Knee Surg Sports Traumatol Arthrosc*.

30. Vega J, Cabestany JM, Golanó P, Pérez-Carro L: Endoscopic treatment for chronic Achilles tendinopathy. *Foot Ankle Surg* 2008;14:204-210.

31. Ortmann FW, McBryde AM: Endoscopic bony and soft-tissue decompression of the retrocalcaneal space for the treatment of Haglund deformity and retrocalcaneal bursitis. *Foot Ankle Int* 2007;28:149-153.

32. Lui TH: Arthroscopic release of first metatarsophalangeal arthrofibrosis. *Arthroscopy* 2006;22:906.

33. van Dijk CN, Veenstra KM, Nuesch BC: Arthroscopic surgery of the metatarsophalangeal first joint. *Arthroscopy* 1998;14:851-855.

34. Davies MS, Saxby TS: Arthroscopy of the first metatarsophalangeal joint. *J Bone Joint Surg Br* 1999;81:203-206.

35. Borton DC, Peereboom J, Saxby TS: Pigmented villonodular synovitis in the first metatarsophalangeal joint: Arthroscopic treatment of an unusual condition. *Foot Ankle Int* 1997;18:504-505.

36. Carro LP, Vallina BB: Arthroscopic-assisted first metatarsophalangeal joint arthrodesis. *Arthroscopy* 1999;15:215-217.

37. Pérez Carro L, Echevarria Llata JI, Martinez Agueros JA: Arthroscopic medial bipartite sesamoidectomy of the great toe. *Arthroscopy* 1999;15:321-323.

38. Chan PK, Lui TH: Arthroscopic fibular sesamoidectomy in the management of the sesamoid osteomyelitis. *Knee Surg Sports Traumatol Arthrosc* 2006;14:664-667.

39. Nishikawa S, Toh S: Arthroscopic treatment of a ganglion of the first metatarsophalangeal joint. *Arthroscopy* 2004;20:69-72.

40. Debnath UK, Hemmady MV, Hariharan K: Indications for and technique of first metatarsophalangeal joint arthroscopy. *Foot Ankle Int* 2006;27:1049-1054.

41. Lui TH: Endoscopic resection of the gouty tophi of the first metatarsophalangeal joint. *Arch Orthop Trauma Surg* 2008;128:521-523.

42. Wang CC, Lien SB, Huang GS, et al: Arthroscopic elimination of monosodium urate deposition of the first metatarsophalangeal joint reduces the recurrence of gout. *Arthroscopy* 2009;25:153-158.

43. Lui TH, Chan KB, Chow HT, Ma CM, Chan PK, Ngai WK: Arthroscopy-assisted correction of hallux valgus deformity. *Arthroscopy* 2008;24:875-880.

44. Lui TH: First metatarsophalangeal joint arthroscopy in patients with hallux valgus. *Arthroscopy* 2008;24:1122-1129.

45. Lui TH, Chan KB, Ng S: Arthroscopic Lapidus arthrodesis. *Arthroscopy* 2005;21:1516.

46. Lui TH: Arthroscopy and endoscopy of the foot and ankle: Indications for new techniques. *Arthroscopy* 2007;23:889-902.

Carol C. Frey, MD or a member of her immediate family serves as a board member, owner, officer, or committee member of Arthroscopy Association of North American, Beach Cities Surgery Center, West Coast Sports Medicine Foundation; serves as a paid consultant to or is an employee of Merck and Pfizer; and serves as an unpaid consultant to EMS.

18

Arthroscopic Ankle Arthrodesis

James P. Tasto, MD
Carol Frey, MD
Peter Laimans, MD
Craig D. Morgan, MD
Richard J. Mason, MD
James W. Stone, MD

Arthroscopic Treatment of Osteochondral Lesions of the Talar Dome

Osteochondritis dissecans of the talar dome is a focal abnormality of articular cartilage and the underlying subchondral bone that can result in fragment separation and loose body formation. In their seminal report on the subject, Berndt and Harty[1] suggested that the majority of cases of osteochondritis dissecans of the talar dome occurred secondary to acute or remote trauma and that medial lesions tended to occur in the posterior half of the talar dome, whereas lateral lesions were usually anterior in location. Their study and subsequent investigations suggested that surgical treatment is appropriate for symptomatic lesions. Because these lesions have never been shown to have an inflammatory component, they are better termed osteochondral lesions of the talar dome. Most studies have suggested that osteochondral talar dome lesions are actually posttraumatic transchondral fractures, but etiologies other than trauma have been suggested.

Traditional surgical approaches to these lesions use an anterolateral arthrotomy for the anterolateral lesions, but medial malleolar osteotomy is often necessary to approach the more posteriorly located medial lesions. With the signifi-

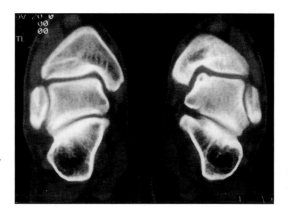

Fig. 1 Computed tomography scan showing a medial talar dome osteochondral lesion of the left ankle.

cant advances in surgical technique that have occurred over the past 10 to 15 years, most of these procedures can be performed arthroscopically with less morbidity than their open counterparts.

After the diagnosis of an osteochondral lesion of the talar dome is confirmed with plain radiographs and/or bone scan, the lesion can be staged using computed tomography (CT) (Fig. 1) or magnetic resonance imaging (MRI)[2,3] (Fig. 2). The CT scan has the advantage of excellent bone imaging, but visualization of articular cartilage is poor in the absence of a contrast agent. Primary views can only be obtained in the coronal and axial planes, with computerized reconstructions for sagittal imaging. MRI has the advantage of imaging without radiation exposure,

adequate imaging of articular cartilage, the ability to detect a fluid or fibrous tissue layer beneath the bony osteochondral lesion, and the ability to detect larger areas of bone edema or other abnormality than that which may be suggested on plain radiographs. We believe that MRI provides the most staging information for a single examination.

Despite the sophistication of radiographic techniques, it is clear that there is no substitute for actual visual inspection and palpation of a lesion when deciding on the most appropriate treatment. Studies have shown significant deviations in appearance from that expected by preoperative radiographic examinations and surgical inspection of the lesion.[4] Arthroscopy therefore

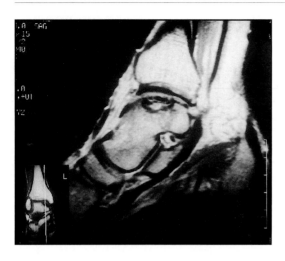

Fig. 2 Magnetic resonance imaging scan showing a medial talar dome osteochondral lesion with loose fragment.

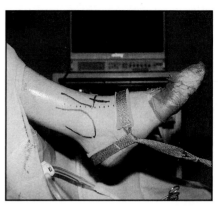

Fig. 3 Noninvasive sterile strap distraction technique.

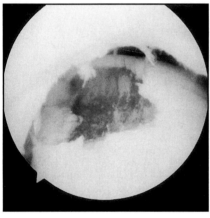

Fig. 4 Arthroscopic photograph of medial talar dome osteochondral lesion after debridement.

becomes both an important diagnostic and staging tool in the treatment of these lesions, in addition to the preferred method of surgical treatment, in most cases.

The decision regarding which surgical technique to use depends on the size and location of the lesion, and the size and quality of the articular cartilage surface and attached subchondral bone. Small lesions with articular cartilage and bone of good quality, especially in skeletally immature patients, are more likely to be salvaged. Options include drilling of the lesion or internal fixation using screws or pins (metal or absorbable). If the lesion

has thin or fragmented articular cartilage or subchondral attached bone, making internal fixation impractical, then the lesion must be debrided and the base of the lesion abraded and/or drilled to create an environment most conducive to the formation of fibrocartilage.

The surgical procedure is performed with the patient under general or spinal anesthesia in the operating room. The patient is positioned supine with the flexed hip and knee supported by a well-padded leg holder. After sterile skin preparation and draping, the noninvasive distractor is placed on the foot and traction applied (Fig. 3). Routine anteromedial, anterolateral, and posterolateral portals are created and a thorough diagnostic examination of the joint is performed. The surgeon must assess the quality of the articular cartilage and the underlying subchondral bone when deciding on the surgical approach to the lesion. The lesion is evaluated visually and is carefully probed to determine whether the bone fragment is separated and loose or firmly attached. A lesion with articular cartilage of poor quality or with fragmented, necrotic subchondral bone must be removed. The lesion most suitable for internal fixation is an acute transchondral fracture with a substantial bony component, in a single fragment.

Lesion Debridement

After visualizing the lesion arthroscopically, the loose fragment is lifted from its bed using an arthroscopic probe, freer elevator, or similar instrument. Loose fragments are carefully removed so as not to create loose bodies that may be difficult to retrieve. Various sizes of straight and angled curettes are helpful to further debride necrotic bone from the base and edge of the lesion. It is very common for medial lesions to extend from their obvious position on the dome of the talus into the medial gutter on the medial side of the talus. Loose articular cartilage and bone in this area must be removed or the patient will likely experience continued symptoms. Debridement must be continued until the articular cartilage is clearly well attached to the subchondral bone at the periphery and all necrotic bone is removed. The bone base of the lesion is further debrided using the curettes or an arthroscopic burr until bleeding from the entire bone bed is demonstrated as the inflow pressure is decreased (Fig. 4). Drilling of the lesion using a smooth Kirschner wire can also be performed, but is not necessary if bleeding bone is clearly demonstrated from the entire surface (Fig. 5). Methods of transmalleolar drilling of medial lesions are generally not necessary and should be avoided because they require placing 1 or more drill holes across the normal articular cartilage of the tibial plafond.

Drilling of Intact Lesions

Lesions with intact articular cartilage surfaces and no motion of the subchondral bone upon palpation may be candidates for drilling. The principle of the procedure is to create potential vascular channels into the lesion for healing, although there is little evidence in the literature regarding its efficacy. Lesions suitable for such treatment are not common, but are most likely seen in skeletally immature patients. Such patients have the greatest chance for healing compared with older patients with more chronic lesions.

Lateral lesions are most commonly located in the anterior portion of the talus and can be approached for drilling from the anterolateral portal while viewing from the anteromedial portal, or by creating an accessory anterolateral portal. A smooth Kirschner wire (approximately 0.062 in) is used to make multiple drill holes into the subchondral bone to a depth of 1 to 1.5 cm. Medial lesions in the posterior part of the talar dome may be impossible to reach from the anteromedial portal even with plantar flexion of the ankle. Under these circumstances the arthroscopic surgeon has 2 choices. The lesion may be drilled by directing the wire across the medial malleolus and into the lesion using a commercially available drill guide, or freehand. Multiple holes can then be placed by alternately dorsiflexing and plantarflexing the ankle. The lesion may be drilled from distal to proximal with a transtalar method as well. The wire is introduced from the sinus tarsi and directed across the talus and into the lesion, either freehand or using a drill guide. Multiple drill holes may be placed in this fashion without drilling through the normal articular cartilage of the medial tibial plafond.

Internal Fixation

Internal fixation is most appropriate for an acute transchondral fracture. These fractures usually occur over the lateral talar dome associated with an inversion injury. Fixation can be achieved using bioabsorbable pins or screws or metal pins or screws. The pins cause less injury to the intact articular cartilage surface but do not provide compression across the lesion. Screws (either lag screws or Herbert screws) can provide compression but cause more injury to the intact articular cartilage and generally require removal after the lesion heals. Medial lesions may be approached by maximum plantar flexion of the ankle. However, an open approach using malleolar osteotomy may be necessary to access the lesion for internal fixation. The surgeon should never hesitate to convert to an open procedure if it will facilitate anatomic replacement of the fragment and decrease injury to the articular cartilage.

Treatment of Large Osteochondral Lesions After Debridement

Patients who undergo debridement of large (greater than 1 cm diameter) osteochondral lesions of the talar dome generally experience significant symptomatic relief and can resume activities of daily living with minimal limitations. However, some patients continue to experience pain despite debridement. In addition, long-term follow-up studies suggest that there is an increased incidence of posttraumatic degenerative arthritis in such patients. Alternatives to simple debridement that attempt to reconstruct an articular cartilage surface have been attempted in such patients. Two general alternatives are available. The first, osteochondral cadaveric allograft using fresh or fresh frozen graft, has been suggested but there is no clinical literature to document its efficacy in the case of talar osteochondral lesions. The other alternative is

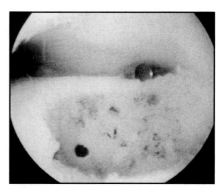

Fig. 5 Medial lesion after debridement and drilling.

to replace the articular surface with an osteochondral autograft using donor material from the patient's own knee joint. An attempt can be made to replace the entire surface using a single graft, or multiple osteochondral "plugs" can be placed.[5] The latter technique has been termed "mosaicplasty," and there are a few studies documenting clinical experience, but no long-term follow-up is as yet available.

At this point the techniques for osteochondral autograft should be considered investigational. The procedure should be reserved for patients who demonstrate debilitating symptoms despite the usual conservative and surgical methods suggested previously, and in whom the only other reasonable alternative to relieve symptoms would be a tibiotalar arthrodesis.

The Role of Arthroscopy in the Treatment of Ankle Instability

Inversion injuries of the ankle are common in athletes and the general population. Though the specific parameters defining this classification are vague and subject to interobserver variation, ankle sprains traditionally have been classified as grade I (mild), grade II (moderate), and grade III (severe). Grade I injuries involve ligaments stretched on a microscopic level with little swelling or tender-

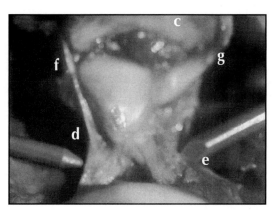

Fig. 6 Anatomic dissection of the ankle. a) talus; b) fibula; c) tibia; d) anterior talofibular ligament; e) posterior talofibular ligament; f) anterior tibiofibular ligament; g) posterior tibiofibular ligament. (Reproduced with permission from Ankle arthroscopic techniques: Recent advances, in Parisien JS (ed): *Current Techniques in Arthroscopy*, ed 3. New York, NY, Thieme Medical Publishers, 1998.)

ness and no mechanical or functional instability. Grade II injuries encompass partial ligament disruption with associated swelling, tenderness, and variable amounts of joint instability. Grade III injuries imply a complete rupture of ligaments, more impressive clinical findings, and increased joint laxity on physical examination. Symptoms of acute or chronic instability also may be apparent.

Most patients who have suffered an ankle sprain, especially grades I and II injuries, recover well with nonsurgical management. With more severe ligament disruption, long-term sequelae may develop, leading to a less than ideal outcome. Common complaints from these patients include persistent pain, swelling, stiffness, muscle weakness, and instability. Indeed, many of these symptoms may be causally interrelated. For this reason, it is important to identify the specific offending pathology responsible for the persistent symptoms.

Anatomy
The lateral ligamentous complex of the ankle consists of 3 ligaments: the anterior talofibular ligament (ATFL), calcaneofibular ligament (CFL), and posterior talofibular ligament (PTFL) (Fig. 6). A study performed by Broström[6] found that isolated tears of the ATFL occurred in 65% of ankle sprains, while a combination of ATFL and CFL disruption occurred in 20%. The PTFL was only

rarely injured. On physical examination of the acute sprain, areas of tenderness may aid in the diagnosis of specific ligament disruption. In chronic injuries with established subjective and objective instability, tenderness may be less distinct. In these cases, dynamic assessment of instability may be aided by the anterior drawer and talar tilt tests. Findings on physical examination may be compared with those noted on stress radiographs. Specific parameters of translation and tilt, which signify ligament disruption, have varied significantly. Many authors have concluded that these maneuvers do not consistently provide reliable diagnostic findings. A prospective study by Johannsen[7] concluded that it is not possible to differentiate between an isolated lesion of the ATFL and a combined lesion of the ATFL and CFL based on these 2 manual tests. In another study, Seligson and associates[8] found that inversion stress testing (talar tilt) was not helpful in the evaluation of the lateral ligaments because of the undetermined contribution of subtalar motion to perceived inversion.

Evaluation
In cases of chronic instability, ankle arthroscopy can provide valuable information and is most useful as a perioperative tool when symptomatic instability requires invasive treatment. Arthroscopic evaluation of the ankle allows inspection

of the anterior and posterior talofibular ligaments, the capsular reflection of the calcaneofibular ligament, the deep deltoid ligament, the syndesmotic ligament complex, and occasionally, the posterolateral ankle and subtalar capsule. Direct observation of the lateral structures during stress testing (talar tilt, translation, and rotation) is possible during arthroscopy as well. In a recent study, Schafer and Hintermann[9] arthroscopically evaluated 110 symptomatic patients and identified ATFL tears in 64%, CFL disruption in 41%, and deltoid ligament injuries in 6%. Early findings in our series (unpublished data) reveal a significant number of partial PTFL tears that had previously been described as a ligament rarely involved in lateral ligamentous injury. A number of studies[9–12] have also identified the association of chronic lateral ankle instability with chondral injury. This is an important point to remember because many of these cartilaginous lesions may go undetected without the aid of direct arthroscopic visualization. It has been reported that stress radiographs and MRI evaluation were normal in more than 50% of cases in which significant intra-articular pathology was subsequently confirmed arthroscopically (unpublished data, 1995).

Technique
Prior to the arthroscopic procedure, both ankles should be examined under anesthesia. Increased talar translation or tilt can be documented with fluoroscopy and compared with the uninvolved side. It is important to determine subtalar motion during fluoroscopic inversion stress testing, because increased motion at this joint can be perceived clinically as increased talar tilt. Using standard anteromedial-anterolateral portals and noninvasive traction of 20 to 25 lb, all ligamentous structures and chondral surfaces can be evaluated. The advantage of noninvasive traction over the use of a fixed ankle distracter is that it allows for

manipulation of the anterolateral portal.

With the camera in the lateral gutter, dynamic assessment of the ankle joint can be performed. With an assistant placing anterior stress on the calcaneus, the amount of anterior-posterior translation of the talus can be identified along with a functional assessment of the lateral ligamentous structures. This maneuver should be repeated with varying degrees of ankle dorsiflexion and plantar flexion. Next, with the assistant placing an inversion force on the calcaneus, the inversion stress test can be evaluated. This position allows direct dynamic observation of the tibiotalar articulation as well as the function of the ligamentous restraints in the lateral gutter. A dynamic assessment of the ankle can be equated to the observation and probing of the anterior cruciate ligament (ACL) during an intraoperative Lachman maneuver in knee arthroscopy.

In cases of more severe lateral ankle injuries, significant disruption of the floor of the lateral gutter will be noted, revealing the underlying subtalar capsule. Though the CFL is an extra-articular structure, its capsular reflection can be visualized in this area. If the CFL has been disrupted, torn or attenuated ligamentous fibers will be seen at the distal tip of the fibula. The PTFL can be seen posteriorly in the lateral gutter, running in a superomedial to inferolateral direction. While inverting the ankle, the camera should be placed deep in the lateral gutter and inferior to the PTFL to view the lateral subtalar area. Moving posteriorly through this region, the posterolateral capsule is encountered. In grade III sprains this portion of the ankle capsule can be disrupted, which creates free communication between the ankle joint and the peroneal sheath (Fig. 7). The camera can easily be passed through the posterolateral capsule in this situation, revealing the peroneal tendons in their sheath.

With the camera returned to the tibiotalar articulation, the talar dome is examined by moving the ankle joint through

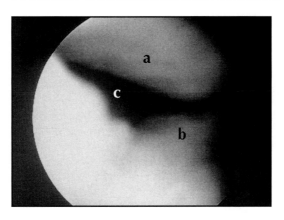

Fig. 7 Arthroscopic view of the left ankle with posterior capsular disruption and exposure of peroneal tendons. a) talus; b) fibula; c) peroneus longus and brevis. (Reproduced with permission from Ankle arthroscopic techniques: Recent advances, in Parisien JS (ed): *Current Techniques in Arthroscopy*, ed 3. New York, NY, Thieme Medical Publishers, 1998.)

dorsiflexion and plantar flexion with careful attention given to the cartilaginous surfaces in case of associated chondral injury. The syndesmotic ligament complex can be probed and dynamically assessed with internal rotation, external rotation, and coronal translation stress.

Placing the camera in the anteromedial portal will make visualization of the medial gutter and deep deltoid ligament possible. Finally, the ATFL can be inspected looking laterally from the anteromedial portal. In most cases of chronic ankle injury, this ligament will be disrupted and a scarred ligament stump will be seen anteriorly near the talar neck.

Hawkins[13] has described an arthroscopic lateral ankle stabilization technique that includes removal of soft tissue and debris from the ATFL insertion site on the talus followed by denuding of articular cartilage with a burr. An accessory portal is created approximately 1 cm distal to the anterolateral portal so that a staple passed through this portal enters the talus at a right angle. After the foot is brought to a neutral position, the tines of the staple gather capsule and ligament tissue while the staple is secured with a mallet. At this time, we do not advocate this procedure.

Our current recommendation is the use of ankle arthroscopy as a perioperative tool in cases of established functional instability. Surgical intervention in the acute ankle sprain, even for a grade III

injury, is not advocated. All patients should have formal physical therapy prior to discussing surgical options. If symptomatic instability persists despite adequate rehabilitative efforts, then an open stabilization procedure should be chosen based on suspected pathology determined through careful history, physical examination, and radiographic studies. Prior to opening the lateral ankle surgically, soft-tissue and chondral injury should be confirmed using evaluation under anesthesia, fluoroscopy, and ankle arthroscopy. In this manner, precise open stabilization techniques can be used to address all areas of ligamentous insufficiency.

The Role of Arthroscopy in the Treatment of Syndesmosis Injuries

Isolated ankle syndesmosis sprains and disruptions are uncommon injuries. More frequently, rupture of the syndesmosis is associated with deltoid ligament injury and fractures of the malleoli. These contributing associated injuries naturally increase the suspicion of syndesmosis involvement based on an understanding of the mechanism of injury. However, an ankle sprain with an undetected syndesmosis injury may lead to a prolonged and complicated recovery from an initially benign injury. A high index of suspicion and early recognition

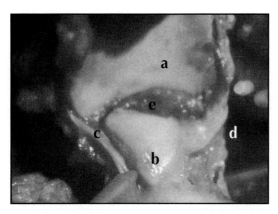

Fig. 8 Prosected anatomic view of distal tibiofibular joint–internal rotation. a) tibia; b) fibula; c) anterior interosseous ligament; d) posterior interosseous ligament; e) interosseous ligament. (Reproduced with permission from Ankle arthroscopic techniques: Recent advances, in Parisien JS (ed): *Current Techniques in Arthroscopy*, ed 3. New York, NY, Thieme Medical Publishers, 1998.)

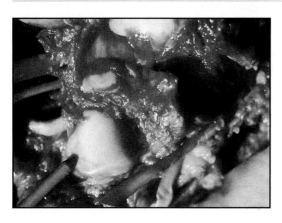

Fig. 9 Prosected anatomic view of distal tibiofibular joint–external rotation.

will lead to improved outcomes in treating this more subtle injury.

The distal tibiofibular syndesmosis consists of 3 separate ligaments: the anterior inferior tibiofibular (AITF) ligament, the posterior inferior tibiofibular (PITF) ligament, and the interosseous ligament (Figs. 8 and 9). A distal fascicle of the PITF ligament has been considered in a separate ligament by some authors and has been named the transverse tibiofibular ligament.[14,15] The mechanism of syndesmosis injury has been described as external rotation of the foot that causes a diastasis of the tibiofibular joint as a result of pressure exerted by the talus. The ankle is likely to be in a position of full dorsiflexion or plantarflexion at the moment of injury as this position places the syndesmosis ligaments under maximal tension.[16] The incidence of ankle diastasis without fracture ranges from 1% to 11% of soft-tissue ankle injuries.[17,18]

Clinical Examination

A careful history and physical examination are essential to confirm the diagnosis of syndesmotic ligament injuries. Although patients may report a variety of mechanisms of injury, trauma that subjects the foot to significant external rotational force should automatically raise suspicion of a syndesmosis injury.[17] Patients may complain of other symptoms including pain over the anterior syndesmosis or medial deltoid, and tenderness or pain with external rotation of the foot. Three manual tests are helpful in isolating a syndesmosis injury. Hopkinson and associates[17] described the squeeze test as compression of the fibula toward the tibia at the distal half of the lower leg that produces pain distally at the syndesmosis. The Cotton test detects increased mediolateral motion of the talus in the mortise. External rotation of the ankle with the knee flexed to 90° will

also produce pain at the anterior syndesmosis indicating either an acute or chronic disruption. Edwards and DeLee[19] have created 2 groups based on radiographic evaluation of syndesmotic diastasis. The latent diastasis group exhibits widening of the diastasis only when external rotation or abduction forces are applied. The frank diastasis group presents with syndesmosis widening a visible on routine radiographs. Additional information can be obtained from CT, MRI, and ankle arthrography.

In many cases, the clinical findings in syndesmotic ligament injuries can be less clear. In the acute setting, physical examination may reveal diffuse, nonspecific tenderness and patients may not be able to tolerate stress radiographs. Marymont and associates[20] suggest the use of radionuclide imaging in these cases, citing a 100% sensitivity. Two cases of positive scans and negative stress radiographs were reported, while Hopkinson and associates[17] identified 6 of 7 patients with similar findings. By maintaining a high index of suspicion in these cases and instituting appropriate treatment, a radiographically occult syndesmosis injury will not be overlooked.

Technique

Ankle arthroscopy has recently become an important tool in the diagnosis and treatment of syndesmotic ligament injuries. Ogilvie-Harris and Reed[21] arthroscopically evaluated 19 patients with chronic symptoms consistent with syndesmosis disruption. A triad of pathologic findings (disruption of both PITF and the interosseous ligaments, and a posterolateral tibial plafond chondral fracture) was identified. Debriding the intra-articular pathology produced good results. In our experience, arthroscopy has been helpful in treating patients who remain symptomatic despite appropriate initial treatment or in cases of a missed diagnosis. Ankle arthroscopy allows static and dynamic inspection of the syndesmotic ligament complex, allowing definitive treatment before the onset of arthritic changes that may result from a chronically incongruent joint. Disruption of the interosseous component of the syndesmotic complex with an intact anterior and PITF ligament has also been observed. The diastasis in the coronal plane is less dramatic than the anterior-posterior and rotational instability patterns noted during direct observation of dynamic stress testing (Figs. 10 and 11). An arthroscopically assisted technique for debridement and stabilization of the disrupted and unstable syndesmosis in early follow-up has led to good results and full return to activity. During second-look arthroscopy at the time of hardware removal, complete healing of the syndesmosis has occurred without evidence of persistent instability during dynamic stress testing (Fig. 12).

The technique uses noninvasive traction of 20 to 25 lb with standard anteromedial and anterolateral portals to examine the ankle joint and syndesmosis. Direct palpation of the syndesmosis is best performed with the arthroscope in the anteromedial portal and a probe in the anterolateral portal. Occasionally the synovium, which overlies the interosseous component of this ligament, may need to be excised to facilitate palpation and visualization of this area. The AITF and PITF ligaments should be inspected for attenuation, partial tears, or complete disruption. With the camera in the anteromedial portal, the syndesmosis should be observed during external rotation of the foot. If the syndesmosis is completely disrupted and a diastasis is present, the anterolateral portal will allow visualization proximal to the distal tibiofibular articulation. The complex and interrelated multiaxial motion of the distal fibula, tibia, and talus can be seen at this time.

After arthroscopic confirmation of syndesmotic ligament disruption and instability, the remainder of the ankle

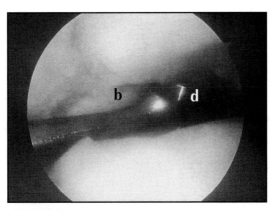

Fig. 10 Arthroscopic view of the right ankle without stress. a) tibia; b) fibula; c) talus; d) interosseous ligament disruption. (Reproduced with permission from Ankle arthroscopic techniques: Recent advances, in Parisien JS (ed): *Current Techniques in Arthroscopy*, ed 3. New York, NY, Thieme Medical Publishers, 1998.)

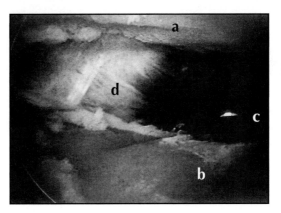

Fig. 11 Arthroscopic view of the right ankle with external rotation stress and significant anterior/posterior patholaxity. a) tibia; b) talus; c) interosseous ligament disruption. (Reproduced with permission from Ankle arthroscopic techniques: Recent advances, in Parisien JS (ed): *Current Techniques in Arthroscopy*, ed 3. New York, NY, Thieme Medical Publishers, 1998.)

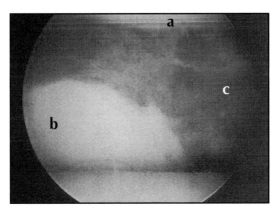

Fig. 12 Arthroscopic view of healed tibiofibular syndesmosis, right ankle. a) tibia; b) fibula; c) healed interosseous ligament. (Reproduced with permission from Ankle arthroscopic techniques: Recent advances, in Parisien JS (ed): *Current Techniques in Arthroscopy*, ed 3. New York, NY, Thieme Medical Publishers, 1998.)

joint should be carefully inspected for associated injuries. Chondral injuries and soft-tissue impingement lesions may not be detected by plain radiographs, CT, or MRI but may be noted arthroscopically. If left untreated, these conditions may cause a poor outcome despite appropriate treatment of the syndesmotic disruption. A systematic inspection of all cartilaginous surfaces should be developed with

the ankle in dorsiflexion and plantarflexion in order to bring the entire weight-bearing portion of the talar dome into view. The most effective way to evaluate the medial gutter and deep fibers of the deltoid ligament is through the anteromedial portal. Although lateral ligamentous injuries are rarely associated with syndesmosis disruption, this area can be inspected and palpated through the

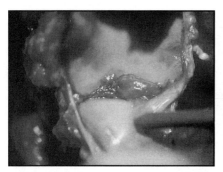

Fig. 13 Curette debriding the interosseous ligament and space.

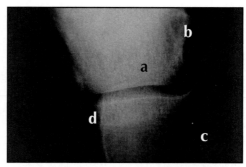

Fig. 14 Preoperative radiograph of the right ankle with diastasis. a) tibia; b) fibula; c) talus; d) diastasis. (Reproduced with permission from Ankle arthroscopic techniques: Recent advances, in Parisien JS (ed): *Current Techniques in Arthroscopy*, ed 3. New York, NY. Thieme Medical Publishers, 1998.)

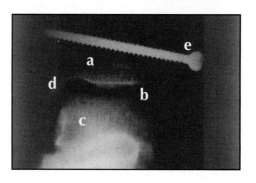

Fig. 15 Postoperative radiograph of corrected diastasis. a) tibia; b) fibula; c) talus; d) closure of medial tibial talar defect; e) syndesmotic screw.

anterolateral portal.

In cases of complete or partial disruption of the syndesmosis with observed instability, stabilization of the syndesmosis is indicated. Arthroscopic debridement and curettage of the interosseous component followed by percutaneous screw fixation has led to promising early results though various open repair and stabilization techniques.[16,19,22] Torn fibers of the interosseous ligament can be removed with a synovial resector. Care should be taken to avoid careless debridement of intact portions of the AITF or PITF ligaments. Next, a curette can debride the distal tibiofibular articulation of remaining interosseous fibers and fibroosseous debris (Fig. 13). The curette is advanced approximately 1 cm proximal to create a bed of cancellous bone throughout the course of the interosseous ligament disruption from anterior to posterior. By placing the camera in the anteromedial portal and looking proximal, the area of debridement between the distal tibia and fibula can be visualized to assure complete removal of residual ligamentous or cartilaginous debris. Finally, a syndesmotic screw is placed percutaneously while the ankle is held in neutral dorsiflexion (Figs. 14 and 15). Fluoroscopy is used to assure anatomic closure of the diastasis, maintenance of an intact mortise, and proper placement of the screw.

Cast immobilization is used in the acute setting of syndesmosis injury without diastasis. Ankle arthroscopy is used for many reasons, including treatment of patients who remain symptomatic after appropriate conservative treatment, for syndesmosis disruption and instability requiring fixation, and for the chronic high ankle sprain with clinical evidence o persistent syndesmosis symptoms. Data accumulated over the last 2.5 years show very promising results with almost complete return to full activity. There has been 1 failure in 9 patients whose diastasis recurred after not adhering to the protocol and resuming weightbearing immediately. This subset of individuals is difficult to treat. As experience builds, it is apparent that the distal tibiofibular articulation and syndesmotic ligaments are complex structures with poorly understood biomechanics.

Arthroscopic Ankle Arthrodesis

There are multiple techniques described in the modern surgical literature for fusion of the tibiotalar joint.[23–36] Complication rates, to include nonunion and infection, range as high as 60% in some series.[27–43] The technique of maintaining the normal stable contour of the mortise and using transarticular compression screw fixation has significantly lowered the nonunion rate.[30,44,45]

As the open technique became more refined, surgeons sought to recreate this technique arthroscopically. Although the first description of a successful arthroscopically assisted ankle fusion was in 1983,[32] only recently have interim and long-term results of this technique in large groups of patients been reported.[46–51] These results compare very favorably to popular open techniques. Furthermore, if the lower morbidity, more rapid mobilization, and shorter time to fusion reported with the arthroscopic technique are considered, it would appear that this technique has many advantages over the open approach.

Indications

The most common indication for arthroscopic ankle fusion is posttraumatic tibiotalar arthritis that has not responded to a

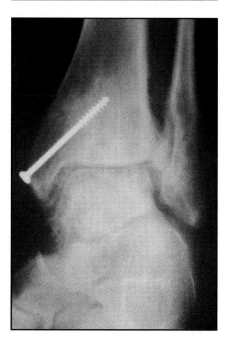

Fig. 16 Preoperative radiograph of a patient with posttraumatic arthritis of the left ankle.

trial of nonsurgical management (Fig. 16). Patients with other disease processes leading to arthritis or instability may be candidates for arthroscopic arthrodesis.[48,49] These conditions are summarized in Outline 1. The arthroscopic technique is also well suited for patients with ankle arthritis and coexisting systemic problems that result in poor wound healing, including diabetes, peripheral vascular disease, rheumatoid arthritis, coagulopathies, long-term steroid use, and previous skin grafts or soft-tissue flaps.[48,49]

The arthroscopic approach does have limitations. It is a very tedious and technically demanding procedure. The surgeon attempting ankle arthroscopy should be experienced in open techniques of ankle fusion should this become necessary during the course of the procedure. Contraindications to arthroscopic ankle fusion are active infection and a neuropathic joint. There are many relative contraindications to arthroscopic fusion (Outline 2). Varus or valgus malalignment of greater than 15° requires significant bone debridement

and is very difficult and time-consuming to do arthroscopically. Tibiotalar joint translation of greater than 1 cm anteriorly or posteriorly is also difficult to correct because of the limited soft-tissue dissection performed arthroscopically. Finally, severe bone loss resulting from trauma, osteonecrosis, or failed arthroplasty cannot easily be corrected arthroscopically and should be dealt with via an open approach.[48,49]

Surgical Technique

Open techniques for fusion of the tibiotalar joint are well described. In 1985, the long-term results of a simple open approach to ankle fusion that maintained the stable configuration of the talus in the mortise and used crossed intra-articular compression screw fixation were reported.[31] The arthroscopic technique was developed to recreate the high success rate of this open procedure while maintaining the advantages of arthroscopy. The challenge in using arthroscopy for this procedure is to reproduce the 3 essential technical steps necessary to obtain a solid fusion: (1) debridement of all hyaline cartilage and subchondral bone; (2) reduction of the tibiotalar joint to a neutral position; and (3) internal fixation with transmalleolar compression screws to maintain the reduction while fusion occurs.

The standard 4-mm arthroscope and 30° foreoblique lens with camera and

video monitor are used in this technique. Motorized suction shavers, abraders, and angled arthroscopic curettes are also necessary. Distraction, by either invasive or noninvasive devices, is used for visualization and instrumentation as needed. Finally, an image intensifier and large (6.5 or 7.0 mm) cannulated screws are needed.

The patient is placed supine on a standard surgical table with a radiolucent distal extension. A pad is placed under the ipsilateral buttock to keep the ankle in neutral rotation. A tourniquet is placed on the upper thigh and standard preparation and draping performed. A sterile bump is then placed under the distal calf to allow free access to the posterior aspect of the ankle joint and to facilitate intraoperative fluoroscopy. The image intensifier is sterilely draped and positioned to allow smooth, rapid access for imaging (Fig. 17).

The next step is application of distraction. The need for this is dependent on ligamentous laxity and remaining joint space. We prefer medially-based invasive distraction because it allows dorsiflexion of the foot while maintaining parallel separation of the joint surfaces. Medially based distraction does not interfere with the arthroscope or instrumentation (Fig. 18). Laterally-based distraction is well described;[52] however, it produces lateral talar tilt, which can lead to difficulties in debridement and obtaining appropriate fusion position. Lateral distraction can

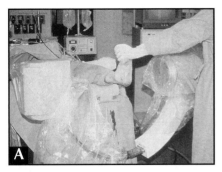 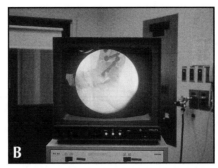

Fig. 17 Positioning for surgery. **A,** Note position of distal calf on sterile bump and location of C-arm. **B,** Fluoroscopy image immediately postfusion.

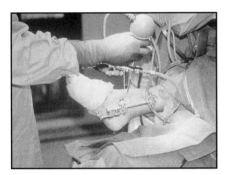 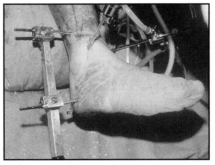

Fig. 18 Intraoperative photo showing use of medial distraction instrumentation on the right ankle. Note the free access to anterior portals.

Fig. 19 Laterally based distraction instrumentation right ankle. Note the position of the device over area where the posterolateral portal is made.

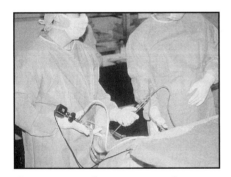 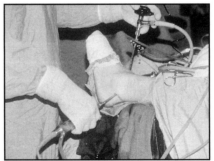

Fig. 20 Position of instrumentation for debridement of the medial side of left ankle joint. Arthroscope is in the anterolateral portal and abrader in anteromedial portal.

Fig. 21 Posterolateral placement of the abrader for debridement of posterior joint space in the left ankle.

also interfere with instrumentation through the posterolateral portal (Fig. 19). Application of invasive distraction devices is not without complications. The surgeon must have a thorough understanding of the neurovascular structure at risk and be familiar with the application technique of the device chosen. These techniques are well described[49,52] and will not be reviewed here. Noninvasive distraction is also used successfully for this procedure. The most commonly used device is a sterile clove-

hitch type apparatus that avoids some of the potential complications associated with invasive distraction, but can limit access to the posterior aspect of the ankle.[47]

Once appropriate distraction is obtained, the arthroscopic portals are established. The anterolateral portal is established first. Then, using the arthroscope to illuminate the subcutaneous location of the saphenous vein and nerve, the anteromedial portal is established. Good visualization is obtained and then the posterolateral portal is made. A large-bore cannula is placed in this portal and is used for fluid inflow and instrumentation of the posterior compartment. A motorized abrader is then used to debride all hyaline cartilage and subchondral bone from the articular surfaces of the talus, tibial plafond, and medial and lateral talomalleolar surfaces. Angled curettes are particularly useful in removing subchondral cysts and excessively sclerotic areas. Debridement of the medial half of the joint is facilitated by placing the arthroscope anterolaterally and the abrader anteromedially (Fig. 20). The reverse position is best for debridement of the lateral side of the joint (Fig. 18). The posterior talus and posterior malleolus are best described by placing the abrader in the posterolateral portal while viewing from either the anteromedial or anterolateral portal (Fig. 21). The goal of debridement is to expose viable cancellous bone while maintaining the normal bony contour of the plafond and talar dome (Fig. 22). Varus and valgus deformities must also be corrected at the time of debridement. Care must be taken to avoid squaring the surfaces and resecting too much bone medially because this produces a varus deformity that can lead to painful postoperative lateral metatarsalgia.[31,49] If an anterior tibial osteophyte is present it is debrided as well. This can be done with an abrader or a small osteotome placed through the anteromedial portal. Once the debridement is complete, the ankle should easily dorsiflex to neutral. If neutral dorsiflexion is not achieved and the Achilles tendon is tight, a percutaneous lengthening can be performed at this time.[48,53]

After debridement is complete, distraction is released and the joint surfaces reduced by applying a compressive force on the hindfoot and dorsiflexing the talus to the neutral position. The ideal position for fusion is 0° to 5° of valgus, neutral dorsiflexion, and external rotation matching the normal contralateral ankle (usually 0° to 5°). This position is verified radiographically and then held either manually or by using the previously applied invasive distraction device to provide compression. The guide wires for the cannulated screw system are then placed. The medial pin is drilled percutaneously from the medial malleolus just above the joint line and angled 40° anteriorly into the talus (Fig. 23). The lateral guide pin is started percutaneously over the fibula, proximal to the joint and also angled anteriorly. Other authors recommend angling the lateral screw posteriorly;[44,50] however, by placing it anteriorly into the talus, maximum bony purchase is obtained without the risk of entering the subtalar joint.[45,49] The position of the guide is assessed by image intensification. The proper drilling and tapping is then performed to place the 6.5- or 7.0-mm cannulated cancellous lag screws (Fig. 24). If the bone is osteopenic or if there is any question as to the stability of the reduction, a third screw can be added. This screw is started in the lateral tibia either anterior or posterior to the fibula and directed to gain maximum purchase and compression. Final radiographic confirmation of the reduction and hardware placement is confirmed and the distraction device removed.

The portals are closed with simple nylon sutures and a well-padded posterior splint is applied, keeping the foot and ankle in neutral dorsiflexion. This splint is converted to a cast at the first office

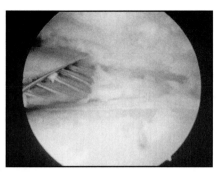

Fig. 22 Intra-articular view of arthroscopic debridement. Removal of hyaline cartilage from talar dome and the tibial plafond to reveal cancellous bone.

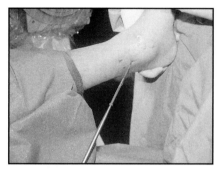

Fig. 23 Placement of guide pin for medial screw right ankle. Note the proximal percutaneous position and anterior angulation.

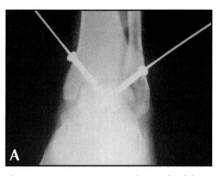
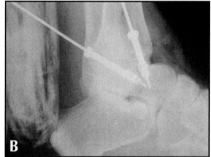

Fig. 24 A, Anteroposterior radiograph of the postreduction fusion position of the left ankle with lag screws in place over guide pins. **B,** Lateral view.

visit and the patient is kept nonweightbearing for 6 weeks. At this point the patient is progressively advanced to full weightbearing in a removable fracture boot. Radiographs and clinical examinations are performed at 3- to 4-week intervals until clinical and radiographic evidence of solid fusion is seen (Fig. 25).

Clinical Results

The short-term results of arthroscopically-assisted ankle fusion are very favorable compared with the open technique. Unfortunately, only a few centers perform a significant number of techniques, and long-term follow-up studies are lacking. In 1991, Myerson and Quill[50] compared the results of open and arthroscopic fusion in patients followed for an average of 23 months postoperatively. They found a shorter time to fusion for the

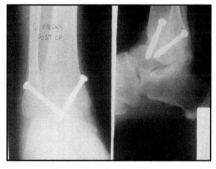

Fig. 25 Radiographs of right ankle at 6 weeks status post procedure showing solid fusion in neutral position.

arthroscopic technique as compared to the open procedure (8.7 weeks versus 14.5 weeks) and a similar complication rate for the 2 procedures. Corso and Zimmer[46] performed arthroscopic ankle arthrodesis on 16 patients with idiopathic, posttraumatic, or rheumatoid arthritis.

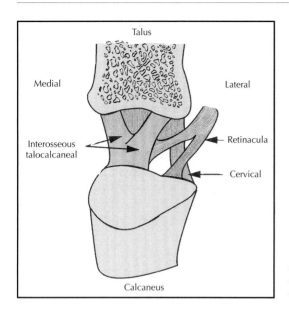

Fig. 26 The subtalar joint can be divided into anterior and posterior sections by the sinus tarsi and tarsal canal.

They noted fusion in all 16 patients at an average of 9.5 weeks and complete resolution of pain in 14 of the 16 patients. Ewing and associates[47] reported on a group of 30 patients who underwent arthroscopically-assisted tibiotalar arthrodesis. This group comprised patients with the diagnosis of either posttraumatic or rheumatoid arthritis, or osteoarthritis. Fusion was achieved in 27 of the 29 patients available for follow-up and nonunion occurred in 2 patients. Ogilvie-Harris and associates[51] noted an 89% fusion rate in 19 patients treated with arthroscopic fusion. This patient population was chosen for the arthroscopic procedure based on osteoarthritis of the ankle with minimal or no deformity. At 2-year follow-up, 84% of the patients had good or excellent results based on a clinical rating scale.

In the longest-term follow-up study to date, 34 patients who underwent arthroscopically assisted ankle fusion between 1983 and 1989 were evaluated.[48] All patients had ankle arthritis with significant pain and failed at least 6 months of conservative treatment. The average age of the patients was 50 years and they were followed for an average of 7.7 years.

Successful fusion was obtained in 33 of 34 ankles (97%). Clinical results were rated as excellent or good in 86% of the patients. The average time to clinical and radiographic union was 63.5 days. Significant subtalar pain occurred in 3 patients, leading to a fair result. The poor results (2 patients) were caused by a malunion and a nonunion that were attributed to surgical errors.

Summary

These studies highlight the high success rate of arthroscopic tibiotalar arthrodesis. Clinical outcome ratings and fusion rates are high, while overall complications are low. Moreover, time to union appears to be significantly reduced as compared to the open technique, most likely because the soft-tissue stripping performed during the arthroscopic procedure is minimal. Another advantage of the limited soft-tissue stripping is decreased postoperative pain.

In fact, most patients are discharged the day of surgery or within 23 hours after surgery. When performed for the proper indications by a skilled surgeon, arthroscopic ankle arthrodesis can yield excellent long-term results.

Subtalar Arthroscopy

The subtalar joint is a complex and functionally important joint of the lower extremity, playing a major role in effecting inversion and eversion of the foot. The complex anatomy of the subtalar joint makes radiographic and arthroscopic examination difficult.[54–62] However, with the introduction of small instruments and precise techniques, arthroscopy of the subtalar joint has expanded. Despite an expansion in techniques, however, the number of reports dealing with subtalar arthroscopy remains small and even fewer deal with clinical applications and results.

Gross Anatomy

The subtalar joint can be divided into anterior and posterior sections by the sinus tarsi and tarsal canal (Fig. 26). Contents of the tarsal canal include the cervical ligament, talocalcaneal interosseous ligament, medial root of the inferior extensor retinaculum, fat pad, and blood vessels (Fig. 27).

The anterior portion of the subtalar joint, also known as the talocalcaneonavicular joint, includes its anterior and middle articulating facets. It also contains the talonavicular articulation and the spring ligament. The anterior subtalar joint is generally thought to be inaccessible to arthroscopic visualization because of the thick interosseous ligament, which fills the tarsal canal. Because of this, the region normally has no connection with the posterior joint complex.

The posterior subtalar joint has a long axis that is located obliquely 40° to the midline of the foot, facing laterally. It consists of the convex posterior facet of the calcaneus and the concave posterior facet of the talus. The capsule of the posterior subtalar joint is reinforced laterally by the cervical ligament and the calcaneofibular ligament, and possesses a posterior pouch and a small lateral recess.

Portal Anatomy

Few studies have been published in the literature dealing with arthroscopy of the subtalar joint. Parisien[59] and Parisien and Vangsness[60] described an anterior and posterior portal, Frey and associates[55] described the middle portal, and Mekhail and associates[63] described the medial portal (Fig. 28).

The posterior portal is described as being approached from the lateral side. A trocar is inserted in an upward and slightly anterior manner approximately 2 cm posterior and just proximal to the tip of the lateral malleolus, making sure it is behind the saphenous vein and nerve and anterior to the Achilles tendon.[60] In an anatomic study of portal placement and safety, the posterior portal was located an average of 25 mm (range 20 to 28 mm) posterior and 6 mm (range 0 to 10 mm) proximal to the tip of the fibula.[55] The posterior portal represents the portal with the greatest risk of causing nerve or vessel damage. Structures endangered with posterior portal placement include the sural nerve, lesser saphenous vein, peroneal tendons, and the Achilles tendon. Great care must be taken during posterior portal placement to avoid injury, especially to the sural nerve and lesser saphenous vein. After the skin incision is made, a hemostat clamp should be used to gently spread the subcutaneous tissue down to the capsular level before insertion of the arthroscope.

In more detail, the sural nerve and lesser saphenous vein run parallel to each other along the posterolateral aspect of the ankle, the nerve lying posterior to the vein at the level of the ankle joint. In 7 of 10 cases reported by Frey and associates[55] the posterior portal was located posterior to the sural nerve, while in 2 cases it was found to be anterior. The average distance of the sural nerve from the posterior portal was 4 mm (range 8 mm posterior, 6 mm anterior). During portal placement in 1 case, the sural nerve was transected; in another, a small laceration was made in

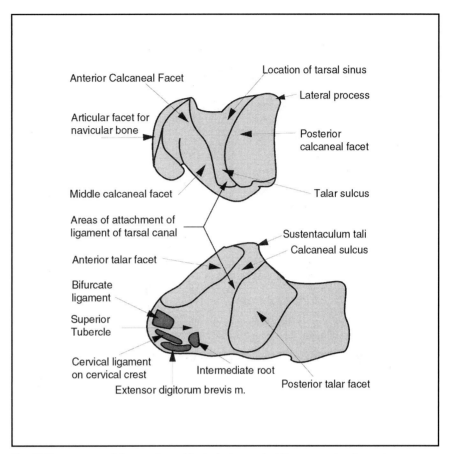

Fig. 27 The contents of the tarsal canal include the cervical ligament, talocalcaneal interosseous ligament, medial root of the inferior extensor retinaculum, fat pad, and blood vessels.

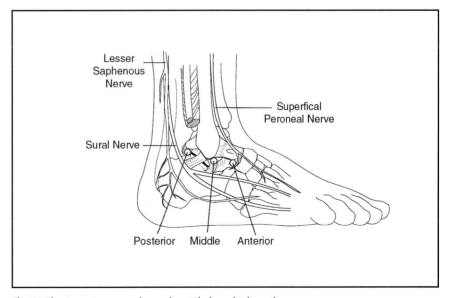

Fig. 28 The 3 most commonly used portals for subtalar arthroscopy.

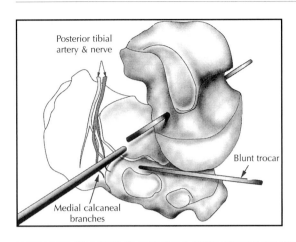

Posterior tibial
artery & nerve

Blunt trocar

Medial calcaneal
branches

Fig. 29 A medial portal is established by placing a blunt-ended trocar into the sinus tarsi and then pushing it through the tarsal canal in a posteromedial and slightly cephalad direction.

the lesser saphenous vein. The peroneal tendon sheath was located an average of 11 mm (range 6 to 16 mm) anterior to the portal, and the Achilles tendon an average of 15 mm posterior (range 10 to 20 mm) to the portal. Neither of these tendons was ever damaged in this series, but their proximity should be noted.

The point of entry for the anterior portal is described as being 2 cm anterior and 1 cm distal to the tip of the distal fibula, directing the instrument slightly upward and about 40° posterior.[10,11] In the study by Frey and associates[55] the point of entry was located an average distance of 28 mm (range 23 to 35 mm) anterior to the tip of the fibula. Structures at risk with placement of this portal include the dorsal intermediate cutaneous branch of the superficial peroneal nerve, the dorsal lateral cutaneous branch of the sural nerve, the peroneus tertius tendon, and a small branch of the lesser saphenous vein. The dorsal intermediate cutaneous branch of the superficial peroneal nerve is located an average distance of 17 mm (range 0 to 28 mm) anterior to the portal. The dorsolateral cutaneous branch of the sural nerve, identified in 8 of 15 specimens reported by Frey and associates[55] was located an average distance of 8 mm (range 2 to 12 cm) inferior to the anterior portal. The peroneus tertius tendon was located an average distance of 21 mm (range 8 to 33 mm) anterior to the portal.

A small branch of the lesser saphenous vein consistently coursed along the anterolateral aspect of the foot in the vicinity of the anterior portal. It is located an average of 2 mm (range 0 to 5 mm) from the anterior portal and was actually lacerated in 20% of the cases reported. With use of the anterior portal, therefore, care must be taken to avoid injury to the dorsal intermediate cutaneous branch of the superficial peroneal nerve as it divides on the dorsum of the foot. A small branch of the lesser saphenous vein is also at risk, although damage to this structure is unlikely to cause significant problems.

The middle portal is described as being about 1 cm anterior to the tip of the fibula, directly over the sinus tarsi.[54] The middle portal was located an average of 10 mm (range 10 to 11 mm) anterior to the tip of the fibula. It is located directly over the sinus tarsi, and placed on structures at risk during the course of its placement. The middle portal is therefore considered relatively safe.

Mekhail and associates[63] described establishment of a medial portal by placing a blunt-ended trocar into the sinus tarsi and then pushing it through the tarsal canal in a postmedial and slightly cephalad direction (Fig. 29). The trocar should be angled about 45° to the lateral border of the foot until exiting the skin. The ankle is in equinus and the foot

inverted during placement of this portal. This position relaxes and slightly displaces the posteromedial neurovascular bundle posteriorly to decrease their risk of injury. Using blunt dissection, portal entry lies along a line joining the tip of the medial malleolus to the medial calcaneal tubercle. The desired cannulation site exists where the anterosuperior three fourths joins the posteroinferior fourth of that line. The authors used skeletal distraction to facilitate the use of this portal. It is believed that the posteromedial and anterolateral aspects of the posterior subtalar joint are better viewed from this portal as opposed to the anterior or posterior portals, respectively. Specifically, the following intra-articular structures were thought to be better visualized: the articular cartilage of the transverse portion and anterolateral slope of the posterior subtalar joint, the calcaneofibular ligament, the posterior pouch of the joint with its synovial lining, the synovium covering the posterior aspect of the interosseous ligament, and the joint capsule. One should be reminded, however, that these findings are the result of a cadaveric study, and no clinical trials have been reported using this portal. The authors also warned that in feet with a great deal of edema or adipose tissue, the exit point for the trocar would be more posterior than usual. This scenario would potentially situate the portal closer to the posterior neurovascular bundle.

Arthroscopic Anatomy

The posterior subtalar joint is divided into 4 compartments: lateral, medial, anterior, and posterior (Fig. 30). The anterior and middle facets are located anterior and medial to the posterior facet, separated from it by the thick interosseous ligaments. It is difficult to visualize the middle and anterior facets unless there is a defect in the interosseous ligament structures. As the arthroscope enters the sinus tarsi, these ligaments block all access to the anterior joint and

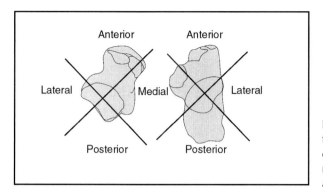

Fig. 30 The posterior sub-talar joint lends itself to division into 4 compartments: lateral, medial, anterior and posterior.

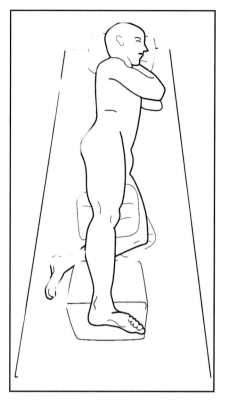

Fig. 31 The patient is placed in the lateral decubitus position with the surgical extremity up. Padding should be placed between the legs.

almost completely fill the tarsal canal. Only if the ligament is removed or torn can the anterior joint be accessed from laterally placed portals.

The best portal combination for access to the cartilaginous posterior facet of the subtalar joint involves placement of the arthroscope through the anterior portal and instrumentation through the posterior portal. This allows direct visualization and instrumentation of nearly the entire cartilaginous surface of the posterior facet, the posterior aspect of the interosseous ligament, the lateral capsule and its small recess (where it is possible to access the calcaneofibular and lateral talocalcaneal ligaments), and the posterior pouch of the posterior joint with its synovial lining. Instrumentation through the anterior portal provided access to the lateral compartment of the posterior facet. The medial, anterior, and posterior compartments cannot be reached through the anterior portal. In addition, significant risk of iatrogenic damage to the underlying subchondral bone exists; therefore, use of the anterior portal for instrumentation of the posterior facet is not recommended.

Access to the anterior and lateral compartments of the posterior facet, as well as structures located in the extra-articular sinus tarsi, is best obtained by placing the arthroscope through the anterior portal and instrumentation through the middle portal. By avoiding posterior portal placement, potential damage to the sural nerve

is averted. In addition, excellent visualization of the medial and posterior compartments of the posterior facet is possible, even though they cannot be instrumented via the middle portal. Therefore, this portal combination is recommended for visualization and instrumentation of the sinus tarsi and anterior and lateral compartments of the posterior subtalar joint, as well as when only visual inspection of the medial and posterior compartments is necessary.

Indications

Indications for subtalar arthroscopy include arthrofibrosis, calcaneonavicular coalition, osteochondral lesions, fractures of the anterior process of the calcaneus, fractures of the lateral process of the talus, degenerative joint disease, synovitis, interosseous ligament tears, instability, capsulitis, chronic pain in the sinus tarsi, subtalar impingment lesions (STIL), and arthrodesis of the subtalar joint.[55,56,59,60]

Arthroscopic Technique

The arthroscopic technique follows the initial description of Parisien[59,60] of an anterior and posterior portal. Frey and associates[55] noted the importance of adding a third middle portal. Local, general, spinal, or epidural anesthesia can be used for this procedure. The patient is placed in the lateral decubitus position with the operative extremity up (Fig. 31). Padding should be placed between the

lower extremities, as well as under the contralateral extremity to protect the peroneal nerve. The contralateral extremity to protect the peroneal nerve. The contralateral extremity should be bent to 90° at the knee. A bolster should be placed distally under the operative extremity to suspend the foot and the leg. A tourniquet is recommended for hemostasis. An invasive or noninvasive distracter can be added if necessary for visualization but usually is not required.

Three portals are available for visualization and instrumentation of the subtalar joint. The anterior portal is placed 2 cm anterior and 1 cm distal to the tip of the lateral malleolus. The middle portal is placed just distal and inferior to the tip of the lateral malleolus. The posterior portal is placed 1 cm proximal to the tip of the fibula and anterior to the Achilles tendon.

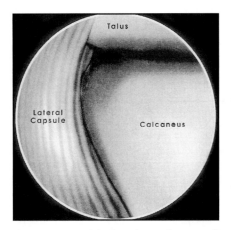

Fig. 32 A view of the lateral capsule, its small recess and the articular cartilage of the posterior facets of the talus and calcaneus. The arthroscope is in the anterior portal.

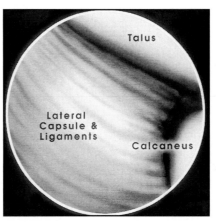

Fig. 33 The interosseous talocalcaneal ligaments. The arthroscope is in the posterior portal.

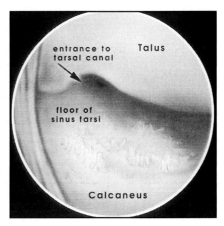

Fig. 34 The posterior facets of the talus and the calcaneus. The arthroscope is in the middle portal. There is an excellent view of the contents of the sinus tarsi.

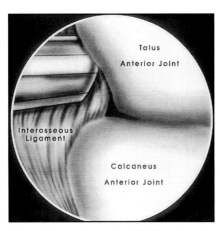

Fig. 35 The anterior and middle facets can be visualized if the interosseous ligament is torn and the arthroscope is passed through the ligament into the anterior compartment of the subtalar joint.

If the posterior portal is placed too proximal, it will inadvertently enter the posterior ankle joint. If the posterior portal is placed too anterior, the sural nerve and saphenous vein are at risk for injury.

The anterior portal is identified first with an 18-gauge spinal needle and the joint is inflated using a 50-ml syringe. If the needle is in the joint, backflow will be observed.

The needle is removed and a small skin incision made. The subcutaneous tis-sue is gently spread using a mosquito clamp. Using the same path, an interchangeable cannula with a semiblunt trocar is placed, followed by the 2.7-mm, 30° oblique arthroscope. An arthroscopic pump is recommended, but continued inflation of the joint with a 50-mm syringe is an alternative method to distend the joint until a second portal is established and gravity inflow is provided.

The middle portal is now placed under direct visualization using an 18-gauge needle and outside-in technique. Once visualized, the needle is removed and replaced with an interchangeable cannula. The lateral aspect of the posterior facet and the interosseous ligament are well visualized from the anterior portal with instrumentation in the middle portal. If there is synovitis or scar tissue present, the middle portal can be used for debridement. The posterior portal can be placed at this time using the same outside-in technique.

A diagnostic arthroscopic examination is performed, viewing from distal to proximal: the posterolateral aspect of the interosseous talocalcaneal ligament, the lateral capsule and its small recess, the articular cartilage of the posterior facets of the talus and calcaneus, and the poste-rior pouch of the joint with its synovial lining (Fig. 32). The arthroscope may now be moved to the posterior portal for examination of the interosseous talocalcaneal ligaments, lateral recess, the reflection of the calcaneofibular ligament, the lateral talocalcaneal ligament, the posterior facet articular cartilage, and the os trigonum and lateral porcess of the talus (Fig. 33).

The middle portal can be used for visualization. If the arthroscope is pointed distally, the interosseous ligament is seen; if the arthroscope is pointed proximally, the posterior facet is seen (Fig. 34).

It is rare to see the anterior and middle facets of the subtalar joint. They can, however, be visualized if the interosseous ligament is torn or the arthroscope is passed through the ligament into the anterior compartment of the subtalar joint (Fig. 35).

Postoperative Care

If the subtalar arthroscopy is performed alone, a bulky dressing is applied and the patient is kept nonweightbearing for 4 to 5 days. A cryotherapy unit is helpful to control postoperative edema. On postoperative day 5, the patient begins weightbearing as tolerated and range of motion exercises. The sutures are removed on postoperative day 10 to 14 and formal physical therapy is begun with range of motion, progressive resistive exercise, proprioception training, and modalities to decrease inflammation including interferential emergency medical services and ice. The patient should be able to return to full activities at 6 to 12 weeks postoperatively.

Results

In a recent report reviewing 49 subtalar arthroscopies performed on joints, the following conditions were present: interosseous ligament injuries (74%), arthrofibrosis (14%), degenerative joint disease (8%), and fibrous coalitions of the calcaneonavicular articulation (4%).

Of the 36 feet with interosseous ligament tears, 27 demonstrated scar formation and hyalinization of the torn ligament ends and subsequent impingement of this material into the anterior aspect of the posterior subtalar joint (Fig. 36). This lesion is referred to as the STIL.

A subjective scale was designed to evaluate the postoperative results in this study. Excellent results indicated that there were no pain or lifestyle restrictions.

Good results indicated that there was improvement but some pain and lifestyle restrictions. Poor results indicated that the patient had not improved or was worse. With an average follow-up of over 4 years, the following results were observed: 47% excellent results, 47% good results, and 6% poor results. Of the patients with poor results, all subsequently had a successful subtalar fusion.

There were 5 reported complications, which included 3 cases of neuritis involving branches of the superficial peroneal nerve, 1 case of sinus tract formation, and 1 case of a superficial wound infection that occurred in the patient with the sinus tract formation. The 3 cases of neuritis were treated successfully with cortisone injections and physical therapy. The patient with the sinus tract formation and

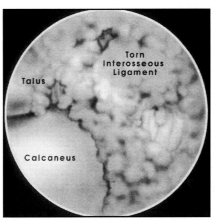

Fig. 36 The torn ends of ligaments can hyalinize and thicken. This material can subsequently impinge into the anterior aspect of the posterior subtalar joint. This lesion is referred to as the subtalar impingement lesion.

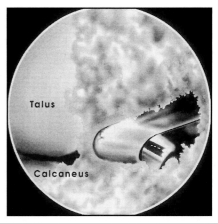

Fig. 37 Instability of the subtalar joint may be viewed arthroscopically as a lateral glide of the posterior calcaneal facet laterally from under the talus.

superficial wound infection was treated successfully with antibiotics, wound care, and subsequent total contact casting.

It should be noted that this study demonstrated that sinus tarsi syndrome is an inaccurate term that should be replaced with a more accurate diagnosis when possible. Arthroscopy is the tool that will allow the orthopaedic surgeon to make a more accurate diagnosis. The authors noted in that study, that of the 14 feet with a preoperative diagnosis of sinus tarsi syndrome, all diagnoses were changed at the time of arthroscopy. The postoperative diagnoses were 10 interosseous ligament tears, 2 cases of arthrofibrosis, and 2 degenerative joints. Clearly, with the more accurate diagnosis that can be made arthroscopically, the general term of "sinus tarsi syndrome" can be dropped. As a result, treatment plans can become more exact and outcomes will hopefully improve. Subtalar instability was also evaluated in this study. Although subtalar instability is most commonly associated with ankle instability, it can exist on its own. Several techniques have been reported[57,62–66] for evaluating subtalar instability, including

fluoroscopy, stress tomograms, subtalar stress radiographs, subtalar arthrograms, and evaluation of the subtalar joint on ankle stress views. Subtalar arthroscopy and direct visualization of the joint may be the most accurate way of evaluating the unstable joint. Because motion occurs in a screw-like fashion[67] about an axis of rotation that forms an angle of 10° to 15° with the sagittal plane and an angle of 45° with the horizontal plane of the foot,[68] it may be that evaluating the joint with varus stress, as done in the above radiographic tests, is not accurate. What was seen at arthroscopy was a lateral glide of the posterior calcaneal facet laterally from under the talus (Fig. 37) which may represent part of the screw motion of the subtalar joint.

Further experience with observing normal motion of the subtalar joint during arthroscopy may lead to greater confidence in recommending arthroscopic stress tests in the evaluation of subtalar joint instability in the future.

Summary

Arthroscopic surgery of the subtalar joint is technically difficult and should only be performed by an arthroscopist experienced in advanced techniques. However, arthroscopy of the subtalar joint and sinus tarsi is a valuable tool in the investigation of hindfoot pathology when conservative treatment fails and a subtalar fusion is not indicated.

Arthroscopic Subtalar Arthrodesis

Surgical procedures designed for subtalar fusion have been in existence for over 90 years. The first subtalar arthrodesis was performed in 1905. There have been numerous techniques reported in the literature that have used both intra-articular as well as extra-articular methods.[69–77] Results have generally been favorable, with a variety of complications reported.[78–80] Data on rate of fusion, time until union, complications, and long-term follow-up is noticeably absent in the older as well as the more recent literature. Several other procedures for subtalar pathology, including arthroplasty, triple arthrodesis, and sinus tarsi exploration, have been described. Surgical open reduction of calcaneal fractures has gained acceptance as a way to restore the normal anatomic alignment of the joint surfaces. This is an effort to avoid the sequelae of posttraumatic degenerative arthritis of the subtalar joint. Both surgical and conservative care of calcaneal fractures continue, however, to be plagued with long-term symptomatic degenerative changes in the subtalar joint.

Arthroscopic subtalar arthrodesis as a surgical procedure was developed in 1992 and first reported at the Arthroscopy Association of North America (AANA) 1994 Annual Meeting in a preliminary review. The procedure was designed to improve traditional methods by using a microinvasive technique. The decision to proceed with this surgical technique grew out of the success with arthroscopic ankle arthrodesis.[81] Subtalar arthroscopy has been described in several studies, but no reported cases or attempts at arthroscopic subtalar fusion have been published.[82] Recent work by Solis (VH Solis, MD, personal communication, 1996) has paralleled some of our earlier work.

The development of an arthroscopic technique was intended to yield less morbidity if it could be performed using the same techniques and principles as an arthroscopic ankle fusion. It was hypothesized that perioperative morbidity could be reduced, blood supply preserved, and proprioceptive and neurosensory input enhanced. A prospective study was initiated to document the effectiveness of the procedure as well as determine the time until complete fusion, the incidence of delayed union and nonunion, and the prevalence of complications.

Indications and Workup

The indications for arthroscopic subtalar arthrodesis are intractable subtalar pain secondary to rheumatoid arthritis, osteoarthritis, and posttraumatic arthritis. Other indications include neuropathic conditions, gross instability, paralytic conditions, and posterior tibial tendon rupture. Most of the earlier literature in subtalar surgery was centered on the stabilization of paralytic deformities secondary to poliomyelitis. The majority of patients encountered in today's medical environment that require this procedure have posttraumatic and arthritic disorders.

Patients must have failed conservative management in order to qualify for arthroscopic subtalar fusion. Conservative treatment includes a variety of modalities including orthotics, nonsteroidal anti-inflammatory agents, activity modification, and occasional cortisone injections into the subtalar joint. They must also be apprised of the possibility of requiring an open procedure should arthroscopic subtalar fusion not be technically feasible.

The patient's history is usually one of lateral hindfoot pain that can be confused quite easily with ankle pathology. An increased symptom with weightbearing on uneven ground is a classic complaint. History of a previous calcaneal fracture should immediately cause suspicion of subtalar pathology. The clinical findings consist of pain over the sinus tarsi and the posterolateral subtalar joint. A reproduction of the symptoms on inversion and eversion of the subtalar joint with the ankle locked in dorsiflexion is also noted.

The clinical workup for this patient profile is quite simple. Often a good history and physical, confirmed by plain radiographs will be sufficient to confirm the diagnosis. On occasion, CT or plain tomography may be necessary.[83] There is little need for MRI or arthrography.[84] Differential injections continue to be a valuable diagnostic aid to confirm as well as distinguish ankle pain from subtalar pain. Radiographic changes do not have to show profound degenerative changes, as only small alterations in the biomechanics of this joint can produce significant symptoms.

The contraindications to this procedure are previously failed subtalar fusions, gross malalignment requiring correction, infection, and significant bone loss. On occasion, a patient with gross malalignment will be a candidate for in situ stablilization. Although significant bone loss has not been encountered frequently, it has not presented a serious problem in a series of arthroscopic ankle arthrodesis.[81]

Each patient was seen in an ambulatory surgery center environment and discharged on the same day. The only exception was the occasional patient seen at the Veterans Administration Hospital affiliated with our teaching institution.[85] Patients were given preoperative, intraoperative, and postoperative antibiotics for a total of 3 doses because of the use of internal fixation. General anesthesia was used in the majority of the cases.

Technique Patients were placed in the lateral decubitus position with the patient lying on the unaffected side. Two pillows were placed between the legs while the affected ankle and subtalar joint were allowed to hang over a blanket roll in a natural position of plantar flexion and inversion. After thoroughly prepping and draping the patient, anatomic landmarks and portal sites are identified and marked with a surgical pen. The tourniquet is then elevated. In general, the surgical procedure was completed within 1 tourniquet time (1 hour and 45 minutes). Establishing the portal sites is one of the more difficult portions of the procedure. To determine an accurate location for the anterolateral portal, the surgeon places his or her thumb in the sinus tarsi while attempting to invert and evert the subtalar joint. The portal is in line with the tip of the fibula, approximately 1 cm distal to the anterior border of the fibula. The needle is placed slightly posterior to the sinus tarsi and angled cephalad 20° to 30° and posteromedially approximately 45°. The posterolateral portal is approximately 1 cm superior to the tip and 1 cm posterior to the border of the fibula. The portal may be established at this time, but can also be established under direct vision once the arthroscope is placed in the anterolateral portal via transillumination. It is critical to predetermine the angles of the subtalar joint because its unique geometry and limited access leaves little room for error. If necessary, fluoroscopy can be used for this procedure to confirm portal location.

These are the 2 conventional portals. If necessary, an accessory portal may be established approximately 1 cm posterior to the anterolateral portal. The accessory portal can be used for debridement or for flow or drainage enhancement; it cannot be used for visualization. Both the anterolateral and posterolateral portals are used in an alternating fashion during the procedure for viewing and for instrumentation. Occasionally, there is significant arthrofibrosis present, making entry and visualization difficult. In these cases, the accessory anterolateral portal is quite useful.

A 2.7-mm, wide angle, shortened small joint arthroscope should be used

for this procedure. It should be equipped with a choice of sheaths to accommodate limited or increased flow. The blunt trocar and sheath are introduced through the anterolateral portal, and the posterolateral portal can be established at this time. In the initial cases, a small laminar spreader was used in the anterolateral portal to increase access, but was later abandoned as a routine; however, it may still be used if distraction is a significant problem. Arthroscopic resection of the interosseous ligament may also be used for additional distraction, but has not been used to date by our group.

It is important to be certain that the arthroscope is in the subtalar joint and that the ankle joint or the fibular talar recess have not been inadvertently entered. All debridement and decortication is performed posterior to the interosseous ligament because only the posterior facet is fused. The middle and anterior facets are not visualized under normal circumstances unless the interosseous ligament is absent. The majority of the procedure is done with the arthroscope in the anterolateral portal and the instruments in the posterolateral portal. The remaining and final debridement will be accomplished alternating these 2 portals.

A primary synovectomy and debridement are necessary for visualization as with other joints. Debridement of the articular surface makes the joint more capacious and makes instrumentation easier. Complete removal of the articular surface down to subchondral bone is the next phase of the procedure. The talocalcaneal geometry is quite unique and will require a variety of instruments. In general, multiangular curettes as well as a complete set of burrs will suffice.

Once the articular cartilage has been resected, approximately 1 to 2 mm of subchondral bone is removed to expose the highly vascular cancellous bone. Care must be taken not to alter the geometry or remove excessive bone, which will

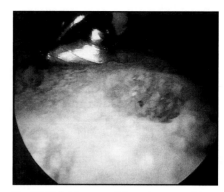

Fig. 38 Debridement of the calcaneus with spot-weld vascular channel.

lead to poor coaptation of the joint surfaces. Once the subchondral plate is removed, small spot-weld holes measuring approximately 2 mm in depth are created on the surfaces of the calcaneus and talus to create vascular channels (Fig. 38). Careful assessment of the posteromedial corner must be made, as residual bone and cartilage can be left there that can interfere with coaptation. Often the curette will safely break down this corner and also provide the surgeon with additional tactile feedback. The neurovascular bundle which is directly posteromedial and has to be taken into consideration at all times and protected.

After viewing from both portals to assure complete debridement and decortication, the tourniquet is released and careful assessment of the vascularity of the calcaneus and talus is made. The joint is then thoroughly irrigated of bone fragments and debris. No autogenous bone graft or bone substitute is needed for this procedure.

The fixation of the fusion is performed with a large cannulated 7-mm screw. The guide pin is started at the dorsal anteromedial talus and angled posterior and inferior to the posterolateral calcaneus, but does not violate the calcaneal cortical surface. Under fluoroscopy, the guide wire is placed with the ankle in maximum dorsiflexion to avoid any possible screw head encroachment or

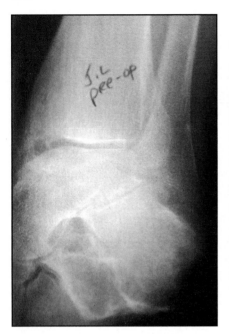

Fig. 39 Preoperative radiograph of the subtalar joint with osteoarthritis.

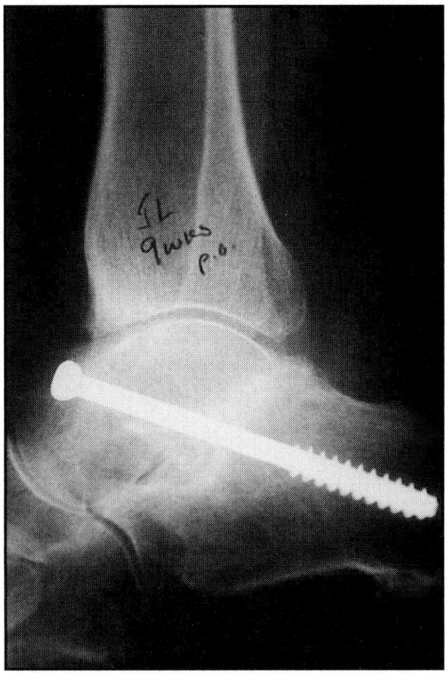

Fig. 40 Postoperative radiograph of subtalar fusion at 9 weeks.

impingement on the anterior lip of the tibia. Once the guide wire is placed under these conditions, the ankle can then be relaxed, the screw inserted under fluoroscopic control, and the fusion site compressed. The screw will run along the natural axis of rotation of the subtalar joint using this technique. Starting the screw from the dorsal and medial aspect of the talus avoids painful screw head prominence over the calcaneus and avoids a second procedure for screw removal. To date, there have been no fractures or complications with this particular fixation technique (Figs. 39 and 40).

Steri-strips are used instead of sutures to allow adequate drainage. A bulky dressing and a short leg bivalve cast are applied. The patient is discharged to home after appropriate circulatory checks in the recovery room. The first clinical evaluation takes place in the office within 48 hours. In approximately 1 week, the cast is removed and the patient is fitted immediately with an ankle-foot orthosis (AFO) if the swelling is minimal. Full

weightbearing is allowed as tolerated at any time following surgery. In general, patients can tolerate full weightbearing without crutch support within 7 to 14 days after surgery. Although patients wear the AFO almost 24 hours a day, they are able to bathe as well as to take the ankle and foot through a range of motion without the brace. It is removed when full union has been achieved. The standard 3 views of the ankle, plus a Browden view, are the radiographs of choice used in follow-up assessment.

Results

Since September 1992, 24 patients have undergone arthroscopic subtalar fusion with sufficient follow-up time to determine the effectiveness of this procedure. Fusion rate, time until complete union, surgical technique, and complications were analyzed. One standard surgical procedure was used and the method of internal fixation was not altered during this entire series. The posterior subtalar joint was the only joint fused during this procedure. Three of the 24 patients

underwent a combined arthroscopic ankle and subtalar fusion. In this series, there were 8 patients with osteoarthritis, 9 patients with posttraumatic arthritis and 2 with rheumatoid arthritis, 4 with posterior tibial tendon ruptures, and 1 with a tarsal coalition.

Every patient had a radiographic evaluation at 2-week intervals to determine the rate and quality of fusion. For an arthrodesis to be considered completely fused, it requires both clinical and radiographic support. The parameters required for a successful arthrodesis are evidence of bone consolidation across the subtalar joint, no motion at the screw, the clinical absence of pain with weightbearing, and pain-free forced inversion and eversion. The average mean follow-up time is 31 months (range, 7 to 64 months). All 24 patients have united clinical and radiographic union, and the average time until complete fusion was 8.9 weeks (range, 6 to 16 weeks).

There are considerable advantages to this technique when compared with open procedures. It is a minimally invasive technique that theoretically preserves the blood supply of the calcaneus and talus. This is especially important considering that many of these patients have had previous invasive surgery. Conventional open procedures by definition interrupt the blood supply and compromise vascular ingrowth and eventual fusion. Avoidance of incisions coupled with early range of motion and weightbearing helps avoid stress deprivation and enhance proprioception, therefore reducing the devastating effects of reflex sympathetic dystrophy.

There have been no reoperations with the exception of a screw removal. One patient had a painful screw at the calcaneus that penetrated the cortex, and the possibility of a stress fracture was entertained. Symptoms resolved after screw removal. Two patients had some residual anterolateral pain with some radiographic changes and clinical evidence of minor degenerative joint disease in the ankle.

Both patients responded with complete relief to a diagnostic xylocaine injection into the ankle joint. Valgus tilting of the ankle joint following subtalar arthrodesis has been reported (unpublished data, 1995), but it is unclear if this is secondary to the fusion of merely a natural progression of the disease. Two cases not included in this series could not be completed arthroscopically because of significant malformation of the calcaneus and arthrofibrosis of the subtalar joint. These patients underwent a modified mini-open posterior subtalar arthrodesis. Identical screw fixation and postoperative protocol was used in these 2 patients. Skin problems about the hindfoot can be catastrophic and are obviously avoided using this technique. There were no superficial or deep infections in this series. All arthroscopic procedures have had reported reductions in infection and it is hoped that this procedure would also fall into that same category. There have not been sufficient cases, however, to validate this hypothesis.

Most open series show a longer time until union, with some prevalence of nonunions. Although too early to validate, preliminary observations would indicate a more rapid time until union as well as an increased rate of union. There has been a paucity of literature over the past 25 years on isolated subtalar arthrodesis with adequate follow-up statistics.

Summary

The obvious socioeconomic advantages are quite dramatic, with early weight-bearing and AFO immobilization allowing patients an early return to work. Outpatient surgery is a cost-effective benefit. Patient satisfactions as well as comfort are greatly enhanced, requiring only oral pain medication. All patients have tolerated their postoperative regimen and same-day discharge.

Arthroscopic subtalar arthrodesis is a technically demanding procedure that requires some rather advanced arthro-scopic skills to perform. Joint access is tight, restricted, and requires small instrumentation. Deformities cannot be corrected; therefore, at this stage, a fusion in situ must be considered. The learning curve is certainly far steeper because of the smaller patient population available for enhancing surgical skills.

Overall, this procedure has stood the test of time and follow-up. The results appear to be excellent in terms of patient satisfaction, fusion rate time until union, and postoperative morbidity. The recognition and enhancement of this technique as well as the development of more advanced technology will certainly allow this arthroscopic subtalar arthrodesis technique to mature even further over time.

References

1. Berndt AL, Harty M: Transchondral fractures (osteochondritis dissecans) of the talus. *J Bone Joint Surg* 1959;41A:988–1020.

2. Ferkel RD, Sgaglione NA: Arthroscopic treatment of osteochondral lesions of the talus: Long term results. *Orthop Trans* 1993-1994;17:1011.

3. Anderson IF, Crichton KJ, Grattan-Smith T, Cooper RA, Brazier D: Osteochondral fractures of the dome of the talus. *J Bone Joint Surg* 1989;71A:1143–1152.

4. Pritsch M, Horoshovski H, Farine I: Arthroscopic treatment of osteochondral lesions of the talus. *J Bone Joint Surg* 1986;68A:862–865.

5. Hangody L, Kish G, Karpati Z, Szerb I, Eberhardt R: Treatment of osteochondritis dissecans of the talus: Use of the mosaicplasty technique—a preliminary report. *Foot Ankle Int* 1997;18:628–634.

6. Broström L: Sprained ankles. *Acta Chir Scand* 1964;128:483–495.

7. Johannsen A: Radiological diagnosis of lateral ligament lesion of the ankle: A comparison between talar tilt and anterior drawer sign. *Acta Orthop Scand* 1978;49:295–301.

8. Seligson D, Gassman J, Pope M: Ankle instability: Evaluation of the lateral ligaments. *Am J Sport Med* 1980;8:39–42.

9. Schafer D, Hintermann B: Arthroscopic assessment of the chronic unstable ankle joint. *Knee Surg Sports Traumatol Arthrosc* 1996;4:48–52.

10. Kibler WB: Arthroscopic findings in ankle ligament reconstruction. *Clin Sport Med* 1996;15:799–804.

11. Lundeen RO: Ankle arthroscopy in the adolescent patient. *J Foot Surg* 1990;29:510–515.

12. Taga I, Shino K, Inoue M, Nakata, Maeda A: Articular cartilage lesions in ankles with lateral ligament injury: An arthroscopic study. *Am J Sport Med* 1993;21:120–126.

13. Hawkins RB: Arthroscopic stapling repair for chronic lateral instability. *Clin Podiatr Med Surg* 1987;4:875–883.

14. Stiehl JB: Complex ankle fracture dislocations with syndesmotic diastasis. *Orthop Rev* 1990;19:99–507.

15. Taylor DC, Englehardt DL, Bassett FH III: Syndesmosis sprains of the ankle: The influence of heterotopic ossification. *Am J Sport Med* 1992;20:146–150.

16. Fritschy D: An unusual ankle injury in top skiers. *Am J Sport Med* 1989;17:282–285.

17. Hopkinson WJ, St. Pierre P, Ryan JB, Wheeler JH: Syndesmosis sprains of the ankle. *Foot Ankle* 1990;10:325–330.

18. Cedell CA: Ankle lesions. *Acta Orthop Scand* 1975;46:425–445.

19. Edwards GS Jr, DeLee JC: Ankle diastasis without fracture. *Foot Ankle* 1984;4:305–312.

20. Marymont JV, Lynch MA, Henning CE: Acute ligamentous diastasis of the ankle without fracture: Evaluation by radionuclide imaging. *Am J Sport Med* 1986;14:407–409.

21. Ogilvie-Harris DJ, Reed SC: Disruption of the ankle syndesmosis: Diagnosis and treatment by arthroscopic surgery. *Arthroscopy* 1994;10:561–568.

22. Katznelson A, Lin E, Militiano J: Ruptures of the ligaments about the tibio-fibular syndesmosis. *Injury* 1983;15:170–172.

23. Baciu CC: A simple technique for arthrodesis of the ankle. *J Bone Joint Surg* 1986;68B:266–267.

24. Campbell P: Arthrodesis of the ankle with modified distraction-compression and bone-grafting. *J Bone Joint Surg* 1990;72A:552–556.

25. Carrier DA, Harris CM: Ankle arthrodesis with vertical Steinmann's pins in rheumatoid arthritis. *Clin Orthop* 1991;268:10–14.

26. Johnson EE, Weltmer J, Lian GJ, Cracchiolo A III: Ilizarov ankle arthrodesis. *Clin Orthop* 1992;280:160–169.

27. Malarkey RF, Binski JC: Ankle arthrodesis with the Calandruccio frame and bimalleolar onlay grafting. *Clin Orthop* 1991;268:44–48.

28. Mann RA, Van Manen JW, Wapner K, Martin J: Ankle fusion. *Clin Orthop* 1991;268:49–55.

29. Marcus RE, Balourdas GM, Heiple KG: Ankle arthrodesis by chevron fusion with internal fixation and bone-grafting. *J Bone Joint Surg* 1983;65A:833–838.

30. Mears DC, Gordon RG, Kann SE, Kann JN: Ankle arthrodesis with an anterior tension plate. *Clin Orthop* 1991;268:70–77.

31. Morgan CD, Henke JA, Bailey RW, Kaufer H: Long-term results of tibiotalar arthrodesis. *J Bone Joint Surg* 1985;67A:546–550.

32. Shneider, D: Arthroscopic ankle fusion. *Arth Video J* 1983;3.

33. Scranton PE Jr: Use of internal compression in arthrodesis of the ankle. *J Bone Joint Surg* 1985;67A:550–555.

34. Sowa DT, Krackow KA: Ankle fusion: A new technique of internal fixation using a compression blade plate. *Foot Ankle* 1989;9:232–240.

35. Weltmer JB Jr, Choi SH, Shenoy A, Schwartsman V: Wolf blade plate ankle arthrodesis. *Clin Orthop* 1991;268:107–111.

36. White AA III: A precision posterior ankle fusion. *Clin Orthop* 1974;98:239–250.

37. Campbell CJ, Rinehart WT, Kalenak A: Arthrodesis of the ankle: Deep autogenous inlay grafts with maximum cancellous-bone apposition. *J Bone Joint Surg* 1974;56A:63–70.

38. Frey C, Halikus NM, Vu-Rose T, Ebramzadeh E: A review of ankle arthrodesis: Predisposing factors to nonunion. *Foot Ankle Int* 1994;15:581–584.

39. Johnson EW Jr, Boseker EH: Arthrodesis of the ankle. *Arch Surg* 1968;97:766–773.

40. Moran CG, Pinder IM, Smith SR: Ankle arthrodesis in rheumatoid arthritis: 30 cases followed for 5 years. *Acta Orthop Scand* 1991;62:538–543.

41. Morrey BF, Wiedeman GP Jr: Complications and long-term results of ankle arthrodeses following trauma. *J Bone Joint Surg* 1980;62A:777–784.

42. Scranton PE Jr, Fu FH, Brown TD: Ankle arthrodesis: A comparative clinical and biomechanical evaluation. *Clin Orthop* 1980;151:234–243.

43. Stuart MJ, Morrey BF: Arthrodesis of the diabetic neuropathic ankle joint. *Clin Orthop* 1990;253:209–211.

44. Holt ES, Hansen ST, Mayo KA, Sangeorzan BJ: Ankle arthrodesis using internal screw fixation. *Clin Orthop* 1991;268:21–28.

45. Maurer RC, Cimino WR, Cox CV, Satow GK: Transarticular cross-screw fixation: A technique of ankle arthrodesis. *Clin Orthop* 1991;268:56–64.

46. Corso SJ, Zimmer TJ: Technique and clinical evaluation of arthroscopic ankle arthrodesis. *Arthroscopy* 1995;11:585–590.

47. Ewing JW, Tasto JA, Tippett JW: Arthroscopic surgery of the ankle, in Jackson DW (ed): *Instructional Course Lectures 44*. Rosemont, IL, American Academy of Orthopaedic Surgeons, 1995, pp 325–340.

48. Glick JM, Morgan CD, Myerson MS, Sampson TG, Mann JA: Ankle arthrodesis using an arthroscopic method: Long-term follow-up of 34 cases. *Arthroscopy* 1996;12:428–434.

49. Morgan CD: Arthroscopic tibiotalar arthrodesis, in McGinty JB (ed): *Operative Arthroscopy*. New York, NY, Raven Press, 1991, pp 695–701.

50. Myerson MS, Quill G: Ankle arthrodesis: A comparison of an arthroscopic and an open method of treatment. *Clin Orthop* 1991;268:84–95.

51. Ogilvie-Harris DJ, Lieberman I, Fitsialos D: Arthroscopically assisted arthrodesis for osteoarthrotic ankles. *J Bone Joint Surg* 1993;75A:1167–1174.

52. Guhl JF: Portals and techniques—mechanical distraction, in Guhl JF (ed): *Ankle Arthroscopy, Pathology and Surgical Techniques*. Thorofare, NJ, Slack Inc, 1988, pp 52–53.

53. Hatt RN, Lamphier TA: Triple hemisection: A simplified procedure for lengthening the Achilles tendon. *N Engl J Med* 1947;236:166–170.

54. Cahill DR: The anatomy and function of the contents of the human tarsal sinus and canal. *Anat Rec* 1965;153:1–17.

55. Frey C, Gasser S, Feder K: Arthroscopy of the subtalar joint. *Foot Ankle Int* 1994;15:424–428.

56. Frey C, Feder KS, DiGiovanni C: Arthroscopic evaluation of the subtalar joint: Does sinus tarsi syndrome exist? *Foot Ankle Int* 1999;20:185–191.

57. Kjaersgaard-Andersen P, Wethelund JO, Helmig P, Soballe K: The stabilizing effect of the ligamentous structures in the sinus and canalis tarsi on movements in the hindfoot. *Am J Sports Med* 1988;16:512–516.

58. Lehman WB, Lehman M: The surgical anatomy of the interosseous ligament of the subtalar joint as it relates to clubfoot surgery. *Bull Hosp Jt Dis Orthop Inst* 1981;41:19–27.

59. Parisien JS (ed): *Arthroscopic Surgery*. New York, NY, McGraw-Hill, 1988.

60. Parisien JS, Vangsness T: Arthrosocopy of the subtalar joint: An experimental approach. *Arthroscopy* 1985;1:53–57.

61. Perry J: Anatomy and biomechanics of the hindfoot. *Clin Orthop* 1983;177:9–15.

62. Resnick D: Radiology of the talocalcaneal articulations: Anatomic considerations and arthrography. *Radiology* 1974;3:581–586.

63. Mekhail AO, Heck BE, Ebraheim NA, Jackson WT: Arthroscopy of the subtalar joint: Establishing a medial portal. *Foot Ankle Int* 1995;16:427–432.

64. Brantigan JW, Pedegana LR, Lippert FG: Instability of the subtalar joint: Diagnosis by stress tomography in three cases. *J Bone Joint Surg* 1977;59A:321–324.

65. Clanton TO: Instability of the subtalar joint. *Orthop Clin North Am* 1989;20:583–592.

66. Zell BK, Shereff MJ, Greenspan A, Liebowitz S: Combined ankle and subtalar instability. *Bull Hosp Jt Dis Orthop Inst* 1986;46:37–46.

67. Manter JT: Movements of the subtalar and transverse tarsal joints. *Anat Rec* 1941;80:397–410.

68. Wright DG, Desai SM, Henderson WH: Action of the subtalar and ankle-joint complex during the stance phase of walking. *J Bone Joint Surg* 1964;46A:361–382.

69. Thomas FB: Arthrodesis of the subtalar joint. *J Bone Joint Surg* 1967;1:93–97.

70. Dick LL: Primary fusion of the posterior subtalar joint and the treatment of fractures of the calcaneus. *J Bone Joint Surg* 1953;35B:375.

71. Gallie WE: Subastragalar arthrodesis and fractures of the os calcis. *J Bone Joint Surg* 1943;25:731.

72. Grice DS: An extra-articular arthrodesis of the subastragalar joint for correction of paralytic flat feet in children. *J Bone Joint Surg* 1952;34A:927.

73. Grice DS: Further experience with extra-articular arthrodesis of the subtalar joint. *J Bone Joint Surg* 1955;37A:246.

74. Hall MC, Pennal GF: Primary subtalar arthrodesis in the treatment of severe fractures of the calcaneus. *J Bone Joint Surg* 1960;42B:336.

75. Geckler EO: Comminuted fractures of the os calcis. *Arch Surg* 1943;61:469.

76. Harris RI: Fractures of the os calcis. *Ann Surg* 1946;124:1082.

77. Wilson PD: Treatment of fractures of the os calcis by arthrodesis of the subtalar joint. *JAMA* 1927;89:1676.

78. Gross RH: A clinical study of bachelor subtalar arthrodesis. *J Bone Joint Surg* 1976;58:343–349.

79. Mallon WJ, Nunley JA: The Grice procedure: Extra-articular arthrodesis. *Orthop Clin N Am* 1989;20:649–654.

80. Moreland JR, Westin GW: Further experience with Grice subtalar arthrodesis. *Clin Orthop* 1986;;207:113–121.

81. Tasto JP: *Arthroscopic Ankle Arthrodesis: A Seven Year Followup*. Rosemont, IL, American Academy of Orthopaedic Surgeons, 1997.

82. Ferkel RA: *Arthroscopic Surgery: The Foot & Ankle*. Philadelphia, PA, Lippencott-Raven, 1996.

83. Seltzer SE, Weisman B: CT of the hindfoot with rheumatoid arthritis. *J Arthritis Rheumatol* 1985;28:12–42.

84. Goosens M, et al: Posterior subtalar joint arthrograpy: A useful tool in the diagnosis of hindoot disorders. *Clin Orthop* 1989;248:255.

85. Thomas FB: Arthrodesis of the subtalar joint. *J Bone Joint Surg* 1967;1:93–97.

Arthroscopy of the Subtalar Joint and Arthroscopic Subtalar Arthrodesis

James P. Tasto, MD

Abstract

Subtalar arthroscopy has become a valuable adjunct to the tools used in lower extremity surgery. For the past 25 years, ankle arthroscopy has been in vogue for treating a variety of conditions. Subtalar arthroscopy has more treatment limitations and is more technically difficult to perform than ankle arthroscopy because of the anatomic confines and structure of the subtalar joint. Most procedures are performed on the posterior aspect of the subtalar joint. The subtalar joint is composed of three articulations (posterior, middle, and anterior facets) and is surrounded by a variety of intra-articular and extra-articular ligaments, whose anatomy must be fully understood before attempting this procedure. Subtalar arthroscopy may be indicated for diagnostic purposes and for débridement of synovial impingement syndromes in the sinus tarsi. It may be used to examine loose bodies or osteochondral lesions, to address fractures of the lateral process of the talus, and to evaluate subtalar instability to determine appropriate stabilization methods. Arthroscopic subtalar arthrodesis also has gained credibility over the past 10 years as an acceptable surgical procedure. Arthroscopic evaluation of subtalar instability is useful in planning the appropriate stabilization.

Subtalar arthroscopy is usually performed with the patient in the lateral decubitus position without traction. Anterior and posterior portals as well as an accessory anterior portal are usually necessary to perform all of the above procedures. Because of the limited confines of the joint, care must be taken to prevent any articular cartilage damage. When performing subtalar arthroscopy in conjunction with ankle arthroscopy, the subtalar arthroscopy should be performed first to avoid excessive extravasation from the ankle arthroscopy, which could obscure entry to the subtalar joint. Complications of subtalar arthroscopy are similar to those encountered in ankle arthroscopy, such as damage to the sural and superficial peroneal nerves.

Arthroscopy of the subtalar joint was originally described by Parisien and Vangsness in 1985.[1] The subtalar joint is a complex joint that is functionally responsible for inversion and eversion of the hindfoot.[2-9] Most arthroscopic procedures are performed in the posterior compartment of this joint. The use of smaller instrumentation and optics has made subtalar arthroscopy a more widely accepted procedure.

Anatomy and Biomechanics

The subtalar joint is composed of three articulations: the posterior, middle, and anterior joints or facets (Figures 1 and 2). There are many extra-articular ligaments that stabilize the subtalar joint. The major ligaments encountered during subtalar arthroscopy are the intra-articular components, which consist of the interosseous, lateral, and anterior talocalcaneal ligaments (Figure 3). These components coalesce to form the division between the posterior and the middle facets of the subtalar joint. The interosseous ligament is a broad, stout structure measuring approximately 2.5 cm in breadth from medial to lateral. It marks the arthroscopic boundary for posterior subtalar arthroscopy. The subtalar joint is a single axis joint that acts like a mitered hinge connecting the talus and calcaneus.[10,11] The axis of movement about this joint is backward, downward, and lateral running from the dorsal medial talus to the posterolateral calcaneus. The subtalar joint is a determinative joint that influences the biomechanics of the distal portion of the midfoot and forefoot. The more horizontal the hinge, the greater the influence that torque and rotation will have

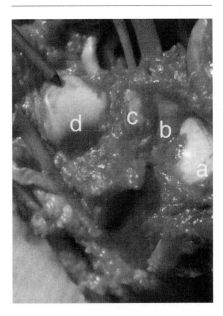

Figure 1 Topographic view of a prosected posterior subtalar joint showing the undersurface of talus (a), the middle facet of talus (b), the anterior facet of talus (c), and the superior surface of calcaneus (d). (Reproduced with permission from Tasto JP: Subtalar arthroscopy, in McGinty JB (ed): *Operative Arthroscopy*, ed 3. Philadelphia, PA, Lippincott Williams & Wilkins, 2003, pp 944-952.)

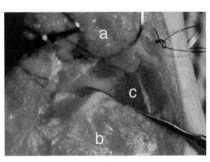

Figure 2 Anatomic dissection of the lateral posterior subtalar joint: talus (a), calcaneus (b), subtalar joint (c). (Reproduced with permission from Tasto JP: Subtalar arthroscopy, in McGinty JB (ed): *Operative Arthroscopy*, ed 3. Philadelphia, PA, Lippincott Williams & Wilkins, 2003, pp 944-952.)

on the midfoot and forefoot. Anatomic studies on cadavers have determined the range of motion of the subtalar joint to be from 20° to 60° of combined inversion and eversion.[10-12]

The three articulations of the subtalar joint simultaneously provide rotation between the talus and calcaneus about a common axis of rotation.[10-12] At the end of its normal range of motion, the curves of the three articulations suddenly become incongruous and no longer provide motion about a common axis of rotation; further motion will disarticulate the subtalar joint.[10-12] This disrupting force must be rotational and must exceed the compressive forces that hold the talus and calcaneus together.[10,11]

At the end of its normal range of motion, the subtalar joint will stop rotating and the ligaments will continue to be relaxed. Only when the transverse rotational force is increased to the extent that it exceeds the compressive force do the ligaments tighten. The ligaments therefore become taut only at the beginning of an imminent dislocation or subluxation.[10,11] The subtalar joint is separated into both an anterior and posterior compartment by the sinus tarsi and the tarsal canal. The contents of the tarsal canal include the cervical ligament, talocalcaneal interosseous ligament, the medial root of the inferior extensor retinaculum, the fat pad, and a variety of blood vessels. The anterior portion of the subtalar joint includes both the anterior and middle facets. It also contains the talonavicular articulation and the spring ligament. The posterior subtalar joint has a long axis that is located obliquely about 40° to the midline of the foot, faces laterally, and consists of a convex posterior facet of the calcaneus and a concave facet of the talus. The capsule of the posterior subtalar joint is reinforced laterally by the cervical ligament and the calcaneofibular ligament.

Indications for Use

As with most arthroscopic surgery, subtalar arthroscopy can be used for diagnostic purposes if there are clinical indications that the suspected disorder is isolated to the subtalar joint. Indications of a subtalar joint disorder include synovitis and partial disruptions of the interosseous ligament in the sinus tarsi, arthrofibrosis, residual posttraumatic scar formation, and the presence of unstable chondral or osteochondral lesions. Subtalar arthroscopy also may be useful in the treatment of fractures of the lateral process of the talus, loose bodies, subtalar impingement, and subtalar arthrodesis. It can be used in combination with an ankle arthroscopy in the evaluation and treatment of combined ankle and subtalar instability for diagnostic and therapeutic treatment.[1,3,4,7]

Contraindications for Use

The subtalar joint is a relatively tight joint, which may prevent easy access. In a patient with a previous fracture and restricted joint access with concomitant arthrofibrosis, arthroscopy may be contraindicated, particularly if the articular surfaces are malaligned. The presence of internal fixation devices may obscure either the anterior or the posterior portal and can make an arthroscopic procedure impossible to perform. Infection around the foot and ankle is a clear contraindication to any elective arthroscopic procedure.

Imaging

Conventional radiographic studies should include a routine AP, lateral, and mortise view of the ankle. A Broden view is helpful in isolating

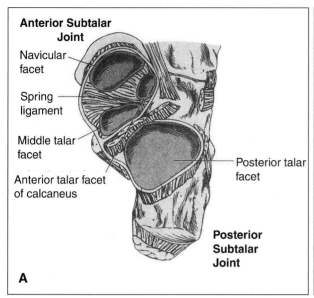

Anterior Subtalar Joint
- Navicular facet
- Spring ligament
- Middle talar facet
- Anterior talar facet of calcaneus
- Posterior talar facet
- **Posterior Subtalar Joint**

A

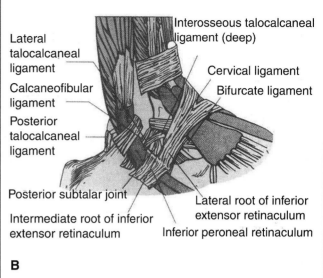

- Lateral talocalcaneal ligament
- Calcaneofibular ligament
- Posterior talocalcaneal ligament
- Interosseous talocalcaneal ligament (deep)
- Cervical ligament
- Bifurcate ligament
- Posterior subtalar joint
- Intermediate root of inferior extensor retinaculum
- Lateral root of inferior extensor retinaculum
- Inferior peroneal retinaculum

B

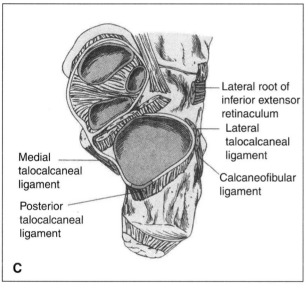

- Lateral root of inferior extensor retinaculum
- Lateral talocalcaneal ligament
- Calcaneofibular ligament
- Medial talocalcaneal ligament
- Posterior talocalcaneal ligament

C

Figure 3 **A,** The subtalar joints. **B,** Lateral view of the right ankle showing the peripheral ligaments. **C,** Axial view of the ankle showing the peripheral ligaments. (Reproduced with permission from Tasto JP: Subtalar arthroscopy, in McGinty JB (ed): *Operative Arthroscopy*, ed 3. Philadelphia, PA, Lippincott Williams & Wilkins, 2003, pp 944-952.)

the posterior subtalar joint to see subtle changes; it is usually taken with the ankle and forefoot in full plantar flexion and internally rotated approximately 40°. MRI is often useful to differentiate intra-articular pathology from the soft-tissue causes of lateral hindfoot pain. If subtle arthritis is suspected, a CT scan may be helpful to define the osseous morphology more accurately.

Currently, arthrography is seldom used in the diagnostic workup for ankle and subtalar pain. Differential injections, however, have proved to be an excellent adjunct for differentiating lateral ankle pain from subtalar pain.

Surgical Technique

The technique for subtalar arthroscopy has been described previously by several authors.[1,3,7] The patient is placed in the lateral decubitus position with the legs and hips appropriately padded. The surgical procedure is generally done with the aid of an inflated thigh tourniquet. In contrast to ankle arthroscopy, no traction is applied to the extremity. The application of a soft-tissue distraction device actually obliterates the portal. Only a slight amount of ankle inversion is allowed because extreme inversion can cause the surrounding soft tissues to obliterate the portals and make the arthroscopic procedure more difficult.

If ankle arthroscopy also is being performed, subtalar arthroscopy should be done first (Figure 4). This sequence will avoid the normal ex-

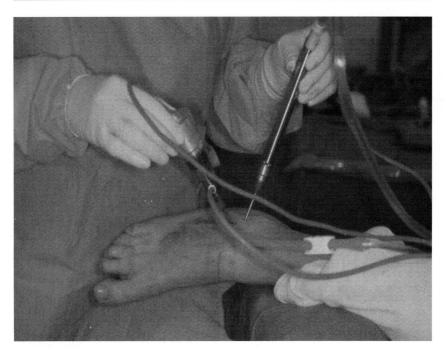

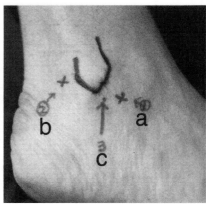

Figure 5 Portal sites for subtalar arthrodesis: anterolateral portal (a), posterolateral portal (b), accessory lateral portal (c). (Reproduced with permission from Tasto JP: Subtalar arthroscopy, in McGinty JB (ed): *Operative Arthroscopy*, ed 3. Philadelphia, PA, Lippincott Williams & Wilkins, 2003, pp 944-952.)

Figure 4 Surgical positioning of the foot for subtalar arthroscopy with the camera in the anterolateral portal and the shaver in the accessory portal. (Reproduced with permission from Tasto JP: Arthroscopic subtalar arthrodesis, in Miller MD, Cole BJ (eds): *Textbook of Arthroscopy*. Philadelphia, PA, WB Saunders, 2004, pp 794-801.)

travasation that occurs with ankle arthroscopy that could hinder a subsequent subtalar procedure. A marking pen is used to outline the fibula, the superficial peroneal nerve, and the sural nerve. All three portals are marked (Figure 5).

The subtalar joint is preinjected with approximately 7 mL of saline. Care must be taken to prevent injection into the subcutaneous tissue. Injection using a large bore needle can provide reassurance that the joint has been entered and will provide the surgeon with an appropriate angle for the initial placement of the arthroscopic sheath and trocar.

The anterolateral portal is established first with a nick and spread technique using a No. 11 blade. This portal is usually located in the region of the sinus tarsi and approximately 1.5 to 2 cm anterior and 1 cm distal to the tip of the lateral

malleolus. Only the skin is incised and further dilation and spreading is done with a small mosquito clamp. The 2.7-mm dull trocar and sheath are then placed in the anterior portal. The arthroscope is then located posterior to the interosseous ligament. If better visualization is initially required, an 18-gauge needle can be placed in juxtaposition to the arthroscope to establish appropriate flow. The posterolateral portal is then established by palpating the soft tissues and establishing the entry site with an 18-gauge needle using an outside-in technique while visualizing the posterolateral portal placement through the anterior portal. The posterolateral portal is usually located approximately 1 cm proximal and 1 cm posterior to the distal tip of the fibula. Care is taken to avoid the sural nerve and the small saphenous vein while estab-

lishing this portal. The nick and spread technique is used in a vertical fashion to avoid damaging these structures. If a large amount of synovium and scar tissue is encountered in the anterior portal and visualization is impaired, then an accessory portal is established and a small shaver is used to débride this area.

Initially, visualization is done from the anterolateral portal with outflow established in the posterior portal. Later in the procedure these portals may be reversed. A pump is used to maintain complete control over the pressure and to avoid excessive extravasation and potential compartment syndrome. The pressure is usually maintained at approximately 35 mm Hg.

A complete diagnostic subtalar arthroscopy is then performed (Figures 6 and 7). The interosseous talocalcaneal ligaments are located distal to the anterolateral portal and the talocalcaneal joint is located proximal to the portal. The lateral recess,

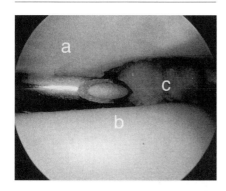

Figure 6 Arthroscopic view of a right posterior subtalar joint: talus (a), calcaneus (b), posteromedial corner (c). (Reproduced with permission from Tasto JP: Subtalar arthroscopy, in McGinty JB (ed): *Operative Arthroscopy*, ed 3. Philadelphia, PA, Lippincott Williams & Wilkins, 2003, pp 944-952.)

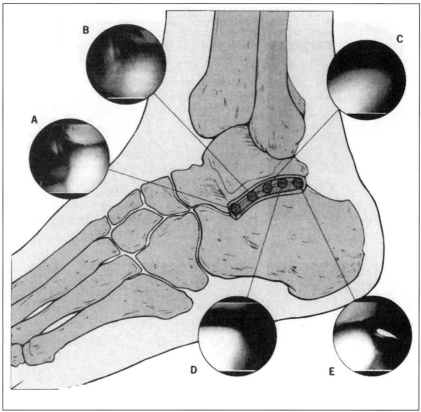

Figure 7 Arthroscopic view of various areas of the posterior subtalar joint in a patient with subtalar instability. Shown are interosseous ligament area (A), anterior aspect of the joint (B), midaspect of the joint (C), posterior aspect of the joint (D), and posterior pouch of the subtalar joint (E). (Reproduced with permission from Tasto JP: Subtalar arthroscopy, in McGinty JB (ed): *Operative Arthroscopy*, ed 3. Philadelphia, PA, Lippincott Williams & Wilkins, 2003, pp 944-952.)

the reflection of the calcaneofibular ligament, the lateral talocalcaneal ligament, the os trigonum, and the lateral process of the talus can now be visualized. The anterolateral portal allows viewing of the posterior compartment, but the anterior and middle facets or the anterior compartment of the subtalar joint are not seen. However, complete disruption of the interosseous ligaments can be seen. It is possible to use the arthroscope to view these compartments if a portal is extended distally through the interosseous ligament.

Conventional 2.0- and 3.5-mm shavers can be used to perform a débridement and synovectomy at the beginning of the procedure to improve visualization. Small loose body forceps can be used to remove loose bodies, and occasionally radiofrequency can be used to perform ablation and modulation of the synovium and abnormal soft tissue.

Results and Complications

Favorable results have been reported using the described technique for subtalar arthroscopy when appropriate indications are defined and there

is adherence to meticulous detail in performing the procedure. In a study of 49 subtalar arthroscopies, Frey and associates[4] reported 94% good to excellent results. Patients in this study had injuries to the interosseous ligament, arthrofibrosis, degenerative joint disease, and fibrous coalitions of the calcaneonavicular joint.

Complications after subtalar arthroscopy included neurapraxia, involving both the sural nerve and the superficial branch of the peroneal nerve, sinus tract infections, and wound infections.[4,13-15] As is the case with ankle arthroscopy, the most common complication is neurapraxia of the superficial pero-

neal nerve or sural nerve. This complication can be avoided if the surgeon has a thorough knowledge of subtalar joint anatomy and carefully uses a nick and spread technique when establishing portals.

Arthroscopic Subtalar Arthrodesis

Surgical procedures designed for subtalar fusion have been in existence for nearly 100 years. Subtalar arthrodesis was first performed in 1905 and numerous techniques using both intra-articular and extra-articular methods have been reported in the literature.[16-24] Results have generally been favorable; however, various complications have been reported.[25-27] Data on rate of fusion, time until union, complications, and long-term follow-up are noticeably missing in the literature. Several other procedures for subtalar pathology have been described, including arthroscopy, arthroplasty, triple arthrodesis, and sinus tarsi exploration. Surgical open reduction of calcaneal fractures has gained acceptance because the procedure aims to restore the normal anatomic alignment of the joint surfaces in an effort to avoid the sequelae of post-traumatic degenerative arthritis of the subtalar joint. Both surgical and nonsurgical care of calcaneal fractures continues to be plagued with long-term symptomatic degenerative changes in the subtalar joint.

Arthroscopic subtalar arthrodesis was developed as a surgical procedure in 1992 and was first reported on in a preliminary review at the 1994 annual meeting of the Arthroscopy Association of North America. The procedure was designed to improve traditional methods by using a minimally invasive technique. The decision to adopt this surgical technique grew out of the success experienced with arthroscopic ankle arthrodesis.[15] Subtalar arthroscopy has been described by several authors, but few reports of arthroscopic subtalar fusion have been published.[28] Work by Solis (VH Solis, MD, personal communication, 1996) has paralleled some of the author's earlier work on arthroscopic subtalar arthrodesis.

The development of an arthroscopic technique for subtalar arthrodesis was intended to lower morbidity using similar techniques and principles as arthroscopic ankle fusion. It was hypothesized that perioperative morbidity could be reduced, blood supply preserved, and proprioceptive and neurosensory input enhanced. A prospective study was initiated to document the effectiveness of the procedure and to determine the time until complete fusion, the incidence of delayed unions and nonunions, and the prevalence of complications.[15]

Indications and Workup

Arthroscopic subtalar arthrodesis is indicated for patients with intractable subtalar pain secondary to rheumatoid arthritis, osteoarthritis, and post-traumatic arthritis. Other indications include neuropathic conditions, gross instability, paralytic conditions, and posterior tibial tendon rupture. Most of the earlier literature on subtalar surgery addressed the stabilization of paralytic deformities secondary to poliomyelitis. Currently, most patients requiring this procedure have post-traumatic and arthritic disorders. A small number of patients have posterior tibial tendon dysfunction or a talocalcaneal coalition.

Patients who have not been successfully treated with nonsurgical management should be considered for arthroscopic subtalar fusion. Nonsurgical treatment includes orthotics, nonsteroidal anti-inflammatory drugs, activity modification, and cortisone injections into the subtalar joint. Patients should be advised of the need for an open procedure if arthroscopic subtalar fusion is found to be technically infeasible.

The patient usually has a history of lateral hindfoot pain that can be easily confused with ankle pathology. An increase in symptoms with weight bearing or from ambulating on uneven terrain is often reported. A patient with a previous calcaneal fracture should immediately alert the physician to the possibility of subtalar pathology. Clinical findings consist of pain over the sinus tarsi and the posterolateral subtalar joint.

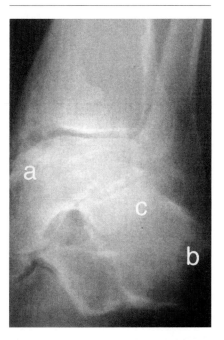

Figure 8 Broden view of an arthritic posterior subtalar joint showing the talus (a), the calcaneus (b), and the subtalar joint (c). (Reproduced with permission from Tasto JP: Subtalar arthroscopy, in McGinty JB (ed): *Operative Arthroscopy*, ed 3. Philadelphia, PA, Lippincott Williams & Wilkins, 2003, pp 944-952.)

Patients also report a reproduction of the symptoms on inversion and eversion of the subtalar joint with the ankle locked in dorsiflexion.

A thorough patient history and physical examination confirmed by plain radiographs are often sufficient to confirm the diagnosis (Figure 8). In some instances, CT or MRI scans may be necessary; however, there is seldom need for a bone scan or arthrography.[29,30] Differential injections continue to be a valuable diagnostic tool to confirm and distinguish ankle pain from subtalar pain. Profound degenerative radiographic changes in the joint are not needed to confirm a diagnosis because only small alterations in the biomechanics of this joint can produce significant symptoms.

The contraindications to arthroscopic subtalar arthrodesis are previously failed subtalar fusions, gross malalignment requiring correction, the presence of infection, and significant bone loss. A patient with moderate malalignment may be a candidate for in situ stabilization. Although significant bone loss has not frequently been encountered, it has not presented a serious problem in a study of arthroscopic ankle arthrodesis.[15]

In a study by Tasto and associates,[15] most patients were treated in an ambulatory surgery center and discharged on the same day. A few patients in the study were treated at a Veterans Administration medical center. Patients were given a total of three doses of preoperative, intraoperative, and postoperative antibiotics because of the use of internal fixation. General anesthesia was used for most patients.

Technique

Patients in the study were placed in the lateral decubitus position lying on the unaffected side.[15] Two pillows were placed between the legs while the affected ankle and subtalar joint were allowed to hang over a blanket roll in a natural position of plantar flexion and inversion. After thoroughly preparing and draping the patient for surgery, anatomic landmarks and portal sites were identified and marked with a surgical pen. The tourniquet was then elevated. The surgical procedure usually was completed within one tourniquet time (1.75 hours).

Establishing the portal sites is one of the more challenging aspects of the procedure and has been previously described. It is critical to predetermine the angles of the subtalar joint because its unique geometry and limited access requires precise determination to prevent error. Fluoroscopy should be used to confirm portal location if necessary.

The anterolateral and the posterolateral portals are the two portals that are conventionally used. If necessary, an accessory portal may be established approximately 1 cm posterior to the anterolateral portal. This portal can be used for débridement or for outflow enhancement and may occasionally be used for visualization. Both the anterolateral and posterolateral portals are used in an alternating manner for viewing and for instrumentation. If significant arthrofibrosis makes entry and visualization difficult, the accessory anterolateral portal is quite useful.

A 2.7-mm, wide-angle, short and small joint arthroscope should be used for this procedure. It should be equipped with a choice of sheaths to accommodate limited or increased flow. The blunt trocar and sheath is introduced through the anterolateral portal; the posterolateral portal can be established at this time. In patients who were initially treated with this procedure, a small laminar spreader was used in the anterolateral portal to increase access. This technique is no longer routinely used, but may be useful if subtalar joint distraction is a problem. Arthroscopic resection of the interosseous ligament also may provide additional distraction.

It is important to confirm that the arthroscope is in the subtalar joint and that the ankle joint or the fibular talar recess have not been inadvertently entered. All débridement and decortication is done posterior to the interosseous ligament because only the posterior facet is fused. The middle and anterior facets are not seen under normal circumstances unless the interosseous ligament is absent. Most of the procedure is

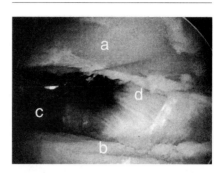

Figure 9 The posterior subtalar joint viewed from the posterolateral portal showing talus (a), calcaneus (b), sinus tarsi (c), and interosseous ligament (d). (Reproduced with permission from Tasto JP: Subtalar arthroscopy, in McGinty JB (ed): *Operative Arthroscopy*, ed 3. Philadelphia, PA, Lippincott Williams & Wilkins, 2003, pp 944-952.)

performed with the arthroscope in the anterolateral portal and the instruments in the posterolateral portal. The remaining débridement is accomplished by alternating these two portals.

At the beginning of the procedure, a primary synovectomy and débridement is necessary for visualization. The articular surface is débrided, making the joint more capacious and making the use of instrumentation easier. Complete removal of the articular surface down to subchondral bone is done next (Figure 9). The unique talocalcaneal geometry requires a variety of instruments, including multiangle curets and a complete set of burrs.

After the articular cartilage has been resected, approximately 1 to 2 mm of subchondral bone is removed to expose the highly vascular cancellous bone. Care must be taken not to alter the geometry and not to remove excessive bone because this would lead to poor coaptation of the joint surfaces. After the subchondral plate is removed, small "spot-weld" holes measuring approximately 2 mm in depth are fashioned on the

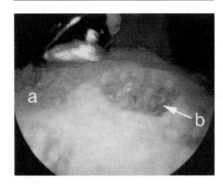

Figure 10 Superior surface of calcaneus following removal of articular surface, decortication, and "spot-welding" showing the calcaneus (a) and a "spot-weld" (b). (Reproduced with permission from Tasto JP: Subtalar arthroscopy, in McGinty JB (ed): *Operative Arthroscopy*, ed 3. Philadelphia, PA, Lippincott Williams & Wilkins, 2003, pp 944-952.)

surfaces of the calcaneus and talus to create vascular channels (Figure 10). Careful assessment of the posteromedial corner must be made because residual bone and cartilage can interfere with talocalcaneal coaptation. The curet often will safely break down this corner and also will provide the surgeon with tactile feedback. The neurovascular bundle located directly posteromedially must be protected throughout the procedure.

After viewing from both portals to ensure complete débridement and decortication, the tourniquet is released and careful assessment of the vascularity of the calcaneus and talus is made. The joint is then thoroughly irrigated to remove bone fragments and debris. Autogenous bone graft or bone substitute are not needed for this procedure.

The fusion is fixed with a large cannulated 7.3-mm screw. The guide pin is started at the dorsal anteromedial talus and angled posterior and inferior to the posterolateral calcaneus; however, it does not violate the calcaneal cortical surface.

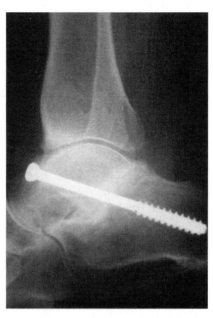

Figure 11 Lateral radiograph of a fused subtalar joint with a single cancellous screw across the posterior facet. (Reproduced with permission from Tasto JP: Subtalar arthroscopy, in McGinty JB (ed): *Operative Arthroscopy*, ed 3. Philadelphia, PA, Lippincott Williams & Wilkins, 2003, pp 944-952.)

Using fluoroscopy, the guide wire is placed with the ankle in maximum dorsiflexion to avoid screw head encroachment or impingement on the anterior lip of the tibia. After the guide wire is placed, the ankle can be relaxed, the screw inserted under fluoroscopic control, and the fusion site compressed. The screw will run along the natural axis of rotation of the subtalar joint using this technique. Starting the screw from the dorsal and medial aspect of the talus avoids painful screw head prominence over the calcaneus and avoids a second procedure for screw removal. To date, there have been no fractures or complications with this particular fixation technique[15] (Figure 11).

Sterile adhesive wound closure strips are used instead of sutures to allow adequate drainage. A bulky

dressing and a short leg bivalved cast are applied. The patient is discharged from the surgical center and may return home after appropriate circulatory checks are completed in the recovery room. The first clinical evaluation takes place in the physician's office within 48 hours. In approximately 1 week, the cast is removed and the patient is fit immediately with an ankle-foot orthosis if swelling is minimal. Full weight bearing is allowed as tolerated at any time after surgery. In general, patients can tolerate full weight bearing without crutch support within 7 to 14 days after surgery. Although patients should wear the ankle-foot orthosis almost 24 hours a day, they are able to bathe and take the ankle and foot through a range of motion movement without the brace. The brace is removed when full union has been achieved. For follow-up assessment, the standard three views of the ankle plus a Broden view are the radiographs of choice.

Results and Complications

Since September 1992, 25 patients have been treated by the author using arthroscopic subtalar fusion with sufficient follow-up time to determine the effectiveness of this procedure. Fusion rate, time until complete union, surgical technique, and the complication rate were analyzed. One standard surgical procedure was used and the method of internal fixation was consistent throughout this study. The posterior subtalar joint was the only joint fused during this procedure. Three of the 25 patients had a combined arthroscopic ankle and subtalar fusion. In this study, 8 patients had osteoarthritis, 10 had posttraumatic arthritis, 4 had posterior tibial tendon dysfunction, 2 had rheumatoid arthritis, and 1 patient had talocalcaneal coalition. Every patient had a radiographic evaluation at 2-week intervals to determine the rate and quality of fusion. Both clinical and radiographic evidence was required to categorize an arthrodesis as completely fused. The parameters required for a successful arthrodesis are evidence of bone consolidation across the subtalar joint, no motion at the screw, the absence of pain with weight bearing, and pain-free forced inversion and eversion. The mean follow-up time was 22 months (range, 6 to 92 months). The subtalar joint of all 25 patients had united clinically and radiographically; the average time until complete fusion was 8.9 weeks (range, 6 to 16 weeks).[15]

Arthroscopic subtalar fusion has many advantages compared with open procedures. It is a minimally invasive technique that theoretically preserves the blood supply of the calcaneus and talus, which is especially important because many of these patients have had previous open surgery. Conventional open procedures by definition interrupt the blood supply and compromise vascular ingrowth and eventual fusion. Avoidance of incisions coupled with early range of motion and weight bearing helps to avoid stress deprivation and enhance proprioception, therefore reducing the devastating effects of complex regional pain syndrome.

There have been no additional surgeries with the exception of screw removals. Two patients had some residual anterolateral pain with some radiographic and clinical evidence of minor degenerative joint disease in the ankle. These findings were noted on preoperative films. One patient had complete pain relief after a diagnostic and therapeutic steroid and lidocaine injection into the ankle joint. One patient eventually underwent arthro-scopic ankle arthrodesis because of preexisting osteoarthritis of the ankle. Valgus tilting of the ankle joint following subtalar arthrodesis has been reported, but it is unclear if this is secondary to the fusion or merely a natural progression of the disease (TC Fitzgibbons, MD, Dublin, Ireland, personal communication, 1995).

Two patients are not included in this study because the procedure could not be completed arthroscopically because of significant malformation of the calcaneus and arthrofibrosis of the subtalar joint. These patients underwent a modified mini-open posterior subtalar arthrodesis. Identical screw fixation and postoperative protocol was used in these two patients. Skin complications about the hindfoot can be catastrophic and are obviously minimized using the arthroscopic technique. No patients in this study had superficial or deep infections. All arthroscopic procedures have been associated with reduced rates of infection. It is believed that subtalar arthroscopic arthrodesis would also produce a low incidence of infection. More study will be needed to validate this hypothesis.

Most studies of open procedures show a longer time until union with some prevalence of nonunion. Although this study was relatively small (25 patients), preliminary observations suggest a more rapid union and an increased rate of union. Because there is, however, a paucity of literature on isolated open subtalar arthrodesis with adequate follow-up statistics over the past 25 years, this comparison is not available.

Summary

An advantage of arthroscopic subtalar fusion with immobilization with an ankle-foot orthosis is early weight bearing, which allows patients an early return to work. Outpatient surgery also is a cost-effective benefit. Patient satisfaction as well as comfort is greatly enhanced, with oral pain medication usually required. All patients treated by the author have tolerated their postoperative regimen and same-day discharge.

Arthroscopic subtalar arthrodesis is a technically demanding procedure that requires advanced arthroscopic skills to perform. Joint access is tight and restricted and requires the use of small instrumentation. Because deformities cannot be corrected at this stage, this procedure must be considered a fusion in situ. Because there are relatively few patients who qualify for this procedure, the learning curve for improving surgical skills is steep. Cadaveric surgical skills workshops are the most efficacious method of mastering this technique.

The results of arthroscopic subtalar arthrodesis appear to be excellent in terms of patient satisfaction, fusion rate, time until union, and postoperative morbidity. The recognition and enhancement of this technique and the development of more advanced technology will allow arthroscopic subtalar arthrodesis to continue to mature and improve in the future.

References

1. Parisien JS, Vangsness T: Arthroscopy of the subtalar joint: An experimental approach. *Arthroscopy* 1985;1:53-57.

2. Cahill DR: The anatomy and function of the contents of the human tarsal sinus and canal. *Anat Rec* 1965;153:1-17.

3. Frey C, Gasser S, Feder K: Arthroscopy of the subtalar joint. *Foot Ankle Int* 1994;15:424-428.

4. Frey C, Feder S, DiGiovanni D: Arthroscopic evaluation of the subtalar joint: Does sinus tarsi syndrome exist? *Foot Ankle Int* 1999;20:185-191.

5. Kjaersgaard-Andersen P, Wethelund JO, Helmig P, Soballe K: The stabilizing effect of the ligamentous structures in the sinus and canalis tarsi on movements of the hindfoot: An experimental study. *Am J Sports Med* 1988;16:512-516.

6. Lehman WB, Lehman M: The surgical anatomy of the interosseous ligament of the subtalar joint as it relates to clubfoot surgery. *Bull Hosp Jt Dis Orthop Inst* 1981;41:19-27.

7. Parisien JS (ed): *Arthroscopy Surgery*. New York, NY, McGraw-Hill, 1988.

8. Perry J: Anatomy and biomechanics of the hindfoot. *Clin Orthop* 1983;177:9-15.

9. Resnick D: Radiology of the talocalcaneal articulations: Anatomic considerations and arthrography. *Radiology* 1974;111:581-586.

10. Inman VT, Mann RA, Duvries HL (eds): *Surgery of the Foot*. St. Louis, MO, CV Mosby, 1973, pp 19-27.

11. Root M, Orien WP, Weld J: Normal and abnormal functions of the foot. *Clin Biomech (Bristol, Avon)* 1977;2:79.

12. Hicks JH: The mechanics of the foot, Vol. 1: The joints. *J Anat* 1953;87:345-357.

13. Williams MM, Ferkel RD: Subtalar arthroscopy: Indications, technique, and results. *Arthroscopy* 1998;14:373-381.

14. Ferkel RA (ed): Subtalar arthroscopy, in *Arthroscopy Surgery: The Foot and Ankle*. Philadelphia, PA, Lippincott-Raven, 1996, pp 231-254.

15. Tasto JP, Frey C, Laimans P, Morgan CD, Mason RJ, Stone JW: Arthroscopic ankle arthrodesis. *Instr Course Lect* 2000;49:259-280.

16. Thomas FB: Arthrodesis of the subtalar joint. *J Bone Joint Surg Br* 1967;49:93-97.

17. Dick IL: Primary fusion of the posterior subtalar joint and the treatment of fractures of the calcaneus. *J Bone Joint Surg Br* 1953;35:375.

18. Gallie WE: Subastragalar arthrodesis and fractures of the os calcis. *J Bone Joint Surg* 1943;25:731.

19. Grice DS: An extra-articular arthrodesis of the subastragalar joint for correction of paralytic flat feet in children. *J Bone Joint Surg Am* 1952;35:927.

20. Grice DS: Further experience with extra-articular arthrodesis of the subtalar joint. *J Bone Joint Surg Am* 1955;37:246.

21. Hall MC, Pennal GF: Primary subtalar arthrodesis in the treatment of severe fractures of the calcaneus. *J Bone Joint Surg Br* 1960;42-B:336-343.

22. Geckler EO: Comminuted fractures of the os calcis. *Arch Surg* 1943;61:469.

23. Harris RI: Fractures of the os calcis. *Ann Surg* 1946;124:1082.

24. Wilson PD: Treatment of fractures of the os calcis by arthrodesis of the subtalar joint. *JAMA* 1927;89:1676.

25. Gross RH: A clinical study of Batchelor subtalar arthrodesis. *J Bone Joint Surg Am* 1976;58:343-349.

26. Mallon WJ, Nunley JA: The Grice procedure, extra-articular subtalar arthrodesis. *Orthop Clin North Am* 1989;20:649-654.

27. Moreland JR, Westin GW: Further experience with Grice subtalar arthrodesis. *Clin Orthop* 1986;207:113-121.

28. Ferkel RA (ed): *Arthroscopic Surgery: The Foot and Ankle*. Philadelphia, PA, Lippencott-Raven, 1996.

29. Seltzer SE, Weissman BN, Braunstein EM, Adams DF, Thomas WH: Computed tomography of the hindfoot with rheumatoid arthritis. *Arthritis Rheum* 1985;28:1234-1242.

30. Goossens M, De Stoop N, Claessens H, Van der Straeten C: Posterior subtalar joint arthrography: A useful tool in the diagnosis of hindfoot disorders. *Clin Orthop* 1989;249:248-255.

Hindfoot Endoscopy for Posterior Ankle Pain

C. Niek van Dijk, MD, PhD

Abstract

Hindfoot pain can be caused by a variety of pathologies, most of which can be diagnosed and treated with endoscopy. The main indications are posterior tibial tenosynovectomy, diagnosis of a longitudinal peroneus brevis rupture, peroneal tendon adhesiolysis, flexor hallucis longus release, os trigonum removal, endoscopic treatment of retrocalcaneal bursitis, endoscopic treatment of Achilles (peri)tendinopathy, and treatment of ankle joint or subtalar joint pathology. The advantages of endoscopic hindfoot surgery over open surgery are less morbidity, reduction of postoperative pain, outpatient treatment, and functional postoperative treatment. Optimal portal placement for each indication has been identified in a cadaver study. The approach for the flexor hallucis longus and os trigonum is particularly challenging because of the adjacent neurovascular bundle. A two-portal hindfoot approach with the patient in the prone position offers excellent access to the flexor hallucis longus. The posterior ankle compartment, os trigonum, and subtalar joint can be visualized and treated through this approach. In 240 consecutive procedures, no major complications were reported. The two-portal hindfoot endoscopy approach is a safe, reliable, and exciting method to diagnose and treat a variety of posterior ankle problems. Endoscopic calcaneoplasty for retrocalcaneal bursitis offers a good alternative to open resection. Experienced arthroscopic surgeons will find this technique rewarding.

Arthroscopy of the ankle joint has become an important diagnostic and therapeutic procedure for chronic and posttraumatic ankle pain. Burman,[1] in 1931, regarded the ankle joint as unsuitable for arthroscopy because of its anatomy. Tagaki,[2] in 1939, described systematic arthroscopic assessment of the ankle joint. Watanabe[3] reported a series of 28 ankle arthroscopies in 1972 followed by Chen and Wertheimer.[4] In the 1980s several publications followed.[5-11] Some authors recommend routine placement of a postero-lateral portal in ankle arthroscopy.[7,8] Because of the potential for serious complications, most authors believe that the posterolateral portal is contraindicated in all but the most extreme situations.[7,8,12-14]

History of the Technique

Arthroscopy of the subtalar joint was first described by Parisien and Vangsness in 1985.[11] Endoscopic access to the posterior tibial tendons, including treatment of pathology, was first described in 1997,[15] followed by tendon sheath endoscopy (tendoscopy) of the peroneal tendons in 1998,[16] and endoscopic release of the flexor hallucis longus tendon in 2000.[17]

Hindfoot endoscopy gives excellent access to the posterior ankle compartment, the subtalar joint, and extra-articular structures such as the os trigonum, the deep portion of the deltoid ligament, the posterior syndesmotic ligaments, the tendons of the tarsal tunnel, the retrocalcaneal bursa, and the Achilles tendon.[17]

Nagai[18] was the first author to use the arthroscope to access the retrocalcaneal recess. He reported on a case in which he identified the Achilles tendon and an avulsed portion of its insertion on the calcaneus. A description of the entry portals and the surgical approach to the retrocalcaneal bursa appeared in 1997 (RO Lundeen, MD, ASFAS Annual Meeting, Palm Springs, FL, unpublished data). The results of a first cohort of 22 consecutive patients with a minimal follow-up of 2 years were published in 2000.[17]

Indications

A variety of soft-tissue pathologies can be present around the ankle joint. In the absence of intra-articular damage, posteromedial ankle symptoms are caused most often by disorders of the posterior tibial tendon.[19] If conservative treatment fails, posterior tibial tendon disorders can be treated with open surgery.[20] Posteromedial overuse and posttraumatic injuries in ballet dancers and soccer players most often are caused by tenosynovitis of the flexor hallucis longus tendon and/or a posterior impingement syndrome. Posterolateral ankle symptoms are caused most often by disorders of the peroneal tendons such as tenosynovitis, partial rupture, and tendon subluxation.

Endoscopic surgery for the treatment of hindfoot pathology offers the advantages of less morbidity, reduction in postoperative pain, and outpatient treatment.[21]

Articular Pathology
Posterior Compartment Ankle Joint The main indications are the débridement and drilling of posteriorly located osteochondral defects of the ankle joint; removal of loose bodies, ossicles, posttraumatic calcifications, or avulsion fragments; resection of posterior tibial rim osteophytes; treatment of chondromatosis; and treatment of chronic synovitis.

Posterior Compartment Subtalar Joint The main indications are osteophyte removal, removal of loose bodies, subtalar arthrodesis, and treatment of an intraosseous talar ganglion by drilling, curetting, and bone grafting.

Periarticular Pathology
Posterior Ankle Impingement Posterior ankle impingement is a source of pain; the patient experiences posterior ankle pain aggravated by forced plantar flexion. Posterior ankle impingement can be caused by overuse or trauma. The distinction between overuse and trauma is important because posterior impinge-

ment caused by overuse has a better prognosis.[22] A posterior ankle impingement syndrome resulting from overuse is found most often in ballet dancers and runners.[23-25] Running that involves forced plantar flexion (such as running downhill) can place repetitive stress on the posterior aspect of the ankle joint;[26] in ballet dancers, the forceful plantar flexion during the en-pointe or the demi-pointe position produces compression. The ankle joint mobility and range of motion gradually increase through exercise. In the presence of a prominent posterior talar process or an os trigonum, this increase can lead to compression of these structures.

In 1995 van Dijk and associates[23] reported the results of ankle and subtalar joint examination in a group of 19 retired dancers. The mean length of a ballet dancer's professional career was 37 years. All of the dancers had been dancing en-pointe, and none of them had encountered a posterior ankle impingement syndrome. A hypertrophic posterior talar process or an os trigonum was present in 18 of the 38 ankle joints. The presence of an os trigonum itself does not seem to be relevant.[23] This anatomic anomaly must be combined with a traumatic event such as a supination trauma, a hyperplantar flexion trauma, dancing on hard surfaces, or pushing beyond anatomic limits for a posterior ankle impingement syndrome to occur.

The forced hyperplantar flexion test is most important for the diagnosis of posterior ankle impingement. In this test the examiner applies repetitive, quick, passive forced hyperplantar flexion movements to the ankle. The test can be repeated in slight outward or slight inward rotation of the foot relative to the

tibia. The examiner should apply this rotation movement on the point of maximal plantar flexion, thereby "grinding" the posterior talar process/os trigonum between the posterior tibial rim and the calcaneus.

A negative test rules out a posterior impingement syndrome. A positive test is followed by a diagnostic infiltration on the os trigonum or posterior talar process. If the pain on forced hyperplantar flexion disappears, the diagnosis of posterior ankle impingement is confirmed.

Deep Portion of the Deltoid Ligament Eversion or hyperdorsiflexion trauma can result in avulsion fragments of the insertion of the deep portion of the deltoid ligament from the talus. Posttraumatic calcifications, or ossicles in the deep portion of the deltoid ligament, can also occur as a result of an eversion trauma.

Flexor Hallucis Longus Flexor hallucis longus tendinitis often is present in patients with a posterior ankle impingement syndrome. The pain is located posteromedially. In ballet dancers, the pain is experienced during plié and especially grand plié positions. The flexor hallucis longus tendon can be palpated in its gliding channel behind the medial malleolus by asking the patient to repetitively flex the big toe with the ankle in 10° to 20° of plantar flexion. The tendon glides up and down under the palpating finger of the examiner. In the presence of stenosing tendinitis or chronic inflammation, crepitus may be palpated, and pain can be provoked. Sometimes a nodule in the flexor hallucis longus tendon can be felt to move up and down under the palpating finger.

Peroneal Tendons Tenosynovitis and dislocation, rupture, and snapping of the peroneal tendons account for most of the symptoms.[27,28] These problems must be differentiated from (fatigue) fractures of the fibula, lesions of the lateral ligament complex, and posterolateral impingement (os trigonum syndrome).

Peroneal tendon disorders often are secondary to chronic lateral ankle instability. Because the peroneal muscles act as lateral ankle stabilizers in chronic lateral instability, increased strain is placed on the peroneal tendons, resulting in hypertrophic tendinopathy, tenosynovitis, and, ultimately, (partial) tendon tears.[29-31] Postsurgery and postfracture adhesions and irregularities in the posterior aspect of the fibula (sliding channel) can be responsible for symptoms in this region.[16]

Posterior Tibial Tendon The posterior tibial tendon plays an important role in normal hindfoot function.[32] Several investigators have described development of posterior tibial tendon dysfunction as the disease progresses from peritendinitis to elongation, degeneration, and rupture.[30-34] Tenosynovitis is often seen in association with flat feet, psoriatic arthritis, and rheumatic arthritis. In the early stage of posterior tibial tendon dysfunction, tenosynovitis is the main symptom. Tenosynovectomy can be performed if conservative treatment fails.[35] Postsurgery and postfracture adhesions and irregularity of the posterior aspect of the tibia (sliding channel) can be responsible for symptoms in this region.

Achilles Tendon and Retrocalcaneal Bursa Chronic retrocalcaneal bursitis is accompanied by deep pain and swelling of the posterior soft tissue just in front of the Achilles tendon. The prominent bursa can be palpated medial and lateral from the tendon at its insertion. The lateral radiograph demonstrates the characteristic prominent superior calcaneal deformity. Surgical treatment involves removal of the bursa and resection of the lateral and medial posterosuperior aspect of the calcaneus. Retrocalcaneal bursitis often is accompanied by midportion insertional tendinosis. The midportion of the tendon is often partially ruptured at its insertion. In the presence of insertional tendinosis, pain is worse after exercise and occurs at the bone-tendon junction. The tenderness is specifically located directly posterior in the midline at the bone-tendon junction.

Neurovascular Bundle Entrapment of the posterior tibial nerve within the tarsal tunnel is commonly known as a tarsal tunnel syndrome.[36] Clinical examination is sufficient to differentiate tarsal tunnel syndrome from an isolated posterior tibial tendon disorder (numbness on neurologic examination).

Surgical Techniques
Posterior Ankle Arthroscopy
The procedure is performed as outpatient surgery with the patient under general or epidural anesthesia. The patient is placed in a prone position. A tourniquet is applied around the upper leg, and a small support is placed under the lower leg, making it possible to move the ankle freely. A soft-tissue distraction device can be used when indicated when the ankle joint has to be entered for the diagnosis and treatment of an osteochondral defect, the removal of loose bodies from the joint synovectomy, and other intra-articular pathology.[37] For irrigation a single bag of normal saline with gravity flow can be used, although glycerine or lactated Ringer's solution can also be used. A 4.0-mm arthroscope with a 30° angle is routinely used for posterior ankle arthroscopy. Apart from the standard excisional and motorized instruments for treatment of osteophytes and ossicles, a 4-mm chisel and a periosteal elevator can be useful.

The landmarks on the ankle are the lateral malleolus, medial and lateral border of the Achilles tendon, and the sole of the foot. The ankle is kept in a neutral position. A line is drawn from the tip of the lateral malleolus to the Achilles tendon, parallel to the sole of the foot.

The posterolateral portal is made just above this line and just in front of the Achilles tendon. After making a vertical stab incision, the subcutaneous layer is split by a mosquito clamp that is directed anteriorly, in the direction of the interdigital webspace between the first and second toes. When the tip of the clamp touches the bone, it is exchanged for a 4.5-mm arthroscope shaft with the blunt trocar pointing in the same direction. The level of the ankle joint and subtalar joint can be distinguished by palpating the bone in the sagittal plane because the prominent posterior talar process or os trigonum can be felt as a posterior prominence between the two joints. The trocar is situated extra-articularly at the level of the ankle joint. The trocar is exchanged for the 4-mm arthroscope; the direction of view is 30° to the lateral side.

The posteromedial portal is made at the same level, just above the line from the tip of the lateral malleolus, and just in front of the medial aspect of the Achilles tendon. After making a vertical stab incision, a mosquito clamp is introduced and directed toward the arthroscope shaft at a 90° angle. When the mosquito clamp touches the shaft of the arthroscope, the shaft is used as a guide for the clamp to move anteriorly in the direction of the ankle joint, touching the arthroscope shaft until it reaches the bone. The arthroscope is now withdrawn slightly and slides over the mosquito clamp until the tip of the mosquito clamp comes to view. The clamp is used to spread the extra-articular soft tissue in front of the tip of the lens. In situations where scar tissue or adhesions are present, the mosquito clamp is exchanged for a 5-mm full radius shaver.[17] The tip of the shaver is directed in a lateral and slightly plantar direction toward the posterolateral aspect of the subtalar joint. When the tip of the shaver has reached this position, shaving can begin. The joint capsule and adipose tissue can be removed. After removal of its very thin joint capsule, the posterior compartment of the subtalar joint can be inspected. At the level of the ankle joint, the posterior tibiofibular and talofibular ligaments are recognized. The posterior talar process can be freed of scar tissue, and the flexor hallucis longus tendon, which is an important landmark, is identified. The shaver should never be used medial from the flexor hallucis longus tendon. After removal of the thin joint capsule of the ankle joint, the ankle joint is entered and inspected.

On the medial side, both the tip of the medial malleolus and the deep portion of the deltoid ligament are visualized. By opening the joint capsule from inside out at the level of the medial malleolus, the tendon sheath of the posterior tibial tendon can be opened.

Applying manual distraction to the os calcis will cause the posterior compartment of the ankle to open, and the shaver can be introduced into the posterior ankle compartment. A soft-tissue distractor can be applied.[37] A total synovectomy and/or capsulectomy can be performed. Almost the entire surface of the talar dome and the complete tibial plafond can be inspected. An osteochondral defect or subchondral cystic lesion can be identified, débrided, and drilled. The posterior syndesmotic ligaments are inspected and, if hypertrophic, partially resected.

Removal of a symptomatic os trigonum, an ununited fracture of the posterior talar process, or a symptomatic large posterior talar prominence requires partial detachment of the posterior talofibular ligament and release of the flexor retinaculum, both of which attach to the posterior talar prominence. Release of the flexor hallucis longus tendon involves detachment of the flexor retinaculum from the posterior talar process by means of a punch.

A tight, thick crural fascia, if present, can hinder the free movement of instruments. It is helpful to enlarge the hole in the fascia by means of a punch or shaver. Bleeding is controlled by electrocautery at the end of the procedure.

After removal of the instruments, the stab incisions are closed with No. 3.0 nylon to prevent sinus formation. A sterile compression dressing is applied.

Postoperative treatment consists of weight bearing, as tolerated, on crutches for 2 or 3 days. The dressing can be removed after 3 days. As soon as possible after the surgery, the patient is advised to start range-of-motion exercises as tolerated.

Posterior Tibial Tendoscopy

The procedure usually is performed as outpatient surgery with the patient under either general or epidural anesthesia. The patient is placed in the lateral decubitus position, with the nonsurgical side up. A tourniquet is applied to the upper leg, and a small support is placed under the lower leg, making it possible to move the ankle freely. The important landmarks are the medial malleolus and the posterior tibial tendon.

Access to the posterior tibial tendon can be obtained throughout the length of the tendon. The two main portals for posterior tibial tendoscopy are located directly over the involved tendon 2 cm distal and 2 cm proximal to the posterior edge of the medial malleolus. In the distal portal an incision is made through the skin. After blunt dissection with a mosquito clamp, the trocar is introduced and then is exchanged for a 2.7-mm arthroscope with an inclination angle of 30°. After introduction of a spinal needle under direct vision, an incision is made through the skin into the tendon sheath to create a proximal portal. Instruments such as a probe, disposable cutting knife, scissors, or shaver can be introduced through this portal. A complete overview of the posterior tibial tendon from its insertion (navicular bone) to some 6 cm above the level of the tip of the medial malleolus can be obtained. The complete tendon sheath can be inspected by rotating the arthroscope over the tendon.

Results from a cadaver study[15] found that a vincula was present in all specimens. During tendoscopy a pathologically thickened vincula can be excised, the tendon sheath can be released, and adhesions can be removed. When a total synovectomy is to be performed, a third portal is created more distal from the previously described portals. To prevent sinus formation, the portals are sutured. Postoperative treatment consists of a pressure bandage and partial weight bearing for 2 to 3 days. Active range of motion is advised in the immediate postoperative period.[15,16]

Peroneal Tendoscopy

The procedure generally is performed in the same way as posterior tibial tendoscopy; however, the important landmarks are the lateral malleolus and the peroneal tendons. Access to the peroneal tendons can be obtained throughout their length. The two main portals for the peroneal tendoscopy are located directly over the involved tendons 2 cm distal and 2 cm proximal to the tip of the lateral malleolus. In the distal portal, an incision is made through the skin. After blunt dissection with a mosquito clamp, the blunt trocar is introduced into the tendon sheath, and a 2.7-mm arthroscope with an inclination angle of 30° is introduced. The proximal portal is made under direct vision after introduction of a spinal needle. Instruments such as a probe, disposable cutting knife, scissors, or shaver system can be introduced. A complete overview of both peroneal tendons can be obtained through the distal portal. The inspection starts some 6 cm proximal from the posterior tip of the lateral malleolus, where a thin membrane splits the tendon compartment into two separate tendon chambers. Both tendons lie in one compartment more distally. The complete compartment can be inspected by rotating the endoscope over and between both tendons.

A vincula attaching both tendons to each other and to the tendon sheath is consistently present in both peroneal tendons over their full length.[16] A pathologically thickened vincula or tendon sheath can be released by tendoscopy. Adhesions can be removed, and a symptomatic prominent tubercle can be resected. A rupture of the peroneal longus or brevis tendon can be su-

tured. When a total synovectomy of the tendon sheath is to be performed, it is advisable to create a third portal either distal or proximal to the usual two portals. To treat recurrent peroneal tendon dislocation, it is possible to deepen the groove of the peroneal tendons with a burr.[35] To prevent sinus formation, the portals are closed. Postoperative treatment consists of a pressure bandage and partial weight bearing for 2 to 3 days. Active range of motion is advised immediately after surgery.

Retrocalcaneal Endoscopy

The procedure is performed with the patient in the prone position.[38] A tourniquet is applied on the upper leg, and a small support is placed under the lower leg.

Two portals are created, one on the medial and one on the lateral side of the Achilles tendon at the level of the superior border of the os calcis. After a vertical stab incision is made at the posterolateral side, a blunt trocar is introduced for blunt dissection and opening of the retrocalcaneal space. The trocar is exchanged for a 4-mm arthroscope with a 30° angle. After localization of the posteromedial portal with a needle, a stab incision is made under direct vision. A probe and subsequently a 5-mm full-radius resector are introduced through the posteromedial portal. After the removal of the bursa and inflamed soft tissue, the calcaneal prominence is removed using the full-radius resector and small acromionizer. Portals should be changed to remove the posterolateral side of the superior calcaneal rim and for final inspection.

Achilles Tendon Tendoscopy

In patients with peritendinitis of the Achilles tendon, the portals are created 2 cm proximal and 2 cm distal

of the lesion. The distal portal is made first; an incision is made through the skin only, the crural fascia is penetrated by the arthroscope shaft with a blunt trocar, and a 2.7-mm arthroscope with an inclination angle of 30° is introduced. After introduction of a spinal needle under direct vision, an incision is made at the location of the proximal portal. The pathologic paratenon is removed with a shaver. The Achilles tendon can be inspected by rotating the scope over the tendon. The plantaris tendon can be recognized and released or resected when indicated.

To prevent sinus formation, the portals are closed. Postoperative treatment consists of a pressure bandage and partial weight bearing for 2 to 3 days. Active range of motion is advised immediately postoperatively.

Technical Alternatives and Pitfalls

Peroneal Tendons

A 2.7-mm arthroscope can be used for routine tendoscopy of the peroneal tendons. It is possible, however, to use a 4-mm arthroscope. The larger diameter scope facilitates better flow of the irrigation fluid that is introduced through the arthroscope shaft into the tendon sheath, which is an advantage when a lot of debris is to be expected, such as during osseous groove deepening procedures for recurrent peroneal tendon dislocation.

Tendoscopy for the Posterior Tibial Tendon

It is important to identify the location of the posterior tibial tendon before creating the portals. The patient should be asked to actively invert the foot, and the physician can identify the tendon and mark the location of the portals on the skin. The tendon sheath between the posterior tibial tendon and the flexor digitorum longus is quite thin. The flexor digitorium can be identified by passively moving the patient's toes.

Achilles Tendon Tendoscopy and Endoscopic Calcaneoplasty

Endoscopic calcaneoplasty may be performed using a 2.7-mm arthroscope instead of a 4-mm arthroscope; however, the 4.0-mm arthroscope is preferable because it provides better flow. By placing the arthroscope between the Achilles tendon and the calcaneus, the arthroscope shaft lifts the tendon off the bone, creating a working space. Fluoroscopy can be useful to check whether enough bone has been removed. It is important to check all the way down to the insertion of the Achilles tendon.

Hindfoot Endoscopy and Posterior Ankle Arthroscopy

The crural fascia in the hindfoot can be quite thick. This local thickening, which is called the ligament of Rouvière, can be attached to the posterior talar process. An arthroscopic punch or scissors can be used to enlarge the entry through the crural fascia. The position of the arthroscope is important. The direction of view should always be lateral. If the arthroscope points into the direction of the webspace of the first and second toes, it is in a safe area. The arthroscope should be positioned lateral to the flexor hallucis longus tendon, using the tendon as a landmark. The arthroscope should be positioned medial from the flexor hallucis longus tendon only when a release of the neurovascular bundle is required (posttraumatic tarsal tunnel syndrome). When removing a hypertrophic posterior talar process by chisel, care should be taken not to place the chisel too far anterior. The procedure should start at the posterosuperior edge of the posterior talar process, and the inferoposterior part of the process chiseled away. The remnant of the process can be removed with a shaver (bone cutter). If the chisel is placed too far anterior, the subtalar joint can be entered.

The advantage of a two-portal procedure with the patient in the prone position is the working space available between the Achilles tendon and the back of the ankle and subtalar joint. The position is ergonomic for the orthopaedic surgeon. Soft-tissue distraction can easily be applied.[37] An alternative is to use two posterolateral portals with the patient in the lateral decubitus position.[39]

Subtalar Arthroscopy

An alternative access to the subtalar joint has been described by several authors.[11,12,14,40] The patient is in the lateral decubitus position, and a combination of anterolateral and posterolateral portals is used. Other authors prefer a supine position.[41]

Rehabilitation

The postoperative treatment of most arthroscopic procedures is functional. Most patients are advised to begin active range of motion immediately after surgery, as tolerated, and protected weight bearing for the first 3 days. One week postoperatively the patient is reevaluated in the outpatient department. If necessary, physiotherapy can be prescribed for range of motion, strengthening, and stability. In a patient in whom a peroneal tendon rupture has been treated with suture repair, a plaster can be applied for 4 weeks, 1 week with non–weight-bearing plaster and 3 weeks of full weight bearing plaster.

Patients

Between 1994 and 2002, 240 endoscopic soft-tissue procedures were performed in 229 consecutive patients at the Academic Medical Center in Amsterdam. The main indication was a posterior ankle impingement syndrome. In 52 patients, a bony impediment (os trigonum or hypertrophic posterior talar process) was removed. In 28 of those patients, a posterior ankle impingement syndrome was combined with flexor hallucis longus tendinitis. Release of the flexor hallucis longus was performed in addition to removal of the bony impediment (Table 1). In eight patients the cause of the posterior ankle impingement syndrome was a soft-tissue impediment that was removed by shaver. A total of 44 patients had flexor hallucis longus tendinitis. The tendinitis was isolated in only seven patients; it was combined with a bony impingement syndrome in 28 patients, an avulsion fracture of the posteromedial tibial rim or an ossicle near the flexor hallucis longus tendon in four patients, and a posteromedial talar osteochondral defect in five patients.

The main indications for endoscopic treatment of Achilles tendon pathology were retrocalcaneal bursitis (39 patients) and peritendinitis (23 patients). The indication for treating the bursitis with endoscopic calcaneoplasty was failure of 6 months of conservative treatment consisting of an inlay, physiotherapy, and at least one injection of cortisone into the retrocalcaneal bursa (Table 2).

The indication for endoscopic release of chronic peritendinitis was failure of at least 1 year of conserva-

Table 1
Endoscopy for Periarticular Hindfoot Pathology: Indications and Procedures*

Number of Patients	Diagnosis	Treatment
8	Soft-tissue impingement	Resection soft-tissue impediment
24	Bony impingement	Resection OT
28	BI+FHL tendinitis	Resection OT + release FHL
7	FHL tendinitis	Release FHL
4	FHL tendinitis + ossicle	Release FHL + ossicle removal
5	FHL tendinitis + OD	Release FHL + OD drilling
2	Tarsal tunnel syndrome	Release tarsal tunnel

* BI = bony impingement, OT = os trigonum, FHL = flexor hallucis longus,
OD = osteochondral defect

Table 2
Endoscopic Treatment of Achilles Tendon Pathology: Indications and Procedures

Number of Patients	Diagnosis	Treatment
39	Retrocalcaneal bursitis	Endoscopic calcaneoplasty
23	Peritendinitis (+ tendinosis)	Resection peritendineum

Table 3
Tendoscopy of the Posterior Tibial Tendon: Indications and Procedures

Number of Patients	Diagnosis	Treatment
8	Tenosynovitis in rheumatoid arthritis	Tenosynovectomy
1	Medial malleolar fracture	Screw removal
1	Exostosis sliding channel	Exostosis removal
21	Tenosynovitis of unknown cause	Various*

* In this diagnostic group, 4 patients had a pathologic thickened vincula that was resected,
6 patients had a length rupture that was sutured using a mini open approach, 4 patients
had degenerative tendon changes that were débrided, 3 patients had adhesions that were
removed, and 3 patients had synovitis that required synovectomy.

tive treatment in a patient with localized symptoms and a structurally intact tendon. The diagnosis of peritendinitis was confirmed on MRI in all patients. Degenerative changes in the Achilles tendon did not exceed more than 30% of its diameter. Conservative treatment consisted of modification of activity level and shoe wear, stretching, ice application, and eccentric calf muscle training.[42]

Tendoscopy of the posterior tibial tendon was performed in 31 patients (Table 3). For the peroneal tendons, the main indication was detection of a longitudinal rupture in the pero-

neus brevis tendon. All patients had a history of an acute lateral ankle ligament rupture. Five of the eight patients with tenosynovitis experienced pain and swelling over the posterior aspect of the lateral malleolus, and three patients presented with a snapping sensation at the level of the lateral malleolus. Seven patients had a chronic tenosynovitis after surgical treatment of a lateral malleolar fracture or a lateral ankle ligament reconstruction (Table 4).

Hindfoot endoscopy for treatment of posterior ankle joint pathology was performed in 36 patients (Table 5). In 13 patients an osteo-

chondral defect was débrided and drilled. The osteochondral defect was located at the posteromedial talar dome in seven patients, in the tibial plafond in four patients, and in the posterolateral talar dome in two patients. Posttraumatic calcifications in the posteromedial capsule or the posteromedial deltoid ligament were present in five patients. Two patients had a Cedell fracture (flexor retinaculum avulsion). All calcifications were removed endoscopically.

A total synovectomy was performed in nine patients. The posterior synovectomy was performed first. The knee was then flexed and an anterior synovectomy was performed using the standard anterolateral and anteromedial approaches. The indications for total synovectomy were chondromatosis (two patients), pigmented villonodular synovitis (three patients), rheumatoid arthritis (two patients), and crystal synovitis (two patients).

A two-portal hindfoot endoscopy for subtalar pathology was performed for degenerative articular changes (10 patients) or removal of a loose body (1 patient), and a large talar intraosseous ganglion was treated in three patients. These multicystic ganglion lesions originated from the subtalar joint. The chondral defect (origin of the ganglion) in the subtalar joint was identified using the two-portal hindfoot approach. The ganglion then was drilled through the posterior talar process, the drill hole was enlarged to 4.5 mm to make introduction of a curet possible and, after curetting and drilling, the cystic defect was filled with cancellous bone from the iliac crest.

Results

Three patients experienced a small area of diminished sensation over the posterior aspect of the hindfoot.

Table 4
Tendoscopy of the Peroneal Tendon: Indications and Procedures

Number ofPatients	Diagnosis	Treatment
5	Snapping tendon	Suture length ruptures (3)*
1	Calcaneal exostosis	Removal exostosis
7	Posttraumatic tenosynovitis	Suture length rupture (5)*

* When a longitudinal rupture of the peroneus brevis tendon was detected, an open repair was performed by means of a small incision

Table 5
Hindfoot Endoscopy for Posterior Ankle/Subtalar Joint Pathology: Indications and Procedures

Number ofPatients	Diagnosis	Treatment
13	Osteochondral defect ankle joint	Débridement + drilling
5	Loose body ankle joint	Removal of loose body
7	Calcification/avulsion	Removal of ossicles
2	Osteophyte posterior tibial rim	Resection of osteophytes
2	Chondromatosis	Anterior + posterior removal
7	Chronic synovitis	Anterior + posterior synovectomy
10	Degenerative changes subtalar joint	Osteophyte removal + débridement
1	Loose body subtalar joint	Removal
3	Intraosseous talar ganglion	Drill, curetting + grafting

Tenosynovectomy, screw removal, and exostosis removal were successfully performed using posterior tibial and peroneal tendoscopy.[15,16] When a longitudinal rupture was detected, a small incision was made, and the rupture was sutured. A symptomatic pathologic thickened posterior tibial vincula was successfully removed in four patients. Removal of an inflamed retrocalcaneal bursa together with removal of the prominent posterosuperior part of the calcaneus (endoscopic calcaneoplasty) was associated with a good or excellent result in 80% of patients.[38] Resection of an inflamed peritendinium in a patient with localized Achilles tendinitis gave promising early results. Removal of a pathologic os trigonum or a painful posterior soft-tissue impediment did not cause any technical problems and was successful in most patients.

None of the patients who underwent a total synovectomy experienced recurrence of synovitis. All loose bodies were successfully removed. Nine of the 13 patients with débrided/drilled osteochondral defects had a good or excellent result. The three patients who were treated for an intraosseous talar ganglion were symptom-free at the last follow-up. All patients who were treated for degenerative changes in the subtalar joint experienced a clear improvement of their symptoms, which did not deteriorate over time.

Summary

The balance between peroneal tendons and posterior tibial tendon plays an important role in normal hindfoot function. Posttraumatic posterior tibial tendon dysfunction can lead to peritendinitis. Tenosynovitis is often associated with flatfoot deformity. When conservative measures fail in an early stage, tenosynovectomy can be performed. Postoperative treatment consists of plaster immobilization for several weeks. Endoscopic release in combination with synovectomy has several advantages including reduced pain, outpatient treatment, good function after treatment, and rapid return to work and sports activities. Posttraumatic and postsurgical symptoms at the posterior margin of the lateral and medial malleolus often are difficult to diagnose and treat. Adhesions between the tendon and tendon sheath or an irregularity of the tendon sliding channel can give rise to pain. Open tendon release requires postoperative plaster immobilization with subsequent chance of new adhesion formation. Endoscopic release has the advantage of a diagnostic and therapeutic procedure that can be performed under local anesthesia and is associated with postoperative patient function.

A new finding in cadaver specimens as well as in all endoscopic procedures involving the posterior tibial tendon was the role of the posterior tibial vincula. Posttraumatic or postsurgery damage to this vincula can cause thickening and scarring of its distal free edge. This thickened vincula can be palpated at the posterior edge of the distal tibia, 3 to 5 cm above the posterior tip of the medial malleolus. Active movement of the tendon and hyperdorsiflexion cause pain as a result of traction between the shortened thickened vincula and its attachment. Endoscopic resection was successful in these patients.

An important cause of posterior ankle pain in athletes, especially ballet dancers and soccer players, is chronic tenosynovitis of the flexor hallucis longus tendon. Open surgery involves opening the tendon sheath, débriding the tendon, and resecting the flexor retinaculum. Postoperative treatment usually requires plaster immobilization. The patient is expected to take up to 6 months for a full recovery. Endoscopic release is associated with a reduction in recovery time and is performed as an outpatient procedure.

The reported results of open treatment of chronic retrocalcaneal bursitis have not been favorable. Nesse and Finsen[43] reported persisting symptoms and complications in 22 out of 35 patients. Angermann and associates[44] reported a failure rate of 50%. Myersen and McGarvey[30] reported favorable results.

Endoscopic calcaneoplasty offers a good alternative to open resection. Surgeons skilled in using the arthroscope will find this endoscopic technique a rewarding experience. Advantages of the endoscopic technique are related to the small incisions.

Complications such as wound dehiscence, painful scars, unsightly scars, and nerve entrapment within the scar are minimized. Because endoscopic surgery allows for excellent visualization from both the medial and lateral sides, the Achilles tendon, its insertion, and the calcaneus can be inspected and subsequently treated, minimizing the chance of removing and disturbing the Achilles attachment. Because of function after treatment, late complications such as stiffness and pain are avoided. With this technique, 80% good to excellent results have been reported.

Reported results for conventional surgical treatments of chronic peritendinitis have been favorable. The percentage of good or excellent results varies between 78% and 96%.[45-49] This same positive out-come has been experienced with endoscopic treatment. The tolerance to this type of outpatient surgery with minimal scarring is favorable. The procedure can be performed under local anesthesia.

The two-portal posterior endoscopic ankle approach with the patient in the prone position offers excellent access to the posterior compartment of the ankle joint, the posterior subtalar joint, and the flexor hallucis longus tendon and os trigonum.[50]

When combined with anterior ankle arthroscopy, most surgeons regard the posteromedial portal to be contraindicated in all but the most extreme situations because of the potential of serious complications. The posterolateral portal, however, is advocated as a routine portal by most authors. When the arthroscope shaft is in place through this posterolateral portal, the instruments inserted through the posteromedial portal must be directed toward the arthroscope shaft. The arthroscope shaft subsequently is used as a guide to orient and direct the medial instruments toward the joint. The neurovascular bundle is thus passed without problem. When performed by a surgeon experienced in the technique, posterior ankle arthroscopy is a safe and reliable method to diagnose and treat a variety of posterior ankle conditions.

References

1. Burman MS: Arthroscopy of direct visualization of joints: An experimental cadaver study. *J Bone Joint Surg* 1931;13:669-695.

2. Tagaki K: The arthroscope. *Jpn J Orthop Assoc* 1939;14:359.

3. Watanabe M: Selfoc-Arthroscope (Watanabe no 24 arthroscope). Monograph. Tokyo, Japan, Teishin Hospital, 1972.

4. Chen DS, Wertheimer SJ: Centrally located osteochondral fracture of the talus. *J Foot Surg* 1992;31:134-140.

5. Biedert R: Anterior ankle pain in sports medicine: Etiology and indications for arthroscopy. *Arch Orthop Trauma Surg* 1991;110:293-297.

6. Feder KS, Schonholtz GJ: Ankle arthroscopy: Review and long-term results. *Foot Ankle* 1992;13:382-385.

7. Ferkel RD, Scranton PE: Arthroscopy of the ankle and foot. *J Bone Joint Surg Am* 1993;75:1233-1242.

8. Guhl JF: *Foot and Ankle Arthroscopy*. New York, NY, Slack, 1993.

9. Jerosch J, Schneider T, Strauss JM, Schurmann N: Arthroscopy of the upper ankle joint: List of indications from the literature–realistic expectations–complications. *Unfallchirurg* 1993;96:82-87.

10. Martin DF, Baker CL, Curl WW, Andrews JR, Robie DB, Haas AF: Operative ankle arthroscopy: Long-term followup. *Am J Sports Med* 1989;17:16-23.

11. Parisien JS, Vangsness T: Arthroscopy of the subtalar joint: An experimental approach. *Arthroscopy* 1985;1:53-57.

12. Guhl JF, Parisien JS, Boyton MD (eds): *Foot and Ankle Arthroscopy*, ed 3. Heidelberg, Germany, Springer-Verlag, 2004.

13. Andrews JR, Timmerman LA (eds): *Diagnostic and Operative Arthroscopy*. Philadelphia, PA, WB Saunders, 1997.

14. Ferkel RD: Arthroscopic surgery, in Whipple TI (ed): *The Foot and Ankle*. New York, NY, Lippincott-Raven, 1996.

15. van Dijk CN, Kort N, Scholten P: Tendoscopy of the posterior tibial tendon. *Arthroscopy* 1997;13:692-698.

16. van Dijk CN, Kort N: Tendoscopy of the peroneal tendons. *Arthroscopy* 1998;14:471-478.

17. van Dijk CN, Scholten PE, Krips R: A 2-portal endoscopic approach for diagnosis and treatment of posterior ankle pathology. *Arthroscopy* 2000;16:871-876.

18. Nagai H: Tunnel endoscopy, in Watanabe M (ed): *Arthroscopy of Small Joints*. New York, NY, Igaku-Shoin, 1986, pp 163-164.

19. Anderson RB, Hodges Davis W: Management of the adult flatfoot deformity, in Myerson M (ed): *Foot and Ankle Disorders*. Philadelphia, PA, WB Saunders, 2000, vol 2, pp 1017-1040.

20. Lapidus PW, Seidenstein H: Chronic non-specific tenosynovitis with a fusion

about the ankle. *J Bone Joint Surg Am* 1950;32A:175-179.

21. van Dijk CN, Scholten PE, Kort NP: Tendoscopy (tendon sheath endoscopy) for overuse tendon injuries. *Oper Tech Sports Med* 1997;5:170-178.

22. Stibbe AB, van Dijk CN, Marti RK: The os trigonum syndrome. *Acta Orthop Scand* 1994;(suppl 262):59-60.

23. van Dijk CN, Lim LS, Poortman A, Strubbe EH, Marti RK: Degenerative joint disease in female ballet dancers. *Am J Sports Med* 1995;23:295-300.

24. Hamilton WG, Geppert MJ, Thompson FM: Pain in the posterior aspect of the ankle in dancers. *J Bone Joint Surg Am* 1996;78:1491-1500.

25. Hedrick MR, McBryde AM: Posterior ankle impingement. *Foot Ankle Int* 1994;15:2-8.

26. Funk DA, Cass JR, Johnson KA: Acquired adult flatfoot secondary to posterior tibial tendon pathology. *J Bone Joint Surg Am* 1986;68:95-102.

27. Roggatz J, Urban A: The calcareous peritendinitis of the long peroneal tendon. *Arch Orthop Trauma Surg* 1980;96:161-164.

28. Schweitzer GJ: Stenosing peroneal tenovaginitis: Case reports. *S Afr Med J* 1982;61:521-523.

29. Yao L, Tong JF, Cracchiolo A, Seeger LL: MR findings in peroneal tendopathy. *J Comput Assist Tomogr* 1995;19:460-464.

30. Myerson MS, McGarvey W: Disorders of the insertion of the Achilles tendon and Achilles tendinitis. *Instr Course Lect* 1999;48:211-218.

31. Richardson EG: Disorders of tendons, in Grenshaw AH (ed): *Campbell's Operative Orthopaedics*. St. Louis, MO, Mosby, 1992, pp 2851-2873.

32. Cozen L: Posterior tibial tenosynivitis secondary to foot strain. *Clin Orthop Relat Res* 1965;42:101-102.

33. Johnson KA, Strom DE: Tibialis posterior tendon dysfunction. *Clin Orthop Relat Res* 1989;239:196-206.

34. Williams R: Chronic non-specific tendovaginitis of tibialis posterior. *J Bone Joint Surg Br* 1963;45:542-549.

35. Trevino S, Gould N, Korson R: Surgical treatment of stenosing tenosynovitis at the ankle. *Foot Ankle* 1981;2:37-45.

36. Coughlin MJ, Mann RA: Tarsal tunnel syndrome, in *Surgery of the Foot and Ankle*, ed 6. St. Louis, MO, Mosby, 1993.

37. van Dijk CN, Verhagen RA, Tol HJ: Technical note: Resterilizable noninvasive ankle distraction device. *Arthroscopy* 2001;17:E12.

38. van Dijk CN, van Dyk GE, Scholten P, Kort NP: Endoscopic calcaneoplasty. *Am J Sports Med* 2001;29:185-189.

39. Lundeen RO: Arthroscopic excision of the os trigonum, in Guhl JF, Parisien JS, Boyton MD (eds): *Foot and Ankle Arthroscopy*, ed 3. Heidelberg, Germany, Springer-Verlag, 2004, pp 191-199.

40. Frey C, Gasser S, Feder K: Arthroscopy of the subtalar joint. *Foot Ankle Int* 1994;15:424-428.

41. Parisien JS: Posterior subtalar joint arthroscopy, in Guhl JF, Parisien JS, Boyton MD (eds): *Foot and Ankle*

Arthroscopy, ed 3. Heidelberg, Germany, Springer-Verlag, 2004; pp 175-182.

42. Alfredson H, Pietila T, Jonsson P, Lorentzon R: Heavy-load eccentric calf muscle training for the treatment of chronic Achilles tendinosis. *Am J Sports Med* 1998;26:360-366.

43. Nesse E, Finsen V: Poor results after resection for Haglund's heel: Analysis of 35 heels in 23 patients after 3 years. *Acta Orthop Scand* 1994;65:107-109.

44. Angermann P, Hovgaard D: Chronic Achilles tendinopathy in athletic individuals: Results of nonsurgical treatment. *Foot Ankle Int* 1999;20:304-306.

45. Kvist H, Kvist M: The operative treatment of chronic calcaneal paratenonitis. *J Bone Joint Surg Br* 1980;62:353-357.

46. Leach RE, Schepsis AA, Takai H: Long-term results of surgical management of Achilles tendinitis in runners. *Clin Orthop Relat Res* 1992;282:208-212.

47. Nelen G, Martens M, Burssens A: Surgical treatment of chronic Achilles tendinitis. *Am J Sports Med* 1989;17:754-759.

48. Schepsis AA: Leach RE: Surgical management of Achilles tendinitis. *Am J Sports Med* 1987;15:308-315.

49. Williams JG: Achilles tendon lesions in sport. *Sports Med* 1986;3:114-135.

50. van Dijk CN, Scholten PE, Krips R: A two-portal endoscopic approach for diagnosis and treatment of posterior ankle pathology. *Arthroscopy* 2000;16:871-876.

Arthroscopy of the Great Toe

Carol Frey, MD
C. Niek van Dijk, MD

Open surgery about the first metatarsophalangeal (MTP) joint can result in stiffness, prolonged swelling, poor wound healing, and trouble with shoewear. However, advancements in small joint instrumentation and arthroscopic technique have expanded the application of arthroscopy in the first MTP joint and helped improve the treatment of many forefoot disorders. Along with the advancements in technique, however, it is important that the surgeon understand the pertinent gross and arthroscopic anatomy of the first MTP joint. A better understanding of the difficult anatomy surrounding the forefoot should help in the performance of arthroscopic surgery as well as in proper recognition of abnormal pathology when present. It should also be recognized that arthroscopy of this joint is a relatively new application, therefore, indications for the procedure are still developing, and no long-term clinical studies have been published. For these reasons, the procedure should be considered investigational at this time.

Gross Anatomy and Biomechanics

Minimal stability is provided by the shallow ball and socket articulation between the proximal phalanx and the metatarsal head. The soft tissues,

including the capsule, ligaments, and musculotendinous structures, provide most of the support to the first MTP joint.

The extensor hallucis longus tendon divides the dorsum of the first MTP joint in half. The branches of the deep peroneal nerve innervate the lateral half and the branches of the superficial peroneal nerve innervate the medial half of the joint. The terminal branches of the saphenous nerve innervate the medial aspect of the great toe (Fig. 1).

On the plantar aspect of the first MTP joint, the sesamoids are within the medial and lateral portions of the flexor hallucis brevis tendon. The sesamoids are enveloped by the split tendon of the flexor hallucis brevis, which sends fibers to the plantar plate and subsequently attaches to the proximal aspect of the proximal phalanx. The plantar plate is a strong fibrous structure that inserts on either side of the MTP joint. The flexor hallucis longus tendon is both superficial and between the 2 heads of the flexor hallucis brevis tendon (Fig. 2).

Biomechanically, the instant centers of motion for the first MTP joint fall within the metatarsal head. Motion occurs between the metatarsal head and the proximal phalanx via a sliding action at the joint surface. In full extension or flexion, this slid-

ing action gives way to compression of the dorsal or plantar articular surfaces of the metatarsal head and the proximal phalanx.

Arthroscopic Anatomy and Portals

The dorsal medial, dorsal lateral, and straight medial portals are the most commonly used portals for arthroscopy of the first MTP joint (Fig. 3). The dorsal medial and dorsal lateral portals are placed at the joint line and on either side of the extensor hallucis longus tendon. The straight medial portal is placed through the medial capsule midway between the dorsal and plantar aspect of the joint, usually under direct visualization.

Intra-articular examination includes visualization of 10 major areas: the lateral gutter; the lateral corner of the metatarsal head; the central portion of the metatarsal head; the medial corner of the metatarsal head; the medial gutter; the medial portion of the proximal phalanx; the central portion of the proximal phalanx; the lateral portion of the proximal phalanx; the medial sesamoid; and the lateral sesamoid.

Technique

The patient is placed in the supine position on the operating room table. General, spinal, epidural, or local

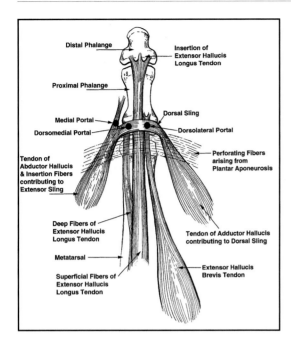

Fig. 1 Musculotendinous anatomy surrounding the first metatarsophalangeal joint. (Reproduced with permission from Frey C: Gross and arthroscopic anatomy of the foot, in Guhl J (ed): *Foot and Ankle Arthroscopy*, ed 3. New York, NY, Springer-Verlag, in press.)

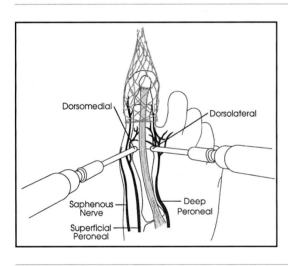

Fig. 2 Anatomic structures at risk with portal placement for first metatarsophalangeal joint arthroscopy. (Reproduced with permission from Frey C: Arthroscopy of the great toe, in Chow J (ed): *Advanced Arthroscopy*. New York, NY, Springer-Verlag, in press.)

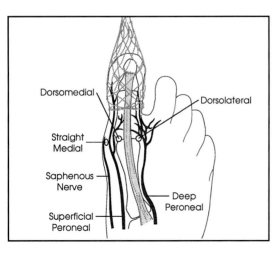

Fig. 3 The dorsal medial, dorsal lateral, and straight medial portals are the most commonly used portals for arthroscopy of the first metatarsophalangeal joint. (Reproduced with permission from Feder K: Arthroscopy and endoscopy of the foot, in Pfeffer G, Frey C (eds): *Current Practices in Foot and Ankle Surgery*. New York, NY, McGraw-Hill, 1994, vol 2.)

anesthesia can all be used. A sterile finger trap is placed on the toe to suspend the lower extremity, with traction applied at the level of the ankle if necessary (Fig. 4).

The dorsal medial or dorsal lateral portal is established first. The joint line is palpated just medial or lateral to the extensor hallucis longus tendon. A 19-gauge spinal needle is used to inflate the MTP joint with 5 ml of normal saline. A 4-mm longitudinal skin incision is made, the subcutaneous tissue is spread with a mosquito clamp to prevent neurovascular injury, and the joint is entered with an interchangeable cannula with a semiblunt trochar. Once visualization of the joint is accomplished through the initial portal, the remaining 2 portals can be established with a spinal needle under direct vision. Use of interchangeable cannulas allows rotation of the video arthroscope and instrumentation so that the entire joint and its pathology can be fully evaluated and treated.

The arthroscopic examination of the great toe is performed through the dorsal lateral portal. The dorsal medial portal provides superior visualization of the dorsal aspect of the metatarsal head and proximal phalanx. The medial and lateral sesamoids can be well visualized from the medial portal (Figs. 5 through 7).

Indications

Indications for surgical arthroscopy of the first MTP joint include osteophytes, hallux rigidus, chondromalacia, osteochondritis dissecans, loose bodies, arthrofibrosis, and synovitis secondary to hyperextension and hyperflexion injuries of the great toe. Evolution of surgical arthroscopic techniques may soon allow arthrodesis of the first MTP joint. Diagnostic arthroscopy may be indicated in cases of recurrent swelling and locking, persistent pain, and stiffness recalci-

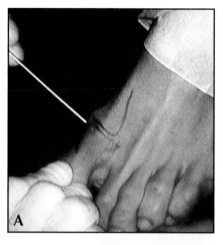
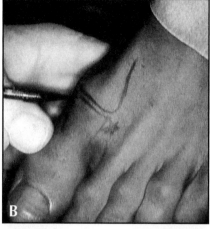
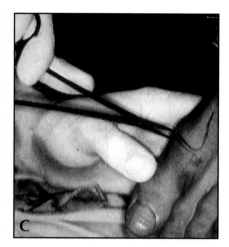
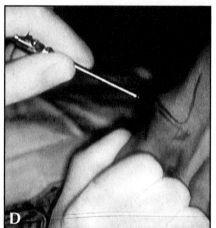
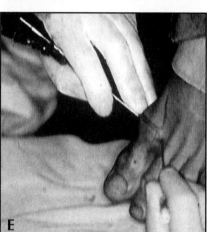

Fig. 4 Using manual traction or a sterile finger trap, the first metatarsophalangeal (MTP) joint can be palpated and a spinal needle introduced through the anteromedial portal site (**A**). Once the joint space is located, a longitudinal skin incision is made through the skin (**B**). Blunt dissection with a hemostat is used to enter the first MTP joint (**C**). The arthroscope with a blunt trocar is introduced through the anteromedial portal (**D**). The location of the anterolateral portal is made under direct visualization by introducing a spinal needle through the portal site (**E**). A skin incision is made for the anterolateral portal and the arthroscope is introduced. (Courtesy of C. Niek van Dijk.)

trant to a full regimen of conservative treatment.

The most common indications for arthroscopy of the great toe include treatment of hallux rigidus with a dorsal osteophyte, and chondromalacia. Dorsal osteophytes may be removed if they are mild to moderate in size. If the osteophyte is large, an open cheilectomy is recommended.

An arthroscopic cheilectomy can be performed through 2 or 3 portals. The arthroscopic shaver and burr are placed in the dorsal medial or medial portal and the arthroscope is placed in the dorsal lateral portal. The osteophyte is removed from distal to proximal and medial to lateral. Up to one third of the articular surface may be removed using this technique and

will help improve range of motion. If a finger trap is used for distraction, it is best to release it prior to removing the osteophytes because the traction may cause the capsule to pull tightly against the osteophyte. Postoperatively, the patient is placed on crutches for 5 days and range of motion exercises begun immediately.

In the presence of chondromalacia or osteochondral lesions, the pathology may be evaluated, loose fragments excised, and bone drilled or abraded to a bleeding surface. The patient is not allowed to bear weight for 2 weeks postoperatively, and early range of motion is encouraged at 5 days.

For evaluation and surgery of the medial sesamoid, the dorsal lateral portal is used for the arthroscope and

the instrumentation is placed in the medial portal. For the lateral sesamoid, the arthroscope is introduced through the dorsal medial portal and the instrumentation is placed in the dorsal lateral portal. To evaluate the sesamoid compartment, it is helpful to release the toe traction and place the great toe in plantar flexion.

Postoperative Care and Rehabilitation

Small portal wounds are closed with interrupted nylon sutures. To prevent fistula formation, a bulky compression dressing is applied for 4 to 7 days. Direct weightbearing is avoided. Sutures are removed at approximately 7 to 10 days after surgery and the patient is started on range of motion

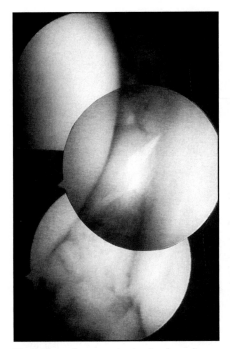

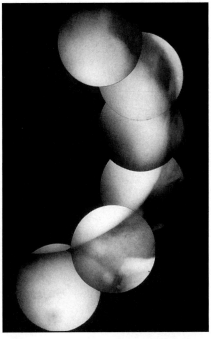

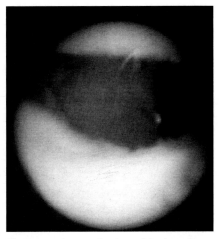

Fig. 7 An arthroscopic view of the lateral sesamoid. At the top is the plantar surface of the metatarsal head and on the bottom is the plantar capsule and the middle part of the lateral sesamoid. (Courtesy of C. Niek van Dijk.)

Fig. 5 The arthroscope is viewing from the anteromedial portal. The metatarsal head is on the left side, the base of the proximal phalanx is on the right side. Between the 2 structures is the plantar capsule and synovium. (Courtesy of C. Niek van Dijk.)

Fig. 6 The arthroscope is viewing from the medial portal. The metatarsal head is to the left and the medial sesamoid is seen plantar to the metatarsal head.

Summary

The few available reports of arthroscopic treatment of the first MTP joint in the literature indicate favorable outcome. However, arthroscopy of the great toe is an advanced technique and should only be undertaken by experienced surgeons.

References

1. Watanabe M: *Selfox-Arthroscope (Watanabe No 24 Arthroscope)*. Tokyo, Japan, Teishin Hospital, 1972.
2. Yovich JV, McIlwraith CW: Arthroscopic surgery for osteochondral fractures of the proximal phalanx of the metacarpophalangeal and metatarsophalangeal (fetlock) joints in horses. *J Am Vet Med Assoc* 1986;188:273–279.
3. Lundeen RO: Arthroscopic approaches to the joints of the foot. *J Am Podiatr Med Assoc* 1987;77:451–455.
4. Bartlett DH: Arthroscopic management of osteochondritis dissecans of the first metatarsal head. *Arthroscopy* 1988;4:51–54.

and strengthening exercises. A wooden shoe is used until postoperative swelling and pain have resolved.

Results

In 1972, Watanabe described the first arthroscopic examination of the MTP joint.[1] In 1986, Yovich and McIlwraith[2] showed that osteochondral fractures of the first MTP (fetlock) joint of the horse could be successfully treated with arthroscopic debridement. In the podiatric literature, Lundeen[3] reported the performance, but no clinical results, of 11 great toe arthroscopies. In 1988, Bartlett[4] reported his technique of first MTP joint surgical arthroscopy and the successful treatment of osteochondritis dissecans of the first metatarsal head. Ferkel and Van Breuken reviewed 12 surgical arthroscopies of the great toe in 1991 (personal communication, San Diego, 1991). The series treated multiple types of pathology of the MTP joint, and good results were reported in 83%.

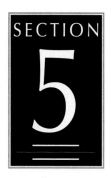

SECTION 5

Forefoot Conditions

Forefoot Conditions

This section provides a review of diverse forefoot conditions that are commonly encountered in an orthopaedic practice. The chapter by Sammarco provides a detailed and well-referenced overview of the correction of severe hallux valgus deformity with proximal first metatarsal osteotomy and distal soft-tissue correction or first metatarsophalangeal joint arthrodesis. Ludloff, proximal crescentic, proximal chevron, scarf, and Mau osteotomies are discussed. These procedures correct metatarsophalangeal joint alignment and the first-second intermetatarsal angle.

A recent study confirmed the success of the Ludloff procedure.[1] Recent studies on proximal chevron osteotomies documented stable fixation with a medial locking plate,[2] and found (in a cadaver model) that fixation with a dorsal L-plate was more stable than with a single screw.[3] Proximal opening wedge first metatarsal osteotomies with plate fixation may be successful and may avoid the potential risk of metatarsal shortening.[4] Furthermore, distal first metatarsal osteotomies may have a role in the management of moderate and severe hallux valgus deformities. A recent, randomized, prospective study showed no difference in correction of average hallux valgus, first-second intermetatarsal, and distal metatarsal articular angles after treatment with scarf or *distal* chevron osteotomies, except in patients with severe hallux valgus; those patients had better correction of the average hallux valgus angle with a *distal* chevron osteotomy.[5]

The chapters by Sammarco and Marks provide reviews of the indications for first metatarsophalangeal joint arthrodesis, including inflammatory conditions, neuromuscular disease, salvage of severe hallux valgus deformity (hallux valgus angle

≥ 40°), failed bunion surgery, infection, and degenerative joint disease. Surgical techniques, proper joint positioning for fusions, and complications also are reviewed. A recent study showed that first metatarsophalangeal joint arthrodesis for the correction of hallux valgus deformity is associated with concurrent correction of the first-second intermetatarsal angle and tibial sesamoid position; an additional first metatarsal osteotomy is not required.[6]

In chapter 24, Richardson reviews the causes and treatments of complications after hallux valgus surgery, including recurrent deformity; hallux varus deformity; transfer lesions; osteonecrosis of the first metatarsal head; and first metatarsal malunion, nonunion, and shortening. A useful table, which lists the numerous clinical considerations in hallux valgus treatment, is included. Research to prevent and treat these complications is ongoing. A recent study of distal chevron osteotomy showed decreased blood flow to the first metatarsal head during each stage of the procedure (medial capsulotomy, 45% decrease; adductor tenotomy and lateral release, 13% decrease; and chevron osteotomy, 13% decrease; total, 71% decrease); however, no osteonecrosis was observed in the 20 patients in this study.[7] Dorsal malunion from proximal crescentic first metatarsal osteotomy may be minimized by attention to the coronal plane orientation of the osteotomy saw blade.[8] Successful correction of iatrogenic hallux varus deformity has been reported with a new method, consisting of static ligamentoplasty of the lateral soft tissues of the first metatarsophalangeal joint with an abductor hallucis tendon transfer, without an interphalangeal joint fusion.[9]

The chapter by Coughlin reviews the evaluation and treatment of lesser toe deformities and other forefoot conditions including mallet toe, hammer toe, claw toe, lesser metatarsophalangeal joint instability, interdigital neuroma, fifth toe deformities, lateral fifth toe corns, and interdigital corns. A recent study reported that a capital oblique lesser metatarsal osteotomy can be complicated by a floating toe deformity.[10] A recently described modification of the capital oblique osteotomy, consisting of a segmental resection osteotomy, also has been reported to have a high complication rate, including transfer metatarsalgia (19%), floating toe (27%), and toe weakness (35%).[11] In a 2007 study that characterized patients surgically treated for crossover second toe deformity, the authors reported that most patients (86%) were women, the mean age at surgery was 59 years, 66% of patients had a positive drawer sign, and there was no correlation between the deformity and second metatarsal length.[12] In another study, some patients treated with interdigital neurectomy had residual pain and functional limitation at an average of 5.5 years after surgery, with 40% of patients having poor results.[13] A follow-up study of the treatment of lateral fifth toe corns (lateral condylectomy and flexor tenotomy or complete condylectomy) and interdigital corns (single condylectomy, double condylectomy of adjacent corns, or complete condylectomy) showed that pain was relieved in most feet (93%) and the results were rated by patients as excellent or good in 97% of feet.[14]

The chapter by Mann and Mann on keratotic disorders of the plantar skin is a well-illustrated review of the evaluation and treatment of common conditions including intractable plantar keratosis (discrete or diffuse) under the metatarsal heads or tibial sesamoid bone. A detailed description of nonsurgical and surgical treatments is provided. Possible complications of a DuVries metatarsal condylectomy are residual postoperative pain and stiffness of the metatarsophalangeal joint; interpositional arthroplasty has been described to improve postoperative pain and limited dorsiflexion.[15] Tibial sesamoid shaving can preserve the integrity of the sesamoid apparatus and hallux alignment; however, a recent study also showed that treatment of sesamoiditis with complete excision of the tibial sesamoid and meticulous repair of the soft-tissue defect and flexor hallucis brevis complex was not associated with any increase in the hallux valgus or first-second intermetatarsal angles.[16]

This section on forefoot conditions concludes with a chapter by Mann and Mann about the classification and surgical treatment of bunionette deformity. A bunionette resulting from lateral prominence of the fifth metatarsal head (type 1) can be treated with a distal chevron or oblique metatarsal osteotomy. A bunionette resulting from lateral bowing of the fifth metatarsal (type 2) or an increased fourth-fifth intermetatarsal angle (type 3) can be treated with a fifth metatarsal diaphyseal osteotomy and soft-tissue repair. Recent follow-up studies of distal metatarsal osteotomies have shown satisfactory results in most patients,[17-19] and a follow-up study of diaphyseal osteotomy confirmed previously reported satisfactory results in more than 90% of patients.[20]

William H. Gondring, MD
Department of Orthopedics
Heartland Health Systems
St. Joseph, Missouri

References

1. Trnka HJ, Hofstaetter SG, Easley ME: Intermediate-term results of the Ludloff osteotomy in one hundred and eleven feet: Surgical technique. *J Bone Joint Surg Am* 2009;91(suppl 2 pt 1):156-168.

2. Gallentine JW, DeOrio JK, DeOrio MJ: Bunion surgery using locking-plate fixation of proximal metatarsal chevron osteotomies. *Foot Ankle Int* 2007;28:361-368.

3. Varner KE, Matt V, Alexander JW, et al: Screw versus plate fixation of proximal first metatarsal crescentic osteotomy. *Foot Ankle Int* 2009;30:142-149.

4. Randhawa S, Pepper D: Radiographic evaluation of hallux valgus treated with opening wedge osteotomy. *Foot Ankle Int* 2009;30: 427-431.

5. Deenik A, van Mameren H, de Visser E, de Waal Malefijt M, Draijer F, de Bie R: Equivalent correction in scarf and chevron osteotomy in moderate and severe hallux valgus: A randomized controlled trial. *Foot Ankle Int* 2008;29:1209-1215.

6. Pydah SK, Toh EM, Sirikonda SP, Walker CR: Intermetatarsal angular change following fusion of the first metatarsophalangeal joint. *Foot Ankle Int* 2009;30:415-418.

7. Kuhn MA, Lippert FG III, Phipps MJ, Williams C: Blood flow to the metatarsal head after chevron bunionectomy. *Foot Ankle Int* 2005;26:526-529.

8. Jones C, Coughlin M, Villadot R, Golanó P: Proximal crescentic metatarsal osteotomy: The effect of saw blade orientation on first ray elevation. *Foot Ankle Int* 2005;26:152-157.

9. Leemrijse T, Hoang B, Maldague P, Docquier PL, Devos Bevernage B: A new surgical procedure for iatrogenic hallux varus: Reverse transfer of the abductor hallucis tendon. A report of 7 cases. *Acta Orthop Belg* 2008;74:227-234.

10. Migues A, Slullitel G, Bilbao F, Carrasco M, Solari G: Floating-toe deformity as a complication of the Weil osteotomy. *Foot Ankle Int* 2004;25:609-613.

11. Garg R, Thordarson DB, Schrumpf M, Castaneda D: Sliding oblique versus segmental resection osteotomies for lesser metatarsophalangeal joint pathology. *Foot Ankle Int* 2008;29:1009-1014.

12. Kaz AJ, Coughlin MJ: Crossover second toe: Demographics, etiology, and radiographic assessment. *Foot Ankle Int* 2007;28:1223-1237.

13. Womack JW, Richardson DR, Murphy GA, Richardson EG, Ishikawa SN: Long-term evaluation of interdigital neuroma treated by surgical excision. *Foot Ankle Int* 2008;29:574-577.

14. Coughlin MJ, Kennedy MP: Operative repair of fourth and fifth toe corns. *Foot Ankle Int* 2003;24:147-157.

15. Myerson MS, Redfern DJ: Technique tip: Modification of DuVries's lesser metatarsophalangeal joint arthroplasty to improve joint mobility. *Foot Ankle Int* 2004;25:278-279.

16. Lee S, James WC, Cohen BE, Davis WH, Anderson RB: Evaluation of hallux alignment and functional outcome after isolated tibial sesamoidectomy. *Foot Ankle Int* 2005;26: 803-809.

17. Legenstein R, Bonomo J, Huber W, Boesch P: Correction of tailor's bunion with the Boesch technique: A retrospective study. *Foot Ankle Int* 2007;28:799-803.

18. Weitzel S, Trnka HJ, Petroutsas J: Transverse medial slide osteotomy for bunionette deformity: Long-term results. *Foot Ankle Int* 2007;28:794-798.

19. Giannini S, Faldini C, Vannini F, Digennaro V, Bevoni R, Luciani D: The minimally invasive osteotomy "S.E.R.I." (simple, effective, rapid, inexpensive) for correction of bunionette deformity. *Foot Ankle Int* 2008;29:282-286.

20. Vienne P, Oesselmann M, Espinosa N, Aschwanden R, Zingg P: Modified Coughlin procedure for surgical treatment of symptomatic tailor's bunion: A prospective followup study of 33 consecutive operations. *Foot Ankle Int* 2006;27:573-580.

William H. Gondring, MD or a member of his immediate family serves as a board member, owner, officer, or committee member of the American Orthopaedic Foot & Ankle Society, St. Joseph Imaging and Breast Center, Offsite Image Management Systems Inc, and Arthroscopy Association of North America.

Surgical Correction of Moderate and Severe Hallux Valgus: Proximal Metatarsal Osteotomy With Distal Soft-Tissue Correction and Arthrodesis of the Metatarsophalangeal Joint

*V. James Sammarco, MD

Abstract

Hallux valgus correction by distal soft-tissue release and proximal metatarsal osteotomy is the procedure of choice for most patients with moderate and severe hallux valgus deformity. Complications can be avoided by selecting a procedure that provides adequate correction of the intermetatarsal angle and ensuring proper balancing of the metatarsophalangeal joint though lateral soft-tissue releases and medial joint plication. Arthrodesis should be considered when revision of failed surgery is planned, degenerative joint disease is present, and where the likelihood of failure of a bunion procedure is high (such as in elderly individuals with osteoporosis, severe deformity with significant involvement of the lesser metatarsophalangeal joint, and when spasticity is present). A review of biomechanical data, clinical studies, and surgical techniques is important for successful treatment of moderate and severe hallux valgus deformity.

The painful bunion deformity is a common and relatively disabling condition that affects individuals of all ages. More than 150 procedures have been described for the treatment of hallux valgus, and the orthopaedic literature has focused predominantly on surgical management of this condition; however, successful treatment is often achieved with simple, off-the-shelf orthotic devices and appropriate shoe wear modifications. Given the potential for surgical complications, the substantial recovery period associated with bunion surgery, and patients' occasional dissatisfaction with the results of otherwise technically successful procedures, it is recommended that nonsurgical treatment be initiated before proceeding with surgery. It is not uncommon for a patient with an asymptomatic bunion to actively seek surgical correction because of cosmetic concerns or because of an inability to wear fashionable shoes comfortably. Although pain alone is not the only indication for surgery, it is not recommended that surgery be performed for cosmetic reasons alone. The American Orthopaedic Foot and Ankle Society (AOFAS) has issued a position statement reflecting this.[1]

Pain resulting from hallux valgus deformity is mechanical in nature and can have extrinsic and intrinsic causes. Most commonly, extrinsic pain is related to mechanical irritation of the prominent medial eminence by shoe wear or is due to impingement of the hallux on the second digit. A painful callus may develop on the medial border of the hallux as a result of pronation of the digit, and pain beneath the second metatarsal head is also common as a result of the transfer of forces as the weight-bearing function of the hallux is compromised by increasing deformity. Most extrinsic pain can

*V. James Sammarco, MD, or the department with which he is affiliated has received research or institutional support from Smith & Nephew.

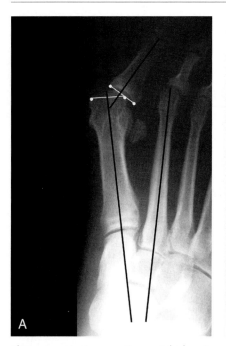
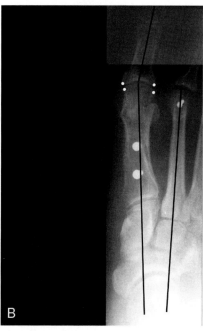

Figure 1 **A,** Preoperative weight-bearing radiograph showing hallux valgus with an incongruent joint. Note the lateral subluxation of the proximal phalanx and the sesamoid complex. **B,** Weight-bearing radiograph made 1 year postoperatively. The intermetatarsal angle was corrected with a proximal osteotomy of the first metatarsal, and the hallux valgus angle was corrected distally with lateral soft-tissue release and medial capsular plication.

be alleviated with nonsurgical treatment, including extra-depth shoes with a wide toe box and soft leather uppers. A silicone toe spacer between the hallux and the second toe decreases pain from impingement, and an accommodative shoe insert with a metatarsal bar can be used to diminish pain beneath the lesser metatarsal heads. Intrinsic pain is caused by abnormal joint mechanics that cause increased joint contact stresses and synovitis and can lead to cartilage degeneration. Pain intrinsic to the joint is typically reproduced with axial loading and motion of the joint and can also manifest as plantar pain with palpation of the sesamoids. Intrinsic pain is less amenable to conservative treatment but can be managed with an orthotic device that incorporates a stiff Morton extension. Corrective devices

may prevent progression of a deformity, but they will not permanently correct it. An in-depth review of conservative treatment of painful bunion deformities is beyond the scope of this chapter, and the reader is referred to a recent article in which current concepts of nonsurgical management are reviewed in greater detail.[2]

The primary indication, for surgical treatment of hallux valgus is pain that fails to respond to conservative treatment, usually within 6 to 12 months. Some conditions may not cause substantial pain but may require surgical correction because of functional problems or rapid progression. Substantial progression of a deformity by one grade or more over a 6- to 12-month period may be an indication for surgical correction, even if pain is not a major symptom.

These conditions are uncommon in patients with idiopathic hallux valgus and typically are related to neuromuscular disease or trauma.

Selection of the proper procedure for hallux valgus surgery is critical to achieving an adequate result and durable correction of the deformity. Bunion deformity has been classified, and the algorithm developed by Mann and Coughlin defines modern decision making in hallux valgus surgery.[3] The metatarsophalangeal joint should be examined radiographically for congruency (Figure 1). If the joint is congruent, surgery must be planned so that it does not alter the congruency. When the metatarsophalangeal joint is incongruent, surgery is planned to restore joint congruency. Bunion deformity is classified as mild, moderate, or severe on the basis of the radiographic findings. Other considerations are the presence of metatarsophalangeal arthritis, hypermobility of the tarsometatarsal joint complex, and the presence of hallux valgus interphalangeus. This chapter is limited to a review of two procedures: bunion correction by proximal metatarsal osteotomy with distal soft-tissue rebalancing and bunion correction by arthrodesis of the metatarsophalangeal joint. Bunion correction by proximal metatarsal osteotomy with distal soft-tissue rebalancing is indicated primarily for moderate and severe bunions when the intermetatarsal angle must be corrected by more than 5° to achieve the desired postoperative position of less than 10°. The hallux valgus angle in these cases is typically more than 30°. Mild bunion deformities with an intermetatarsal angle of 14° or less can typically be corrected with a distal osteotomy; however, in elderly individuals or those with osteoporosis, a more proximal osteotomy may be

Table 1
General Indications for Proximal Metatarsal Osteotomy With Distal Soft-Tissue Rebalancing

Bunion Grade	Hallux Valgus Angle	Intermetatarsal Angle	Other Factors	Notes
Moderate	< 40°	≥ 14°	Incongruent joint	Congruent joint may require double osteotomy
Severe	≥ 40°	≥ 16°	Incongruent joint	Fusion should be considered for an elderly patient, one with osteoporotic bone, and one with multiple lesser toe deformities

Table 2
Indications for Fusion in Patients With Hallux Valgus

Arthritis associated with hallux valgus

Neuromuscular disease/spasticity

Inflammatory arthritis

Severe deformity with osteoporosis

Salvage after failed bunion surgery or failed arthroplasty

Salvage after infection (staged reconstruction)

considered to improve the available bone stock for fixation of the osteotomy site and to lessen the chances of osteonecrosis of the first metatarsal head. Fusion is most commonly done for the treatment of hallux valgus associated with arthritis or as a salvage procedure following failed previous bunion surgery and attempted arthroplasty. Other indications include neuromuscular conditions that cause spasticity, such as cerebral palsy and stroke, because of the high recurrence rate associated with standard procedures and the tendency for progression of the deformity with time.[4] Primary arthrodesis may also be considered for patients with severe deformity who are at high risk for failure of an osteotomy because of osteoporosis or an inability to comply with weight bearing and other activity restrictions during the postoperative period. The indications for these procedures are outlined in Tables 1 and 2.

Proximal Osteotomy With Distal Soft-Tissue Rebalancing

Traditionally, the complication rates associated with proximal osteotomies have been higher than those associated with distal osteotomies. Many authors have noted a high prevalence of dorsal malunion following proximal metatarsal osteotomies, and this is primarily due to either loss of fixation or fracture of the metatarsal once weight bearing is initiated.[5-9] Factors that may contribute to complications include patient age, bone density, and the degree of stability of the osteotomy site. The development of newer (and more expensive) fixation devices has not necessarily improved the situation. A thorough understanding of the anatomy and biomechanics of the first ray is key to avoiding complications.

Anatomic and Biomechanical Factors Associated With Bunion Correction Surgery

The biomechanics of the metatarsals in the human are unique in that they are the only long bones that support load perpendicular to their axis during most phases of gait and standing. The forces acting on the first metatarsal during gait were defined in the classic article by Stokes and associates,[10] who described the factors responsible for the forces in the metatarsal during gait; these include the inclination of the first metatarsal to the ground, the lengths of the first metatarsal and phalanges, the forces generated by the plantar muscles and soft tissues through the windlass mechanism, and the weight of the individual. These factors directly affect the forces that act on the first metatarsal: bending moment, shear, and axial load. For a given load, bending moment and shear forces increase with increasing metatarsal length and decreasing metatarsal inclination. Conversely, axial load increases and bending moment decreases as the metatarsal inclination increases.

Stokes and associates also calculated the effects of the tension generated by the plantar soft tissues on these forces.[10] Force at the metatarsal head is a combination of direct force through the plantar aspect of the foot and sesamoids and joint reaction forces across the metatarsophalangeal joint. This is an intrinsic mechanism whereby part of the force of weight bearing is transferred to axial load rather than shear and bending. Functionally, this is known as the "windlass mechanism" whereby dorsiflexion of the metatarsophalangeal joints causes increased tension in the longitudinal arch and raises the longitudinal arch of the foot. Increasing pull from the short and long toe flexors and increasing tension within the plantar fascia as the metatarsophalangeal joint rolls into dorsiflexion diminish bending moment and shear forces across the metatarsal while increasing axial load and the joint reaction force at the metatarsophalangeal joint. It should be noted that the calculations by Stokes and associates were based on an ideal model with a normal first metatarsophalangeal joint. Diminished motion at the metatarsophalangeal joint from arthritis or other pathologic conditions can decrease the function of the windlass mechanism and increase shear and bending forces through the metatarsal.[11]

The osseous anatomy must also be considered in the planning of a first metatarsal osteotomy. Metaphyseal osteotomies have the advantage of a larger surface area for osseous healing and screw fixation. Diaphyseal osteotomies involve less surface area and may be subject to higher strains due to disruption of the cortical architecture of the bone. A computerized finite-element analysis was performed by Kristen and associates[12] using a three-dimensional model derived from digitized cadaveric data to calculate stress and strain patterns in the first metatarsal. Simulated weight-bearing loads were applied across this model from 30° to 70° of dorsal extension, and stress and strain were visualized with use of von Mises stress analyses. Stresses were concentrated along the plantar aspect of the diaphysis and at the dorsolateral diaphyseal-metaphyseal junction, and slight dorsomedial deformation occurred. The authors suggested that, when performing an osteotomy, the surgeon should avoid violating these areas to minimize the chance for displacement.

In hallux valgus deformity, the anatomy of the first metatarsophalangeal joint becomes distorted and the subluxated joint capsule causes deforming forces that pull the hallux into further valgus and displace the first metatarsal head medially. This problem is primarily related to lateralization of the flexor hallucis longus, flexor hallucis brevis, and adductor hallucis tendons, which

occurs as the joint subluxates laterally and the hallux pronates.[13,14] Lateral and plantar migration of the abductor hallucis tendon and attenuation of the dorsomedial aspect of the joint capsule diminish the normal resistant forces to valgus deviation.[15] These changes, while flexible early in the disease process, tend to become rigid and fixed as time progresses. Contractures of the lateral aspect of the joint are accompanied by permanent shortening and fibrosis of those tissues and require meticulous surgical release for adequate correction. The combination of the lateralized moment across the metatarsophalangeal joint and loss of the normal balancing structures medially creates a medial deforming vector on the first metatarsal head. Saltzman and associates[16] performed a force vector analysis of these moments in a cadaveric model and noted an increase in medializing forces on the first metatarsophalangeal joint with increasing hallux valgus and supination. Translational and derotational osteotomies had minimal effect on these vectors. These authors concluded that normalization of these vectors through soft-tissue reconstruction was as important as realignment of the osseous structures in the prevention of recurrence of the deformity in the frontal plane. In a cadaver study, Coughlin and associates[17] demonstrated the importance of restoring the axial alignment of the osseous structures and that correction of the intermetatarsal angle with an osteotomy increased the stability of the first ray.

Principles Governing First Metatarsal Osteotomies

Osteotomy of the first metatarsal has been studied extensively. The geometric principles used in determin-

ing correction were explored by Kummer and Jahss.[18-20] Correction of the intermetatarsal angle is increased per degree of rotation or lateral translation as the osteotomy is moved more proximally. One degree of correction is achieved on average for each millimeter of lateral translation in distal osteotomies of the metatarsal head, and only about 5° of correction can be achieved with a distal chevron-type osteotomy because further translation will result in instability of the final construct. Moving the osteotomy more proximally moves the center of rotation, and more correction is achieved per degree of rotation. Kummer and Jahss also noted that a degree of shortening and elevation of the first metatarsal head is inherent in these osteotomies. Nyska and associates[21] performed a geometric analysis of the Ludloff, Mau, Scarf, proximal chevron, proximal crescentic, and wedge osteotomies. They noted the best correction was achieved by the Ludloff osteotomy angled 16° to the shaft; however, this caused elevation and shortening. The 8° Ludloff osteotomy provided angular corrections similar to those provided by the basilar wedge and crescentic osteotomies, but with less elevation and shortening.

The stability of first metatarsal osteotomies has been studied extensively, and these osteotomies have been classified according to their geometry[11] (Figure 2). Complete osteotomies are those that divide the metatarsal into two separate fragments. These osteotomies can achieve correction through multiplanar manipulation of the distal fragment. Incomplete opening and closing wedge osteotomies leave one cortex intact to act as a hinge, which adds stability but decreases the freedom of correction. Complete osteotomies may be classified as intrinsically stable or as intrinsically unstable (Figure 3). Intrinsic stability is present when an osteotomy incorporates the direct transfer of deforming forces from the distal fragment into the proximal fragment by nature of its geometry. For displacement into dorsiflexion, which is the primary force that causes early failure, stability is related to the sagittal orientation of the osteotomy. A limb of the osteotomy that is oriented from proximal-plantar to dorsal-distal will impart intrinsic stability to the distal fragment. Osteotomies that are intrinsically unstable are those that have no osseous resistance to deforming forces and that are entirely dependent on internal fixation for maintenance of position during osseous healing. These include any osteotomy that has a single plane oriented from dorsal-proximal to plantar-distal or is perpendicular to the shaft of the metatarsal.

Consideration should be given to the method of fixation of the metatarsal osteotomy site. Fixation of all metatarsal osteotomy sites is recommended regardless of inherent stability or instability. Distal osteotomies have intrinsic stability of great enough magnitude that Kirschner wire fixation is often adequate. Because of the increased moment arm present with proximal osteotomies, simple Kirschner wire fixation is usually inadequate for definitive fixation. Screw fixation of osteotomy sites has been proven to be biomechanically superior to pin fixation in several studies and can provide rigid fixation of some otherwise unstable constructs.[22,23] The bending strength of the screw is much greater than that of a Kirschner wire because of the screw's increased diameter, and stability to rotation can be achieved through compression of

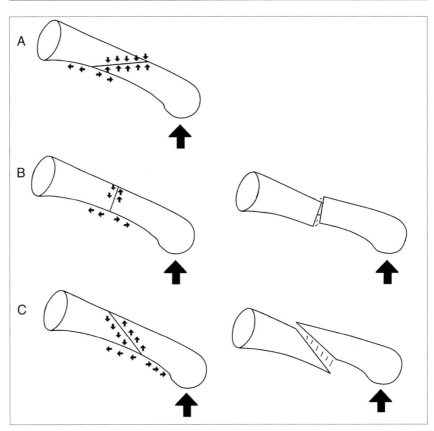

Figure 2   The effect of the orientation of the osteotomy on intrinsic stability. **A,** Sagittal orientation from dorsal-distal to proximal-plantar imparts inherent stability as a result of direct transfer of forces from the distal fragment into the proximal fragment. **B** and **C,** A vertical or a proximal-dorsal to distal-plantar orientation affords no intrinsic stability. (Reprinted with permission from Sammarco VJ, Acevedo J: Stability and fixation techniques in first metatarsal osteotomies. *Foot Ankle Clin* 2001;6:409-432.)

the osteotomy site itself. The predominant mechanical disadvantage of screw fixation is the stress risers created by their application. Fracture can occur through these stress risers once weight bearing is initiated. Use of a plate for primary fixation in bunion surgery is relatively uncommon despite mechanical and clinical data that show that they provide more stability than simple screw fixation.[24,25] Technically, application of small plates designed for fracture fixation can be quite time-consuming because of the need for finely adjusted contouring of the devices. Rigid fixation can be achieved, but this technique is

usually reserved for cases in which standard fixation is deemed inadequate intraoperatively because of osteoporosis or fracture. New, procedure-specific devices, including wedge plates and locking plates, have recently been marketed, but there are no published clinical data supporting their use and justifying their expense.

Proximal Crescentic Osteotomy
To perform a proximal crescentic osteotomy, as popularized by Mann and associates,[26-28] the surgeon uses a curved oscillating saw to create an osteotomy from the proximal-dorsal aspect of the metaphysis to the plan-

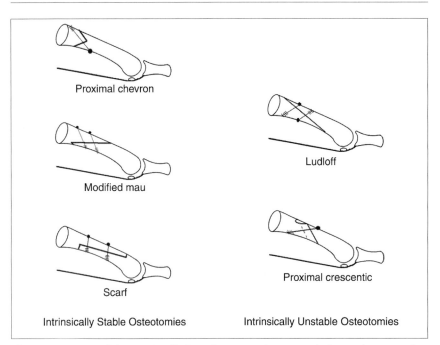

Figure 3   Some of the proximally based osteotomies currently in use for correction of varus angulation of the first metatarsal associated with hallux valgus.

tar aspect of the proximal part of the diaphysis. The intermetatarsal angle is corrected by rotating the distal fragment in the trough created in the base of the first metatarsal. Rather than simply rotating in a single plane, the distal fragment rolls in the inclined trough created by the saw blade, and medial or lateral angulation of the osteotomy will cause elevation or depression of the metatarsal head, respectively, as the distal fragment is rotated laterally.[29] The osteotomy site is fixed with a single compression screw from the dorsal cortex of the distal fragment to the plantar aspect of the metaphysis of the proximal fragment. Single-screw fixation provides little resistance to rotation about its axis, and some have found it necessary to augment fixation with an additional Kirschner wire or plate if fixation is questionable.[24,30] Failure tends to occur through fracture of the dorsal bone bridge at the screw head or by loosening of the fixation screw, allowing loss of correction and elevation of the distal fragment.[21,31] Regardless of the fixation technique, the proximal crescentic osteotomy remains one of the most unstable first metatarsal osteotomies. Biomechanical studies have shown the loads to failure following a crescentic osteotomy to be lower than those following Ludloff, proximal chevron, proximal closing wedge, Scarf, and Mau osteotomies.[22,32,33] Fatigue studies have shown stability to cyclic loading after crescentic osteotomies to be relatively inferior as well.[31] Modifying this osteotomy with a proximal crescentic shelf (a dorsal dome cut and an inferior oblique cut) does not appear to improve the relative loads to failure.[34] Stability can be improved by fixing the osteotomy site with a new procedure-specific plate.[35]

Clinical data have varied widely among studies of the proximal cres-

centic osteotomy. Brodsky and associates[36] prospectively evaluated plantar pressure measurements at a mean of 29 months after proximal crescentic osteotomy in 32 patients. Twelve patients had first metatarsal elevation of more than 2 mm, and a transfer lesion developed under the second metatarsal head in five of those patients. These authors found control of the crescentic osteotomy to be unpredictable in the sagittal plane. In a prospective, randomized study, Easley and associates[6] compared proximal chevron osteotomy with proximal crescentic osteotomy for hallux valgus correction in 84 feet followed for a minimum of 1 year. Although the clinical results were good in both groups, the sites of the proximal chevron osteotomies healed faster and a higher prevalence of dorsal malunion was seen in the group treated with the proximal crescenotic osteotomy. Thordarson and Leventen[9] reported the results of 33 proximal crescentic osteotomies done to treat hallux valgus deformity. After a minimum of 2 years of follow-up, these authors reported good clinical results but noted an average dorsiflexion malunion of 6.2° through the osteotomy site. Staple fixation was noted to be more unstable and to result in more dorsiflexion. In a retrospective study of 50 patients who had undergone hallux valgus correction with either a proximal chevron or a proximal crescentic osteotomy, Markbreiter and Thompson[37] noted equivalent good results in the two groups. Okuda and associates[38] reported excellent correction of radiographic parameters and good clinical results in a study of 47 feet followed for an average of 48 months after proximal crescentic osteotomy done to treat hallux valgus. Okuda and associates[39] also reported that the

1-year results of this procedure were predictive of the 3-year results.

Proximal Chevron Osteotomy

The distal chevron osteotomy was first described by Austin and Leventen[40] and refers to a horizontally directed V pattern that imparts inherent stability to the distal fragment. The chevron osteotomy pattern has also been used in the proximal part of the metatarsal for correction of moderate and severe metatarsus primus varus.[41,42] Biomechanically, the osteotomy site derives stability as forces are directly transferred from the distal fragment to the proximal fragment through the dorsal shelf. The osteotomy should be directed with the apex distal, as directing the apex proximally creates a stress riser in the proximal fragment adjacent to the articular surface and may result in a fracture into the first tarsometatarsal articulation.[6] Directing the apex distally moves the stress riser distally and into the distal fragment, thus diminishing the moment arm and eliminating the risk of intra-articular fracture should failure occur. The osteotomy site is fixed from plantar to proximal-dorsal, which provides compression on the tension side of the osteotomy. The screw should not be applied from dorsal to plantar because that concentrates stresses at the apex of the osteotomy and predisposes the bone to fracture under low loads.[32]

The chevron osteotomy has been studied biomechanically to determine its corrective potential and stability. Nyska and associates[21] found that less correction was achieved with the proximal chevron osteotomy than with the Ludloff, crescentic, and closing wedge osteotomies; however, correction was achieved by lateral translation only, without rota-

tion. According to Kummer's analysis, the proximal chevron osteotomy can achieve high levels of correction if the distal fragment is rotated with translation, as is commonly done in clinical practice.[18] McCluskey and associates[33] compared stiffness and load to failure between cadaveric models of proximal crescentic and proximal chevron osteotomies and noted greater stability with the proximal chevron technique. In a study of the Ludloff, Scarf, biplanar closing wedge, Mau, proximal chevron, and proximal crescentic osteotomies in cadaveric preparations, Trnka and associates[32] noted less stability with the proximal chevron osteotomy than with the others tested except for the proximal crescentic osteotomy; however, the fixation screw was placed dorsally rather than plantarly, which allows distraction of the plantar cortex during loading. It is possible that this study demonstrated the importance of using a plantar-based screw rather than identifying an inherent problem with the osteotomy. Acevedo and associates[31] studied five osteotomies in a cyclic loading model and found the site of the proximal chevron osteotomy to be stronger than all others tested in both Sawbones and cadaveric models with a screw placed from plantar to dorsal.

Correction of hallux valgus with the proximal chevron osteotomy has reportedly yielded good clinical results with few complications. Sammarco and associates[41] reported on 43 patients who had undergone surgical correction of hallux valgus with a proximal chevron osteotomy for correction of the intermetatarsal angle.[41] No malunions were found, and the AOFAS score improved significantly. Sammarco and Russo-Alesi[43] reported the results of 72 consecutive procedures after an av-

erage duration of follow-up of 41 months. Again, dorsal malunion was not observed, and improvement in the AOFAS scores was noted. Easley and associates[6] reported good clinical results after both the proximal chevron and the proximal crescentic osteotomy but noted a lower complication rate and faster healing of the osteotomy site after the proximal chevron osteotomy. Those authors thought that improved stability of the osteotomy site was responsible for these outcomes. Markbreiter and Thompson[37] reported the results in 50 feet in which either a proximal crescentic or a chevron osteotomy had been done for the correction of hallux valgus. Excellent results were reported in both groups, but the proximal chevron osteotomy was thought to be technically easier to perform because of its inherent stability.

Scarf Osteotomy

The Scarf osteotomy was introduced to the surgical community by Zygmunt and associates,[44] and its use for the correction of moderate and severe metatarsus primus varus has steadily increased in Europe and elsewhere. As originally described, the osteotomy is horizontal in the distal part of the diaphysis, with a limb exiting superiorly at the distal end of the metatarsal and a limb exiting proximally at the midpart of the diaphysis. The osteotomy provides tremendous inherent stability to displacement as a result of the long dorsal shelf afforded with the horizontal saw cut. The originally described osteotomy achieved correction by lateral translation of the distal fragment. Barouk[45] and Weil[46] proposed numerous modifications, including lengthening or shortening of the metatarsal, rotation of the distal fragment, raising or lowering of the metatarsal head, and correction of the distal metatarsal articular angle by rotation of the distal fragment. Nyska and associates[21] noted less correction of the intermetatarsal angle with the Scarf osteotomy than with the Ludloff, closing wedge, and crescentic osteotomies.

Barouk's modifications extend the osteotomy proximally, which allows greater correction of the intermetatarsal angle but also increases the moment arm on the dorsal shelf, and fracture of the metatarsal has been reported as a complication.[47,48] Trnka and associates[32] performed static load-to-failure testing in cadavers in which the Scarf osteotomy had been performed and compared the results with those after five other osteotomies of the first metatarsal. They found that the osteotomy site was stable and concluded that it should be acceptable for patients with normal bone density to immediately bear weight in a postoperative shoe. In their study, however, the osteotomy did not include the proximal extension that is currently used to achieve greater corrections of the intermetatarsal angle. Acevedo and associates[31] performed cyclic loading of the sites of Scarf osteotomies in Sawbones models and found substantial problems with fracture of the metatarsal at the proximal part of the dorsal limb. There may also be problems with positioning of the final construct as a result of the diaphyseal nature of the osteotomy. Because the osteotomy divides the metatarsal horizontally along its length, the distal fragment may rotate axially as the medial cortex of the distal fragment slides into the medullary canal of the proximal fragment, causing undesired elevation and supination of the distal articular surface (so-called troughing).[11,47]

Clinical studies of the Scarf osteotomy have demonstrated mixed results. Aminian and associates[49] evaluated the results of 27 consecutive Scarf osteotomies at an average of 16 months. The complication rate was low, and the AOFAS scores improved. Fracture of the metatarsal was not noted. Jones and associates[50] reviewed the results at a mean of 20 months after 35 Scarf osteotomies were done for hallux valgus correction. Excellent correction was achieved, as demonstrated radiographically and clinically, and pedobarographic measurements made after more than 1 year were noted to be normalized. One intraoperative fracture was noted, but no postoperative stress fractures occurred. The authors concluded that the procedure is effective, with reproducible results, for correction of moderate and severe deformity. Coetzee[47] reported less promising clinical results after 20 Scarf osteotomies. Malunion from troughing, malrotation, and fracture were responsible for major complications despite postoperative immobilization in a short leg cast for 6 weeks. Forty-five percent of the patients were dissatisfied with the result of the surgery after 1 year. At an average of 22 months following 84 Scarf osteotomies, Crevoisier and associates[51] noted improvement in radiographic parameters and AOFAS scores, although 11% of the patients were not satisfied and required additional procedures. Problems with the fixation of the osteotomy site and stiffness of the first metatarsophalangeal joint occurred. Fracture was not reported.

Ludloff Osteotomy

The metatarsal osteotomy described by Ludloff extends from the dorsal aspect of the metaphysis proximally to the plantar aspect of the diaphysis distally. Despite the inherent instability of its geometry, the Ludloff osteotomy affords a broad surface for screw fixation, which substantially increases the relative strength of the construct. Some biomechanical studies have shown the load-to-failure values after the Ludloff osteotomy to be superior to those after the proximal chevron or crescentic osteotomies. Lian and associates[22] noted that a Ludloff osteotomy site fixed with two screws was 82% stronger than the site of a crescentic osteotomy fixed with a single screw. Using a cadaver model, Trnka and associates[32] noted that, compared with five other constructs, the Ludloff osteotomy provided excellent stability and stiffness. Acevedo and associates[31] noted that the Ludloff osteotomy resulted in excellent fatigue endurance under cyclic loading in both a cadaver and a Sawbones model. The osteotomy site is fixed with two screws, which compress the proximal and distal fragments in diaphyseal bone. When loaded to failure, the osteotomy site fails either by fracture of the metatarsal at the proximal screw head or from pullout of the screw threads. In a Sawbones model, Nyska and associates[21] noted that the sagittal inclination of the Ludloff osteotomy plays a large role in the amount that the intermetatarsal angle can be corrected.[52] A 16° angulation allowed the most correction but also caused shortening and elevation of the first metatarsal head, whereas an 8° angulation afforded correction comparable with that provided by other proximal osteotomies without substantial shortening or elevation. Beischer and associates[53] noted that 10° is the ideal orientation for correction without shortening or elevation.

The Ludloff osteotomy with

screw fixation for correction of hallux valgus has had excellent clinical results to date. Chiodo and associates[54] reviewed the results of 70 procedures for correction of moderate and severe hallux valgus. After an average duration of follow-up of 30 months, the satisfaction rate was 94% and few complications had developed. The authors noted that fixation was inadequate in two patients who had required a steeper osteotomy in the sagittal plane. These two osteotomy sites healed with callus formation and slight shortening, and elevation of the first metatarsal was noted on the final follow-up radiographs. Improved fixation methods may negate these issues.[30,55-57] Petroutsas and Trnka[58] reported the results in 70 patients at a minimum of 2 years after they had undergone a Ludloff osteotomy for hallux valgus repair. Radiographic measurements had improved. Evaluation with a four-point clinical scale showed that 81% of the patients were satisfied or very satisfied, but 5% had continued pain.

Mau Osteotomy

The osteotomy described by Mau and Lauber[59] is an oblique diaphyseal osteotomy that is directed from proximal-plantar to distal-dorsal. With this procedure, as originally described, the angular correction that can be achieved by rotation of the distal fragment is less than that possible with the more proximal osteotomies. Nyska and associates[21] showed that both the 8° and the 16° Mau osteotomies provide angular correction without substantial elevation but the correction is greater with the Ludloff osteotomy, probably because of the more proximal center of rotation. Although clinical comparison studies of the Mau osteotomy are lacking, mechanical

testing has shown that it provides superior stability. Both static and dynamic fatigue studies have shown Mau osteotomy sites to be more stable than the sites of other proximal and shaft osteotomies, including the Scarf and the Ludloff procedures.[31,32] In one clinical study with a short follow-up (18 weeks), Neese and associates[60] noted a low prevalence of shortening and malunion. More long-term prospective trials are needed to determine the clinical efficacy of the procedure. This osteotomy was modified with a second cut through the plantar metaphyseal cortex, which allows it to be extended more proximally to gain more substantial correction while taking advantage of its superior biomechanical properties (Figure 4). A detailed description of the author's preferred surgical technique for the modified Mau osteotomy was recently published.[61]

Arthrodesis of the Hallux Metatarsophalangeal Joint for Treatment of Hallux Valgus

Arthrodesis of the first metatarsophalangeal joint for the treatment of hallux valgus is a salvage procedure that is primarily used when more standard bunion correction procedures will not provide durable results or pain relief or have a high risk of early failure. Coughlin and associates[62] reported the results of arthrodesis for the treatment of 21 moderate or severe cases of idiopathic hallux valgus. Arthrodesis was considered for moderate bunions if degenerative changes of the first metatarsophalangeal joint were seen radiographically or if there was advanced deformity of the lesser metatarsophalangeal joints. Primary arthrodesis was considered for severe deformity in which the hallux valgus angle was more than 40°, re-

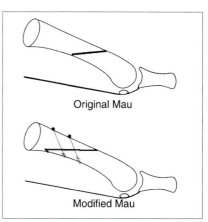

Figure 4 Modification of the Mau osteotomy moves the osteotomy proximally into the metaphysis and the proximal part of the diaphysis of the bone. This allows greater correction of the intermetatarsal angle and provides more predictable healing. (Reprinted with permission from Sammarco VJ: Surgical strategies: Mau osteotomy for correction of moderate and severe hallux valgus deformity. *Foot Ankle Int* 2007;28:857-864.)

gardless of the presence of degenerative changes or involvement of the lesser metatarsophalangeal joints. Three nonunions occurred; two were asymptomatic and one was revised to a fusion, which was successful. All patients were considered to have a good or excellent result at the time of final follow-up, at an average of 8.2 years (range, 24 to 272 months). Similarly, Riggs and Johnson[63] noted that in most cases arthrodesis for the treatment of hallux valgus was successful at the time of short- or long-term follow-up (range, 1 to 15 years), with resolution of pain in 92% of patients. Overall satisfaction was rated at 86%, although hardware frequently had to be removed (in 30% of the cases) and the rate of complications, including infection and failure, was 8%. Tourné and associates[64] suggested that arthrodesis of the metatarsophalangeal joint was a predict-

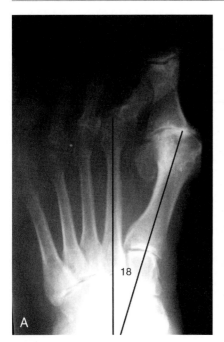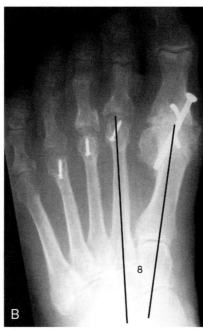

Figure 5 **A,** Correction of hallux valgus deformity with an arthrodesis should be considered if there is substantial arthritis of the metatarsophalangeal joint. **B,** Note the correction of the intermetatarsal angle without osteotomy of the first metatarsal.

able method for managing hallux valgus deformity in elderly individuals. Arthrodesis should also be considered the primary treatment of hallux valgus in patients with clinically relevant osteoarthritis or inflammatory arthritis of the metatarsophalangeal joint, as reconstructive procedures designed to restore axial alignment do not address the underlying loss of cartilage or destruction of the normal supporting structures.[65,66] Hallux valgus associated with spasticity, as is commonly seen in patients with cerebral palsy, has a high recurrence rate when treated with standard techniques. Davids and associates[4] reviewed 26 cases of hallux valgus managed with arthrodesis of the first metatarsophalangeal joint in children with cerebral palsy. They noted high satisfaction among both patients and caregivers, with excellent radiographic and clinical correction. They recommended fusion for pri-

mary treatment in children with a spastic foot deformity.

Salvage following failed bunion surgery is technically demanding, and attempts at revision are associated with increased failure rates. If a specific cause for the failure can be identified, it may be possible to revise the previous bunion surgery successfully, but arthrodesis can usually be used for salvage in difficult cases in which nonunion, osteonecrosis, or extensive arthritis is present. Grimes and Coughlin[67] reported 33 cases in which a failure of hallux valgus surgery was treated with arthrodesis of the metatarsophalangeal joint. Four nonunions resulted, three of which were asymptomatic. Radiographic correction was excellent in all cases. Although the patients with failed bunion surgery had improvement following the arthrodesis, the final results were worse than the final results of successful primary bunion

surgery. Kitaoka and Patzer[68] noted that, compared with successful primary procedures, arthrodeses done to revise failed bunion surgery resulted in similar improvements in scores but less patient satisfaction. These authors also observed that the results of the arthrodeses were slightly better than those of resection arthroplasties for salvage following failed bunion surgery. Myerson and associates[69] described staged arthrodesis for the management of failed bunion surgery associated with osteomyelitis. Several studies have shown that arthrodesis of the first metatarsophalangeal joint will correct an even substantially increased intermetatarsal angle, and metatarsal osteotomy is typically not necessary[70] (Figure 5).

Biomechanical studies may help surgeons to select the appropriate technique for arthrodesis of the metatarsophalangeal joint. A more stable construct theoretically allows a higher fusion rate and permits earlier weight bearing. Joint preparation is usually done through a dorsal or medial incision. Preparation with matched cuts made with a straight or crescentic saw or a "cup-in-cone" arthrodesis bed prepared with a high-speed burr or with matched conical reamers has been reported. In cadaveric models of arthrodeses of the first metatarsophalangeal joint, Curtis and associates[71] noted that machined conical reaming followed by fixation with interfragmentary screws provided more strength than preparation with matched planar cuts regardless of the fixation technique, including the use of a dorsal plate. In a study involving mechanical testing of five fusion models in cadavers, Politi and associates[72] similarly noted that conical reaming provided improved strength compared with that provid-

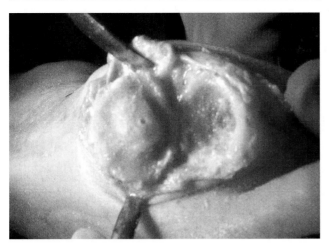

Figure 6 The cup-in-cone arthrodesis bed is created by denuding cartilage and subchondral bone with a 5-mm burr to create matching fusion surfaces.

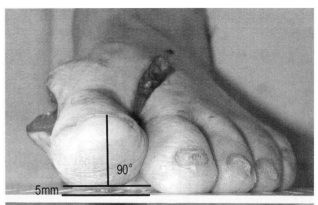

Figure 7 A lid from an instrument set can be used to gauge dorsiflexion intraoperatively. Approximately 5 mm of clearance of the pulp of the digit from the floor is desired to allow roll-off of the hallux. Care should be taken to fix the toe rotation so that it is neutral to the axis of the foot.

ed by planar excision. The strongest construct in this study was created by matched conical reaming and use of a dorsal compression plate and a single oblique lag screw. A review of the available mechanical data shows plate-and-screw fixation to be the most stable, followed by interfragmentary or intramedullary screw fixation, both of which are superior to fixation with Kirschner wires or compression staples.[73-75]

Author's Preferred Technique: Cup-in-Cone Arthrodesis With Crossed Screws

The preferred technique is based on an attempt to balance the available biomechanical data with current constraints imposed by implant cost and the surgical time required for the procedure. The costs of specialized plates, compression staples, and cannulated screws must be balanced against the surgeon's ability to achieve successful results with less expensive, generic solid screws and fracture plates. It has been my experience that even the use of precontoured plates substantially increases

operating room time and can be associated with incorrect alignment of the arthrodesis. At least three commercially manufactured conical reaming systems are currently available for this procedure, but they must usually be rented or purchased or are paired with an implant system. Surgeons must take care when learning to use these systems because fractures of both the metatarsal head and the proximal phalanx have been seen with use of these reamers. The cup-in-cone preparation described by Myerson is done through a dorsal incision and with use of a standard, inexpensive 5-mm burr[76] (Figure 6). The first metatarsal head is denuded of any remaining cartilage and subchondral bone until the underlying cancellous bone is exposed. The proximal phalanx is similarly prepared to create the recipient "cup," following removal of cartilage and subchondral bone. Final adjustments are made with the burr for positioning, and the metatarsophalangeal joint is stabilized with a Kirschner wire and checked for alignment. The arthro-

desis site can be secured with two 4.0-mm cannulated or noncannulated cancellous screws. If stability is poor secondary to osteoporosis or bone loss, a contoured one-third tubular plate will substantially improve fixation.

Final positioning should consist of 10° to 20° of hallux valgus, but care must be taken to allow clearance of the second toe by 1 to 2 mm. Dorsiflexion should be 15° to 30° from the first metatarsal, or 5° to 10° from the floor. A good way to assess the final position intraoperatively is to press the foot flat on a sterile plate (an instrument case lid) (Figure 7). The hallux should not impinge on the second toe, rotation should be neutral with the axis of the floor, and there should be approximately 5 mm of space between the plate and the pulp of the hallux. Malpositioning is the most common complication associated with this surgery. Plantar flexion and malrotation are associated with secondary arthritis of the interphalangeal joint. Excessive dorsiflexion may cause difficulty with shoe wear and transfer lesions at the lesser metatarsophalangeal joints. After the surgery, the patient wears a postoperative shoe with weight bearing on the heel for 4 to 6 weeks or until fusion is evident radiographically.

Summary

Hallux valgus correction with distal soft-tissue release and proximal metatarsal osteotomy is the procedure of choice for most patients with a symptomatic moderate or severe hallux valgus deformity. Complications can be avoided by selecting a procedure that provides adequate correction of the intermetatarsal angle and ensuring proper balancing of the first metatarsophalangeal joint through lateral soft-tissue releases and medial joint plication. Arthrodesis of the first metatarsophalangeal joint should be considered when revision of failed bunion surgery is planned or when degenerative joint disease is present. Arthrodesis should also be considered if the likelihood of failure of a standard bunion procedure is high, such as in elderly individuals with osteoporosis, patients with severe deformity and substantial involvement of the lesser metatarsophalangeal joints, and those with neuromuscular spasticity.

References

1. Position statement on cosmetic foot surgery. American Orthopaedic Foot and Ankle Society; Rosemont, Illinois. 2003. Available at: http://www.aofas.org/i4a/pages/index.cfm?pageid=367 2. Accessed August 8, 2007.

2. Sammarco VJ, Nichols R: Orthotic management for disorders of the hallux. *Foot Ankle Clin* 2005;10:191-209.

3. Mann RA, Coughlin MJ (eds): *Surgery of the Foot and Ankle*. St. Louis, MO, Mosby, 1993, pp 167-296.

4. Davids JR, Mason TA, Danko A, Banks D, Blackhurst D: Surgical management of hallux valgus deformity in children with cerebral palsy. *J Pediatr Orthop* 2001;21:89-94.

5. Acevedo JI: Fixation of metatarsal osteotomies in the treatment of hallux valgus. *Foot Ankle Clin* 2000;5: 451-468.

6. Easley ME, Kiebzak GM, Davis WH, Anderson RB: Prospective, randomized comparison of proximal crescentic and proximal chevron osteotomies for correction of hallux valgus deformity. *Foot Ankle Int* 1996;17:307-316.

7. Gill LH: Distal osteotomy for bunionectomy and hallux valgus correction. *Foot Ankle Clin* 2001;6:433-453.

8. Pearson SW, Kitaoka HB, Cracchiolo A, Leventen EO: Results and complications following a proximal curved osteotomy of the hallux metatarsal. *Contemp Orthop* 1991;23:127-132.

9. Thordarson DB, Leventen EO: Hallux valgus correction with proximal metatarsal osteotomy: Two-year follow-up. *Foot Ankle* 1992;13: 321-326.

10. Stokes IA, Hutton WC, Stott JR: Forces acting on the metatarsals during normal walking. *J Anat* 1979;129: 579-590.

11. Sammarco VJ, Acevedo J: Stability and fixation techniques in first metatarsal osteotomies. *Foot Ankle Clin* 2001;6:409-432.

12. Kristen KH, Berger K, Berger C, Kampla W, Anzböck W, Weitzel SH: The first metatarsal bone under loading conditions: A finite element analysis. *Foot Ankle Clin* 2005;10:1-14.

13. Alvarez R, Haddad RJ, Gould N, Trevino S: The simple bunion: Anatomy at the metatarsophalangeal joint of the great toe. *Foot Ankle* 1984;4:229-240.

14. Jahss MH: Hallux valgus: Further considerations: The first metatarsal head. *Foot Ankle* 1981;2:1-4.

15. Scranton PE Jr, Rutkowski R: Anatomic variations in the first ray: Part II. Disorders of the sesamoids. *Clin Orthop Relat Res* 1980;151:256-264.

16. Saltzman CL, Aper RL, Brown TD: Anatomic determinants of first metatarsophalangeal flexion moments in hallux valgus. *Clin Orthop Relat Res* 1997;339:261-269.

17. Coughlin MJ, Jones CP, Viladot R, et al: Hallux valgus and first ray mobility: A cadaveric study. *Foot Ankle Int* 2004;25:537-544.

18. Kummer FJ: Mathematical analysis of first metatarsal osteotomies. *Foot Ankle* 1989;9:281-289.

19. Jahss MH, Troy AI, Kummer F: Roentgenographic and mathematical analysis of first metatarsal osteotomies for metatarsus primus varus: A comparative study. *Foot Ankle* 1985;5: 280-321.

20. Kummer F, Jahss M: Mathematical analysis of foot and ankle osteotomies, in Jahss M (ed): *Disorders of the Foot and Ankle: Medical and Surgical Management*. Philadelphia, PA, WB Saunders, 1991, pp 541-563.

21. Nyska M, Trnka HJ, Parks BG, Myerson MS: Proximal metatarsal osteotomies: A comparative geometric analysis conducted on sawbone models. *Foot Ankle Int* 2002;23:938-945.

22. Lian GJ, Markolf K, Cracchiolo A III: Strength of fixation constructs for basilar osteotomies of the first metatarsal. *Foot Ankle* 1992;13:509-514.

23. Shereff MJ, Sobel MA, Kummer FJ: The stability of fixation of first metatarsal osteotomies. *Foot Ankle* 1991;11: 208-211.

24. Rosenberg GA, Donley BG: Plate augmentation of screw fixation of proximal crescentic osteotomy of the first metatarsal. *Foot Ankle Int* 2003;24: 570-571.

25. Campbell JT, Schon LC, Parks BG, Wang Y, Berger BI: Mechanical comparison of biplanar proximal closing wedge osteotomy with plantar plate fixation versus crescentic osteotomy with screw fixation for the correction of metatarsus primus varus. *Foot Ankle Int* 1998;19:293-299.

26. Mann RA, Rudicel S, Graves SC: Repair of hallux valgus with a distal soft-tissue procedure and proximal meta-

tarsal osteotomy: A long-term follow-up. *J Bone Joint Surg Am* 1992;74: 124-129.

27. Mann RA: Distal soft tissue procedure and proximal metatarsal osteotomy for correction of hallux valgus deformity. *Orthopedics* 1990;13: 1013-1018.

28. Mann RA: Hallux valgus. *Instr Course Lect* 1986;35:339-353.

29. Jones C, Coughlin M, Villadot R, Golanó P: Proximal crescentic metatarsal osteotomy: The effect of saw blade orientation on first ray elevation. *Foot Ankle Int* 2005;26:152-157.

30. Jung HG, Guyton GP, Parks BG, et al: Supplementary axial Kirschner wire fixation for crescentic and Ludloff proximal metatarsal osteotomies: A biomechanical study. *Foot Ankle Int* 2005;26:620-626.

31. Acevedo JI, Sammarco VJ, Boucher HR, Parks BG, Schon LC, Myerson MS: Mechanical comparison of cyclic loading in five different first metatarsal shaft osteotomies. *Foot Ankle Int* 2002;23:711-716.

32. Trnka HJ, Parks BG, Ivanic G, et al: Six first metatarsal shaft osteotomies: Mechanical and immobilization comparisons. *Clin Orthop Relat Res* 2000; 381:256-265.

33. McCluskey LC, Johnson JE, Wynarsky GT, Harris GF: Comparison of stability of proximal crescentic metatarsal osteotomy and proximal horizontal "V" osteotomy. *Foot Ankle Int* 1994;15:263-270.

34. Earll M, Wayne J, Caldwell P, Adelaar R: Comparison of two proximal osteotomies for the treatment of hallux valgus. *Foot Ankle Int* 1998;19: 425-429.

35. Jones C, Coughlin M, Petersen W, Herbot M, Paletta J: Mechanical comparison of two types of fixation for proximal first metatarsal crescentic osteotomy. *Foot Ankle Int* 2005;26: 371-374.

36. Brodsky JW, Beischer AD, Robinson AH, Westra S, Negrine JP, Shabat S: Surgery for hallux valgus with proximal crescentic osteotomy causes vari-

able postoperative pressure patterns. *Clin Orthop Relat Res* 2006;443: 280-286.

37. Markbreiter LA, Thompson FM: Proximal metatarsal osteotomy in hallux valgus correction: A comparison of Crescentic and Chevron procedures. *Foot Ankle Int* 1997;18:71-76.

38. Okuda R, Kinoshita M, Morikawa J, Jotoku T, Abe M: Distal soft tissue procedure and proximal metatarsal osteotomy in hallux valgus. *Clin Orthop Relat Res* 2000;379:209-217.

39. Okuda R, Kinoshita M, Morikawa J, Yasuda T, Abe M: Proximal metatarsal osteotomy: Relation between 1- to greater than 3-years results. *Clin Orthop Relat Res* 2005;435:191-196.

40. Austin DW, Leventen EO: A new osteotomy for hallux valgus: A horizontally directed "V" displacement osteotomy of the metatarsal head for hallux valgus and primus varus. *Clin Orthop Relat Res* 1981;157:25-30.

41. Sammarco GJ, Brainard BJ, Sammarco VJ: Bunion correction using proximal Chevron osteotomy. *Foot Ankle* 1993;14:8-14.

42. Sammarco GJ, Conti SF: Proximal Chevron metatarsal osteotomy: Single incision technique. *Foot Ankle* 1993;14:44-47.

43. Sammarco GJ, Russo-Alesi FG: Bunion correction using proximal chevron osteotomy: A single-incision technique. *Foot Ankle Int* 1998;19: 430-437.

44. Zygmunt KH, Gudas CJ, Laros GS: Z-bunionectomy with internal screw fixation. *J Am Podiatr Med Assoc* 1989; 79:322-329.

45. Barouk LS: Scarf osteotomy for hallux valgus correction: Local anatomy, surgical technique, and combination with other forefoot procedures. *Foot Ankle Clin* 2000;5:525-558.

46. Weil LS: Scarf osteotomy for correction of hallux valgus: Historical perspective, surgical technique, and results. *Foot Ankle Clin* 2000;5:559-580.

47. Coetzee JC: Scarf osteotomy for hallux valgus repair: The dark side. *Foot Ankle Int* 2003;24:29-33.

48. Miller JM, Stuck R, Sartori M, Patwardhan A, Cane R, Vrbos L: The inverted Z bunionectomy: Quantitative analysis of the scarf and inverted scarf bunionectomy osteotomies in fresh cadaveric matched pair specimens. *J Foot Ankle Surg* 1994;33:455-462.

49. Aminian A, Kelikian A, Moen T: Scarf osteotomy for hallux valgus deformity: An intermediate followup of clinical and radiographic outcomes. *Foot Ankle Int* 2006;27:883-886.

50. Jones S, Al Hussainy HA, Ali F, Betts RP, Flowers MJ: Scarf osteotomy for hallux valgus: A prospective clinical and pedobarographic study. *J Bone Joint Surg Br* 2004;86:830-836.

51. Crevoisier X, Mouhsine E, Ortolano V, Udin B, Dutoit M: The scarf osteotomy for the treatment of hallux valgus deformity: A review of 84 cases. *Foot Ankle Int* 2001;22:970-976.

52. Nyska M, Trnka HJ, Parks BG, Myerson MS: The Ludloff metatarsal osteotomy: Guidelines for optimal correction based on a geometric analysis conducted on a sawbone model. *Foot Ankle Int* 2003;24:34-39.

53. Beischer AD, Ammon P, Corniou A, Myerson M: Three-dimensional computer analysis of the modified Ludloff osteotomy. *Foot Ankle Int* 2005;26:627-632.

54. Chiodo CP, Schon LC, Myerson MS: Clinical results with the Ludloff osteotomy for correction of adult hallux valgus. *Foot Ankle Int* 2004;25: 532-536.

55. Schon LC, Dom KJ, Jung HG: Clinical tip: Stabilization of the proximal Ludloff osteotomy. *Foot Ankle Int* 2005;26:579-581.

56. Bae SY, Schon LC: Surgical strategies: Ludloff first metatarsal osteotomy. *Foot Ankle Int* 2007;28:137-144.

57. Stamatis ED, Navid DO, Parks BG, Myerson MS: Strength of fixation of Ludloff metatarsal osteotomy utilizing three different types of Kirschner wires: A biomechanical study. *Foot Ankle Int* 2003;24:805-811.

58. Petroutsas J, Trnka HJ: The Ludloff osteotomy for correction of hallux

valgus. *Oper Orthop Traumatol* 2005; 17:102-117.

59. Mau C, Lauber HJ: Die operative behandlung des hallux valgus. *Deutsche Zeit Orthop* 1926;197:361-377.

60. Neese DJ, Zelichowski JE, Patton GW: Mau osteotomy: An alternative procedure to the closing abductory base wedge osteotomy. *J Foot Surg* 1989;28:352-362.

61. Sammarco VJ: Surgical strategies: Mau osteotomy for correction of moderate and severe hallux valgus deformity. *Foot Ankle Int* 2007;28: 857-864.

62. Coughlin MJ, Grebing BR, Jones CP: Arthrodesis of the first metatarsophalangeal joint for idiopathic hallux valgus: Intermediate results. *Foot Ankle Int* 2005;26:783-792.

63. Riggs SA Jr, Johnson EW Jr: McKeever arthrodesis for the painful hallux. *Foot Ankle* 1983;3:248-253.

64. Tourné Y, Saragaglia D, Zattara A, et al: Hallux valgus in the elderly: Metatarsophalangeal arthrodesis of the first ray. *Foot Ankle Int* 1997;18: 195-198.

65. Mann RA, Thompson FM: Arthrodesis of the first metatarsophalangeal joint for hallux valgus in rheumatoid arthritis: 1984. *Foot Ankle Int* 1997;18: 65-67.

66. Lipscomb PR: Arthrodesis of the first metatarsophalangeal joint for severe bunions and hallux rigidus. *Clin Orthop Relat Res* 1979;142:48-54.

67. Grimes JS, Coughlin MJ: First metatarsophalangeal joint arthrodesis as a treatment for failed hallux valgus surgery. *Foot Ankle Int* 2006;27:887-893.

68. Kitaoka HB, Patzer GL: Salvage treatment of failed hallux valgus operations with proximal first metatarsal osteotomy and distal soft-tissue reconstruction. *Foot Ankle Int* 1998;19: 127-131.

69. Myerson MS, Miller SD, Henderson MR, Saxby T: Staged arthrodesis for salvage of the septic hallux metatarsophalangeal joint. *Clin Orthop Relat Res* 1994;307:174-181.

70. Cronin JJ, Limbers JP, Kutty S, Stephens MM: Intermetatarsal angle after first metatarsophalangeal joint arthrodesis for hallux valgus. *Foot Ankle Int* 2006;27:104-109.

71. Curtis MJ, Myerson M, Jinnah RH, Cox QG, Alexander I: Arthrodesis of the first metatarsophalangeal joint: A biomechanical study of internal fixation techniques. *Foot Ankle* 1993;14: 395-399.

72. Politi J, John H, Njus G, Bennett GL, Kay DB: First metatarsal-phalangeal joint arthrodesis: A biomechanical assessment of stability. *Foot Ankle Int* 2003;24:332-337.

73. Neufeld SK, Parks BG, Naseef GS, Melamed EA, Schon LC: Arthrodesis of the first metatarsophalangeal joint: A biomechanical study comparing memory compression staples, cannulated screws, and a dorsal plate. *Foot Ankle Int* 2002;23:97-101.

74. Molloy S, Burkhart BG, Jasper LE, Solan MC, Campbell JT, Belkoff SM: Biomechanical comparison of two fixation methods for first metatarsophalangeal joint arthrodesis. *Foot Ankle Int* 2003;24:169-171.

75. Rongstad KM, Miller GJ, Vander Griend RA, Cowin D: A biomechanical comparison of four fixation methods of first metatarsophalangeal joint arthrodesis. *Foot Ankle Int* 1994;15: 415-419.

76. Myerson MS (ed): Foot and ankle disorders, in *Arthrodesis of the Midfoot and Forefoot Joints*. Philadelphia, PA, WB Saunders, 2000, pp 972-998.

Arthrodesis of the First Metatarsophalangeal Joint

Richard M. Marks, MD

Abstract

Arthrodesis of the first metatarsophalangeal joint is indicated in patients with symptomatic arthrodesis or advanced hallux valgus deformities that are unresponsive to nonsurgical treatment. Several fixation techniques have been described, including interfragmentary compression screws and/or dorsal plate fixation. Using these modern fixation techniques, the rate of fusion is between 94% to 98%, with high patient satisfaction. Appropriate positioning of the fusion is important for satisfactory outcome.

Fusion or arthrodesis of the first metatarsophalangeal (MTP) joint is performed principally to treat advanced hallux rigidus with concomitant symptoms secondary to arthritis (Figure 1). Patients with symptomatic arthrosis of the first MTP joint will report discomfort while walking and during activities such as squatting, and inflammation is noted at rest. Motion of the first MTP joint is limited and symptoms are exacerbated by axial loading and compression (grind test).

Indications

Arthrodesis of the first MTP joint is also indicated in patients with advanced hallux valgus deformities not amenable to standard surgical correction of the bunion, or those patients with hallux valgus with concomitant arthrosis and/or limited motion. Failed bunion surgery that results in recurrence, pain, and stiffness is also a relative indication for fusion of the joint (Figure 2). In patients with inflammatory arthritides with concomitant hallux valgus, fusion of the first MTP joint[1,2] is often needed because of the high recurrence rate of hallux valgus deformity after standard bunion corrective procedures, secondary to incompetency of the soft-tissue envelope (Figure 3). Similarly, those individuals with hallux valgus deformity secondary to stroke, cerebral palsy, or head injury should undergo fusion of the joint because of spasticity and the unreliable outcome of standard hallux valgus correction.

A failed Keller resection arthroplasty[3] (Figure 4) or failed MTP joint arthroplasty with either a Silastic implant or metal prosthesis[4] (Figure 5) are additional indications for surgery. These patients often have shortening of the hallux, cock-up deformity, and transfer metatarsalgia. Varying degrees of bone loss may coexist, which may require an interpositional bone graft to restore appropriate hallux length.

Nonsurgical options for the treatment of symptomatic arthrosis include the use of a Morton's extension, which provides rigidity to the medial column as well as stiffening of the patient's shoe sole, with or without the use of a forefoot rocker. The use of nonsteroidal anti-inflammatory drugs and modalities may be beneficial.

Surgical Technique

Fusion of the first MTP joint is performed under an ankle block combined with intravenous sedation. A 4-inch bandage is used to exsanguinate the foot and ankle and is wrapped at the level of the ankle over a 4-inch sterile pad, which serves as a tourniquet. Several incisions for approach to the joint have been described. The medial approach, while cosmetically pleasing, tends to make mobilization of the lateral soft tissues more difficult. The dorsomedial approach is to be avoided because of the potential for damage to the dorsomedial cutaneous branch of the superficial peroneal nerve. The author's preference is to approach the joint through the dorsal approach.

The dorsal approach is performed over the dorsal midline of the joint, just medial to the extensor hallucis longus (EHL) tendon. In advanced stages of hallux valgus, the incision should follow the

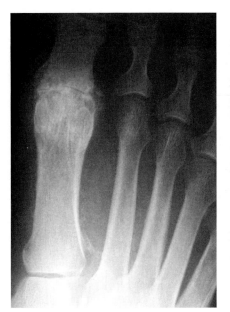

Figure 1 AP radiograph of a patient with advanced degenerative changes of the first MTP joint.

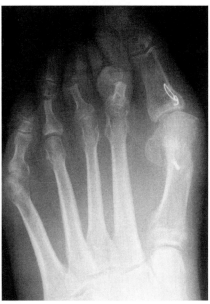

Figure 2 AP radiograph of recurrent hallux valgus deformity with concomitant arthrosis.

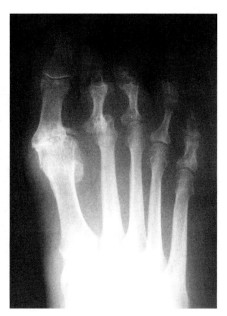

Figure 3 AP radiograph of a patient with inflammatory arthritis, hallux valgus, and advanced degenerative changes of the first MTP joint.

dorsal contours of the base of the proximal phalanx and distal metatarsal joint. The incision is started at the midportion of the proximal phalanx and carried 4 cm proximal to the joint to allow for adequate exposure of the medial, lateral, and plantar soft tissues while avoiding soft-tissue compromise.

The incision is carried down to the level of the EHL tendon, which is protected laterally with a retractor. The joint capsule is sharply entered dorsally and soft tissues reflected medially and laterally. The medial and lateral collateral ligaments should be fully released in a subperiosteal fashion, taking care to fully release their plantar attachments. It is often necessary to resect dorsal, medial, and lateral osteophytes with the use of a rongeur. If a prominent medial eminence exists, this is resected with the use of a chisel and mallet; however, care must be taken to maintain a sufficient medial shelf of bone to allow for screw placement.

The proximal phalanx is then placed in plantar flexion and the plantar plate attachment to the base of the proximal

phalanx is mobilized, taking care to avoid injury to the long or short flexor tendons. Pronation and supination of the proximal phalanx assist in full mobilization of the lateral and medial soft tissues. Once the exposure is completed, the full extent of the articular surface of the proximal phalanx should be visualized. Osteophytes from the base of the proximal phalanx may need to be resected to determine the true extent of the articular surface. If advanced hallux valgus is present, a Z-lengthening of the EHL tendon may be necessary to relieve valgus tension.

Preparation of the joint should be performed in a meticulous fashion with rongeurs, curets, and chisels to remove cartilage and subchondral bone to a bleeding cancellous surface on both sides of the joint. This process will maximize fusion incorporation. Several techniques for joint preparation can be used. Flat cuts performed with a microsagittal saw are less forgiving, as the exact amount of valgus and dorsal angulation must be created with the saw cuts. Additionally, flat cuts have the potential to lead to shorten-

ing of the hallux, with subsequent transfer metatarsalgia.

Concentric or in situ preparation of the joint minimizes shortening and provides for greater ease of positioning of the fusion. With this technique, initial joint preparation is performed with a rongeur for preparation of the first metatarsal head, and a combination of a small chisel and curets are used to prepare the base of the proximal phalanx. Creation of congruent joint surfaces may be performed manually or with the use of reciprocating hand or power reamers.[5-7]

In the author's clinical experience, concentric preparation of the joint allows for the greatest ease of positioning in all planes, because of the ability to "dial in" the degree of correction. If reciprocating reamers are used, the surgeon must take care to remove all subchondral bone before their usage. Failure to do so will result in a higher nonunion rate.

Fusion Position

Proper positioning of the first MTP joint requires correction in the AP and sagittal planes as well as correction of any rotational deformity. Positioning in the AP plane should range between 10° to 15° of valgus orientation. Concomitant hallux interphalangeus may require less valgus correction at the MTP joint, and if there is a valgus windswept deformity of the lesser toes, a slightly larger valgus orientation is preferable. If associated surgery is required on the second toe, it should be stabilized before positioning of the first MTP joint to serve as a guide for hallux positioning. Excessive valgus orientation may result in lateral impingement, whereas insufficient valgus orientation will lead to an increased incidence of interphalangeal joint arthrosis, and the sensation of "vaulting-off" the forefoot at terminal stance.

Correction in the sagittal plane should result in 5° to 10° of dorsiflexion relative to the ground, or 20° to 30° of dorsiflexion relative to the first metatarsal shaft. Intraoperatively, this is best performed by placing the foot on a flat surface, and allowing for 2 to 5 mm of clearance. Similarly, a functional toe-off position can be simulated by placing the foot on a flat surface and applying pressure on the plantar aspect of the foot to dorsiflex the ankle and tarsometatarsal joint while maintaining the resting position of the hallux on the flat surface.[8] In rare instances, additional dorsiflexion of the joint is performed to accommodate women's shoe wear; however, patients must be counseled that this decision may lead to excessive dorsiflexion while walking barefoot or when wearing low-heeled shoes. Therefore, this procedure is not standardly recommended. Excessive dorsiflexion of the joint can lead to a cock-up deformity with development of callosity over the interphalangeal joint, and may also create increased pressure under the sesamoids. Inadequate dorsiflexion of the joint will create problems at toe-off with subsequent interphalangeal joint hyperextension and arthrosis.

The joint should be maintained in a

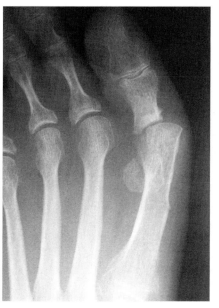

Figure 4 Recurrent hallux valgus deformity following failed Keller resection arthroplasty.

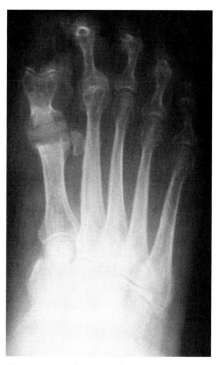

Figure 5 AP radiograph of a patient with a failed Silastic implant. Note cystic changes about the joint and shortening of the first MTP joint relative to the second MTP joint.

neutral position relative to the coronal plane. Residual pronation will result in medial callosity and increased medial nail pressure, whereas supination of the joint will create lateral nail pressure.

Fixation Techniques

Several fixation techniques have been described for fusion of the first MTP joint. The use of chromic catgut in one British series demonstrates a 90% union rate,[9] whereas intraosseous wiring in other studies revealed a 56% to 96% union rate.[10,11] Historically, threaded Steinmann pins[2,3] placed in an antegrade position distally across the interphalangeal joint then brought retrograde across the MTP joint showed a high incidence of union; however, the 40% incidence of interphalangeal arthrosis noted radiographically, as well as the requirement for Steinmann pin removal, has caused this technique to fall out of favor. Similarly, the use of smooth Kirschner wires is reserved for those patients with extremely poor bone quality.

Modern fixation techniques involve the use of interfragmentary compression

screws, dorsal plate fixation ($^1/_3$ or $^1/_4$ tubular), or a combination thereof[5,12,13] (Figure 6). Cannulated headless variable compression screws may also be used[14] with the advantage of lack of prominent hardware while avoiding the possibility of dorsal cortex breakout from head impingement (Figure 7). Experimentally, the strength of fixation of various constructs has been evaluated. In one study,[15] an AO 4.0-mm compression screw was compared to a dorsal miniplate, a 4.5-mm Herbert screw, and a Steinmann pin, with a derotation Kirschner wire added for stability. It was found that the miniplate and Herbert screw were stronger than the 4.0-mm screw, which was comparable to the Steinmann pin. Another study compared the combination of flat cuts for bone preparation with the use of crossed Kirschner wires, crossed compression screws, or dorsal plate to the conical preparation of the joint with the use of

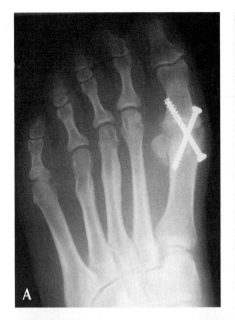
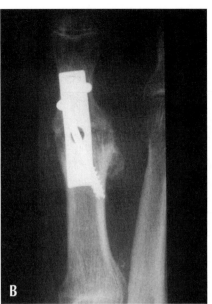
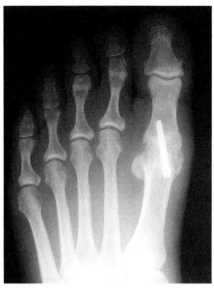

Figure 7 Use of a headless variable compression screw may help prevent prominent hardware and dorsal cortex breakout secondary to head impingement.

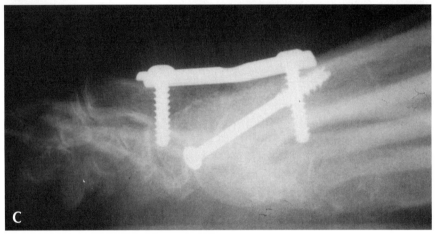

Figure 6 Several methods for fusion of the first MTP joint may be used, including crossed interfragmentary compression screws (**A**) or a combination of interfragmentary compression screws and dorsal plate (**B** and **C**).

crossed screws.[16] It was found that conical preparation of the bone combined with crossed compression screws provided the strongest fixation. The cost-effectiveness of fusion fixation has also been evaluated.[17] Small fragment compression screws were compared with a variable pitch headless compression screw (Herbert) as well as a dorsal compression plate. Factors such as cost, patient-reported outcomes, and outcome incidences or complications were taken into account. The small fragment screws were found to

have the lowest average cost of use, which was most strongly influenced by union rate and the cost of the fixation systems.

In the author's practice, crossed cannulated 4-0 screws, or a cannulated headless screw with the addition of a temporary derotation Kirschner wire is standardly used. The screws are placed from a medial proximal to lateral distal direction, and a medial distal to lateral proximal direction, in a crossed fashion. The screw must be initially placed in a

slightly plantar position to maximize bone purchase, as the fusion position is one of slight dorsiflexion. A dorsal compression plate, with or without a separate compression screw, is used in those patients with poor bone quality that will not provide sufficient fixation strength with screws alone.

After fluoroscopic verification of appropriate fusion position, closure is performed with 2-0 absorbable sutures for the capsule, 4-0 absorbable sutures for subcutaneous tissues, and 4-0 nylon sutures for skin. If lengthening of the EHL tendon is necessary, tendon repair is performed with a 3-0 absorbable suture, and the repair is reinforced with a 0.062-inch Kirschner wire placed across the interphalangeal joint to protect the repair. The Kirschner wire can be advanced proximally across the MTP joint to serve as a derotation device.

A soft dressing and postoperative wooden-soled shoe are applied in the operating room, and patients are instructed to elevate the foot during the first week. Heel weight bearing with the assistance of crutches is allowed. At 10 days after surgery, non-weight-bearing radiographs are obtained, sutures are removed, and a repeat soft dressing is applied. The dressings are changed every 10 days to 2 weeks. At 6 weeks postoperatively, weight-bearing radiographs are obtained, and if sufficient fusion incorporation is noted, the Kirschner wire is removed and full weight bearing in the postoperative shoe is started. Patients progress from the postoperative shoe to a comfortable sneaker over 2 weeks, as swelling and discomfort allow. Patients are counseled that it may take 10 weeks to 4 months for swelling to completely resolve.

Complications

Fusion nonunion, when all fixation techniques are considered, occurs in approximately 10% of patients. The use of modern rigid internal fixation techniques increases fusion rates to 94% to 98%.[5,12] A fibrous nonunion is generally well tolerated, especially in patients with rheumatoid arthritis. Surgical correction of a symptomatic nonunion is treated with repreparation of the fusion surfaces to create a bleeding cancellous bed. Care must be taken to resect all fibrous tissue and avascular bone. Revision is performed with rigid internal fixation. For patients in whom a Keller resection arthroplasty was previously performed, there may be inadequate length for application of a dorsal plate.

If bone loss is present before surgery secondary to prior excessive bone resection, or the preparation of the nonunion site additionally shortens the hallux, or the patient had previously undergone a Keller resection arthroplasty and is experiencing transfer metatarsalgia, then interpositional bone grafting may be necessary.[18,19] If no transfer metatarsalgia is present before revision, the fusion often can be revised in situ, without lengthening. If transfer metatarsalgia is present, it must be determined if it is diffuse, or

limited to the second metatarsal. If transfer metatarsalgia is diffuse, a lengthening fusion with either tricortical iliac crest or allograft bone is performed with a dorsal plate or compression screw. An alternative method is to rheumatoid forefoot-type reconstruction with fusion of the joint and resection of the lesser metatarsal heads. If transfer metatarsalgia is limited to the second metatarsal head, consideration can be given toward fusion combined with a second metatarsal shortening osteotomy. If shortening of the second metatarsal places the patient at risk for developing third metatarsalgia, a lengthening fusion is indicated.

Malunion of the first MTP joint may occur in all three planes. Excessive dorsiflexion will result in a cock-up deformity of the interphalangeal joint, creating a dorsal corn and sesamoiditis. Inadequate dorsiflexion will result in interphalangeal hyperextension, arthrosis, and problems with toe-off. Excessive valgus positioning will result in lesser toe impingement and problems with shoe wear. Inadequate valgus creates problems with toe-off, and can lead to interphalangeal arthrosis and the creation of hallux interphalangeus. Correction of malunions requires the use of a corrective closing or opening wedge or concentric rotational osteotomy.

Interphalangeal joint arthrosis occurs in 6% to 15% of patients, and may represent the natural progression of arthritic changes adjacent to the fused MTP joint, or as a result of inadequate dorsiflexion or valgus positioning. This condition is also seen as a result of threaded pins placed across the interphalangeal joint, or from excessive valgus pull from the EHL tendon.

Summary

Symptomatic arthritis of the first MTP joint requires arthrodesis when nonsurgical methods such as the use of an orthotic device with Morton's extension does not adequately relieve symptoms. Symptomatic arthritis may occur as a

result of idiopathic arthritis, inflammatory arthritis, failed bunion correction, or failed implant of the first MTP joint. A dorsal incision is used to ensure full exposure and adequate visualization of the joint. Care must be taken to prepare the joint surfaces down to bleeding cancellous bone in order to maximize the fusion success rate. Shortening of the metatarsals should be avoided to prevent transfer metatarsalgia. The fusion position should allow for 10° to 15° of valgus orientation in the AP plane, with 5° to 10° of dorsiflexion relative to the ground. Modern fusion techniques include the use of interfragmentary compression screws and/or dorsal plating. These modern fixation techniques result in a 94% to 98% fusion rate.

References

1. Coughlin MJ: Rheumatoid forefoot reconstruction: A long-term follow-up study. *J Bone Joint Surg Am* 2000;82:322-341.

2. Mann RA, Thompson FM: Arthrodesis of the first metatarsophalangeal joint for hallux valgus in rheumatoid arthritis. *Foot Ankle Int* 1997;18:65-67.

3. Coughlin MJ, Mann RA: Arthrodesis of the first metatarsophalangeal joint as salvage for the failed Keller procedure. *J Bone Joint Surg Am* 1987;69:68-75.

4. Hecht PJ, Gibbons MJ, Wapner KL, Cooke C, Hosington SA: Arthrodesis of the first metatarsophalangeal joint to salvage failed silicone implant arthroplasty. *Foot Ankle Int* 1997;18:383-390.

5. Coughlin MJ, Abdo RV: Arthrodesis of the first metatarsophalangeal joint with Vitallium plate fixation. *Foot Ankle Int* 1994;15:18-28.

6. Jeffery JA, Freedman LF: Modified reamers for fusion of the first metatarsophalangeal joint. *J Bone Joint Surg Br* 1995;77-B:328-329.

7. Wilkinson J: Cone arthrodesis of the first metatarsophalangeal joint. *Acta Orthop Scand* 1978;49:627-630.

8. Harper MC: Positioning of the hallux for first metatarsophalangeal joint arthrodesis. *Foot Ankle Int* 1997;18:827.

9. Chana GS, Andrew TA, Cotterill CP: A simple method of arthrodesis of the first metatarsophalangeal joint. *J Bone Joint Surg Br* 1984;66:703-705.

10. O'Doherty DP, Lowrie IG, Magnussen PA, Gregg PJ: The management of the painful first metatarsophalangeal joint in the older patient: Arthrodesis or Keller's arthroplasty? *J Bone Joint Surg Br* 1990;72:839-842.

11. Phillips JE, Hooper G: A simple technique for arthrodesis of the first metatarsophalangeal joint. *J Bone Joint Surg Br* 1986;68:774-775.

12. Holmes GB: Arthrodesis of the first metatarsophalangeal joint using interfragmentary screw and plate. *Foot Ankle* 1992;13:333-335.

13. Turan I, Lindgren U: Compression-screw arthrodesis of the first metatarsophalangeal joint of the foot. *Clin Orthop* 1987;221:292-295.

14. Wu KK: Fusion of the metatarsophalangeal joint of the great toe with Herbert screws. *Foot Ankle* 1993;14:165-169.

15. Rongstad KM, Miller GJ, Vander Griend RA, Cowin D: A biomechanical comparison of four fixation methods of first metatarsophalangeal joint arthrodesis. *Foot Ankle Int* 1994;15:415-419.

16. Curtis MJ, Myerson M, Jinnah RH, Cox OG, Alexander I: Arthrodesis of the first metatarsophalangeal joint: A biomechanical study of internal fixation techniques. *Foot Ankle* 1993;14:395-399.

17. Watson AD, Kelikian AS: Cost-effectiveness comparison of three methods of internal fixation for arthrodesis of the first metatarsophalangeal joint. *Foot Ankle Int* 1998;19:304-310.

18. Brodsky JW, Ptaszek AJ, Morris SG: Salvage first MTP arthrodesis utilizing ICBG: Clinical evaluation and outcome. *Foot Ankle Int* 2000;21:290-296.

19. Myerson MS, Schon LC, McGuigan FX, Oznur A: Result of arthrodesis of the hallux metatarsophalangeal joint using bone graft for restoration of length. *Foot Ankle Int* 2000;21:297-306.

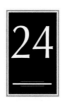

Complications After Hallux Valgus Surgery

E. Greer Richardson, MD

Complications after hallux valgus surgery can occur even after detailed physical and radiographic evaluations, excellent surgical technique, and careful postoperative care.[1-4] Recurrence of the original deformity or development of the opposite deformity, hallux varus; clawed hallux; and transfer keratotic lesions that cause intractable discomfort beneath the lesser metatarsal heads all can compromise the results of surgery[5-7] (Fig. 1).

Prevention of Complications
Careful preoperative evaluation can identify factors that influence both the choice of surgical procedure and the results of treatment (Outline 1). For example, although a bunion typically is present with hallux valgus deformity, this is not always true (Fig. 4); neither is first metatarsal varus always present. The capsulosesamoid apparatus must be evaluated.[3,8-10]

Physical Examination
The feet should be examined with the patient sitting, standing, lying supine, and lying prone, unless there is some reason for not putting the patient in one or more of these positions. Recurrence of hallux valgus deformity is more likely when subluxation or dislocation of the first metatarsophalangeal joint is present. Pronation of the hallux (frequently an indication of severe deformity),

dislocation of the sesamoids laterally, fixed deformity, pes planus, joint hypermobility, and a tight heel cord may contribute to the likelihood of recurrence of the deformity after hallux valgus repair.

Radiographic Evaluation
Not enough emphasis can be placed on a concise, detailed evaluation of the weightbearing radiographs in the preoperative planning of procedures to correct hallux valgus deformity. As in the physical examination, radiographic examination of the feet is incomplete without weightbearing views. The difference in the magnitude of the deformity on nonweightbearing and weightbearing views often is striking.[11-15]

Weightbearing Anteroposterior View On a weightbearing anteroposterior view, the alignment of the first ray should be carefully evaluated and the following noted:[16] (1) varus of the first metatarsal (normal intermetatarsal angle is 9° or less), (2) severity of hallux valgus (normal hallux valgus angle is 15° or less), (3) congruity or incongruity of the first metatarsophalangeal joint (hallux valgus deformity can exist even in a congruous joint), (4) length of the first metatarsal relative to the second (is the second metatarsal more than 6 to 7 mm longer than the first?), (5) subluxation of the sesamoid bones (if present, to what extent?), (6) well-

developed facet between the first and the second metatarsals, suggesting difficulty displacing the first metatarsal laterally at the first metatarsocuneiform joint, (7) sloping of the first metatarsocuneiform articulation laterally to medially at a severe angle, (8) degenerative arthritic changes at the interphalangeal, metatarsophalangeal, or metatarsocuneiform articulations, (9) hallux valgus interphalangeus of 10° or less in neutral flexion and extension of the interphalangeal joint, (10) excessive distal metatarsal articular angle (normal distal metatarsal angle is 15° or less), (11) convex medial bowing of the proximal phalanx.[17]

Weightbearing Lateral View On the weightbearing lateral view of the foot, the following should be evaluated: (1) collapse deformity of the metatarsocuneiform, cuneiform-navicular, or naviculotalar articulation, (2) increased talocalcaneal angle, suggesting a valgus posture of the hindfoot, (3) calcaneal inclination angle (10° or more is normal; a reduced angle is indicative of a valgus hindfoot and possibly pes planus), (4) dorsiflexion of the first metatarsal, indicating incongruous reduction into concavity of the base of the proximal phalanx, (5) angle between the diaphysis of the proximal phalanx and the diaphysis of the first metatarsal (20° or more is normal), (6) delineation of the cortical

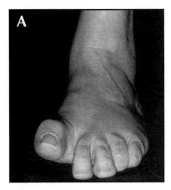 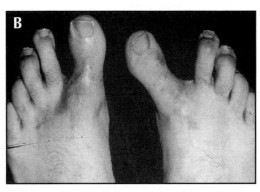

Fig. 1 A, Intrinsic minus hallux (clawtoe deformity) after failed distal metatarsal osteotomy. **B,** Severe hallux varus after a failed McBride bunionectomy and fibular sesamoidectomy.

Outline 1

Clinical considerations in the treatment of hallux valgus deformity

1. Pronation of the hallux and its part in the overall deformity.
2. The location of the sesamoid bones and if and where they are palpable.
3. Large callus formation on the tibial side of the hallux interphalangeal joint.
4. Pronation of the metatarsal head in tandem linkage with the hallux.
5. Pronation of the entire foot and correction of this hallucal pronation.
6. Passive correction of the deformity. If the valgus deformity is not correctable passively, measurement of the degree to which it can be corrected.
7. Passive weightbearing correction compared with passive nonweightbearing correction.
8. Active and passive ranges of motion of the first metatarsophalangeal joint with the hallux congruously reduced on the first metatarsal head and when the hallux deformity is not corrected.
9. Collapsed deformity at the mid- or hindfoot.
10. Contraction of the heel cord.
11. Asymmetry with weightbearing posture of the 2 feet even though both feet have a hallux valgus deformity. Is the prognosis the same after hallux valgus repair for both feet (Fig. 2)?
12. Prominence of the bursa over the medial aspect of the first metatarsal head.
13. With palpation of the medial eminence through the skin, determination of interposition of the capsule between skin and bone.
14. Hypermobile first ray compared with the other foot if the deformity is not bilateral. Can the first metatarsal passively be pushed towards the second metatarsal without restriction?
15. Hypermobility in all the joints of the foot and ankle.
16. First metatarsal head prominence dorsally with weight.
17. Clinical conditions of the lesser toes, particularly the second toe. (A fixed hammer deformity of the second toe with extensor posture of the toe at the second metatarsophalangeal joint or a second toe overlapping the hallux may create a space into which the hallux may rapidly return after hallux valgus repair.) The necessity of second toe realignment to obviate this potential problem (Fig. 3).
18. Previous surgeries that failed to correct the deformity.
19. Condition of the soft tissue.
20. Mobility of the first metarsophalangeal joint.
21. Crepitance of the first metatarsophalangeal joint.
22. Palpable pedal pulses.
23. Intact sensory and motor components of the nerve supply to the foot.

---

outlines of the fifth, fourth, and third metatarsals even if overlapped (if the fifth and fourth metatarsal cortical borders are not clearly outlined on the weightbearing lateral radiograph, pronation of the foot should be suspected).

These observations help determine the degree of valgus thrust on the hallux metatarsophalangeal joint during the stance phase of gait, which influences treatment decisions. For example, correction of a recurrent valgus deformity in a patient with posterior tibial tendon insufficiency may require an arthrodesis. The lateral weightbearing radiograph also is invaluable in evaluating a flat, pronated, valgus foot.[15]

Nonweightbearing Medial Oblique View The nonweightbearing medial oblique view may show arthritic changes in the first metatarsal-medial cuneiform articulation or a calcaneonavicular tarsal coalition, changes that are not visible on other views. Either of these conditions may compromise surgery because they limit midtarsal and subtalar joint motion, increasing the strain on the capsular repair at the metatarsophalangeal joint and the stress across the first metatarsophalangeal and first metatarsal medial cuneiform articulations.

Weightbearing Sesamoid View The weightbearing sesamoid view (Fig. 5) is especially useful in the evaluation of recurrent hallux valgus deformity. Determining where the sesamoid bones lie in relation to their facets on the first metatarsal head often is difficult on an anteroposterior view; the sesamoids may appear markedly subluxed laterally on an anteroposterior view, while a sesamoid view shows them in anatomic position in their facets. Training our technicians to reliably and reproducibly obtain this view has been worth the effort. Repositioning the intrinsic and extrinsic muscles and the capsulosesamoid apparatus into their anatomic positions is the key to correction, and the weightbearing sesamoid view is helpful in planning the best means to accomplish this.[15]

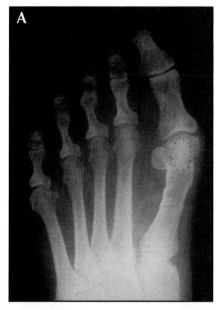

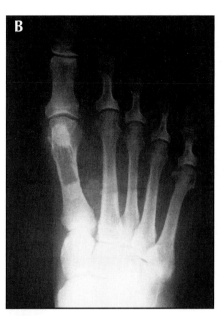

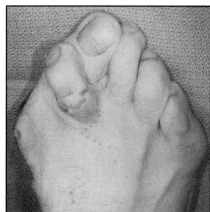

Fig. 3 Hallux valgus with cross-over deformity of the second toe.

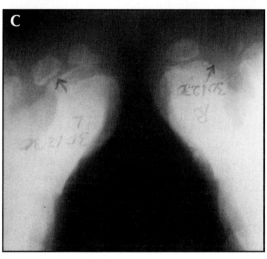

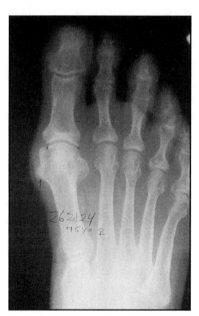

Fig. 2 Bilateral hallux valgus. **A,** Severe hallux valgus deformity failed after McBride procedure. **B** and **C,** Hallux valgus deformity treated with fibular sesamoidectomy. Greater correction is obtained but there is a higher risk for developing hallux varus.

Fig. 4 Prominent bunion with normal hallux valgus angle.

Specific Complications
Recurrent Deformity
Recurrent Valgus Deformity With Normal Distal Metatarsal Articular Angle After Soft-Tissue Procedure Soft-tissue repair alone, given the fact that medial eminence removal is intrinsic to any "bunion repair," is not frequently performed, and its usefulness is controversial.[14,19–23] A first web space dissection and lateral release are essential elements of any soft-tissue repair.

To avoid recurrence of the deformity after simple bunionectomy (medial eminence excision and capsular imbrication) the procedure should be avoided, except in elderly patients who have impending skin breakdown over the medial eminence. Except in these patients, this procedure should not be considered even if the hallux is congruously reduced on the first metatarsal head and the hallux valgus and intermetatarsal angles are normal. Although it is tempting to do a minor procedure for a minor deformity, this is an error of judgment. A first web space dissection and lateral release should be performed with medial eminence removal and medial capsular imbrication.

The magnitude and rigidity of the recurrent deformity are guides to treatment. As a rule, a deformity that occurred after a soft-tissue procedure should not be treated with another soft-tissue procedure unless the deformity is completely flexible (the hallux can be easily reduced into varus and the first metatarsal freely translates laterally by

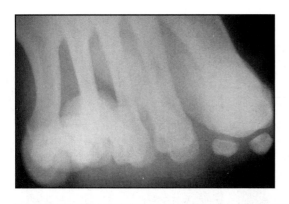

Fig. 5 Weightbearing sesamoid view.

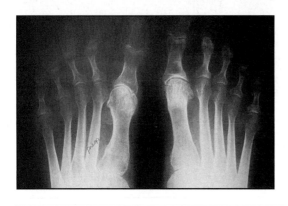

Fig. 6 Increased distal metatarsal articular angle and incongruent first metatarsophalangeal joint after basilar metatarsal osteotomy. Note degenerative changes.

manual pressure). First web space dissection, lateral release, and repeat medial capsular imbrication with manual medial displacement of the first metatarsal are recommended in patients with mild, flexible deformity that is symptomatic despite appropriate shoewear.[15,18,19] The indications include (1) an intermetatarsal 1-2 angle of 13° or less; (2) a hallux valgus angle of 30° or less; (3) a normal distal metatarsal articular angle (less than 10° to 15°); (4) minimal degenerative changes at the first metatarsophalangeal joint; (5) 50° to 60° of passive motion of the first metatarsophalangeal joint; (6) subluxation but not complete dislocation of the sesamoid bones; (7) ability to displace the first metatarsal laterally at the metatarsocuneiform joint from its abnormal varus inclination; (8) some degree of longitudinal arch present when weightbearing, determined clinically and radiographically. If the arch is improved with passive dorsiflexion of the hallux while standing, the patient does not have fixed, structural pes planus, and a soft-tissue repair is likely to endure.

Recurrent Hallux Valgus Deformity With Abnormal Distal Metatarsal Articular Angle After a Soft-Tissue Procedure When an increased distal metatarsal articular angle is present in recurrent hallux valgus, reducing the hallux will place the metatarsophalangeal joint incongruously on the metatarsal head (Fig. 6). The phalanx will rest in varus on the first metatarsal head and will leave the lateral aspect of the first metatarsal head uncovered. Correction of this deformity is accomplished with medial capsulorrhaphy, distal metatarsal displacement osteotomy (chevron), and first web space dissection with lateral soft-tissue release. Osteonecrosis of the first metatarsal head is a risk with distal metatarsal osteotomy and lateral release (Fig. 7), but the extent of necrosis and its clinical significance are unknown.[15,17]

Malunion After Chevron Osteotomy Malunion after a chevron osteotomy (Fig. 8) is uncommon if 3 steps in operative technique are followed: (1) the osteotomy is internally fixed and manually tested, and fixation is changed or augmented with a pin or small fragment screw if any movement occurs; (2) the distal fragment is placed plantar or inferior to the proximal fragment after internal fixation; and (3) weightbearing is guarded if fixation is not rigid.[15,24–27]

The difficulty in correcting a dorsal malunion after chevron osteotomy is preserving length. The initial chevron osteotomy often shortens the hallux 4 to 6 mm, and impaction and necrosis at the osteotomy site can decrease length another 4 to 6 mm, resulting in 1 to 1.5 cm of shortening that causes transfer metatarsalgia beneath the second metatarsal head or prevents relief of existing metatarsalgia. Varus or valgus malunion can occur after a chevron osteotomy, but this is not as common as dorsal malunion. Varus or valgus malunion of a chevron osteotomy, even with mild to moderate incongruity of the first metatarsophalangeal joint, is tolerated better by the patient than a dorsal malunion with transfer metatarsalgia. Regardless of the plane(s) of the malunion, the surgical technique to correct the deformity is basically the same.

Technique for Correcting Distal Malunion After Failed Chevron Osteotomy

The distal metatarsal is exposed from the junction of the middle and distal thirds to the base of the proximal phalanx. The previous osteotomy is inspected, but its "limbs" should not predetermine the plane(s) of the corrective osteotomy. With a 2-mm drill bit (even smaller if available), a semi-circle of unicortical holes is made from dorsal to plantar adjacent to or within the previous osteotomy site (an arc of approximately 60°). These holes are connected by using only the corner of a 5- to 6-mm sharp, straight osteotome as a cutting edge. Care should be taken not to penetrate the lateral cortex with the osteotome. Using the 2-mm (or less) drill bit, numerous holes are made in the lateral cortex and the osteotomy is completed with a thin (1 mm × 9 mm) blade on a small power saw. This technique reduces the amount of shortening. The head is manually rotated plantarward until the dorsal cortex of the capital (distal) fragment is inferior (plantar) to the dorsal cortex of the shaft (proximal) fragment. This will slightly plantarflex the first metatarsal head, allowing it to assume more of the weightbearing load across the metatarsal heads. If the capital fragment has healed in varus or valgus, the deformity is reversed until the capital fragment is reduced to normal anatomic alignment with the shaft. Of course the malunion may be in 2 or more planes, but this "broomstick" osteotomy will allow correction of all planes of deformity. Internal fixation with Kirschner wires (K-wires), small screws, or absorbable pins is necessary. Interfragmentary wires are technically difficult to use in this location but are not contraindicated.

Postoperative Care

Depending on the rigidity of fixation and body habitus of the patient, as well as compliance by the patient, protected weightbearing can begin immediately. A short leg cast that extends distal to the toes and crutches or a walker may be necessary. The patient should be told before surgery that permanent loss of some metatarsophalangeal joint motion can be

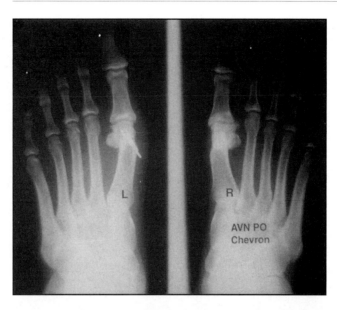

Fig. 7 Osteonecrosis after a distal metatarsal osteotomy (chevron).

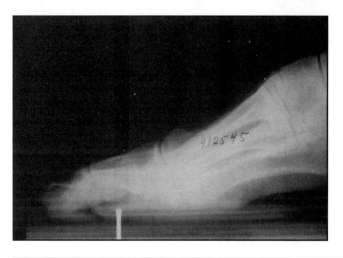

Fig. 8 Dorsal malunion after chevron osteotomy with intractable plantar keratosis beneath the second metatarsal.

expected, but that function should not be compromised. Full unprotected weightbearing is allowed when union of the osteotomy is apparent both clinically and radiographically. Final range of motion is not known until 12 to 18 months postoperatively.

Recurrent Hallux Valgus Deformity After Basilar Metatarsal Osteotomy and First Web Space Dissection or Release Recurrent deformity after basilar metatarsal osteotomy and first web space dissection or release should be treated with a second basilar metatarsal osteotomy, medial capsular imbrication of the

first metatarsophalangeal joint, and first web space dissection with release of the contracted lateral structures.[28-34] Indications for this procedure include: (1) an intermetatarsal angle of 14° or more; (2) hallux valgus angle of more than 30°; (3) normal distal metatarsal articular angle (10° to 15°); (4) splayed forefoot; (5) minimal to mild osteoarthritic changes at the first metatarsophalangeal joint (arthrodesis is indicated if the articular cartilage is damaged); (6) markedly subluxed or dislocated sesamoid bones; (7) 50° to 60° of passive range of motion of the first metatarsopha-

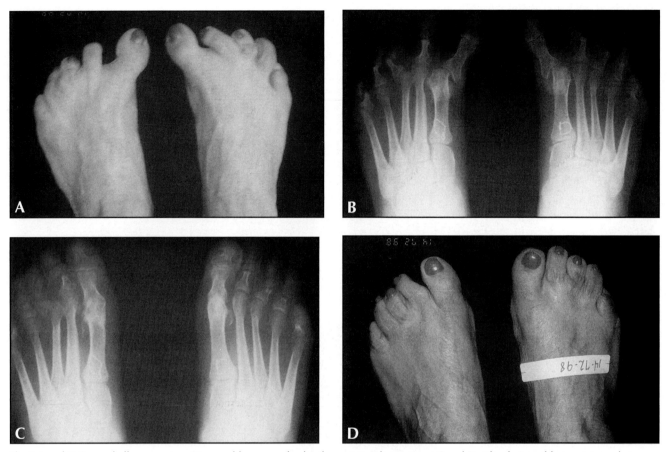

Fig. 9 A and **B,** Severe hallux varus in a 45-year-old woman after basilar metatarsal osteotomy. **C** and **D,** After fusion of first metatarsophalangeal joints.

langeal joint; and (8) arch structures that increase valgus stress on the metatarsophalangeal joint.

A combination of chevron and Akin osteotomies can be used for greater correction of valgus deformity.[15,35,36] Although Mitchell and Baxter[36] reported satisfactory results with this combined procedure, they caution that it should not be used if sesamoid subluxation and a wide intermetatarsal angle are present.

For severe recurrent deformity, arthrodesis of the first metatarsophalangeal joint often is the most appropriate operation[29,37,38] (Fig. 9). The surgical technique varies according to the type of osteotomy and the kind of fixation used.[39] Nonunion, malunion, and degenerative arthritis of

the interphalangeal joint of the hallux are the most frequent complications after arthrodesis of the first metatarsophalangeal joint. Accurate positioning of the hallux is essential during the procedure. Lapidus recommended combining arthrodesis of the first metatarsal medial cuneiform joint with distal soft-tissue release for severe recurrent deformities.[40–42]

Resection and Replacement Arthroplasty of the First Metatarsophalangeal Joint Resection (Keller) arthroplasty can be used for correction of recurrent deformity in elderly patients who have limited physical demands on their feet and who have some degree of osteoarthritis at the first metatarsophalangeal joint.[5,43–56] Its usefulness may be

expanded if the hallux, after resection of its base, is internally fixed to the first metatarsal before it is secured with 2 K-wires.

The results of replacement arthroplasty of the first metatarsophalangeal joint for correction of recurrent hallux valgus have varied[57] (Fig. 10). Cracchiolo and associates[58] recommended replacement arthroplasty of the first metatarsophalangeal joint in patients with rheumatoid arthritis and severe destruction of the metatarsophalangeal joints, but in most patients, resection of the base of the proximal phalanx, temporary internal fixation, and soft-tissue repair provide just as good results as replacement arthroplasty, with less expense and fewer complications (Fig. 11).

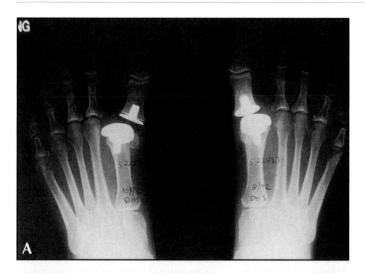

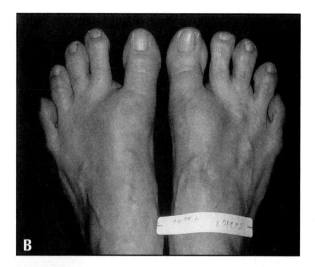

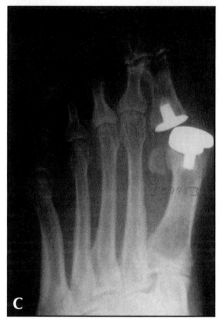

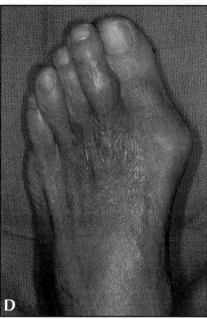

Fig. 10 A and **B,** Hallux varus deformity after replacement arthroplasty. **C** and **D,** Hallux valgus deformity after failed replacement arthroplasty.

Acquired Hallux Varus

Hallux varus[59–64] was not recognized as a complication of hallux valgus surgery until McBride[19] reported this deformity in 5.1% of patients treated with his procedure for hallux valgus (medial eminence removal, medial capsulorrhaphy, and fibular sesamoidectomy). Since then, many authors have reported this complication, with incidences varying from 2% (Peterson and associates[65]) to 17% (Trnka and associates[66]). Surprisingly, few patients with hallux varus complain about appearance (only if varus is greater than 10° to 15°) or discomfort (rare and usually associated with degenerative changes of the first metatarsophalangeal joint).[21]

Hawkins classified hallux varus into two types: static and dynamic.[3,15] Static deformities are uniplanar; dynamic deformities are multiplanar.

Static (Uniplanar) Hallux Varus

Supple, uniplanar, passively correctable hallux varus usually is asymptomatic and is mainly a cosmetic complication[21] (Fig. 12). When the foot is viewed in a weightbearing position, the hallux rests in varus, the metatarsophalangeal joint rests in a normal position in the sagittal plane (10° to the plantar surface of the foot or 20° to 25° to the first metatarsal), and the interphalangeal joint is in a normal position. Most often the hallux is not rotated abnormally in an axial plane and does not assume a "snake-in-the-grass" appearance in the frontal plane.[4] All the deformity occurs at the metatarsophalangeal joint, but only in

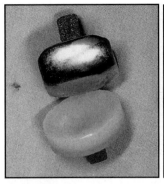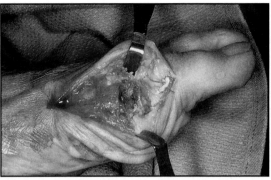

Fig. 11 Large size of prostheses required for replacement arthroplasty leaves large gap, making arthrodesis difficult.

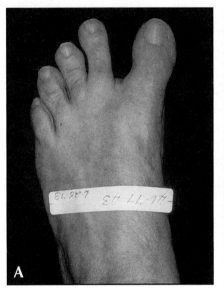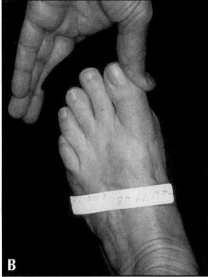

A

B

Fig. 12 A and **B,** Passively correctable hallux varus (static deformity).

the transverse or frontal plane. Uniplanar deformity most commonly occurs when a mild to moderate hallux valgus deformity is treated with a lateral soft-tissue release combined with medial capsular imbrication and medial eminence excision. According to Trnka and associates,[66] excising too much of the medial eminence (within or immediately lateral to the sagittal groove) is a major contributing factor to hallux varus. Excision of the fibular sesamoid and overcorrection of the first intermetatarsal angle to less than 5° also may be causes of hallux varus uniplanar deformity. Normally, the

hallux rests on the first metatarsal head in about 10° of valgus. If the intermetatarsal angle is reduced to less than 5° and the hallux is reduced congruously on the metatarsal head, the necessary valgus angulation must be 15° (5° varus of the first metatarsal plus 10° distal metatarsal articular angle). Often the hallux is aligned parallel to the second toe if that toe is straight, or to the medial border of the foot if it is not, but this clinically straight posture actually places the hallux into varus in relation to the articular surface of the first metatarsal head. When the lateral restraining

structures are released and the medial eminence is removed, the hallux is at risk of drifting farther into varus. Overcorrection of the intermetatarsal angle and removal of the medial eminence at the sagittal groove instead of medial to it may contribute to the development of hallux varus deformity.

The surgical treatment of this deformity is straightforward and results are predictable. A static deformity is easier to correct than a dynamic one[1,3,67] (Fig. 13).

Soft-Tissue Correction
Technique
An incision is made on the medial side of the hallux at the midline in the internervous plane. The incision should extend from the midportion of the diaphysis of the proximal phalanx to 4 to 5 cm proximal to the metatarsophalangeal joint. The dorsal skin flap (on the capsule) is raised 4 to 5 mm, and the plantar flap is raised 2 to 3 mm. Care should be taken not to injure the dorsal sensory nerve near the medial eminence and first metatarsal.

A capsular incision is made in the midline medially. The dorsal and plantar capsular flaps are elevated until the dorsomedial corner of the first metatarsal and the tibial sesamoid plantarward are clearly exposed. After the hallux is adducted to the midline, the first metatarsophalangeal joint is flexed and extended. The soft-tissue release is carried dorsally and plantarward until the hallux can be placed into 10° to 15° of valgus on the metatarsal. The hallux is flexed and extended and passively dorsiflexed 40° to 50° in this valgus position. A small osteotome or periosteal elevator is placed between the articular surface of the tibial sesamoid and the first metatarsal head. If the tibial sesamoid slides back into its facet on

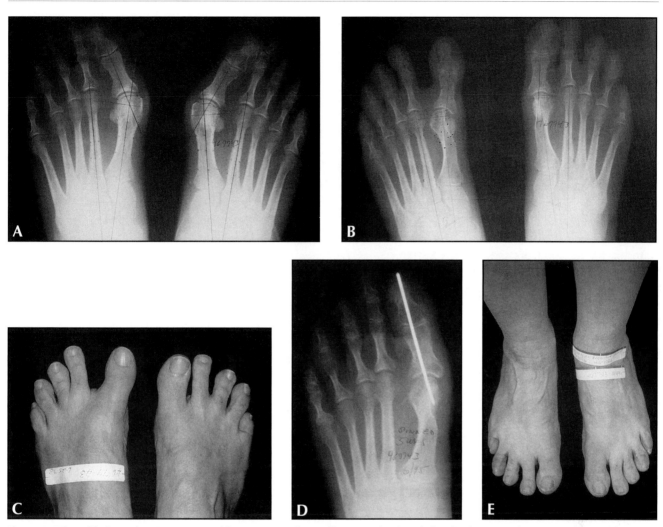

Fig. 13 A, Bilateral hallux valgus in a 62-year-old woman. **B** and **C,** Hallux varus developed after distal metatarsal osteotomy from a valgus malution and increased distal metatarsal articular angle. **D** and **E,** After medial capsulotomy and tibial sesamoid reduction for varus deformity. Pin remained for 5 weeks.

the metatarsal head with passive valgus of the hallux or requires only gentle levering and pushing to reduce and maintain it, the correction will be long-lasting.

With the hallux positioned in 15° valgus, 10° extension, and neutral rotation, a 0.062-in K-wire is placed obliquely from distal medial in the proximal phalanx to proximal lateral in the first metatarsal, starting at the metaphyseal-diaphyseal flair of the proximal phalanx. The wire is cut off beneath the skin where it can be removed in the office under local anesthesia. The tourniquet is released and hemostasis obtained. The capsule should not be closed. The skin is closed with permanent 4-0 monofilament nylon suture. Simple stitches are placed near the wound margins, because the skin is under tension and mattress sutures could further compromise the blood supply to the skin margins. Because neither capsular nor subcutaneous sutures are used, the skin must be closed with more stitches than usual; gaps left between the stitches could cause a synovial fistula or an infection. A forefoot dressing is applied. The dressing does not have to help maintain the reduced position of the hallux because this is done by the articular wire.[15]

Postoperative Care

The patient is allowed touch-down weightbearing in a removable boot with crutches for 3 weeks and then weightbearing to tolerance without crutches for an additional 3 weeks. In the first 3 weeks, the boot can be removed at night and for bathing. The wire is removed in the office in 4 to 6 weeks (6 weeks if the reduction was difficult). If it is necessary to remove the wire earlier than 3 weeks after surgery, the hallux should be taped to the second and third toes until it has no tendency to drift medially.

Although soft-tissue repair generally is a reliable procedure that does not markedly reduce range of motion of the first metatarsophalangeal joint and has minimal perioperative morbidity, occasionally tendon transfer or arthrodesis may be required for severe hallux varus deformity. I prefer arthrodesis to tendon transfer, although Johnson, Mann, Myerson, and others have reported favorable results after tendon transfer or tenodesis.[6,21,68–70]

Transfer of Extensor Hallucis Longus With Arthrodesis of the Interphalangeal Joint of the Hallux [4,6,71]

A dorsal curvilinear incision is made, starting just lateral to insertion of the extensor hallucis longus tendon, and is gently carried laterally toward the first web space in the interval between the first and second metatarsals. The incision is then inclined medially, ending along the lateral aspect of the extensor hallucis longus tendon at the first metatarsocuneiform joint. The extensor hallucis longus tendon is detached distally, and the surfaces of the interphalangeal joint are removed. After the distal phalanx is drilled from its articular surface, the arthrodesis site is placed together, and the drill bit is inserted through the end of the toe into the proximal phalanx. A 4.0-mm, small fragment, partially threaded, cancellous bone screw of the appropriate length is then inserted and the arthrodesis is compressed. A 2-0 absorbable suture is placed through the mobilized extensor hallucis longus tendon. A hole is drilled from dorsal to plantar in the lateral aspect of the base of the proximal phalanx. The drill bit is increased from a 2.5 mm to

3.5 mm. Curettes are used to further enlarge the hole if necessary. Since the "pulley" is the transverse intermetatarsal ligament, the tendon is pulled plantar to it through the drill hole in the proximal phalanx in a plantar to dorsal direction. A K-wire is used to hold the toe in the proper position, and the tendon is reattached so that it is taut. This holds the great toe in proper valgus and plantar alignment.

Dynamic (Multiplanar) Hallux Varus

Dynamic hallux varus is a multiplanar deformity that may rapidly become fixed. Multiplanar deformities often are symptomatic and difficult to correct surgically. I prefer the descriptive term "intrinsic minus deformity of the hallux with a varus component," which emphasizes that the varus is only one part of the deformity. This is an intrinsic-extrinsic muscle imbalance or an intrinsic minus hallux. In this type of hallux varus, the first metatarsophalangeal joint is hyperextended (usually with some degree of fixed soft-tissue contracture) and the interphalangeal joint is acutely flexed. The hallux is rotated and its varus and extension posture makes shoe wear difficult. The most common complaint is that the toe box of the shoe rubs on the dorsomedial surface of the interphalangeal joint. Patients frequently complain of a keratotic lesion beneath the first metatarsal head caused by the extended hallux pushing the first metatarsal head plantarward. Hammertoe deformities develop in the lesser toes (usually 2 and 3) and metatarsalgia develops as the hallux assists less and less in the stance phase of the gait cycle.[72]

Anatomy and Pathogenesis
The intrinsic muscles balance the hallux on the first metatarsal head,

while the extrinsic muscles add gross balance and greatly increase the mobility of the hallux.[3,4,58,73–75] The first metatarsophalangeal joint is a shallow, ball-in-socket joint with little stability from bony configurations. The location of the tendon insertions of the abductor-adductor hallucis, the flexor hallucis brevis (both components), and the extensor hallucis brevis balance the hallux congruently on the first metatarsal head. If the positions of these tendon insertions are altered relative to the axis of rotation in flexion or extension at the metatarsophalangeal joint, this balance is disrupted. In intrinsic minus-varus hallux, the ability of the flexor hallucis brevis to flex the metatarsophalangeal joint is decreased. The abductor hallucis, unencumbered by its antagonist (adductor), pulls the hallux medially, uncovering the metatarsal head laterally. The extensor hallucis brevis hyperextends the hallux against a weakened flexor hallucis brevis, and, as the hallux drifts medially and dorsally, the extrinsic muscle-tendon units begin to exacerbate the deformity. The flexor hallucis longus further flexes the interphalangeal joint, and the forces of the extensor hallucis longus and the extensor hallucis brevis increase the extension deformity. The sesamoid bones sublux medially, carrying the plantar plate, flexor hallucis brevis, and adductor and abductor hallucis tendons of insertion with them, thereby contributing to the pattern and rigidity of the deformity. The components of this deformity quickly become fixed, making passive correction impossible and surgical correction difficult and multifaceted.

Bony and Soft-Tissue Correction
Technique A midline medial incision is made and the metatarsal head is exposed by incising the capsule 2 to 3 mm plantar to where the skin inci-

sion was centered. The capsule is elevated from the head of the metatarsal and the base of the proximal phalanx dorsally and plantarward. The tibial sesamoid is exposed. If the deformity is fixed in extension at the metatarsophalangeal joint, a wider resection of the soft tissue is needed up to the junction of the neck and shaft of the first metatarsal. The hallux is manually reduced into a valgus position and then released to evaluate the tightness. The articular surfaces are examined, and if the head of the first metatarsal shows loss of articular cartilage or unhealthy appearing articular cartilage, presumably from chronic pressure placed against it, then an arthrodesis is indicated. If the articular cartilage appears reasonably normal, then the hallux is held in 10° of valgus and a 0.062-in K-wire is placed across the joint obliquely from the base of the proximal phalanx medially to the head and neck junction of the first metatarsal laterally. The sesamoids are placed beneath the head of the metatarsal. The interphalangeal joint contracture is released through a dorsal inverted L-incision with the transverse limb across the dorsum of the interphalangeal joint and the proximal limb extending 2 to 3 cm proximally along the dorsolateral border of the head and neck of the proximal phalanx.

If the metatarsophalangeal joint requires arthrodeses, the interphalangeal joint flexion contracture should be corrected by releasing the plantar plate and both collateral ligaments, bringing the interphalangeal joint into a corrected position, and holding it with a 0.062-in K-wire. If the metatarsophalangeal joint does not require arthrodeses, the articular surfaces of the interphalangeal joint are removed in preparation for an arthrodesis. This serves two purposes: it will correct a fixed deformity of

the interphalangeal joint, or, if the deformity is supple, it will allow relative shortening of the extensor and flexor hallucis longus muscle-tendon units, thereby decreasing their deforming forces.

The interphalangeal joint arthrodesis is fixed with crossed K-wires or a small intramedullary fragment screw. The technique of Johnson is recommended if a screw is used. A hole is drilled into the distal phalanx from the articular surface through the tip of the hallux just beneath the nail, and then the drill bit is reversed into the proximal phalanx. Usually a 4.0-mm partially threaded, cancellous, small fragment screw (40 to 50 mm) is used. I prefer Kirschner wires, but either technique is acceptable. The tourniquet is removed, and the hallux is held in 10° to 15° of valgus with the interphalangeal joint arthrodesed in neutral position, while the skin is closed with simple, interrupted, small sutures. The stitches are placed close to the skin edge, because bringing the hallux from a varus to a valgus posture places the skin under tension. Some wound necrosis medially frequently occurs after hallux varus repair, and the patient should be advised of this. A forefoot dressing is applied.

Postoperative Care The patient is encouraged to rest and elevate the foot above heart level for several days. For the first 3 weeks after surgery, only nonweightbearing ambulation on crutches is allowed. If the patient is allowed to bear weight, a short leg cast that extends past the toes is recommended. Weightbearing to tolerance in a removable walking boot is allowed for the next 3 weeks. The K-wire is removed between the fourth and sixth weeks, depending on how difficult it was to correct the deformity: the more difficult the deformity correction, the longer the fixation should remain.

References

1. Donley BG: Acquired hallux varus. *Foot Ankle Int* 1997;18:586–592.

2. Edelman RD: Iatrogenically induced hallux varus. *Clin Podiatr Med Surg* 1991;8:367–382.

3. Hawkins F: Acquired hallux varus: Cause, prevention and correction. *Clin Orthop* 1971;76: 169–176.

4. Johnson KA, Saltzman CL, Friscia DA: Hallux varus, in Gould JS, Thompson FM, Cracchiolo A III, et al (eds): *Operative Foot Surgery*. Philadelphia, PA, WB Saunders, 1994, pp 28–35.

5. Johnson KA, Saltzman CL: Complications of resection arthroplasty (Keller) and replacement arthroplasty (silicone) procedures. *Contemp Orthop* 1991;23:139–147.

6. Johnson KA, Spiegl PV: Extensor hallucis longus transfer for hallux varus deformity. *J Bone Joint Surg* 1984;66A:681–686.

7. Joseph B, Jacob T, Chacko V: Hallux varus: A study of thirty cases. *J Foot Surg* 1984;23: 392–397.

8. McElvenny RT: Hallux varus. *Quart Bull Northwest Univ Med Sch* 1941;15:277–280.

9. Antrobus JN: The primary deformity in hallux valgus and metatarsus primus varus. *Clin Orthop* 1984;184:251–255.

10. Scranton PE Jr, Rutkowski R: Anatomic variations in the first ray: Part I. Anatomic aspects related to bunion surgery. *Clin Orthop* 1980; 151:244–255.

11. Austin DW, Leventen EO: A new osteotomy for hallux valgus: A horizontally directed "V" displacement osteotomy of the metatarsal head for hallux valgus and primus varus. *Clin Orthop* 1981;157:25–30.

12. Carr CR, Boyd BM: Correctional osteotomy for metatarsus primus varus and hallux valgus. *J Bone Joint Surg* 1968;50A:1353–1367.

13. Clark HR, Veith RG, Hansen ST Jr: Adolescent bunions treated by the modified Lapidus procedure. *Bull Hosp Jt Dis Orthop Inst* 1987; 47:109–122.

14. Mann RA: Decision-making in bunion surgery, in Greene WB (ed): *Instructional Course Lectures XXXIX*. Park Ridge, IL, American Academy of Orthopaedic Surgeons, 1990, pp 3–13.

15. Richardson EG: Disorders of the hallux, in Crenshaw AH (ed): *Campbell's Operative Orthopaedics*, ed 8. St. Louis, MO, Mosby-Year Book, 1992, vol 4, pp 2615–2692.

16. Sheref MJ, Johnson KA: Radiographic anatomy of the hindfoot. *Clin Orthop* 1983;177: 16–22.

17. Richardson EG, Graves SC, McClure JT, Boone RT: First metatarsal head-shaft angle: A method of determination. *Foot Ankle* 1993;14:181–185.

18. Hansen CE: Hallux valgus treated by the McBride operation: A follow-up. *Acta Orthop Scand* 1974;45:778–792.

19. McBride ED: The conservative operation for "bunions": End results and refinements of technique. *JAMA* 1935;105:1164–1168.

20. Coughlin MJ: Juvenile bunions, in Mann RA, Coughlin MJ (eds): *Surgery of the Foot and Ankle,* ed 6. St. Louis, MO, Mosby-Year Book, 1993, pp 297–339.

21. Mann RA, Coughlin MJ: Adult hallux valgus, in Mann RA, Coughlin MJ (eds): *Surgery of the Foot and Ankle,* ed 6. St. Louis, Mosby-Year Book, 1993, pp 167–296.

22. Franco MG, Kitaoka HB, Edaburn E: Simple bunionectomy. *Orthopedics* 1990;13:963–967.

23. Johnson JE, Clanton TO, Baxter DE, Gottlieb MS: Comparison of chevron osteotomy and modified McBride bunionectomy for correction of mild to moderate hallux valgus deformity. *Foot Ankle* 1991;12:61–68.

24. Hattrup SJ, Johnson KA: Chevron osteotomy: Analysis of factors in patients' dissatisfaction. *Foot Ankle* 1985;5:327–332.

25. Johnson KA: Chevron osteotomy of the first metatarsal: Patient selection and technique. *Contemp Orthop* 1981;3:707–711.

26. Meier PJ, Kenzora JE: The risks and benefits of distal first metatarsal osteotomies. *Foot Ankle* 1985;6:7–17.

27. Pochatko DJ, Schlehr FJ, Murphey MD, Hamilton JJ: Distal chevron osteotomy with lateral release for treatment of hallux valgus deformity. *Foot Ankle Int* 1994;15:457–461.

28. Coughlin MJ: Proximal first metatarsal osteotomy, in Johnson KA (ed): *The Foot and Ankle.* New York, NY, Raven Press, 1994, pp 85–105.

29. Fitzgerald JA: A review of long-term results of arthrodesis of the first metatarsophalangeal joint. *J Bone Joint Surg* 1969;51B:488–493.

30. Mann RA, Rudicel S. Graves SC: Repair of hallux valgus with a distal soft-tissue procedure and proximal metatarsal osteotomy: A long-term follow-up. *J Bone Joint Surg* 1992;74A:124–129.

31. Stokes IA, Hutton WC, Stott JR, Lowe LW: Forces under the hallux valgus foot before and after surgery. *Clin Orthop* 1979;142:64–72.

32. Thordarson DB, Leventen EO: Hallux valgus correction with proximal metatarsal osteotomy: Two-year follow-up. *Foot Ankle* 1992;13:321–326.

33. Trethowan J: Hallux valgus, in Choyce CC (ed): *A System of Surgery.* New York, NY, PB Hoeber, 1923.

34. Truslow W: Metatarsus primus varus or hallux valgus? *J Bone Joint Surg* 1925;7:98–108.

35. Mitchell CL, Fleming JL, Allen R, Glenney C, Sanford GA: Osteotomy-bunionectomy for hallux valgus. *J Bone Joint Surg* 1958;40A:41–60.

36. Mitchell LA, Baxter DE: A Chevron-Akin double osteotomy for correction of hallux valgus. *Foot Ankle* 1991;12:7–14.

37. Henry AP, Waugh W, Wood H: The use of footprints in assessing the results of operations of hallux valgus: A comparison of Keller's operation and arthrodesis. *J Bone Joint Surg* 1975;57B:478–481.

38. Coughlin MJ, Mann RA: Arthrodesis of the first metatarsophalangeal joint as salvage for the failed Keller procedure. *J Bone Joint Surg* 1987;69A:68–75.

39. Mann RA, Thompson FM: Arthrodesis of the first metatarsophalangeal joint for hallux valgus in rheumatoid arthritis. *J Bone Joint Surg* 1984;66A:687–692.

40. Lapidus PW: A quarter of a century of experience with the operative correction of the metatarsus varus primus in hallux valgus. *Bull Hosp Joint Dis* 1956;17:404–421.

41. Lapidus PW: The author's bunion operation from 1931 to 1959. *Clin Orthop* 1960;16:119–135.

42. Mauldin DM, Sanders M, Whitmer WW: Correction of hallux valgus with metatarso-cuneiform stabilization. *Foot Ankle* 1990;11:59–66.

43. Keller WL: The surgical treatment of bunions and hallux valgus. *NY Med J* 1904;80:741–742.

44. Ford LT, Gilula LA: Stress fractures of the middle metatarsals following the Keller operation. *J Bone Joint Surg* 1977;59A:117–118.

45. Friend G: Sequential metatarsal stress fractures after Keller arthroplasty with implant. *J Foot Surg* 1981;20:227–231.

46. Frisch EE: Technology of silicones in biomedical applications, in Rubin LR (ed): *Biomaterials in Reconstructive Surgery.* St. Louis, MO, CV Mosby, 1983, pp 73–90.

47. Johnson KA, Buck PG: Total replacement arthroplasty of the first metatarsophalangeal joint. *Foot Ankle* 1981;1:307–314.

48. Love TR, Whynot AS, Farine I, Lavoier M, Hunt L, Gross A: Keller arthroplasty: A prospective review. *Foot Ankle* 1987;8:46–54.

49. Merkle PF, Sculco TP: Prosthetic replacement of the first metatarsophalangeal joint. *Foot Ankle* 1989;9:267–271.

50. Rogers W, Joplin R: Hallux valgus, weak foot and the Keller operation: An end-result study. *Surg Clin North Am* 1947;27:1295–1302.

51. Shiel WC Jr, Jason M: Granulomatous inguinal lymphadenopathy after bilateral metatarsophalangeal joint silicone arthroplasty. *Foot Ankle* 1986;6:216–218.

52. Turner RS: Dynamic post-surgical hallux varus after lateral sesamoidectomy: Treatment and prevention. *Orthopedics* 1986;9:963–969.

53. Swanson AB, de Groot Swanson G, Maupin BK, et al: The use of a grommet bone-liner for flexible hinge implant arthroplasty of the great toe. *Foot Ankle* 1991;12:149–155.

54. Thomas FB: Keller's arthroplasty modified: A technique to ensure postoperative distraction of the toe. *J Bone Joint Surg* 1962;44B:356–365.

55. Vallier GT, Petersen SA, LaGrone MO: The Keller resection arthroplasty: A 13-year experience. *Foot Ankle* 1991;11:187–194.

56. Maschas A, Cartier P: Radiological results of the Keller operation. *Rev Chir Orthop Reparatrice Appar Mot* 1974;60(suppl 2):146–149.

57. Swanson AB: Implant arthroplasty for the great toe. *Clin Orthop* 1972;85:75–81.

58. Cracchiolo A III, Swanson A, Swanson GD: The arthritic great toe metatarsophalangeal joint: A review of flexible silicone implant arthroplasty from two medical centers. *Clin Orthop* 1981;157:64–69.

59. Banks AS, Ruch JA, Kalish SR: Surgical repair of hallux varus. *J Am Podiatr Med Assoc* 1988;78:339–347.

60. Granberry WM, Hickey CH: Idiopathic adult hallux varus. *Foot Ankle Int* 1994;15:197–205.

61. Miller JW: Acquired hallux varus: A preventable and correctable disorder. *J Bone Joint Surg* 1975;57A:183–188.

62. Mills JA, Menelaus MB: Hallux varus. *J Bone Joint Surg* 1989;71B:437–440.

63. Thomson SA: Hallux varus and metatarsus varus: A five-year study (1954-1958). *Clin Orthop* 1960;16:109–118.

64. Sloane D: Congenital hallux varus: Operative connection. *J Bone Joint Surg* 1935;17:209–211.

65. Peterson DA, Zilberfarb JL, Greene MA, Colgrove RC: Avascular necrosis of the first metatarsal head: Incidence in distal osteotomy combined with lateral soft tissue release. *Foot Ankle Int* 1994;15:59–63.

66. Trnka H-J, Zettl R, Hungerford M, Mühlbauer M, Ritschl P: Acquired hallux varus and clinical tolerability. *Foot Ankle Int* 1997;18:593–597.

67. Tourné Y, Saragaglia D, Picard F, De Sousa B, Montbarbon E, Charbel A: Iatrogenic hallux varus surgical procedure: A study of 14 cases. *Foot Ankle Int* 1995;16:457–463.

68. Juliano PJ, Myerson MS, Cunningham BW: Biomechanical assessment of a new tenodesis for correction of hallux varus. *Foot Ankle Int* 1996;17:17–20.

69. Myerson M: Hallux varus, in Myerson M (ed): *Current Therapy in Foot and Ankle Surgery.* St. Louis, MO, Mosby-Year Book, 1993, pp 70–73.

70. Myerson MS, Komenda GA: Results of hallux varus correction using an extensor hallucis brevis tenodesis. *Foot Ankle Int* 1996;17:21–27.

71. Skalley TC, Myerson MS: The operative treatment of acquired hallux varus. *Clin Orthop* 1994;306:183–191.

72. Poehling GG, DeTorre J: Hallux varus and hammertoe deformity. *Orthop Trans* 1982;6:186.

73. Albreckht E: Pathology and treatment of hallux valgus. *Russki Vrach* 1911;10:14.

74. Jahss MH: Spontaneous hallux varus: Relation to poliomyelitis and congenital absence of the fibular sesamoid. *Foot Ankle* 1983;3:224–226.

75. Reverdin J: Anatomie et operation de l'hallux valgus. *Trans Int Med Cong* 1881;2:408–412.

Lesser Toe Abnormalities

Michael J. Coughlin, MD

Abstract

Lesser toe abnormalities, which can result in significant pain and discomfort, are caused by several intrinsic or extrinsic factors including inflammatory arthritis, trauma, congenital abnormalities, neuromuscular disorders, or poorly fitting shoe wear. Identification of the etiology of the deformity is necessary to determine whether conservative or surgical treatment is warranted and to possibly halt progression of the deformity.

Although the lesser toes appear to be inconsequential because of their size, pain and deformity of the lesser toes may be a disabling condition. The underlying causes are frequently attributed to high-fashion footwear because of the high incidence of these problems in women.[1] In one study, an increased incidence of hammer toes and neuromas was observed in the female population with advancing age; there was a relatively low incidence of similar problems in men.[2] While ill-fitting shoe wear may be the most common cause, other factors associated with lesser toe deformities include inflammatory arthritis, trauma, congenital abnormalities, and neuromuscular disorders. The basic anatomic shape of the toes and metatarsals may play a role in later development of lesser toe deformities. Inflammatory arthropathies including gout, rheumatoid arthritis, psoriatic arthritis, systemic lupus erythematosus, and nonspecific synovial inflammatory disorders may be a precursor to metatarsophalangeal and lesser toe disorders.[3-5]

Isolated or repetitive injury to the interphalangeal or metatarsophalangeal joints may lead to the development of a mallet toe, a hammer toe, or a Freiberg's infraction.[6-8] Congenital deformities associated with the forefoot include a crossover fifth toe, contracted lesser toes, and malalignment of the metatarsophalangeal joint. Neuromuscular diseases including muscular dystrophies, Charcot-Marie-Tooth disease, poliomyelitis, and even lumbar disk disease may lead to a contracture deformity of the metatarsophalangeal and interphalangeal joints of the lesser toes.[5]

Most importantly, the basic anatomy of the forefoot may place a foot at risk for the development of these deformities. A hallux valgus deformity places extrinsic pressure on the second toe and in time may lead to subluxation or dislocation of the metatarsophalangeal joints as well as hammer toe deformities.[9] A toe that is longer in relationship to adjacent toes may lead to curling or contracture because of pressure against the end of the toe box of the shoe, and in time a mallet toe, hammer toe, or corn may develop.[10] An irregularly shaped middle phalanx may lead to medial or lateral deviation of the toe and a mallet toe deformity.[6]

Attention to the patient's description of symptoms and observation of the deformity as well as identification of any underlying causes, whether intrinsic or extrinsic, are important steps as they may determine not only the course of treatment but also possible prevention of progression of disorders.

Often with a lesser toe deformity, pain is exacerbated by constricting shoe wear (Fig. 1). Relief of extrinsic pressure often reduces discomfort. The use of a roomy toe box, a lower heel, and a soft

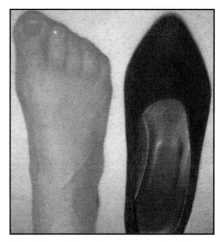

Fig. 1 Constricting shoe wear may lead to pressure and deformity of the lesser toes.

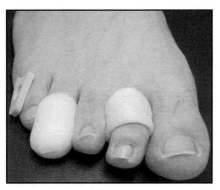

Fig. 2 Various methods of conservative treatment: a soft pad for treatment of a corn on the fifth toe, a toe cap for treatment of a lesion on the tip of the toe, and tube gauze for treatment of a severe hammer toe deformity.

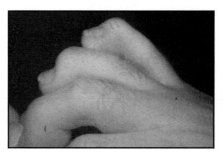

Fig. 3 Mallet toe deformities of the third, fourth, and fifth toes.

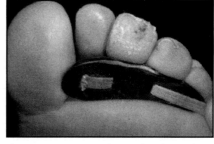

Fig. 4 A toe crest may be used to diminish pressure and to assist with healing of the lesion at the tip of the toe.

leather upper may be combined with padding of the lesion. Tube gauze, lamb's wool, foam corn pads or toe caps, and metatarsal pads are frequently used to relieve pressure areas (Fig. 2). Padding of symptomatic areas without wearing a shoe with a roomy toe box may actually exacerbate symptoms.

The common problems encountered in the forefoot include mallet toes, hammer toes, claw toes, interdigital corns, lateral corns on the fifth toe, and crossover fifth toes. Instability of the lesser metatarsophalangeal joints, Freiberg's infraction, and interdigital neuromas are also commonly seen; they present with the common symptom of pain and may be associated with lesser toe deformities as well.

Mallet Toes
Definition and History
A mallet toe is a fixed deformity of a lesser toe in which the distal phalanx is plantar flexed on the middle phalanx (Fig. 3). It may be deviated as well, either medially or laterally, in relation to the middle phalanx. As the tip of the toe repetitively strikes the ground, pain occurs and a callus develops at the tip of the toe or over the dorsal aspect of the distal interphalangeal joint. Occasionally, a toenail deformity occurs.

Mallet toes occur much less fre-

quently than hammer toes (ratio, 1:9).[5] The deformity occurs most frequently in a toe that is longer than adjacent toes, but it occurs with almost equal frequency in the second, third, and fourth toes.[6]

Physical Examination
With the patient standing, the distal interphalangeal joint is often flexed at a 90° angle, placing weight-bearing pressure on the toe tip and the nail. The proximal interphalangeal joint may be slightly flexed, but there is rarely malalignment of the metatarsophalangeal joint. A callus may be present at the tip of the toe and over the dorsal aspect of the distal interphalangeal joint.

Conservative Treatment
A shoe with a roomy toe box and a low heel will often alleviate symptoms. A toe crest placed beneath the toes may elevate the digit and relieve pressure (Fig. 4). A foam toe pad may also be used to diminish the pressure on the toe tip.

Surgical Treatment
Occasionally with a flexible deformity, a percutaneous release of the flexor digitorum longus tendon may alleviate symptoms[11,12] (Fig. 5). More commonly, the deformity is fixed and osseous decompression of the distal interphalangeal joint is necessary.[6]

A digital block is used for anesthesia, and a Penrose drain may be used as a

tourniquet. An elliptical incision centered over the dorsal aspect of the distal interphalangeal joint is deepened to excise the underlying extensor tendon and capsule. Care is taken to avoid injury to the nail matrix and to the adjacent neurovascular bundles. The collateral ligaments are released, exposing the distal condylar region of the middle phalanx. The bone is transected in the supracondylar region, and the distal fragment is excised. The corresponding articular surface of the distal phalanx is resected as well. In the depths of the wound, the capsule and the flexor digitorum longus tendon are identified and are released, allowing the toe to be straightened without tension. If the toe cannot be correctly aligned, more bone from the middle phalanx is resected. The toe is stabilized with a 0.045-in (0.114-cm) Kirschner wire (K-wire).

Postoperative Care
A gauze-and-tape compression dressing is applied postoperatively and is changed on a weekly basis. The K-wire and sutures are removed 3 weeks following surgery. The toe is then taped in a corrected position for 6 weeks to ensure adequate soft-tissue healing.

Results and Complications
Satisfactory results were reported following 62 of 72 mallet toe repairs performed in 50 patients.[6] Forty-seven of the 50 patients had complete pain relief, and the

deformity was adequately corrected in 65 of the 72 toes. A successful fusion was obtained in 50 of the 72 toes following resection of the condyles of the middle phalanx and the corresponding articular surface of the distal phalanx. The rate of satisfaction following a successful arthrodesis of the distal interphalangeal joint was slightly higher than that following a fibrous union, although the difference was not significant. The rates of satisfaction and maintenance of the corrected position were slightly higher when a flexor tenotomy had been performed.

Complications are uncommon following a mallet toe repair. Persistent swelling invariably resolves with time. Recurrence of a mallet toe deformity is also uncommon and is often associated with failure to release the flexor digitorum longus tendon.[6] An adjacent digital nerve may be injured at the time of surgery, leaving numbness along the medial or lateral border of the toe, but this is rarely a major symptom. The patient should be counseled that a preoperative toenail deformity associated with a mallet toe usually does not resolve following correction of the mallet toe deformity.

Hammer Toes
Definition and History
A hammer toe deformity occurs at the proximal interphalangeal joint of a lesser toe when the middle phalanx is plantar flexed on the proximal phalanx. Frequently, the metatarsophalangeal joint is hyperextended. The distal interphalangeal joint may be flexed, extended, or in a neutral position.[1,5,9] A patient may have a single or multiple hammer toes.[7] The deformity develops most commonly in a longer toe, and a toe with increased length is at increased risk for the development of a hammer toe deformity.[7]

The chief symptom of a hammer toe deformity is pain and pressure over the dorsal aspect of the proximal interphalangeal joint, which is often associated with a hypertrophic callus on the dorsal

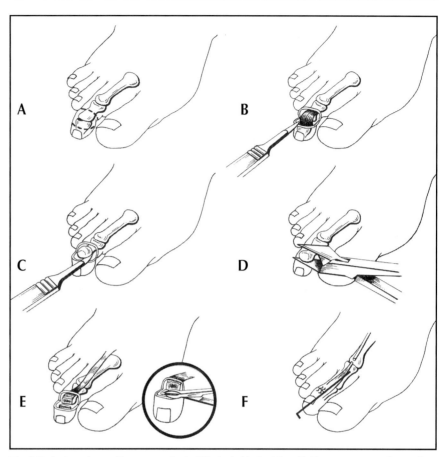

Fig. 5 Technique for mallet toe repair. **A,** Elliptical skin incision. **B,** The extensor tendon and the capsule are excised. **C,** The collateral ligaments are released, exposing the condyles of the middle phalanx. **D,** The distal part of the middle phalanx is removed with bone-cutting forceps. **E,** The exposed articular surface of the distal phalanx is resected with a rongeur. **F,** Fixation with an intramedullary K-wire.

aspect of the digit. It becomes difficult to wear constricting shoes because of pressure against the contracted digit. When the metatarsophalangeal joint becomes hyperextended, a keratotic lesion may develop plantar to the corresponding metatarsal head. Also, with a severe contracture, a callus at the tip of the toe or a nail deformity may develop.

Physical Examination
The patient is examined in both a standing and a sitting position. By definition, flexion of the proximal interphalangeal joint is a universal finding. A variable degree of flexion of the distal interphalangeal joint may be present. The metatarsophalangeal joint may be hyperextended or aligned in a neutral position (Fig. 6). The status of the metatarsophalangeal joint needs to be determined, as a hyperextension deformity of the metatarsophalangeal joint (a complex hammer toe deformity) requires simultaneous realignment. The deformity may be fixed, semiflexible, or flexible; it is important to distinguish the nature of the deformity and its rigidity, as these determine the method of treatment. If the deformity can be passively corrected, it is considered flexible. Moving the ankle from dorsiflexion to plantar flexion determines the tightness of the flexor tendons. A flexible hammer toe deformi-

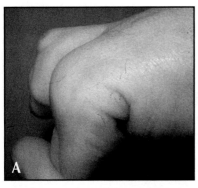 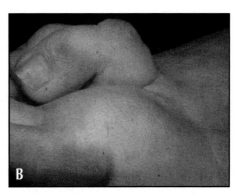

Fig. 6 A, A simple hammer toe deformity with contracture of the proximal interphalangeal joint and no deformity of the metatarsophalangeal joint. **B,** A complex hammer toe deformity characterized by hyperextension of the metatarsophalangeal joint, severe flexion of the proximal interphalangeal joint, and mild flexion of the distal interphalangeal joint.

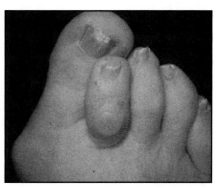

Fig 7 Moderate hallux valgus deformity with a concomitant second hammer toe. Repair of the hammer toe would be difficult without correction of the hallux valgus deformity.

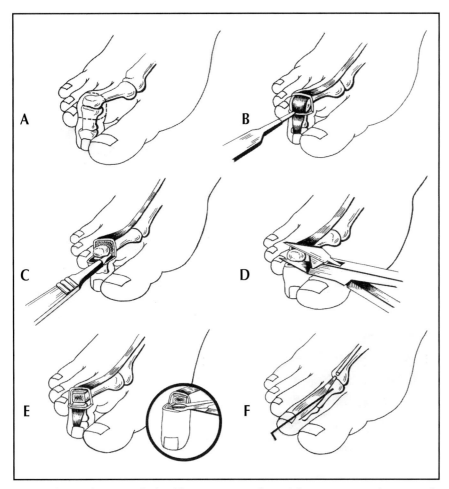

Fig. 8 Technique for repair of a fixed hammer toe. **A,** Elliptical skin incision over the proximal interphalangeal joint. **B,** The dorsal aspect of the capsule and the extensor tendon are excised. **C,** The collateral ligaments are severed, exposing the distal condyles of the proximal phalanx. **D,** The condyles of the proximal phalanx are removed with bone-cutting forceps. **E,** The articular surface of the middle phalanx is removed. **F,** Fixation with a K-wire.

ty corrects as the ankle is brought into plantar flexion. The forefoot should be palpated for adjacent areas of tenderness at the base of the involved toes to identify any pain at the metatarsophalangeal joint or interdigital neuromas. The foot should be inspected for a hallux valgus deformity and other lesser toe deformities, as these may require treatment as well (Fig. 7).

Conservative Treatment

Nonsurgical treatment involves relieving the dorsal pressure over the proximal interphalangeal joint, the pressure beneath the tip of the involved toe, and, when present, the pressure beneath the corresponding metatarsal head by both shoe modifications and padding. When the patient has a fixed deformity, a toe crest or foam toe cap may reduce pressure on the tip of the toe (Fig. 4). Tube gauze may diminish dorsal pressure on the digit as well. When the deformity is refractory to conservative care, surgical intervention may be beneficial.

Surgical Technique for Repair of a Fixed Hammer Toe Deformity

Following administration of a digital block, an elliptical (or longitudinal) incision is centered over the dorsal surface of the proximal interphalangeal joint (Fig. 8).

The skin, extensor tendon, and joint capsule are excised. The collateral ligaments are exposed over the proximal interphalangeal joint and are released, exposing the distal condyles of the proximal phalanx, which are resected transversely in the supracondylar region with bone-cutting forceps. The articular surface of the base of the middle phalanx is removed with a rongeur. A 0.045-in (0.114-cm) K-wire is introduced at the proximal interphalangeal joint and driven distally until it exits the tip of the toe. Then, with the digit aligned in a correct position, the K-wire is driven proximally to stabilize the arthroplasty site. The pin is bent at the tip of the toe to prevent proximal migration (Fig. 9).

Alternative Procedures

Other procedures recommended for the treatment of fixed hammer toe deformities include diaphysectomy,[13,14] partial proximal phalangectomy,[15-17] and even amputation as an ultimate salvage (R VanderWilde, MD and D Campbell, MD, unpublished data, 1993).

If a deformity of the metatarsophalangeal joint exists concomitantly with a hammer toe deformity, realignment of the metatarsophalangeal joint must be performed as well. For a mild deformity, an extensor tendon lengthening may suffice. For a moderate deformity, a release of the metatarsophalangeal joint capsule as well as a flexor tendon transfer may be necessary.[4] For a more severe deformity involving subluxation or frank dislocation, often soft-tissue releases are inadequate and osseous decompression is necessary. (A more complete discussion is presented in the section on metatarsophalangeal joint subluxation and dislocation.) There must be sufficient room for the corrected toe at the conclusion of the hammer toe correction. A concomitant hallux valgus deformity must be corrected or extrinsic pressure from the great toe or pressure from adjacent lesser toes will place the corrected toe at risk for recurrence.

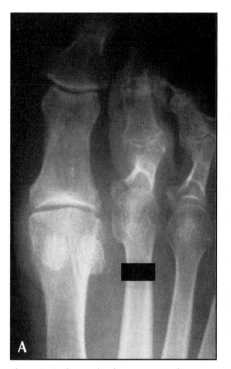 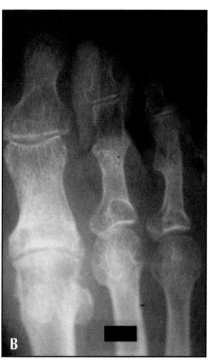

Fig. 9 A, Radiograph of preoperative hammer toe deformity. **B,** Radiograph following hammertoe repair with fusion of the proximal interphalangeal joint. (Reproduced with permission from Coughlin MJ, Dorris J, Polk E: Operative repair of the fixed hammertoe deformity. *Foot Ankle Int* 2000;21:94-104.)

Surgical Technique for a Flexor Tendon Transfer

A flexible or dynamic hammer toe deformity is often reduced with the patient sitting and the foot in an equinus position (Fig. 10). Patients with a flexible hammer toe do not have a classic claw toe deformity because the metatarsophalangeal joint is not involved. A flexible hammer toe is caused by a contracture of the flexor digitorum longus tendon.[1]

After administration of peripheral anesthesia, a transverse incision is made at the proximal plantar flexion crease of the involved digit. The soft tissue is spread, and the flexor tendon sheath is identified and is split longitudinally. A small clamp is used to place tension on the flexor digitorum longus tendon, which is the deepest of the three tendons and is characterized by a midline raphe. A percutaneous release of the distal insertion is carried out through a puncture

wound at the plantar base of the distal phalanx. The tendon is delivered into the more proximal wound and split longitudinally along the decussation, creating two tendon tails. On the dorsal aspect of the digit, a longitudinal incision is centered over the proximal phalanx. A small hemostat is passed from a dorsal to plantar direction on either side of the proximal phalanx, deep to the neurovascular bundle and superficial to the extensor hood. The two tails of the tendon are then passed on either side of the proximal phalanx and sutured in place to the extensor expansion or to the dorsal aspect of the digit. The toe is held in approximately 20° of plantar flexion as the flexor tendon is sutured to the extensor tendon under a moderate amount of tension. (On occasion, a K-wire is used to stabilize the toe. It should be used only to reinforce the repair, as the toe may redeform after it is removed.) Kuwada[18] described transfer

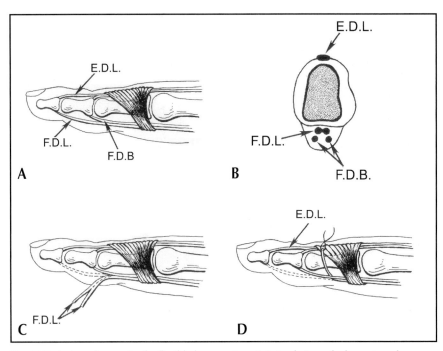

Fig. 10 Technique for repair of a flexible hammer toe. **A,** Lateral view of a lesser toe, demonstrating the anatomy of the flexor and extensor tendons. **B,** Cross-sectional anatomy at the level of the metatarsal head region. The tendon of the flexor digitorum is the deepest tendon and is characterized by a midline raphe. **C,** The flexor digitorum longus tendon has been detached at its insertion in the base of the distal phalanx with a small puncture wound and delivered through the more proximal plantar wound at the base of the toe. The tendon is split longitudinally along its median raphe, producing two segments. **D,** A tail of the flexor digitorum longus is delivered on either side of the proximal phalanx and sutured into the extensor hood. The tendon is transferred through a subcutaneous tunnel and is secured to the extensor expansion with the toe held in approximately 20° of plantar flexion at the metatarsophalangeal joint. E.D.L. = extensor digitorum longus, F.D.L. = flexor digitorum longus, and F.D.B. = flexor digitorum brevis.

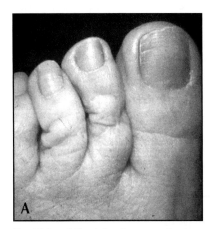 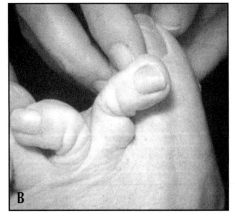

Fig. 11 Instability following excessive bone resection. **A,** Clinical appearance of the second and third digits. **B,** Clinical appearance with stress placed on the digits, demonstrating instability due to excessive bone resection. (Reproduced with permission from Coughlin MJ, Mann RA (eds): *Surgery of the Foot and Ankle*, ed 7. St. Louis, MO, Mosby, 1999.)

of the tendon through a drill hole in the base of the proximal phalanx. Otherwise, the two techniques are similar.

Postoperative Care After Repairs of Fixed and Flexible Hammer Toes

A gauze-and-tape compression dressing is applied at the time of surgery and is changed on a weekly basis. Any sutures and K-wires that were placed are removed 3 weeks following surgery. The involved toes are taped in a corrected position for 6 more weeks, until adequate healing has occurred.

Results and Complications

Both resection arthroplasty[19-21] and arthrodesis[22-25] have been recommended for the treatment of a fixed hammer toe deformity. Repair of a hammer toe creates an ankylosis of the proximal interphalangeal joint. Whether fusion or arthrofibrosis occurs is not critical, as patients are equally satisfied with either result.[7] Coughlin and associates[7] reported acceptable results in 91 of 118 toes that had been operated on in 63 patients. Ohm and associates[26] reported even better results: in a study of 25 patients, 59 of 62 toes that had been operated on had a satisfactory result. Coughlin and associates[7] reported an excellent rate of pain relief (92%) and a high rate of satisfaction (84%) following arthroplasty of the proximal interphalangeal joint. An 81% fusion rate was reported but equal satisfaction was found following fusion or fibrous union. As Kelikian[27] stated, repair of a hammer toe "yielded a satisfactory result if followed by stiffness of the joint." A stable repair is resistant to redeformation or recurrence.

Complications following hammer toe repair are uncommon. Recurrence may be because of inadequate bone resection or a tight flexor tendon, both of which may eventually require a repeat procedure if the recurrence is symptomatic. The digit might become unstable if bone resection is excessive[1] (Fig. 11); however,

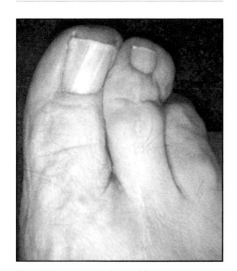

Fig. 12 Postoperatively, molding may occur as the digit conforms to the space between the remaining digits.

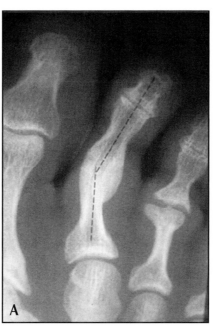

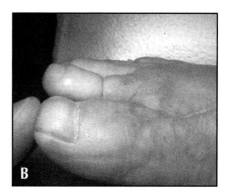

Fig. 13 A, Radiographic evidence of malalignment of the second toe following hammer toe repair. **B,** Hyperextension malalignment as seen clinically on a lateral photograph. (Reproduced with permission from Coughlin MJ, Dorris J, Polk E: Operative repair of the fixed hammertoe deformity. *Foot Ankle Int* 2000;21:94-104.)

no cases of instability were reported following the technique reported above.[7] Swelling is a common finding after correction of a hammer toe,[26,28,29] but it almost always subsides with time.[7] It should be noted that a toe will often swell to fill the space between adjacent toes, a condition referred to as molding of the digit[1] (Fig. 12). Patients should be alerted to the possibility that these conditions will develop. Probably the most common cause of dissatisfaction after surgery is malalignment,[7,29] which can occur in three planes: rotation, varus-valgus, or dorsiflexion-plantar flexion. An overall rate of malalignment of 15% (18 of 118 toes) was reported, although several of these cases were mild and were not bothersome to the patient[7] (Fig. 13). The use of intramedullary K-wire fixation is thought to substantially diminish malalignment; however, use of K-wires for longer than 3 weeks has been associated with both infection and wire breakage.[30]

Results following flexor tendon transfer for the treatment of a flexible hammer toe have generally been good; however, it is important that this procedure not be used alone for a fixed con-

tracture, as it will not produce a satisfactory result. It may be used in association with other procedures to correct alignment of the lesser toes. The rate of satisfactory results of flexor tendon transfer for the treatment of a flexible hammer toe has ranged from 54% to 90%.[31-36] Thompson and Deland[37] reported generally excellent relief of pain following this procedure; however, only 54% of toes with a subluxated metatarsophalangeal joint were noted to have complete correction at the time of final follow-up.

Complications following flexor tendon transfer include transient swelling and numbness, but these problems usually subside with time.[1] Occasionally, a K-wire placed across the metatarsophalangeal joint will break. Postoperative vascular insufficiency of a digit is unusual, but it may require removal of an intramedullary K-wire. It is paramount that adequate alignment be achieved through soft-tissue balancing intraoperatively in the event that it becomes necessary to remove the K-wire early. Following a flexor tendon transfer, patients lose the ability to curl the lesser toes. The theory behind a flexor tendon transfer is

that it enables the flexor digitorum longus tendon to assume intrinsic function and removes a deforming force at the same time. The flexor digitorum longus transfer does realign the toe, but with a loss of prehensile action of the other lesser toes. Frequently, the patient retains passive but not active function of the interphalangeal joints, although the proximal interphalangeal joint may become stiff with time. Patients should be counseled that they will lose dynamic function of the toes following a flexor tendon transfer, but this is usually a reasonable trade-off for stability of the digit.

Claw Toes
Definition and History
Development of a claw toe deformity may be associated with inflammatory arthropathy, postural deformities such as a cavus foot, trauma to the lower extremity, and neuromuscular dysfunction in which there is weakness or loss of intrinsic muscle function.[3,38-43] While many cases are idiopathic, a concerted effort should be made to determine the underlying diagnosis, as it may affect the long-term results and prognosis.[1,31,33,39]

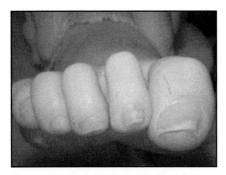

Fig. 14 Clawing of all five digits demonstrated with the push-up test, in which the examiner's hand pushes the foot and ankle into dorsiflexion, causing clawing of the digits.

The major symptom of clawing of the lesser toes is pain associated with a lesser toe contracture. A callosity overlying the proximal interphalangeal joint dorsally and beneath the metatarsophalangeal joint plantarly may be noted. With a severe contracture, a pressure callosity or breakdown may develop on the tip of the toe as it impacts against the sole of the shoe.

While the appearances of a complex hammer toe deformity and a claw toe deformity may be similar,[1] hyperextension of the metatarsophalangeal joint is the key component in differentiating the two diagnoses. A hammer toe may or may not be associated with hyperextension of the metatarsophalangeal joint, but a classic claw toe, by definition, is always associated with such hyperextension.[44,45] The deformity may be flexible or fixed depending on its duration.[1] The hyperextension deformity forces the metatarsal head plantarward, leading to the common symptoms of metatarsalgia, which may progress to a plantar callosity and even ulceration.

Physical Examination
The foot should be inspected with the patient both sitting and standing to assess midfoot and hindfoot deformities, including a cavus deformity, hindfoot varus, or contracture of the Achilles ten-

don, all of which may be associated with neuromuscular abnormalities.[9,10,39,46] To determine whether the toe deformities are fixed or dynamic, the foot is examined with the patient sitting. Absence of clawing with the ankle in plantar flexion and then development of clawing as the ankle is moved into dorsiflexion (a positive push-up test) is a classic finding associated with flexible or dynamic claw toe deformities[40] (Fig. 14). A flexible lesser-toe deformity is most frequently treated with a flexor tendon transfer, a procedure also commonly used to correct a flexible hammer toe deformity.[31,34-36] A metatarsophalangeal soft-tissue release (extensor tenotomy or lengthening with or without metatarsophalangeal capsulotomy) may be necessary depending on the magnitude of the contracture.[31,33,35]

Conservative Treatment
The use of footwear with a soft leather upper and a roomy toe box will often accommodate lesser toe contractures. Padding of the lesser toe deformities can be helpful. A toe crest may decrease pressure on the tips of the toes, and a soft insole with a metatarsal pad may decrease pressure beneath the metatarsal heads.

Surgical Technique for Repair of a Fixed Claw Toe Deformity
The factors determining the appropriate surgical technique used to correct a claw toe deformity are both the magnitude of the deformity and the inherent flexibility. When the digit is completely flexible at both of the interphalangeal joints, a flexor tendon transfer will often adequately correct the contracture and realign the digit. A metatarsophalangeal soft-tissue release may or may not be necessary.

In the presence of a fixed claw toe deformity, a hammer toe repair,[47] as described previously, is performed to align the digit. Adequate decompression is necessary to align the toe. K-wire fixation is used to stabilize the digit. A simul-

taneous contracture of the distal interphalangeal joint is not corrected surgically at the same time; often it is not a severe deformity, and a distal flexor tenotomy and K-wire fixation with concurrent treatment of the hammer toe deformity often will suffice. When only an isolated contracture of the distal interphalangeal joint is present, it may be treated with a mallet toe repair in conjunction with a soft-tissue correction of the metatarsophalangeal joint. The degree of deformity of the metatarsophalangeal joint determines whether an extensor tendon lengthening or release and/or a release of the metatarsophalangeal joint capsule is necessary. A concurrent claw toe contracture of the hallux is typically treated with fusion of the interphalangeal joint and transfer of the extensor hallucis longus to the first metatarsal head.[48]

Release of the Metatarsophalangeal Joint
A 2-cm incision is centered in the interspace between adjacent metatarsophalangeal joints and deepened to the extensor tendon, which is released or lengthened. The metatarsophalangeal joint capsule is exposed, and the dorsal, lateral, and medial aspects of the capsule and the collateral ligaments are released. A 0.045-in (0.114-cm) K-wire that was used to stabilize the proximal interphalangeal joint is then advanced across the metatarsophalangeal joint. It is bent at the tip of the toe to prevent proximal migration, and the remainder of the pin is cut and removed.

Postoperative Care
A gauze-and-tape compression dressing is applied and is changed weekly until drainage has subsided. The patient is allowed to walk while wearing a stiff-soled postoperative shoe. Sutures and the K-wire are removed 3 weeks after surgery. The involved toes are taped for 6 weeks after surgery, until adequate soft-tissue healing has occurred.

Results and Complications

Different procedures have been performed for claw toe repairs, making comparison difficult. Taylor[36] and Pyper[34] both transferred the long and short flexor tendons to the extensor expansion. Taylor[35,36] did not perform a resection arthroplasty at the proximal interphalangeal joint, whereas Pyper did. Taylor[36] reported that 50 of 68 patients had a good result, and Pyper[34] reported that 24 of 40 feet had complete or marked improvement at the time of final follow-up. It is likely that failure to correct fixed deformities of the lesser toes diminished the overall efficacy of the procedures described in these early reports. Furthermore, the authors did not define the underlying diagnoses. Transfer of the short flexor has been abandoned because of the difficulty of the surgical technique. In another series, an 83% rate of good and excellent results was reported; however, many of the deformities that were treated in that study were associated with congenital abnormalities.[33] Barbari and Brevig[31] reported that 28 of their 31 patients (90%) had a satisfactory result, but they noted restriction of motion of both the metatarsophalangeal and the interphalangeal joint in 27 of the 39 feet. This was probably the most comprehensive study reported in the literature, as the authors described preoperative demographic characteristics, performed a detailed range-of-motion analysis, presented detailed results, and carried out in-depth postoperative evaluation. They recommended resection arthroplasty for fixed deformities. A later report by Thompson and Deland[37] noted that complete lesser toe realignment was achieved in only 7 of 12 cases.

The most common complications following a claw toe repair are incomplete correction and recurrent deformity, conditions often associated with an element of fixed deformity. Thus, a soft-tissue release with a flexor tendon transfer should be performed only in the presence of a flexible or dynamic contracture. With a fixed contracture of the proximal interphalangeal joint, an arthroplasty of that joint is necessary to decompress and realign the toe.[41,44] Release of the metatarsophalangeal joint capsule and release or lengthening of the extensor tendon are equally important to balance the digit and to achieve adequate realignment.

Metatarsalgia may continue to be a symptom after lesser toe realignment. Concurrent hindfoot and midfoot deformities may be the cause of these symptoms. Treatment of such symptomatic deformities should precede distal surgical corrections. Furthermore, extensive surgery on a digit should be performed with attention to the vascular status of the toe. Metatarsophalangeal joint release, flexor tendon transfer, and realignment of a severely contracted toe may compromise circulation. Careful postoperative monitoring may be necessary. Removal of a K-wire may be required should the vascular status of the toe become impaired in the perioperative period.

Instability of the Lesser Metatarsophalangeal Joints
Definition and History

Instability of the lesser metatarsophalangeal joints is a common problem[49-51] that may occur with trauma,[1,52-54] synovitis, or inflammatory arthritis.[1,3,38,39,55] Typically, with trauma, the plantar plate and capsule are disrupted, and reduction of a traumatic dislocation may be difficult without a surgical release. Idiopathic subluxation and dislocation are by far the most frequent disorders of the metatarsophalangeal joint, and they almost always occur at the second metatarsophalangeal joint.[46] Excessive length of the second ray is often mentioned as a risk factor,[1,56] as it results in both pressure on the tip of the digit as it strikes the end of the toe box of the shoe and increased pressure from an overuse syndrome with chronic deterioration of the plantar aspect of the capsule[56] (MJ Coughlin, MD, RC Schenck Jr, MD, and D Bloome, MD, unpublished data, 2001). Extrinsic pressure with an associated hallux valgus deformity may lead to pressure on the digit and destabilization of the second metatarsophalangeal joint.

The terms synovitis, capsulitis, crossover second toe, subluxation, and dislocation all describe a continuum of instability of the lesser metatarsophalangeal joint. Depending on the actual structures that deteriorate (the plantar aspect of the capsule and/or the collateral ligaments), the metatarsophalangeal joint may be characterized by a pure hyperextension deformity, a lateral deviation, or, more commonly, a medial deviation. Typically, over time, erosion of the fibular collateral ligament and the plantar lateral aspect of the capsule allows the toe to drift in a dorsomedial direction.[4,56]

The most frequent symptom of early instability of the second metatarsophalangeal joint is ill-defined pain in the forefoot, not dissimilar to that caused by an interdigital neuroma. In fact, the major challenge for the physician is to assist the patient in defining the exact location of the pain. With time and the onset of digital deformity, the diagnosis becomes more obvious. Early on, however, there is typically neither a digital deformity nor a deformity at the metatarsophalangeal joint. With time and with increased deformity, a hammer toe may lead to pain with shoe wear. Frequently, the symptoms of metatarsophalangeal joint subluxation are insidious. The pain occurs with walking and is less severe with rest. Typically, the pain does not radiate to the toes unless there is a concomitant neuroma (MJ Coughlin, MD, RC Schenck Jr, MD, and D Bloome, MD, unpublished data, 2001).

Physical Examination

Localized swelling of the toe and/or metatarsophalangeal joint and tenderness on palpation of the plantar aspect of the metatarsophalangeal joint are early phys-

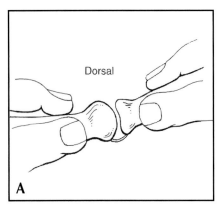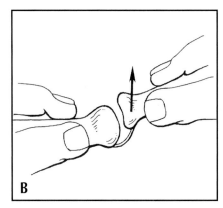

Fig. 15 The drawer test. **A,** The involved toe is grasped between the examiner's thumb and index finger and stressed in a dorsal direction. **B,** This maneuver elicits pain at the metatarsophalangeal joint and is pathognomonic of instability.

ical findings. With time, dorsomedial deviation of the toe at the metatarsophalangeal joint and a progressive hammer toe deformity are noted.

The most useful test for diagnosis of instability of the metatarsophalangeal joint is the drawer test (Fig. 15). In this test, the toe is vertically subluxated, which places a shear stress on the plantar aspect of the capsule and elicits characteristic pain.[8,57,58] Typically, instability of the metatarsophalangeal joint is not associated with neuritic symptoms or numbness unless a concomitant interdigital neuroma has developed. Coughlin and associates (unpublished data, 2001) reported that such neuromas occur in up to 20% of cases. With time, a patient loses the ability to flex the toe or toes of the involved foot.

A radiographic examination is helpful both to assess the magnitude of the malalignment and to rule out confounding diagnoses such as a Freiberg's infraction, degenerative joint disease, and inflammatory arthritis. On AP radiographs, progressive hyperextension of the metatarsophalangeal joint is characterized by gradual diminution of the joint space as the proximal phalanx subluxates dorsally over the metatarsal head. On lateral radiographs, frank dislocation may eventually

be demonstrated (Fig. 16). A bone scan may assist in localizing ill-defined forefoot pain to a specific metatarsophalangeal joint.

Conservative Treatment

Treatment of a symptomatic crossover toe involves use of a well-fitted shoe with sufficient room for the deformity of the second toe. A metatarsal pad placed just proximal to the symptomatic metatarsophalangeal joint may reduce plantar pressure. Taping of the involved toe to an adjacent digit may decrease symptoms, but it will not correct the deformity. Nonsteroidal anti-inflammatory medications may decrease discomfort. The judicious use of an intra-articular steroid injection may diminish symptoms. Trepman and Yeo[59] and Mizel and Michelson[60] reported success with intra-articular steroid injection; however, Reis and associates[61] reported dislocation of the metatarsophalangeal joint following an intra-articular steroid injection.

Surgical Treatment of Mild and Moderate Malalignment of the Lesser Metatarsophalangeal Joint

A deformity of the second metatarsophalangeal joint is frequently associated with a hammer toe deformity. The magnitude

of the deformity and its rigidity determine the procedure required for realignment. A rigid, fixed hammer toe deformity requires an arthroplasty of the proximal interphalangeal joint, whereas a flexible deformity is treated with a flexor tendon transfer. (See the discussion on repair of fixed and flexible hammer toes.) A flexor tendon transfer may be used even in the presence of a fixed deformity, for which it is used to stabilize or realign the metatarsophalangeal joint and may be combined with a repair of the fixed hammer toe.

With progression of metatarsophalangeal joint subluxation, the deviation of the metatarsophalangeal joint may be lateral, medial, or dorsal. The metatarsophalangeal joint is first explored through a curvilinear dorsal incision exposing the joint. A lengthening or release of the extensor tendon is carried out. The dorsal aspect of the capsule is released along with adjacent contractures of either the medial or the lateral aspect of the capsule. Release of the first lumbrical may remove a substantial deforming force. With hyperextension of the metatarsophalangeal joint, adhesions frequently develop between the plantar aspect of the metatarsal head and the plantar aspect of the capsule, which must be released as well to allow reduction of the base of the proximal phalanx. Once the capsule has been released, any remaining deviation can be corrected with tightening of the collateral ligaments (reefing at the metatarsophalangeal joint) on the elongated side.[1] One or two figure-of-8 sutures are placed in the distal lateral aspect of the metatarsophalangeal joint capsule and directed into the plantar lateral aspect of the capsule proximally. Typically, this will correct 5° to 10° of axial malalignment. A flexor tendon transfer will often provide a plantar flexion force to the digit and increase stability as well. Intraoperative plantar flexion-dorsiflexion of the ankle is a provocative test for determining stability of the joint

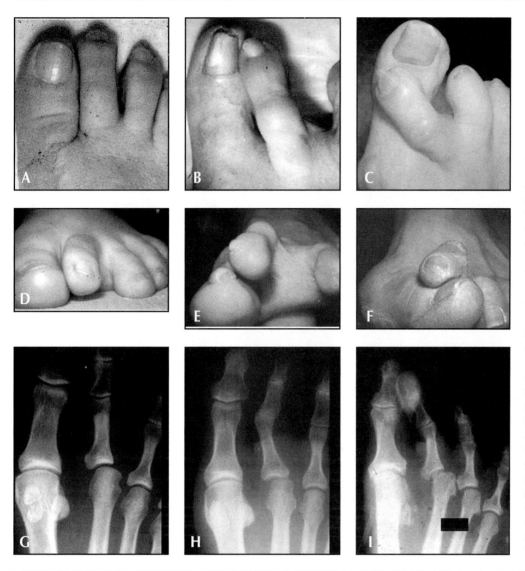

Fig 16 Instability of the second metatarsophalangeal joint with progressive deviation. **A-C,** Clinical views showing mild deformity (**A**), moderate deformity (**B**), and severe deformity (**C**). (**C** reproduced with permission from Coughlin MJ: Crossover second toe deformity. *Foot Ankle* 1987;8:29-39.) **D-F,** End-on views showing mild deformity (**D**), moderate deformity (**E**), and severe deformity (**F**). (**D** reproduced with permission from Coughlin MJ, Mann RA (eds): *Surgery of the Foot and Ankle*, ed 7. St. Louis, MO, Mosby, 1999. **E** reproduced with permission from Coughlin MJ: Crossover second toe deformity. *Foot Ankle* 1987;8:29-39.) **G-I,** Radiographs showing mild deformity (**G**), moderate deformity (**H**), and severe deformity (**I**). (**I** reproduced with permission from Coughlin MJ: Crossover second toe deformity. *Foot Ankle* 1987;8:29-39.)

after realignment has been performed. If the joint is well aligned and stabilized, the repair can be protected with placement of an intramedullary 0.045-in (0.114-cm) K-wire. The toe, however, should be well aligned before the K-wire is placed. The extensor tendon is repaired, and the skin is closed in a routine fashion (Fig. 17).

Postoperative Care

A gauze and tape compression dressing is applied and is changed on a weekly basis. Sutures and K-wires are removed 3 weeks following surgery. The toe is then taped in a slightly overcorrected position with slight plantar flexion for 6 weeks.

Surgical Correction of Moderate and Severe Instability and Malalignment of the Lesser Metatarsophalangeal Joint

A moderate or severe deformity involves both subluxation or dislocation of the metatarsophalangeal joint and a fixed hammer toe deformity. A soft-tissue release (including tendon lengthening and release of the metatarsophalangeal joint capsule) is necessary but often insufficient. Adhesions of the plantar aspect of the capsule are released, and a flexor tendon transfer may help to realign the joint; however, osseous decompression is often necessary. Choices for

osseous decompression include partial proximal phalangectomy,[16,17] arthroplasty of the metatarsal head,[1] and shortening osteotomy of the second metatarsal.[62,63] Shortening osteotomies have been recognized to be effective in achieving joint decompression by lengthening the adjacent soft-tissue structures.

Technique of Capital Osteotomy

A 3-cm incision is placed either in the second interspace or directly over the second metatarsophalangeal joint (Fig. 18). The dorsal, medial, and lateral aspects of the capsule are released. Plantar flexion of the proximal phalanx exposes

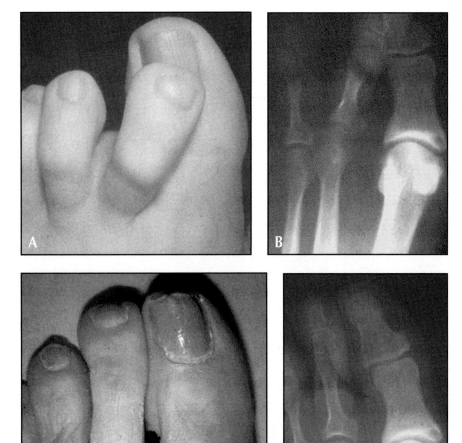

Fig. 17 Soft-tissue realignment for treatment of a crossover second toe. **A,** Preoperative clinical appearance. **B,** Preoperative radiographic appearance. **C,** Postoperative clinical appearance following flexor tendon transfer and soft-tissue realignment. (B and C Reproduced with permission from Coughlin MJ: Crossover second toe deformity. *Foot Ankle* 1987; 8:29-39.) **D,** Postoperative radiographic appearance.

the proximal phalanx and help to realign the metatarsophalangeal joint.

Postoperative Care
A gauze-and-tape compression dressing is applied and changed on a weekly basis. Walking is permitted with a stiff wooden-soled postoperative shoe. Weight-bearing in a soft-soled shoe is permitted at 6 weeks. The toe is supported with taping in a corrected position for 6 weeks after the dressing has been removed.

Results and Complications
The surgical correction of 15 toes with use of a variety of surgical techniques depending on the severity of the deformity has been reported.[51] The techniques included soft-tissue release, flexor tendon transfer, and occasional osseous decompression for the treatment of both chronic and acute subluxation of the metatarsophalangeal joint. Fourteen of the 15 toes had a good or excellent result. In another report, on seven younger, more active patients, a good or excellent result was obtained in five patients.[57] A positive drawer test was pathognomonic of early instability of the metatarsophalangeal joint.

Trnka and associates[63] reported on 15 patients in whom a total of 25 capital oblique osteotomies had been performed. Twenty-one of the 25 metatarsophalangeal joint dislocations were successfully relocated, with an average shortening of 4.4 mm. Twelve of the 15 patients were satisfied with the result. Complications included limited plantar flexion following the osteotomy.

Other procedures reported for the treatment of instability and malalignment of the second metatarsophalangeal joint include transfer of the extensor digitorum brevis. In one study,[64] a high level of successful realignment was reported in toes treated with this procedure. Results of partial proximal phalangectomy or proximal phalangectomy and syndactylization (Fig. 19) were reported by

the metatarsal head. A longitudinal oblique distal metatarsal osteotomy is performed from a distal superior point (2 mm inferior to the dorsal metatarsal superior articular surface), parallel to the plantar surface of the foot, and continued in a proximal direction until the saw blade penetrates the proximal metatarsal cortex. The distal fragment is proximally translated the desired amount (2 to 6 mm) and is stabilized with one or two dorsoplantar lag screws. Care is taken to avoid using excessively long screws. The dorsal surface of the metatarsal head, which now extends beyond the articular surface, is beveled with a rongeur. The extensor tendon is repaired in a lengthened fashion. Frequently, a flexor tendon transfer is performed; this removes a deforming force from the distal aspect of the toe and adds a plantar flexion force to the proximal aspect. Whether a flexor tendon transfer is a dynamic transfer or merely has a tenodesis effect is probably academic. The effect is to stabilize and depress

Conklin and Smith[16] and by Cahill and Connor.[15] Conklin and Smith[16] reported that 31 of 52 patients had complete relief of pain but 15 patients were dissatisfied after partial proximal phalangectomy. Cahill and Connor[15] reported that the procedure resulted in substantial relief of symptoms but a poor cosmetic appearance. Seventeen of 34 patients had a poor result. Daly and Johnson[17] combined a partial proximal phalangectomy of the second and third metatarsophalangeal joints with partial syndactylization in 53 patients (60 feet). Cock-up deformity recurred in 10 patients, residual pain was present in 14, excessive shortening occurred in 3, and moderate or severe cosmetic problems were noted in 15.

On occasion, a digit is amputated because of the severity of the deformity or the age of the patient. VanderWilde and Campbell (unpublished data, 1993) performed 23 amputations on 16 patients. Eleven patients were satisfied at the time of long-term follow-up, but hallux valgus was noted to progress, and one patient had a metatarsophalangeal arthrodesis at a later date.

The magnitude of the surgery performed to correct metatarsophalangeal malalignment and hammer toe deformities is limited by the possibility of vascular compromise. These deformities must be treated in a progressive fashion in order to avoid excessive surgery, which can imperil the vascular status of the digit.

An adequate soft-tissue release is the first step in achieving realignment, and a transfer of an extrinsic tendon may help to remove a deforming force and add a stabilizing force. Adequate osseous decompression is frequently necessary to achieve realignment of toes with more severe deformities. Reduction of pain is the primary objective of surgery, and the patient should expect a passively aligned toe, but typically dynamic function is lost. A certain amount of arthrofibrosis of the metatarsophalangeal joint is present after reconstruction. Recurrence is prob-

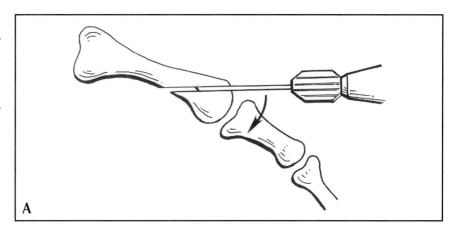

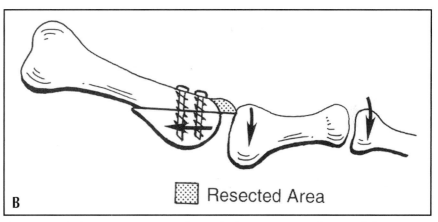

Fig. 18 Capital oblique osteotomy. **A,** A longitudinal osteotomy is made as parallel as possible to the plantar surface of the foot. The amount of displacement is determined before the procedure. **B,** The osteotomy is displaced proximally and fixed with one or two mini-fragment compression screws. The prominent metaphyseal spike is excised.

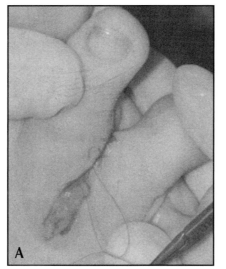
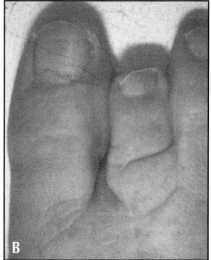

Fig. 19 Mini-syndactylization of the lesser toes. **A,** Surgical technique. **B,** Less than satisfactory cosmetic result (Courtesy of K. Johnson, MD.)

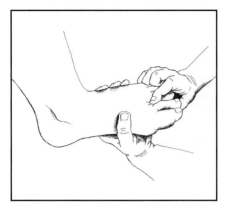

Fig. 20 The Mulder sign. The thumb and index finger of the examiner are used to palpate the symptomatic interspace. With compression of the transverse arch with the other hand, a click may be noted. The click is thought to represent subluxation of the nerve beneath the transverse metatarsal ligament.

ably the most frequent complication of the treatment of a subluxated or dislocated digit. With extensive surgery on a lesser toe, possible complications include vascular compromise and fatigue and breakage of K-wires. Postoperative edema may take months to subside. Unless there is an injury to the digital nerves, numbness or paresthesias often subside with time.

Interdigital Neuroma
Definition and History
An interdigital neuroma presents as ill-defined forefoot pain most typically in the second or third intermetatarsal space. It commonly presents in the fifth decade of life.[2,65,66] Its frequent presentation in women has led to the implication of high-fashion footwear as a cause.[2,67,69] When there is numbness and radiation of neuritic symptoms into the digits, the diagnosis of an interdigital neuroma should be considered when evaluating lesser toe abnormalities, especially those associated with malalignment or pain in the lesser metatarsophalangeal joints. Instability of an adjacent lesser metatarsophalangeal joint and inflammatory arthritis are the major confounding diagnoses (MJ

Coughlin, MD, RC Schenck Jr, MD, and D Bloome, MD, unpublished data, 2001).

The major symptom of an interdigital neuroma is intractable pain, which is most frequently isolated to either the second or the third intermetatarsal space.[67,70] Occurrence in the first or fourth interspace is exceedingly rare.[67,70] Radiation of neuritic pain, numbness in the digits, increased pain with constricting shoe wear, and relief with removal of shoes are common with a symptomatic neuroma.

Physical Examination
On physical examination, pain is isolated to the symptomatic intermetatarsal space. A Mulder sign[70-72] is thought to demonstrate subluxation of the thickened nerve beneath the transverse metatarsal ligament (Fig. 20). In one study,[70] radiation of neuritic pain was found in 35% of 74 patients, numbness of an adjacent digit in 30%, and a positive Mulder sign in 41% on preoperative physical examination. Careful examination revealed decreased sensation in the digits in approximately one third of patients.[70] Radiographs are helpful to rule out confounding diagnoses such as degenerative arthritis, Freiberg's infraction, and inflammatory arthritis as well as instability of the lesser metatarsophalangeal joints. While often a patient has difficulty isolating the exact area of forefoot pain, sequential injections of 1% lidocaine hydrochloride into the symptomatic interspace and adjacent metatarsophalangeal joints may help to localize the painful interspace.[70,73] Only approximately 40% of patients can accurately localize the pain without the use of lidocaine injections.

Conservative Treatment
The use of metatarsal pads, orthotic devices, nonsteroidal anti-inflammatory medication, shoe modifications, diminished activity, and occasionally steroid injection all may help to diminish symptoms.[74-77] Conservative measures relieve symptoms in more than 50% of cases.[78-80]

When these methods are unsuccessful, surgical excision of the symptomatic nerve may be considered.

Surgical Technique for Excision of an Interdigital Neuroma
After administration of peripheral anesthesia, a 3-cm dorsal longitudinal incision is centered over the involved interspace. A dorsal approach has been favored and is associated with a much lower rate of wound complications.[71,76,81,82] The transverse metatarsal ligament is placed under tension with a self-retaining retractor and is then transected. A small Freer elevator is used to delineate the interdigital nerve distally below the bifurcation, and proximally the common digital nerve is identified in the interosseous region. Approximately 3 cm proximal to the bifurcation, the nerve is transected. Then both branches are transected distal to the bifurcation, and the segment is removed. It is important to sever any adjacent capsular branches in order to allow proximal migration of the nerve stump and thus diminish the chance of the neuroma recurring.[68,71,83] The wound is approximated with an interrupted skin closure.

Postoperative Care
A gauze-and-tape compression dressing is applied at the time of surgery and is changed weekly. Weight bearing in a stiff-soled postoperative shoe is immediately allowed as tolerated. Sutures are removed 3 weeks following surgery, and the foot is protected in a compression wrap for 3 more weeks.

Results and Complications
The aim of the clinician is both to educate the patient and to help him or her to define the exact location of the pain. With a careful preoperative clinical evaluation in which confounding clinical diagnoses are eliminated, a high success rate can be expected.[70] In general, results following surgical treatment of a neuroma are satisfactory, with relief of symptoms in

approximately 80% of cases.[68,70,71,81] Nonetheless, it is not uncommon for a patient to have residual tenderness in the involved interspace or pain in an adjacent interspace following such surgery.[69,70] However, this is rarely bothersome to the patient and is usually found only on clinical examination.[70] Mann and Reynolds[71] observed substantial variability in the cutaneous innervation of the distal part of the forefoot. Coughlin and Pinsonneault[70] noted that half of the patients studied had subjective numbness after surgery, but it was bothersome in only 6 of 71 feet. The results of objective evaluation of numbness vary from patient to patient; however, a much wider area of postoperative numbness has been demonstrated following excision of adjacent neuromas.[84] Surgery in adjacent interspaces is infrequently performed and rarely if ever performed simultaneously.[68,70,84] Friscia and associates[67] found a higher dissatisfaction rate following excision of adjacent neuromas in a small series of nine patients.

Complications following neuroma excision include continued pain, wound infection, fat atrophy, and intractable plantar keratoses.[67,69-71,81] Although Coughlin and Pinsonneault[70] noted a positive Tinel sign postoperatively in one third of cases, no patient was aware of this sign prior to their postoperative evaluation. Up to 40% of patients may have postoperative limitations of activity,[70,81] and limitations with regard to the type of shoes that can be worn are frequent as well.[67,69-71]

Deformities of the Fifth Toe
Definition and History
Deformities of the metatarsophalangeal joint of the fifth toe can result in overlapping, underlapping, or a cock-up deformity of the digit. A cock-up deformity is often associated with progressive development of a fixed hammer toe and occurs in older individuals (Fig. 21). Overlapping (Fig. 22) and underlapping fifth toes typically are congenital deformities, and

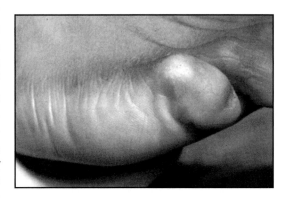

Fig. 21 Cock-up deformity of the fifth toe.

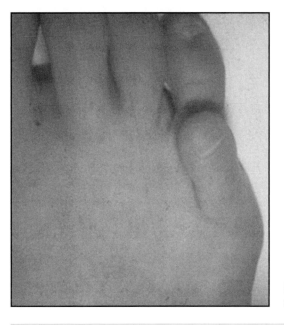

Fig. 22 Preoperative appearance of a crossover fifth-toe deformity.

both are externally rotated. With an overlapping toe, a contracture of the extensor digitorum longus tendon is associated with hyperextension of the metatarsophalangeal joint. An underlapping fifth toe frequently is associated with contracture of both the flexor digitorum longus tendon and the plantar aspect of the metatarsophalangeal joint capsule. Capsular adhesions frequently develop in the area of redundant capsule and resist simple soft-tissue release.[85] A severe cock-up deformity of the fifth toe often consists of a fixed hammer toe deformity coupled with a hyperextension deformity of the metatarsophalangeal joint in which the base of the proximal phalanx articulates

with the metatarsal articular surface at almost a 90° angle.

The major symptom of any of these deformities is pain caused by pressure of the involved toes against the shoe. However, it is not unusual for younger patients to be concerned with the cosmetic appearance of the toe as well. Ascertaining the major problem is important in discerning the patient's expectations of treatment.

Physical Examination
Axial rotation of the digit, varus or medial deviation of the proximal phalanx, and hyperextension or flexion contracture of the metatarsophalangeal joint are the characteristic deformities. A hammer toe

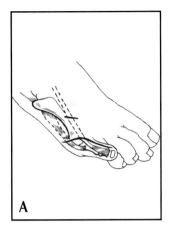 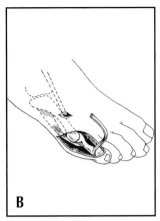 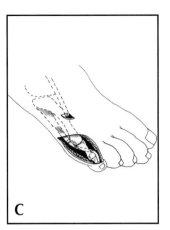 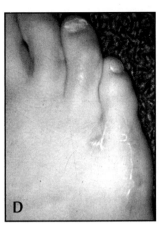

Fig. 23 Technique for repair of an overlapping fifth toe. **A,** Surgical incision to expose the overlapping fifth toe. **B,** Following proximal release of the extensor digitorum longus and metatarsophalangeal capsular release. **C,** Following transfer of the extensor digitorum longus beneath the proximal phalanx to correct both hyperextension and malrotation of the fifth toe. **D,** Postoperative appearance following soft-tissue release and tendon transfer.

also occurs with a cock-up fifth-toe deformity. The severity of the skin and soft-tissue contractures determines the magnitude of the deformity, and the magnitude determines whether a soft-tissue release or an osseous decompression will be necessary to realign the digit.

Conservative Treatment

Often, mild deformities are adequately managed with shoe wear modifications. A shoe with a broad, roomy toe box to decrease pressure on the fourth and fifth toes is often sufficient. Padding with the use of tube gauze or foam pads may diminish extrinsic pressure. When non-surgical treatment is unsuccessful, surgical intervention is tailored to the specific deformities.

Surgical Treatment of an Overlapping Fifth Toe

For less severe deformities, a soft-tissue metatarsophalangeal joint release and correction of skin contractures may allow successful realignment of the digit.[86,87] For more severe contractures, Lapidus[88] advocated a soft-tissue release combined with a transfer of the extensor digitorum longus tendon to the abductor digiti quinti (Fig. 23).

After administration of regional anesthesia, a dorsal curvilinear incision is centered over the fifth metatarsophalangeal joint. The dorsal, medial, and lateral portions of the metatarsophalangeal joint capsule are released. A curved elevator is used to release any plantar adhesions between the plantar aspect of the capsule and the metatarsal head,[85] which, if left intact, may prevent reduction of the metatarsophalangeal joint. The insertion of the extensor digitorum longus tendon is preserved distally, but it is released proximally 3 to 4 cm proximal to the metatarsophalangeal joint through a small puncture incision. If any hyperextension, abduction, or rotation of the digit remains following the soft-tissue capsular release, transfer of the extensor digitorum longus tendon is carried out. The tendon is delivered subcutaneously into the distal wound. It is then carefully transferred circumferentially around the proximal phalanx, from medial to plantar, to the lateral aspect of the fifth toe (deep to the neurovascular bundle). At the conclusion of the transfer, the toe should be in neutral rotation, neutral flexion, and slight valgus. With the toe positioned in correct alignment, the tendon stump is sutured into the abductor digiti quinti.

The skin edges are sutured to minimize tension on the realigned toe.

Alternative Method

Osseous decompression of the metatarsophalangeal joint contracture may be accomplished with a partial or total proximal phalangectomy.[89,90] Syndactylization of the fourth and fifth toes may be necessary to stabilize the digit following phalangectomy.[91-94] Depending on the severity of the contracture and the amount of bone resected, shortening of the fifth toe will occur. A patient should be informed about this prior to surgery.

General Postoperative Care Following Realignment of the Fifth Toe

A gauze-and-tape compression dressing is applied at the time of surgery and is changed weekly to maintain the digit in the correct position. If a K-wire has been placed, the dressing may be changed less frequently. The patient is allowed to walk while wearing a stiff-soled postoperative shoe. Three weeks after surgery, the sutures and the K-wire are removed. The fifth toe is taped to the fourth toe for 6 to 8 weeks, until adequate soft-tissue healing has occurred.

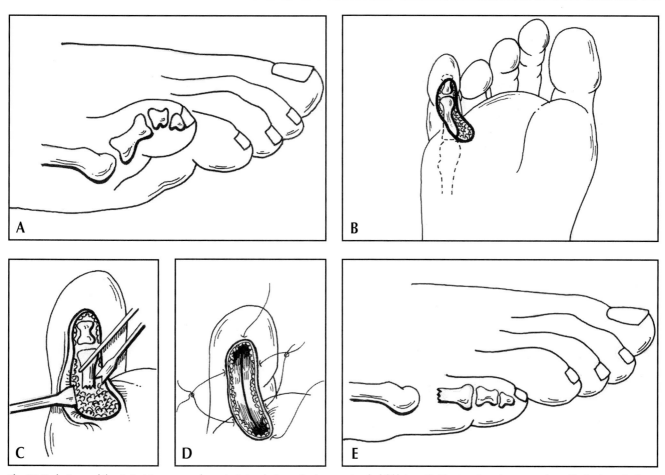

Fig. 24 Technique of the Ruiz-Mora procedure. **A,** Lateral view of a hyperextended fifth toe. **B,** Plantar view demonstrating elliptical surgical excision of the skin and soft tissue. **C,** Subtotal resection of the proximal phalanx. **D,** Technique of skin closure reducing the ellipse. **E,** Final position of the toe following the procedure.

Results and Complications

Frequently, a soft-tissue release and realignment is effective treatment for an overlapping fifth toe; a tendon transfer is reserved for more severe deformities. Cockin,[85] Black and associates,[95] and Lantzounis[86] all reported greater than 80% rates of successful results following soft-tissue realignment.

Complications include undercorrection or recurrence of deformity, which is often caused by inadequate soft-tissue release. Mann and Coughlin[96] estimated that the recurrence rate following this procedure is 10%. Vascular compromise is a risk because of the substantial soft-tissue release necessary to achieve adequate realignment.

Surgical Treatment of Cock-Up Deformity of the Fifth Toe (Modified Ruiz-Mora Procedure)

In a cock-up deformity of the fifth toe, a severe dorsiflexion contracture of the fifth toe is combined with a fixed hammer toe deformity (Fig. 24). While a soft-tissue release of the metatarsophalangeal joint contracture combined with a hammer toe repair of the fifth toe will often suffice for mild to moderate deformities, frequently the fixed nature of a severe deformity requires substantial osseous decompression to successfully realign the digit.

After administration of regional anesthesia, a longitudinal elliptical incision is centered on the plantar aspect of the fifth toe, deviating in a medial direction at the

base of the digit. Following excision of the ellipse of skin and soft tissue, the flexor tendon is released. The proximal phalanx is exposed, and, with a subperiosteal dissection, either the proximal one-half or the entire phalanx is excised, depending on the magnitude of the toe contracture. The goal is to successfully realign the toe without placing tension on the skin or neurovascular bundles. Once the osseous decompression is accomplished, the skin edges of the ellipse are approximated at a right angle to the longitudinal axis of the fifth toe, correcting alignment in both the axial and the sagittal plane.

Janecki and Wilde[90] reported a 23% incidence of bunionette formation and a 32% incidence of formation of a hammer

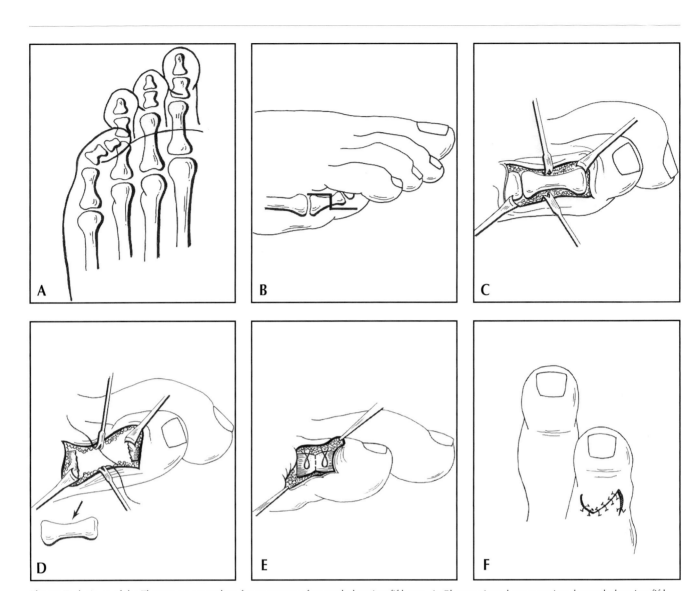

Fig. 25 Technique of the Thompson procedure for treatment of an underlapping fifth toe. **A,** Plantar view demonstrating the underlapping fifth toe. **B,** Lateral view demonstrating the skin incision. **C,** Technique for excision for the proximal phalanx. **D,** After excision of the proximal phalanx. **E,** Intraoperative capsular closure. **F,** Closure of the z-plasty incision.

toe deformity of the fourth toe following a complete phalangectomy. They revised their procedure and recommended a subtotal resection of the proximal phalanx. All of the patients, however, had complete relief of symptoms and correction of the deformity, and the problems seemed to be related to excessive shortening of the fifth toe. Dyal and associates[89] reported that 8 of 12 patients were satisfied after the resection and realignment. None had formation of a bunionette or hammer toe.

Probably the main complication following this procedure is instability of the fifth toe. Dyal and associates[89] noted that some patients were dissatisfied with the severe shortening and poor cosmetic appearance after the operation. The average shortening was slightly more than 1 cm. The difficulty in treating a severe cock-up deformity of the fifth toe is that inadequate soft-tissue release can be associated with either recurrence or vascular compromise and substantial osseous decompression can be associated with unac-

ceptable shortening of the digit. A frank preoperative discussion with the patient is important to both define the patient's expectations and educate him or her regarding the possibility of complications. A subtotal resection of the phalanx appears to be preferable.

Surgical Treatment of an Underlapping Fifth Toe
An underlapping fifth toe, in which the fifth toe lies beneath the fourth toe, is much less common than either of the

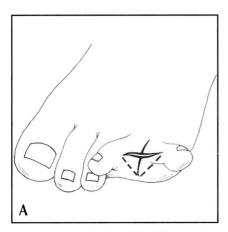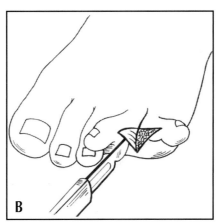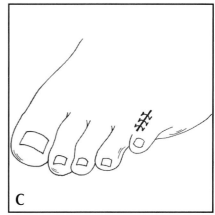

Fig. 26 Syndactylization of the fifth toe. **A,** Proposed skin incision. **B,** Removal of two triangular wedges. **C,** Following closure of the skin with mini-syndactylization of the fifth toe.

previously described deformities[97] (Fig. 25). After administration of regional anesthesia, a z-type incision is centered over the lateral aspect of the proximal phalanx of the fifth toe. The distal limb of the z lies laterally, and the proximal limb lies medially. The dissection is deepened to expose the proximal phalanx. The tendon of the extensor digitorum longus is released. The proximal phalanx is partially or completely excised, depending on the magnitude of the contracture (as is done for the Ruiz-Mora procedure). The digit is derotated, and the capsule is closed to reduce the soft-tissue dead space. (An intramedullary K-wire often is used to stabilize the toe.) The z-type incision is rotated to correct the skin contracture and is approximated with interrupted sutures.

Technique of Syndactylization of the Fourth and Fifth Toes

Syndactylization of the fourth and fifth toes is reserved for severe deformities and as a means of salvage following failed prior surgery, not only for instability of the fifth toe but for that of any of the other lesser toes (Fig. 26). Often, it is coupled with partial proximal phalangectomy of the fourth and fifth toes.

After administration of a regional anesthetic block, the fourth and fifth toes

are separated by a web-bisecting incision. It is flanked by two peridigital triangular skin incisions, which are then resected, and both plantar and dorsal flaps are developed. Partial proximal phalangectomies are performed (either on the fifth toe or on the fourth and fifth toes) through the same incision.[91] Care is taken to protect the neurovascular bundles during the dissection. The dorsal and plantar flaps are apposed and closed with interrupted sutures.

Results and Complications

Kelikian and associates[92] and others[17,93,94] have reported satisfactory results with syndactylization of the lesser toes. Daly and Johnson[17] reported a 75% rate of satisfactory results with syndactylization and partial proximal phalangectomy of the second and third toes. Marek and associates,[94] Jahss,[91] Scrase,[98] and Leonard and Rising[93] all proposed it as an effective treatment for fifth-toe deformities. However, a surgeon must be aware that correcting a deformity by creating a second deformity may not be an acceptable alternative to the patient. The cosmetic results may be troubling. Furthermore, syndactylization does not always stabilize a digit and may actually lead to a deformity of the adjacent digit.

When fifth-toe deformities are treat-

ed, adequate alignment must be achieved at the time of surgery. When a soft-tissue release alone does not sufficiently realign the digit, a tendon transfer or osseous decompression should be considered. Severe deformities characterized by skin contractures may herald neurovascular compromise with only a soft-tissue release. Amputation, on the other hand, is rarely considered as a primary procedure, but it may be considered as a salvage of a previous failure. Associated development of a bunionette, hammer toe deformities of the fourth and fifth toes, or an intractable plantar keratotic lesion beneath the fourth metatarsal head may be the late sequelae of a fifth-toe amputation.

Interdigital and Lateral Fifth-Toe Corns
Definition and History

The term corn is used to describe a callosity overlying an osseous prominence in which keratotic layers of epidermis accumulate in response to extensive pressure or friction.[99] Because of the high prevalence of corn formation in women, high-fashion footwear has frequently been implicated as a cause.[1] The most common location for corns is over the dorsolateral aspect of the fifth toe[9,100] (Fig. 27, *A*) and in the interdigital space between the fourth and fifth toes.[101] A corn

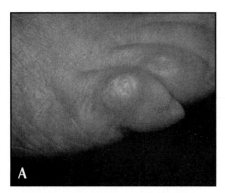 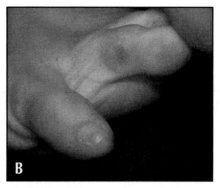 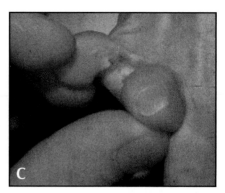

Fig. 27 A, Lateral fifth-toe corn. **B,** Interdigital corn. **C,** Interdigital web-space corn. (Reproduced with permission from Coughlin MJ, Mann RA (eds): *Surgery of the Foot and Ankle*, ed 7. St. Louis, MO, Mosby, 1999.)

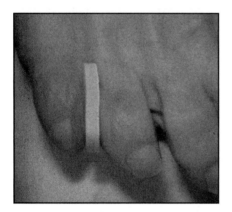

Fig. 28 Pad placed between the fourth and fifth toes to cushion an interdigital corn.

may affect one or several digits. A variety of terms have been used to describe a lateral corn on the fifth toe, including hard corn and heloma durum.[5,102] Likewise, terms such as kissing corn and heloma molle have been used for an interdigital corn.[103,104] All of these terms lead to substantial confusion because, from a histologic standpoint, the keratotic lesions are identical; thus, usually it is preferred that the actual location of the callosity be used to describe the corn. Although Gillett[105,106] found that interdigital corns were much more commonly seen in a distal location (Fig. 27, *B*) than in the web space (Fig. 27, *C*), results from another study found the prevalence of interdigital corns and lateral fifth-toe corns to be approximately equal (M Kennedy, MD and MJ Coughlin, MD, unpublished data, 2002).

When a corn develops in a web space, maceration due to condensation of moisture may make it difficult to differentiate the lesion from a mycotic infection.[10,91,102] The chief symptom of a symptomatic corn is pain associated with the development of a thickened callosity over a lesser toe. An interdigital corn has been noted to be much more painful than a lateral fifth-toe corn.[1] Often a wide foot or splaying of the forefoot has been associated with corn formation, and a concomitant bunionette or hallux valgus deformity is not uncommon. Although it has been hypothesized that a short fifth metatarsal distorts the normal relationship of the phalanges, allowing impingement of interdigital prominences against other prominences,[107] Zeringue and Harkless[108] found no substantial difference in the relative lengths of the fourth and fifth metatarsals in feet with a webspace corn. Likewise, rarely is an exostosis, degenerative joint disease, or a subluxated or hypertrophied condyle the underlying cause of corn formation. A contracted digit is probably the most common deformity associated with corn formation.[108]

Conservative Treatment

Nonsurgical treatment for either type of corn is centered around the relief of pressure. Shoes with a wide, roomy toe box and a lower heel, padding of the sympto-

matic lesion, and shaving of the corn often give symptomatic relief (Fig. 28).

Surgical Treatment of a Lateral Fifth-Toe Corn

When conservative care is unsuccessful, a lateral fifth toe corn may be treated with either a lateral condylectomy and flexor tenotomy or a complete condylectomy (Fig. 29). The procedure for a complete condylectomy is identical to that described for a hammer toe repair. Young patients with a flexible deformity may be treated with a flexor tenotomy.[11,12]

After a digital anesthetic block has been administered, a longitudinal incision is centered over the involved toe just dorsal to the keratotic lesion. Typically, the incision is extended over the midportion of the middle phalanx to the base of the proximal phalanx. (Treatment of a distal lesion on the proximal phalanx does not include excision of the callus.) The incision is deepened to the phalanx, and the capsule and the collateral ligaments are reflected off of the condyles. The condyle is shaved with a rongeur, leaving a substantial portion of the joint intact to avoid instability. When the distal portion of the proximal phalanx and the proximal portion of the distal phalanx are thought to be simultaneously involved, both areas should be shaved. The remaining edges are smoothed with a rongeur. The capsule is closed with a single interrupted

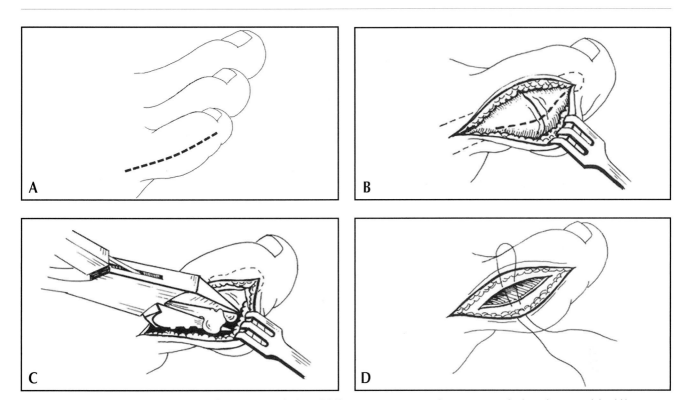

Fig. 29 Technique of partial condylectomy for treatment of a lateral fifth-toe corn. **A,** Surgical incision over the lateral aspect of the fifth toe. **B,** Capsular incision. **C,** Removal of the prominent condyle. **D,** Capsular repair following osseous resection.

absorbable suture. The skin is approximated with interrupted nylon sutures.

Surgical Treatment of an Interdigital Corn

An interdigital corn can be treated with a condylectomy of adjacent corns or a complete condylectomy (hammer toe correction) of one of the digits. Treatment depends on the severity of the deformity.

For a complete condylectomy, a procedure identical to that described for a hammer toe repair is performed (Fig. 8). More typically, an interdigital corn is treated with simultaneous procedures on the medial condyle of the proximal phalanx of the fifth toe and the lateral condyle of the proximal phalanx of the fourth toe.

Following a digital block, a dorsal incision is deepened to the underlying condyle. The capsule is reflected, and the condyle is removed with a fine-tipped rongeur to create a slight concavity. Following resection of the prominent bone, the capsule is approximated with a single interrupted absorbable suture. When a corn has developed in a web space, the resection involves the distal portion of the proximal phalanx of the fifth toe and the lateral aspect of the base of the proximal phalanx of the fourth toe. Care must be taken to avoid any incision in the web space, as delayed healing or a sinus tract may develop as a result of maceration in this area.

An alternate procedure for treatment of web space corns is syndactylization,[109,110] but it is typically reserved as a revision procedure following failure of a more primary procedure. Amputation is rarely performed for treatment of an interdigital corn.

Postoperative Care

A gauze-and-tape compression dressing is applied and is changed weekly until drainage subsides. Walking while wearing a postoperative shoe or sandal is contin-

ued until swelling subsides. The treated toe is taped to an adjacent toe for approximately 6 weeks to promote soft-tissue healing.

Results and Complications

In a series of patients studied, a high level of overall satisfaction was found after surgical treatment of both lateral fifth toe and interdigital corns. At an average of 7 years postoperatively, (M Kennedy, MD and MJ Coughlin, MD, unpublished data, 2001) 60 of 62 feet (97%) had a good or excellent result, and 47 of 51 patients (92%) were pain free. The satisfaction rate was slightly higher after treatment of interdigital corns than it was after treatment of lateral fifth-toe corns. The recurrence rate has ranged from 2% to 5% in this series and others.[104] In the study by Kennedy and Coughlin, complications following surgery were uncommon. Numbness was rare. Stiffness of the involved digit was reported by more than half of the patients and was more commonly associated with a complete condylectomy. Fifth-toe instability is uncommon, and when it occurs it is usually associated with an excessive osseous resection (or a lack of capsular closure). Activity restrictions are infrequent following surgery, but shoe-wear constraints are more common, especially after treatment of a lateral fifth-toe corn. Of the 62 feet studied, 13 of 31 feet had shoe wear restrictions after a repair of a fifth-toe corn and 7 of 31 feet had such restrictions after surgery for an interdigital corn.

Summary

Pain in the digits or the forefoot need not be a difficult diagnostic problem. A careful history should be recorded to help to elicit important information regarding what activities exacerbate symptoms. A careful physical examination will help to identify fixed as well as flexible deformities and the exact location of pain. Conservative treatment of many of these deformities often results in substantial relief of symptoms. When necessary, surgical intervention with attention to careful alignment of the involved digits will often result in a satisfactory resolution of the problem.

References

1. Coughlin M, Mann R: Lesser toe deformities, in Coughlin MJ, Mann RA (eds): *Surgery of the Foot and Ankle*, ed 7. St. Louis, MO, Mosby Yearbook, 1999, pp 320-391.

2. Coughlin MJ, Thompson FM: The high price of high-fashion footwear. *Instr Course Lect* 1995;44:371-377.

3. Coughlin M: Arthritides, in Coughlin MJ, Mann RA (eds): *Surgery of the Foot and Ankle*, ed 7. St. Louis, MO, Mosby Yearbook, 1999, pp 560-650.

4. Coughlin MJ: Subluxation and dislocation of the second metatarsophalangeal joint. *Orthop Clin North Am* 1989;20:535-551.

5. Coughlin MJ: Mallet toes, hammer toes, claw toes, and corns: Causes and treatment of lesser-toe deformities. *Postgrad Med* 1984;75:191-198.

6. Coughlin MJ: Operative repair of the mallet toe deformity. *Foot Ankle Int* 1995;16:109-116.

7. Coughlin MJ, Dorris J, Polk E. Operative repair of the fixed hammertoe deformity. *Foot Ankle Int* 2000;21:94-104.

8. Thompson FM, Hamilton WG: Problems of the second metatarsophalangeal joint. *Orthopedics* 1987;10:83-89.

9. Coughlin MJ: Lesser toe deformities. *Orthopedics* 1987;10:63-75.

10. Coughlin M: Lesser toe abnormalities, in Chapman MW (ed): *Operative Orthopaedics*. Philadelphia, PA, JB Lippincott, 1988, pp 1765-1776.

11. Hamer AJ, Stanley D, Smith TW: Surgery for curly toe deformity: A doubleblind, randomised, prospective trial. *J Bone Joint Surg Br* 1993;75:662-663.

12. Ross ER, Menelaus MB: Open flexor tenotomy for hammer toes and curly toes in childhood. *J Bone Joint Surg Br* 1984;66:770-771.

13. McConnell B: Correction of hammer-toe deformity: A 10-year review of subperiosteal waist resection of the proximal phalanx. *Orthop Rev* 1975;8:65-69.

14. McConnell BE: Hammertoe surgery: Waist resection of the proximal phalanx, a more simplified procedure. *South Med J* 1975;68:595-598.

15. Cahill BR, Connor DE: A long-term follow-up on proximal phalangectomy for hammer toes. *Clin Orthop* 1972;86:191-192.

16. Conklin MJ, Smith RW: Treatment of the atypical lesser toe deformity with basal hemiphalangectomy. *Foot Ankle Int* 1994;15:585-594.

17. Daly PJ, Johnson KA: Treatment of painful subluxation or dislocation at the second and third metatarsophalangeal joints by partial proximal phalanx excision and subtotal webbing. *Clin Orthop* 1992;278:164-170.

18. Kuwada GT: A retrospective analysis of modification of the flexor tendon transfer for correction of hammer toe. *J Foot Surg* 1988;27:57-59.

19. Creer W: Treatment of hammer toe. *Br Med J* 1935;1:527-528.

20. Glassman F, Wolin I, Sideman S: Phalangectomy for toe deformity. *Surg Clin North Am* 1949;29:275-280.

21. Sarrafian SK: Correction of fixed hammertoe deformity with resection of the head of the proximal phalanx and extensor tendon tenodesis. *Foot Ankle Int* 1995;16:449-451.

22. Alvine FG, Garvin KL: Peg and dowel fusion of the proximal interphalangeal joint. *Foot Ankle* 1980;1:90-94.

23. Soule R: Operation for the correction of hammer toe. *NY Med J* 1910;91:649-650.

24. Threthowen W: Treatment of hammertoe. *Lancet* 1925;1:1312-1313.

25. Young CS: An operation for the correction of hammer-toe and claw-toe. *J Bone Joint Surg* 1938;20:715-719.

26. Ohm OW II, McDonell M, Vetter WA: Digital arthrodesis: An alternate method for correction of hammer toe deformity. *J Foot Surg* 1990;29:207-211.

27. Kelikian H: *Hallux Valgus: Allied Deformities of the Forefoot and Metatarsalgia*. Philadelphia, PA, WB Saunders, 1965, pp 292-304.

28. Lehman DE, Smith RW: Treatment of a symptomatic hammertoe with a proximal interphalangeal joint arthrodesis. *Foot Ankle Int* 1995;16:535-541.

29. Pichney GA, Derner R, Lauf E: Digital "V" arthrodesis. *J Foot Ankle Surg* 1993;32:473-479.

30. Reece AT, Stone MH, Young AB: Toe fusing using Kirschner wire: A study of the postoperative infection rate and related problems. *J R Coll Surg Edinb* 1987;32:158-159.

31. Barbari SG, Brevig K: Correction of clawtoes by the Girdlestone-Taylor flexor-extensor transfer procedure. *Foot Ankle* 1984;5:67-73.

32. Cyphers SM, Feiwell E: Review of the Girdlestone-Taylor procedure for claw-toes in myelodysplasia. *Foot Ankle* 1988;8:229-233.

33. Parrish TF: Dynamic correction of clawtoes. *Orthop Clin North Am* 1973;4:97-102.

34. Pyper JB: The flexor-extensor transplant operation for claw toes. *J Bone Joint Surg Br* 1958;40:528-533.

35. Taylor RG: An operative procedure for the treatment of hammer-toe and clawtoe. *J Bone Joint Surg* 1940;22:608-609.

36. Taylor RG: The treatment of claw toes by multiple transfers of flexor into extensor tendons. *J Bone Joint Surg Br* 1951;33:539-542.

37. Thompson FM, Deland JT: Flexor tendon transfer for metatarsophalangeal instability of the second toe. *Foot Ankle* 1993;14:385-388.

38. Mann RA, Coughlin MJ: The rheumatoid foot: Review of literature and method of treatment. *Orthop Rev* 1979;8:105-112.

39. Mann R, Coughlin M: Lesser toe deformities, in Jahss MH (ed): *Disorders of the Foot and Ankle: Medical and Surgical Management*, ed 2. Philadelphia, PA, WB Saunders, 1991, pp 1208-1209.

40. Mann RA, Coughlin MJ: Lesser toe deformities, in Mann RA, Coughlin MJ (eds): *The Video Textbook of Foot and Ankle Surgery*. St Louis, MO, Medical Video Productions, 1991, pp 47-49.

41. McCluskey WP, Lovell WW, Cummings RJ: The cavovarus foot deformity: Etiology and management. *Clin Orthop* 1989;247:27-37.

42. Karlstrom G, Lonnerholm T, Olerud S: Cavus deformity of the foot after fracture of the tibial shaft. *J Bone Joint Surg Am* 1975;57:893-900.

43. Schnepp KH: Hammer-toe and claw foot. *Am J Surg* 1937;36:351-359.

44. Frank GR, Johnson WM: The extensor shift procedure in the correction of clawtoe deformities in children. *South Med J* 1966;59:889-896.

45. Heyman CH: The operative treatment of clawfoot. *J Bone Joint Surg* 1932;14:335-338.

46. Cole WH: The treatment of claw-foot. *J Bone Joint Surg* 1940;22:895-908.

47. DuVries HL: *Surgery of the Foot* ed 1. St Louis, MO, Mosby, 1959, pp 359-660.

48. Jones R: The soldier's foot and treatment of common deformities of the foot: Part II. Clawfoot. *Br Med J* 1916;1:749-751.

49. Branch HE: Pathological dislocation of the second toe. *J Bone Joint Surg* 1937;19:978-984.

50. DuVries H: Dislocation of the toe. *JAMA* 1956;160:728.

51. Coughlin M: When to suspect crossover second toe deformity. *J Musculoskel Med* 1987;4: 39-48.

52. Brunet JA, Tubin S: Traumatic dislocations of the lesser toes. *Foot Ankle Int* 1997;18:406-411.

53. Murphy JL: Isolated dorsal dislocation of the second metatarsophalangeal joint. *Foot Ankle* 1980;1:30-32.

54. Rao JP, Banzon MT: Irreducible dislocation of the metatarsophalangeal joints of the foot. *Clin Orthop* 1979;145:224-226.

55. Mann RA, Mizel MS: Monarticular nontraumatic synovitis of the metatarsophalangeal joint: A new diagnosis? *Foot Ankle* 1985;6: 18-21.

56. Coughlin MJ: Crossover second toe deformity. *Foot Ankle* 1987;8:29-39.

57. Coughlin MJ: Second metatarsophalangeal joint instability in the athlete. *Foot Ankle* 1993;14:309-319.

58. Deland JT, Sobel M, Arnoczky SP, Thompson FM: Collateral ligament reconstruction of the unstable metatarsophalangeal joint: An in vitro study. *Foot Ankle* 1992;13:391-395.

59. Trepman E, Yeo SJ: Nonoperative treatment of metatarsophalangeal joint synovitis. *Foot Ankle Int* 1995;16:771-777.

60. Mizel MS, Michelson JD: Nonsurgical treatment of monarticular nontraumatic synovitis of the second metatarsophalangeal joint. *Foot Ankle Int* 1997;18:424-426.

61. Reis ND, Karkabi S, Zinman C: Metatarsophalangeal joint dislocation after local steroid injection. *J Bone Joint Surg Br* 1989;71:864.

62. Giannestras NJ: Shortening of the metatarsal shaft in the treatment of plantar keratosis: An end-result study. *J Bone Joint Surg Am* 1958;40:61-71.

63. Trnka HJ, Muhlbauer M, Zettl R, Myerson MS, Ritschl P: Comparison of the results of the Weil and Helal osteotomies for the treatment of metatarsalgia secondary to dislocation of the lesser metatarsophalangeal joints. *Foot Ankle Int* 1999;20:72-79.

64. Haddad SL, Sabbagh RC, Resch S, Myerson B, Myerson MS: Results of flexor-to-extensor and extensor brevis tendon transfer for correction of crossover second toe deformity. *Foot Ankle Int* 1999;20:781-788.

65. Bradley N, Miller WA, Evans JP: Plantar neuroma: Analysis of results following surgical excision in 145 patients. *South Med J* 1976;69: 853-854.

66. Keh RA, Ballew KK, Higgins KR, Odom R, Harkless LB: Long-term follow-up of Morton's neuroma. *J Foot Surg* 1992;31:93-95.

67. Friscia DA, Strom DE, Parr JW, Saltzman CL, Johnson KA: Surgical treatment for primary interdigital neuroma. *Orthopedics* 1991;14: 669-672.

68. Youngswick FD: Intermetatarsal neuroma. *Clin Podiatr Med Surg* 1994;11:579-592.

69. Karges DE: Plantar excision of primary interdigital neuromas. *Foot Ankle* 1988;9:120-124.

70. Coughlin MJ, Pinsonneault T: Operative treatment of interdigital neuroma: A long-term follow-up study. *J Bone Joint Surg Am* 2001;83:1321-1328.

71. Mann RA, Reynolds JC: Interdigital neuroma: A critical clinical analysis. *Foot Ankle* 1983;3: 238-243.

72. Mulder JD: The causative mechanism in Morton's metatarsalgia. *J Bone Joint Surg Br* 1951;33:94-95.

73. Thompson FM, Deland JT: Occurrence of two interdigital neuromas in one foot. *Foot Ankle* 1993;14:15-17.

74. Coughlin MJ: Common causes of pain in the forefoot in adults. *J Bone Joint Surg Br* 2000;82:781-790.

75. Graham CE, Graham DM: Morton's neuroma: A microscopic evaluation. *Foot Ankle* 1984;5: 150-153.

76. Greenfield J, Rea J Jr, Ilfeld FW: Morton's interdigital neuroma: Indications for treatment by local injections versus surgery. *Clin Orthop* 1984;185:142-144.

77. Rasmussen MR, Kitaoka HB, Patzer GL: Nonoperative treatment of planta interdigital neuroma with a single corticosteroid injection. *Clin Orthop* 1996;326:188-193.

78. Betts LO: Morton's metatarsalgia: neuritis of the fourth digital nerve. *Med J Australia* 1940;1: 514-515.

79. Hauser ED: Interdigital neuroma of the foot. *Surg Gynecol Obstet* 1971;133: 265-267.

80. Johnson JE, Johnson KA, Unni KK: Persistent pain after excision of an interdigital neuroma: Results of reoperation. *J Bone Joint Surg Am* 1988;70:651-657.

81. Dereymaeker G, Schroven I, Steenwerckx A, Stuer P: Results of excision of the interdigital nerve in the treatment of Morton's metatarsalgia. *Acta Orthop Belg* 1996;62:22-25.

82. McKeever DC: Surgical approach for neuroma of plantar digital nerve (Morton's metatarsalgia). *J Bone Joint Surg Am* 1952;34:490.

83. Amis JA, Siverhus SW, Liwnicz BH: An anatomic basis for recurrence after Morton's neuroma excision. *Foot Ankle* 1992;13:153-156.

84. Benedetti RS, Baxter DE, Davis PF: Clinical results of simultaneous adjacent interdigital neurectomy in the foot. *Foot Ankle Int* 1996;17:264-268.

85. Cockin J: Butler's operation for an over-riding fifth toe. *J Bone Joint Surg Br* 1968;50:78-81.

86. Lantzounis LA: Congenital subluxation of the fifth toe and its correction by periosteocapsuloplasty and tendon transplantation. *J Bone Joint Surg* 1940;22:147-150.

87. Wilson JN: V-Y correction for varus deformity of the fifth toe. *Br J Surg* 1953;41:133-135.

88. Lapidus PW: Transplantation of the extensor tendon for correction of the overlapping fifth toe. *J Bone Joint Surg* 1942;24:555-559.

89. Dyal CM, Davis WH, Thompson FM, Elonar SK: Clinical evaluation of the Ruiz-Mora procedure: Long-term follow-up. *Foot Ankle Int* 1997;18:94-97.

90. Janecki CJ, Wilde AH: Results of phalangectomy of the fifth toe for hammertoe: The Ruiz-Mora procedure. *J Bone Joint Surg Am* 1976;58:1005-1007.

91. Jahss M: Miscellaneous soft tissue lesions, in Jahss M (ed): *Disorders of the Foot*. Philadelphia, PA, WB Saunders; 1982, pp 646-843.

92. Kelikian H, Clayton L, Loseff H: Surgical syndactylia of the toes. *Clin Orthop* 1961;19: 208-229.

93. Leonard MH, Rising EE: Syndactylization to maintain correction of overlapping 5th toe. *Clin Orthop* 1965;43:241-243.

94. Marek L, Giacopelli J, Granoff D: Syndactylization for the treatment of fifth toe deformities. *J Am Podiatr Med Assoc* 1991;81: 248-252.

95. Black GB, Grogan DP, Bobechko WP: Butler arthroplasty for correction of the adducted fifth toe: A retrospective study of 36 operations between 1968 and 1982. *J Pediatr Orthop* 1985;5:439-441.

96. Mann RA, Coughlin MJ: Lesser toe deformities. *Instr Course Lect* 1987;36:137-159.

97. Thompson TC: Surgical treatment of disorders of the forepart of the foot. *J Bone Joint Surg Am* 1964;46:1117-1128.

98. Scrase WH: The treatment of dorsal adduction deformities of the fifth toe. *J Bone Joint Surg Br* 1954;36:146.

99. Bonavilla EJ: Histopathology of the heloma durum: Some significant features and their implications. *J Am Podiatry Assoc* 1968;58: 423-427.

100. McElvenny RT: Corns: Their etiology and treatment. *Am J Surg* 1940;50:761-765.

101. Gillett HG, Du P: Interdigital corns. *Chiropodist* 1952;7:84-86.

102. Brahms MA: Common foot problems. *J Bone Joint Surg Am* 1967;49:1653-1664.

103. Day RD, Reyzelman AM, Harkless LB: Evaluation and management of the interdigital corn: A literature review. *Clin Podiatr Med Surg* 1996;13:201-206.

104. DuVries H: Disorders of the skin, in DuVries HL (ed): *Surgery of the Foot*. St Louis, MO, Mosby, 1959, pp 171-178.

105. Gillett HG: Incidence of interdigital clavus: A note on its location. *J Bone Joint Surg Br* 1974;56:752.

106. Gillett HG: Interdigital clavus: Predisposition is the key factor of soft corns. *Clin Orthop* 1979;142:103-109.

107. Gillett HG, Du P: Etiological factors responsible for cornification of the base of the fourth cleft. *Chiropodist* 1947;2:291-297.

108. Zeringue GN Jr, Harkless LB: Evaluation and management of the web corn involving the fourth interdigital space. *J Am Podiatr Med Assoc* 1986;76: 210-213.

109. Haboush EJ, Martin RV: Painful interdigital clavus (soft corn): Treatment by skin-plastic operation. *J Bone Joint Surg* 1947;29:756-757.

110. Strach EH, Cornah MS: Syndactylopoiesis: A simple operation for interdigital soft corn. *J Bone Joint Surg Br* 1972;54:530-531.

Keratotic Disorders of the Plantar Skin

Roger A. Mann, MD
Jeffrey A. Mann, MD

Abstract

Keratotic lesions on the plantar aspect of the foot develop beneath an osseous prominence and can result in substantial disability. This occurs because, during normal gait, the metatarsal head area is subjected to more prolonged stress than any other area on the plantar aspect of the foot. In the treatment of this disorder, it is imperative to establish the etiology, among many possibilities, and then address the specific pathology accordingly.

A keratotic lesion of the plantar skin is a result of friction or pressure, or both, beneath an osseous prominence. A keratotic lesion, a callus, can form anywhere on the body over an osseous prominence as a result of friction. Its location beneath the osseous prominence helps to distinguish it from other disorders of the skin, such as a wart. A certain amount of thickening of the plantar skin is normal in an active individual and should not be considered to be abnormal. The keratotic lesions discussed in this chapter are those that develop beneath a metatarsal head or the tibial sesamoid or that are occasionally associated with an accessory sesamoid bone.

Biomechanical Considerations

During normal gait, the center of weight-bearing pressure moves along the plantar aspect of the foot and re- mains beneath the metatarsal heads for approximately 50% of the stance phase.[1,2] The windlass mechanism of the foot plantar flexes the metatarsals during the second half of the stance phase, depressing the metatarsal heads into the plantar skin. This mechanism transfers weight to the toes during the last 12% of the stance phase. When an anatomic or structural abnormality disrupts the weight-bearing pattern, abnormal weight transfer occurs, re- sulting in abnormal weight distribu- tion and a keratotic lesion (intractable plantar keratosis).

These abnormalities occur most often when the toes, especially the great toe, are not functioning nor- mally—eg, in a patient with rheuma- toid arthritis or severe hallux valgus. When the pressure of weight bearing is not effectively transferred to the hallux at the end of stance phase, and there is excessive pressure beneath the lesser metatarsal heads, abnormal callus may form. When the callus is painful, the normal mechanisms of gait are disrupted even further.

Anatomic Considerations

The first metatarsal carries approxi- mately 50% of the body weight.[3] The second and third metatarsals are rig- idly attached to their respective cunei- form bones, and, as a result, minimal dorsiflexion or plantar flexion occurs at these articulations. Consequently, when the first metatarsal does not carry its share of the body weight, cal- lus often forms beneath the adjacent metatarsal heads, especially the sec- ond one. Because the fourth and fifth metatarsals are more mobile, a callus rarely develops beneath them unless there is some type of abnormal foot posture such as a plantar flexed fifth metatarsal associated with a tailor's bunion. The windlass mechanism plantar flexes the first metatarsal as the proximal phalanx is drawn dorsally over the metatarsal head. When this mechanism is impaired, as in a patient with a severe hallux valgus deformity, more weight is transferred to the sec- ond and third metatarsals and a kera- totic lesion develops. In 60% of the general population, the first metatar- sal is shorter than the second metatar- sal but the mechanics of gait are

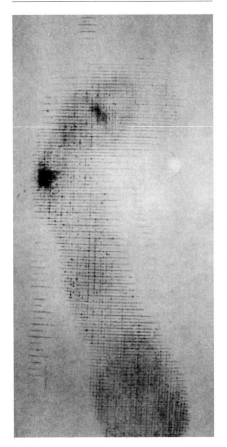

Figure 1 Harris mat print of a patient with varus forefoot deformity. Note that pressure is borne by the lateral aspect of the foot with decreased weight bearing beneath the medial aspect of the foot. (Reproduced with permission from Coughlin MJ, Mann RA (eds): *Surgery of the Foot and Ankle*. St. Louis, MO, Mosby, 1999, p 394.)

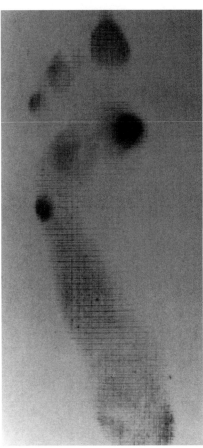

Figure 2 Harris mat print of a patient with a valgus forefoot deformity. Increased weight is borne along the medial side of the foot and, in particular, beneath the first metatarsal head. (Reproduced with permission from Coughlin MJ, Mann RA (eds): *Surgery of the Foot and Ankle*. St. Louis, MO, Mosby, 1999, p 395.)

normal. If there is excessive shortening of the first metatarsal, as may occur following trauma or surgery or in a patient with a Morton foot, the first metatarsal head does not carry its share of the body weight, even with a normally functioning plantar aponeurosis. The excessive pressure is transferred to the second and third metatarsals, resulting in callus formation (a so-called transfer lesion). If the first metatarsal-cuneiform joint has excessive mobility, as is the case in about 3% to 5% of individuals (MJ Coughlin, MD, personal communi-

cation, 2002), the first metatarsal again may not carry its share of the weight, resulting in transfer of pressure to the lesser metatarsals and development of a callus beneath the second, and sometimes the third, metatarsal. Occasionally, correction of a bunionette deformity is followed by the development of a keratotic lesion beneath the fourth metatarsal head when too much dorsiflexion occurs at the site of the osteotomy of the fifth metatarsal.

The posture of the foot must always be considered during the evaluation of a patient with an intractable plantar keratosis. An intractable plantar keratosis may result from an abnormal posture of the foot, and it will persist unless the abnormality is accommodated for with an orthosis or is corrected surgically. This is particularly a problem in an insensate foot as it may result in ulceration.

The various abnormal foot postures that can cause an intractable plantar keratosis include an equinus deformity of the ankle joint, a cavus deformity, a fixed varus deformity of the forefoot, a fixed valgus deformity of the forefoot, abnormal alignment of the metatarsophalangeal joints, and posttraumatic deformity.

Ankle equinus deformity, if severe, results in localized weight bearing on the metatarsal heads, which over time produces a diffuse callus, usually beneath the first, second, and third metatarsal heads. This is occasionally a painful condition and not infrequently results in atrophy of the plantar fat pad.

In a foot with a cavus deformity, the calcaneus is frequently dorsiflexed and the forefoot is in equinus, limiting weight bearing to the area directly beneath the metatarsal heads. Sometimes, the first metatarsal is substantially plantar flexed, resulting in a diffuse lesion. Occasionally, as a result of the rigidity of the foot, a lesion develops beneath the fifth metatarsal head as well.

Flatfoot deformity usually does not lead to the development of a substantial callus beneath the metatarsal heads. If, however, it is associated with a severe hallux valgus deformity, a callus may develop along the plantar medial aspect of the great toe at the level of the interphalangeal joint.

A fixed varus deformity of the forefoot in which the lateral border of the foot is more plantar flexed than the medial border may produce an intractable plantar keratosis beneath the fifth metatarsal head (Figure 1).

A fixed valgus deformity of the forefoot in which the first metatarsal is more plantar flexed in relation to the lesser metatarsals may result in a diffuse intractable plantar keratosis beneath the first metatarsal head (Figure 2). This deformity is usually associated with a cavus deformity in Charcot-Marie-Tooth disease.

Abnormal alignment of the metatarsophalangeal joints secondary to chronic subluxation or dislocation with decreased weight-bearing function of the toes results in abnormal pressures under the metatarsal heads. This often occurs in patients with advanced rheumatoid arthritis (Figure 3). Trauma to the forefoot or hindfoot occasionally is followed by malalignment with excessive plantar flexion or dorsiflexion of a metatarsal head, resulting in abnormal pressure and creating an intractable plantar keratosis.

There are iatrogenic causes of malalignment following hindfoot surgery, such as a malaligned triple arthrodesis, or following forefoot surgery, such as malalignment or shortening of the metatarsals, that can result in an intractable plantar keratosis.

Diagnosis

The evaluation of a patient with a plantar keratotic lesion begins with the recording of a history of the problem, with notation of the precise location of the pain, any previous treatment, and the types of shoes that aggravate and relieve the pain.

The physical examination begins with the patient in a standing position so that the examiner can observe the posture of the longitudinal arch, the hindfoot, and the position

of the toes. The range of motion of the ankle, subtalar, transverse tarsal, and metatarsophalangeal joints is noted. Then, with the patient sitting, the foot is examined to look for any abnormal posture, such as varus or valgus, and the neurovascular status of the foot is noted.

The plantar aspect of the foot is examined to determine the location and characteristics of the lesion. A plantar wart may be confused with an intractable plantar keratosis, but, as a general rule, warts are not located directly beneath a metatarsal head. The intractable plantar keratosis needs to be carefully evaluated to establish which metatarsal head it is beneath. The keratosis may be a localized, discrete callus beneath an osseous prominence; a diffuse callus beneath a single metatarsal head; or a diffuse callus beneath multiple metatarsal heads.

To identify the nature of the lesion, and particularly to be sure that it is not a wart, the lesion should be trimmed with a No. 17 blade. Trimming away its superficial aspects makes it possible to identify the margins of the callus since a well-localized intractable plantar keratosis has very circumscribed edges in contrast to a diffuse callus, which is a generalized thickening of the plantar skin without a specific margin. A wart may have a small amount of keratotic tissue overlying it, but paring very soon results in bleeding, which is sometimes vigorous, from the multiple end arteries within it (Figure 4). An intractable plantar keratosis has no blood vessels, only a keratotic core (Figures 5 and 6).

Radiographs of the foot in the weight-bearing position, including sesamoid views if indicated, should be made. Sometimes, placement of a small radiopaque marker over the center of the lesion may help to identify the offending structure.

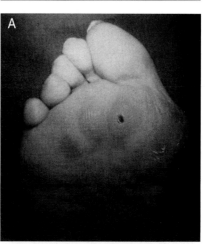

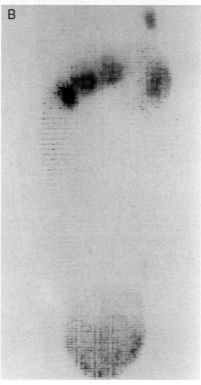

Figure 3 A, The foot of a patient with rheumatoid arthritis and large diffuse plantar callosities beneath the metatarsal heads. (Reproduced with permission from Coughlin MJ, Mann RA (eds): *Surgery of the Foot and Ankle*. St. Louis, MO, Mosby, 1999, p 395.) **B,** Harris mat print demonstrating concentration of pressure beneath metatarsal heads and no weight-bearing by the lesser toes. (Reproduced with permission from Coughlin MJ, Mann RA (eds): *Surgery of the Foot and Ankle*. St. Louis, MO, Mosby, 1999, p 395.)

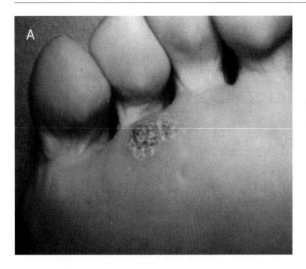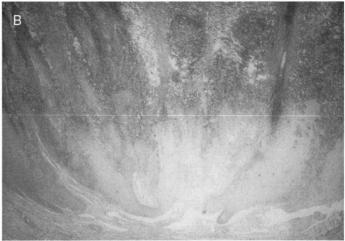

Figure 4 A, A wart on the plantar aspect of the foot usually does not develop in a weight-bearing area. **B,** Histologically, a wart demonstrates considerable vascularity. (Reproduced with permission from Mann RA: Intractable plantar keratosis. *Instr Course Lect* 1984;33:290.)

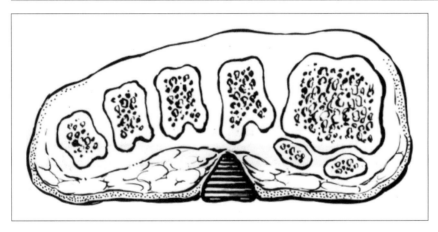

Figure 5 A discrete plantar keratosis beneath the prominent fibular condyle of the second metatarsal head. (Reproduced with permission from Coughlin MJ, Mann RA (eds): *Surgery of the Foot and Ankle.* St. Louis, MO, Mosby, 1999, p 399.)

Conservative Management

When trimming a well-localized intractable plantar keratosis, one should attempt to reduce the keratotic tissue initially and then carefully débride the central keratotic core, which is almost invariably invaginated. Unfortunately, with a deep-seated lesion, it is difficult to remove all of the dense keratotic tissue at the initial débridement, and sometimes several trimmings are necessary to permit the deepest portion of the callus to surface. After the callus is débrided, a soft metatarsal support, such as a Hapad (Bethel Park, PA), is placed in the shoe just proximal to the metatarsal head to relieve the pressure on the involved area. This type of soft support works extremely well, but it is important that the shoe be of adequate size to accommodate the support. As a general rule, for the shoe to be the most effective, it must be wide enough and have laces, a soft insole, and a fairly stiff sole. The stiff sole keeps the foot fairly flat in the shoe, some-

what negating the function of the plantar aponeurosis and thereby diminishing the downward thrust of the metatarsal heads. A cross-trainer type of tennis shoe can be very effective in relieving pressure against an intractable plantar keratosis. The metatarsal support is placed into the shoe just proximal to the area of the lesion (Figure 7). It is very important to inform the patient that the support may at first feel uncomfortable and require a period of "breaking in" of 7 to 10 days. If the foot has a fixed postural deformity, a soft support may not be adequate and an accommodative arch support with a soft upper may be needed. It is important that the patient place the arch support into a shoe that has sufficient room for both the foot and the orthosis.

Once the initial treatment has been provided, the patient is seen periodically to trim the lesion and to adjust or modify the metatarsal support. If the patient is comfortable with the soft support but wishes to have a more permanent device, an orthosis can be ordered. The advantage of using a soft support initially is that one can find out whether such a support will provide the patient with relief at a very low cost before a more expensive orthotic device is ordered.

If the callus persists and remains symptomatic, surgical intervention can be considered.

Determination of Type of Surgical Treatment Indicated

The characteristics of the intractable plantar keratosis usually determine the type of surgical management that is indicated.

Discrete Intractable Plantar Keratosis A discrete intractable plantar keratosis with a central keratotic core is observed beneath the fibular condyle of usually the second, and occasionally the third, metatarsal head as well as beneath the tibial sesamoid (Figure 8). When a person with a well-localized intractable plantar keratosis walks over a Harris mat, the imprint that is created is well localized beneath the prominence that has created the callus (Figure 9). Histologically, this lesion consists of dense keratinized tissue with a central core (Figure 6).

Diffuse Intractable Plantar Keratosis A diffuse intractable plantar keratosis is observed beneath a metatarsal head that does not have a prominent fibular condyle; it is found most frequently beneath the second metatarsal alone or beneath both the second and the third metatarsal heads. When this type of callus is débrided, it is not possible to identify a central core (Figure 10), as is observed in a discrete callus. When a patient with this type of callus walks over a Harris mat, a diffuse print is created beneath the entire metatarsal head or beneath multiple metatarsal heads (Figure 11). This type of lesion may be observed beneath the first metatarsal head of a cavus foot (fixed forefoot valgus) or beneath

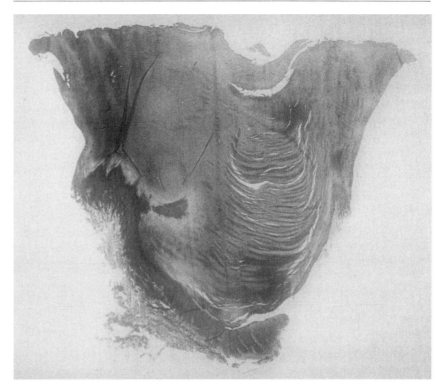

Figure 6 Histologic section of a keratotic lesion, demonstrating layers of keratin with no blood vessels. (Compare with Figure 4, *B*.) (Reproduced with permission from Mann RA: *Du Vries' Surgery of the Foot,* ed 4. St. Louis, MO, CV Mosby, 1978.)

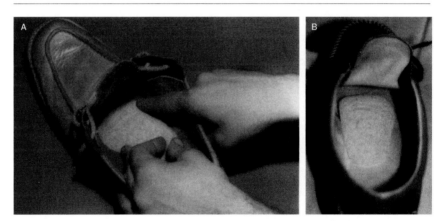

Figure 7 Placement of a soft metatarsal support in the shoe. The shoe should be large enough and preferably have laces. **A,** The metatarsal support is placed just proximal to the lesion to relieve the pressure on it. Usually, it is best to start with a small pad to increase acceptance by the patient. (Reproduced with permission from Coughlin MJ, Mann RA (eds): *Surgery of the Foot and Ankle.* St. Louis, MO, Mosby, 1999, p 397.) **B,** The support can be moved medially or laterally depending on the location of the lesion. (Reproduced with permission from Coughlin MJ, Mann RA (eds): *Surgery of the Foot and Ankle.* St. Louis, MO, Mosby, 1999, p 397.)

the second metatarsal head of a foot with severe hallux valgus, a short or hypermobile first metatarsal, or previous bunion surgery if the joint has been destabilized or the first metatarsal has been elevated or short-

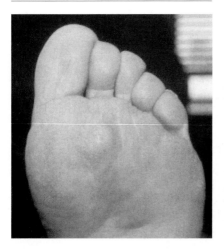

Figure 8 A discrete, localized intractable plantar keratosis beneath the second metatarsal head. Although the keratosis appears somewhat diffuse, a central keratotic core can be identified with débridement.

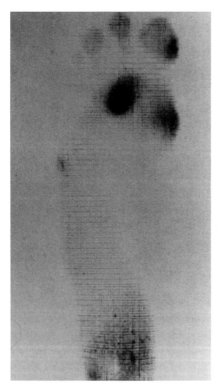

Figure 11 A Harris mat print demonstrating a diffuse keratotic lesion beneath the second metatarsal head. (Compare this pattern with that shown in Figure 9.) (Reproduced with permission from Mann RA: Intractable plantar keratosis. *Instr Course Lect* 1984;33:293.)

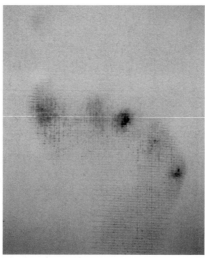

Figure 9 A Harris mat print demonstrating a well-localized area of pressure representing a discrete plantar keratosis beneath the third metatarsal head. (Reproduced with permission from Coughlin MJ, Mann RA (eds): *Surgery of the Foot and Ankle*. St. Louis, MO, Mosby, 1999, p 398.)

ened. A diffuse callus beneath the second, the third, and possibly the fourth metatarsal head is most commonly noted in a foot with an extremely short first metatarsal (a Morton foot), which results in increased weight bearing beneath the middle three metatarsals (Figure 12). On occasion, a diffuse callus may be observed beneath the fifth metatarsal head of a patient with a varus configuration of the forefoot or in association with a tailor's bunion with a plantar flexed fifth metatarsal.

Surgical Treatment of a Localized Intractable Plantar Keratosis

A localized intractable plantar keratosis, which usually develops beneath the prominence of the fibular condyle, is treated with a DuVries metatarsal condylectomy. The procedure was initially described by DuVries[4] as an arthroplasty of the

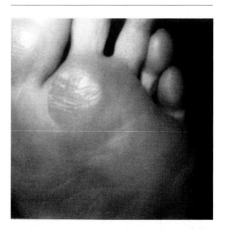

Figure 10 A diffuse keratotic lesion. When this lesion is trimmed, there is no central core, and that finding distinguishes it from a discrete keratotic lesion. (Reproduced with permission from Mann RA: Intractable plantar keratosis. *Instr Course Lect* 1984;33:293.)

metatarsophalangeal joint, involving removal of a portion of the distal articular cartilage from the metatarsal head and the plantar condyle. It has been subsequently modified so that only the plantar condyle is removed. Both procedures produce highly satisfactory results when performed for this specific indication.

Modified DuVries Metatarsal Condylectomy
Surgical Technique
1. The hockey-stick-shaped incision begins dorsally in the second web space. It is carried across the metatarsal head proximally to about the distal third of the metatarsal shaft (Figure 13, *A*).
2. The incision is deepened along the medial and lateral aspects of the extensor hood, and the transverse metatarsal ligament is identified and released.
3. The interval between the extensor digitorum longus tendon and the extensor digitorum brevis tendon is identified, and the tendons are separated, exposing the capsule of the metatarsophalangeal joint.

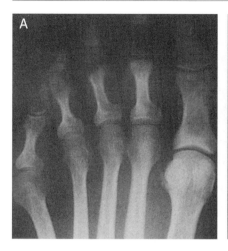 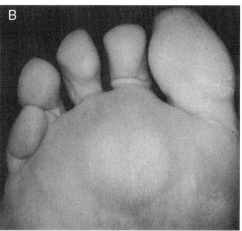 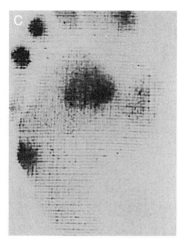

Figure 12 Typical findings with a Morton foot. **A,** Radiograph demonstrating a short first metatarsal and relatively long second and third metatarsals. **B,** A diffuse callus is seen beneath the second and third metatarsal heads. **C,** A Harris mat print demonstrating increased weight bearing beneath the second and third metatarsals, with little or no weight bearing beneath the first metatarsal head. (Reproduced with permission from Coughlin MJ, Mann RA (eds): *Surgery of the Foot and Ankle.* St. Louis, MO, Mosby, 1999, p 401.)

4. The medial and lateral collateral ligaments are transected and, with use of the thumb, the metatarsophalangeal joint is sharply plantar flexed while pressure is applied to the plantar aspect of the foot with the index and long fingers of the same hand (Figure 13, *B* and *C*).

5. As recommended by Mann and Coughlin,[5] the plantar 20% to 30% of the metatarsal head is removed with a 10- to 12-mm thin osteotome (Figure 13, *D*). The osteotome must be angulated slightly plantarward to avoid splitting the metatarsal shaft.

6. Once the osteotomy is completed, the plantar condyle is removed from the wound with utilization of a Freer elevator or a thin rongeur. This portion of the procedure can be somewhat difficult. If adequate exposure has not been gained, it is difficult to remove this plantar fragment because there is a periosteal attachment proximally. Because of the periosteal attachment, the fragment cannot be pulled out directly forward but rather must first be pushed into the adjacent interspace to remove it intact (Figure 14). If the condyle becomes fragmented, it should be carefully reconstructed on the operating table to be sure that all of it has been removed.

7. The osteotomy edges are smoothed, and the joint is reduced. The skin edges are closed in a routine manner.

8. The foot is placed in a compression dressing for the first 18 to 24 hours, during which time the patient is permitted to walk in a postoperative shoe.

Postoperative Care The foot is kept in a circumferential dressing, and the patient wears the postoperative shoe for 3 weeks. After 3 weeks, range-of-motion exercises are started.

Results The results of this procedure are generally satisfactory. It is imperative, however, that it be used only for a keratotic lesion beneath the fibular condyle.

In a review of the results in 100 patients, the rate of satisfaction was found to be 93%.[6] Of the lesions treated in those patients, 42% were beneath the second metatarsal head; 31%, the third metatarsal head; 19%, the fourth metatarsal head; and 8%, the fifth metatarsal head. A transfer lesion occurred in 13% of the patients, and the original lesion failed to resolve in 5%. There was a 5% rate of complications that included one fracture of a metatarsal head, osteonecrosis of a metatarsal head, and clawing of a toe. There were no dislocations of the metatarsophalangeal joint following this procedure. There was rarely more than 25% loss of the postoperative range of motion of the metatarsophalangeal joint.

Vertical Chevron Osteotomy
A vertical chevron osteotomy of the metatarsal head has been described for the treatment of a painful callus beneath the metatarsal head. The article describing the procedure[8] did not categorize calluses as localized or diffuse, but the procedure has been found to be useful mainly for the treatment of a transfer lesion following a fracture of an adjacent metatarsal that has healed in some

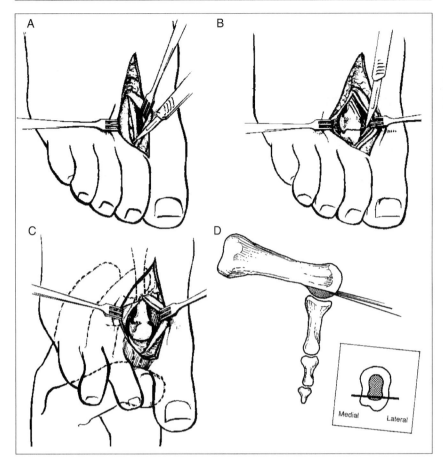

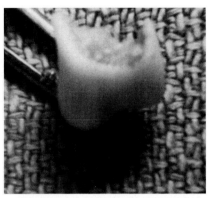

Figure 14 An excised plantar condyle. Note the marked prominence of the fibular portion. (Reproduced with permission from Mann RA: *Du Vries' Surgery of the Foot*, ed 4. St. Louis, MO, CV Mosby, 1978.)

Figure 13 Surgical technique for a modified DuVries plantar condylectomy. **A,** A hockey-stick-shaped incision beginning in the web space is carried proximally to about the distal third of the metatarsal shaft. The skin and extensor tendons are retracted, and the capsule is incised longitudinally. **B,** The capsule and collateral ligaments on both sides of the metatarsal head are sectioned. **C,** The involved toe is plantar flexed with the thumb while pressure is applied to the plantar aspect of the metatarsal shaft by the index and long fingers. **D,** Coughlin's modification of the plantar condylectomy. The plantar 20% to 30% of the condyle is removed, and the distal portion of the metatarsal head is left intact. (**A** through **C** are reproduced with permission from Mann RA: Intractable plantar keratosis. *Instr Course Lect* 1984;33:292. **D** is reproduced with permission from Coughlin MJ, Mann RA (eds): *Surgery of the Foot and Ankle*. St. Louis, MO, Mosby, 1999, p 402.)

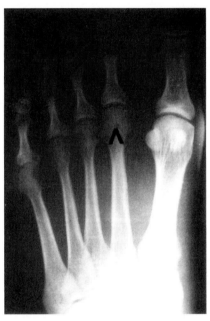

Figure 15 Radiograph demonstrating a vertical chevron osteotomy. The metatarsal head should be elevated approximately 3 mm. (Reproduced with permission from Coughlin MJ, Mann RA (eds): *Surgery of the Foot and Ankle*. St. Louis, MO, Mosby, 1999, p 403.)

dorsiflexion or for the treatment of a transfer lesion following a DuVries plantar metatarsal condylectomy. We have not used the procedure for a transfer lesion associated with a hallux valgus deformity. The vertical chevron osteotomy is performed in the metaphyseal region, and the metatarsal head is elevated approximately 3 mm.

Surgical Technique

1. A 2-cm dorsal incision is centered over the metatarsal head and neck. The incision is carried down to expose the extensor tendons, which are moved aside.
2. The metatarsal neck is exposed along its dorsal aspect, and care is taken not to cut the collateral ligaments. As a rule, the metatar-

sophalangeal joint is not entered.

3. A vertical chevron-type cut with the apex based distally is created just proximal to the dorsal joint capsule (Figure 15).

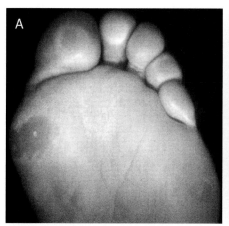 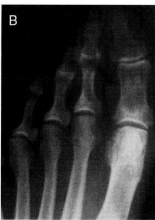 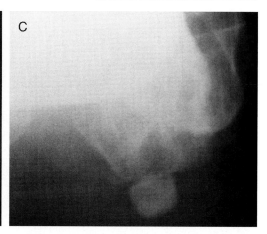

Figure 16 A hyperkeratotic lesion beneath the tibial sesamoid following a bunionectomy. **A,** Although there may be a moderate amount of callus over the lesion, once it is trimmed, a discrete keratotic lesion is usually identified. **B,** Radiograph demonstrating that the tibial sesamoid is centered beneath the metatarsal head. **C,** Axial radiograph demonstrating the sesamoid sitting beneath the crista of the metatarsal head. (Reproduced with permission from Coughlin MJ, Mann RA (eds): *Surgery of the Foot and Ankle.* St. Louis, MO, Mosby, 1999, p 404.)

4. The metatarsal head is displaced dorsally with use of manual pressure. It should be raised approximately 3 mm. An effort should be made to avoid over-displacing the head fragment because doing so may lead to a transfer lesion.

5. The osteotomy site is stabilized with a 0.045-inch (0.114-cm) Kirschner wire, which is introduced through a separate stab wound.

6. The skin is closed in a routine manner, and a compression dressing is applied.

Postoperative Care The patient is permitted to walk in a postoperative shoe with weight bearing as tolerated. The Kirschner wire is removed after 3 weeks, at which time gentle range of motion is begun. The postoperative shoe is used for a total of 6 weeks. Sometimes, the metatarsal head takes on a very osteopenic appearance, but we have not observed osteonecrosis in any of our patients.

Results In a series of 45 feet,[7] 30 (67%) had complete relief of symptoms and 11 (24%) had residual pain. A transfer lesion developed in

four feet (9%). The callus was unchanged in two feet. In another study of 21 feet (mean age of the patients, 59 years), 16 (76%) had a good result; 2 (10%), a fair result; and 3 (14%), a poor result.[8] The callosity persisted in four feet (19%), and a transfer lesion developed in three (14%).

Localized Callus Beneath the Tibial Sesamoid

A discrete callus beneath the first metatarsal head almost always lies beneath the tibial sesamoid. A localized lesion beneath the fibular sesamoid is rare. A diffuse callus may be observed under the entire first metatarsal head in patients with a plantar flexed first metatarsal or a cavus foot deformity, such as occurs in Charcot-Marie-Tooth disease.

The lesion beneath the tibial sesamoid is a discrete callus and, when it is débrided, a small keratotic core is observed. This lesion frequently can be treated effectively by débridement and placement of a soft arch support just proximal to the metatarsal head. It may develop following bunion surgery, when the

tibial sesamoid has not been fully reduced or when there has been some recurrence of the deformity and the tibial sesamoid becomes located beneath the crista of the first metatarsal (Figure 16).

If conservative management fails to resolve the problem adequately, the tibial sesamoid can be shaved, excising its plantar half. Shaving of the tibial sesamoid, rather than excising it completely, is preferred because there is substantially less morbidity after shaving.

Surgical Technique

1. The skin incision is made slightly plantar to the midline and is centered over the medial aspect of the metatarsophalangeal joint. It is carried down to the capsular structures without undermining the skin (Figure 17, *A*).

2. With plantarward dissection along the capsular plane, the insertion of the tendon of the abductor hallucis muscle is identified; just beneath it lies the plantar medial cutaneous nerve. This nerve is almost within a thin fibrous tunnel at this level, lying just along the inferior aspect of the abductor

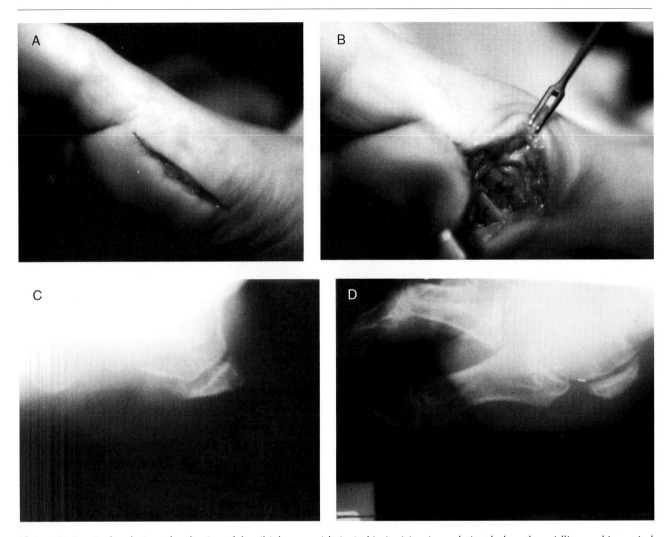

Figure 17 Surgical technique for shaving of the tibial sesamoid. **A,** A skin incision is made just below the midline and is carried down to expose the joint capsule. The plantar medial cutaneous nerve is identified and retracted. **B,** After exposure of the tibial sesamoid, the plantar half is removed. **C** and **D,** Axial and lateral radiographs showing the tibial sesamoid after removal of its plantar half. (**A** and **B** are reproduced with permission from Coughlin MJ, Mann RA (eds): *Surgery of the Foot and Ankle.* St. Louis, MO, Mosby, 1999, p 405. **C** and **D** are reproduced with permission from Mann RA: Intractable plantar keratosis. *Instr Course Lect* 1984;33:296.)

hallucis tendon. If one cannot observe it at the time of surgery, it often can be palpated. The nerve occasionally runs alongside a small blood vessel, which may help to identify it.

3. Once the nerve is identified, it is retracted dorsally and the plantar aspect of the tibial sesamoid is exposed. The periosteum on the plantar aspect of the sesamoid is removed, exposing its plantar two thirds. Because this approach goes beneath the abductor hallucis tendon, care should be taken not to violate that tendon and thus to minimize the possibility of creating a hallux valgus deformity.

4. A small sagittal saw is used to remove the plantar half of the tibial sesamoid (Figure 17, *B*). The edges are smoothed by buffing with the saw.

5. The plantar aspect of the wound is inspected to be sure that the flexor hallucis longus tendon is intact.

6. The wound is closed in a routine manner, and a compression dressing is applied.

Postoperative Care The patient is permitted to walk in a postoperative shoe with the foot in a firm circumferential dressing incorporating the hallux and pulling it into varus for 4 weeks, after which weight bearing is permitted as tolerated.

Results A follow-up study of 14 patients (16 feet) demonstrated an excellent result with no recurrence of the callus in 9 and a good result with slight recurrence of the callus in 4 patients. One patient had a fair result, which required periodic trimming of the plantar callus.[9] All patients maintained a full range of motion of the first metatarsophalangeal joint, and none had a painful scar.

Complications The most important complication following this procedure is an injury to the plantar medial cutaneous nerve. When this complication occurs, consideration should be given to moving the nerve away from the plantar aspect of the foot. The nerve should be transected and brought more proximally, burying it beneath the abductor hallucis muscle to prevent a neuroma from forming along the plantar medial aspect of the foot.

Surgical Treatment of a Diffuse Intractable Plantar Keratosis

A diffuse keratotic lesion may develop as a result of many conditions. It is beyond the scope of this chapter to discuss all of the ramifications of problems involving the metatarsophalangeal joints, such as subluxation and dislocation, that can cause a diffuse intractable plantar keratosis. If subluxation or dislocation is present, it is imperative that it be considered the primary problem and the diffuse intractable plantar keratosis be considered the secondary one. Therefore, only the problems observed will be discussed, with the assumption that there is no malalignment of the involved metatarsophalangeal joint.

In the most common anatomic pattern of the foot, the second metatarsal is the longest. Occasionally, a diffuse intractable plantar keratosis will develop beneath the second metatarsal and become symptomatic. It usually responds to conservative management with a soft metatarsal support. As a result of surgery or trauma, a metatarsal may become dorsiflexed, and a transfer lesion may develop beneath the adjacent metatarsal. When a diffuse intractable plantar keratosis is present beneath multiple metatarsal heads, it is usually attributable to a lack of weight bearing by the first metatarsal and surgery usually is not indicated. The condition can usually be managed with an accommodative orthosis. Our experience has been that attempts to carry out osteotomies of multiple metatarsal heads in the absence of substantial pathologic findings are often less than optimal and such procedures should not be done.

When selecting the proper treatment of a diffuse intractable plantar keratosis following trauma, one must decide whether the problem is being caused by an elevated or a shortened metatarsal. If a metatarsal has been elevated and a diffuse intractable plantar keratosis has developed beneath the adjacent metatarsal, then a dorsiflexion osteotomy may be adequate to resolve the problem. If the metatarsal has been shortened, then shortening of the adjacent metatarsal is the treatment of choice. It is important to remember that any pathologic problem within the metatarsophalangeal joint must be corrected because this may be the cause of, or may contribute to, the lesion.

When a metatarsal is dorsiflexed in relation to the adjacent metatarsal, particularly when the condition involves the second and third metatarsals, a well-planned dorsiflexion osteotomy of the metatarsal associated with the callus can resolve the problem. This osteotomy can be performed either distally, as described previously, or proximally.

Proximal Basal Metatarsal Osteotomy

A proximal osteotomy is used to treat a diffuse intractable plantar keratosis when there is no shortening of the adjacent metatarsal. This condition usually occurs after metatarsal surgery or a fracture.

Surgical Technique

1. The skin incision is made over the dorsal aspect of the proximal half of the involved metatarsal and is carried down through subcutaneous tissue and fat. It is imperative to carefully avoid the dorsal cutaneous nerves. It is also important that the proper metatarsal be identified, which occasionally is difficult. If there is any doubt, an intraoperative radiograph should be made.

2. The dorsal aspect of the metatarsal is identified, the extensor tendon is pulled aside, and the metatarsal is exposd.

3. The osteotomy site should be at the flare of the base of the metatarsal. The bone in this area is usually cancellous. If the osteotomy is performed too far proximally, it is difficult to produce an accurate cut because the saw has a tendency to bounce off the adjacent metatarsals.

4. The size of the wedge that is removed depends on the degree of elevation of the adjacent metatarsal head. The involved metatarsal head usually needs to be elevated 2 to 4 mm; thus, the size of the base of the wedge usually should not exceed 2 to 3 mm. The osteotomy is cut so as to leave a plantar hinge intact (Figure 18).

5. Fixation of the osteotomy site is performed by placing a 2.7-mm screw in the proximal portion of

the base of the metatarsal, drilling a transverse hole through the metatarsal about 1 cm distal to the osteotomy, and then securing the osteotomy site with a 22-gauge wire. When this technique is used, the osteotomy site can be closed and semirigidly fixed, and the metatarsal head can be precisely positioned. If the metatarsal has not been elevated sufficiently, the wire is

removed, more bone is removed, and the osteotomy site is refixed. This is a very precise way to elevate the metatarsal (Figure 19).

6. The skin is closed in a single layer and a compression dressing is applied.

Postoperative Care The patient is encouraged to walk in a postoperative shoe until the site has healed, which occurs in approximately 6 to 8 weeks. With the compression ob-

tained with the surgical method, the osteotomy site usually heals fairly rapidly. We did not review the results in any series of patients treated with this procedure.

Oblique Metatarsal Osteotomy

The oblique metatarsal osteotomy was initially described as a proximal step-cut osteotomy designed to shorten the symptomatic metatarsal.[10] We believe that the original procedure is technically too difficult; therefore, it was modified to a long oblique osteotomy, which is technically simpler and produces a satisfactory result.

Surgical Technique

1. A long dorsal skin incision is centered over the involved metatarsal. It is imperative that the metatarsal be carefully palpated and, if necessary, that a confirmatory radiograph be made to ensure that the correct one has been selected. As the incision is deepened through the subcutaneous tissue and fat, care must be

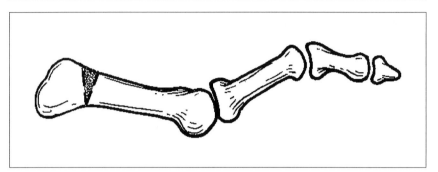

Figure 18 Technique for basal metatarsal osteotomy. Following the osteotomy, a dorsally based wedge of bone is removed from the affected metatarsal, allowing it to dorsiflex. (Reproduced with permission from Coughlin MJ, Mann RA (eds): *Surgery of the Foot and Ankle*. St. Louis, MO, Mosby, 1999, p 410.)

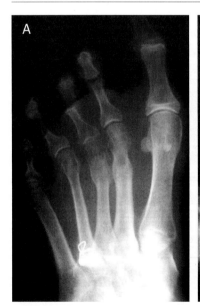
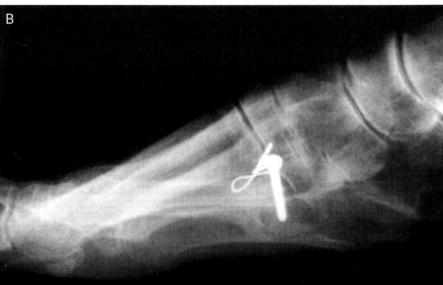

Figure 19 Radiographs of a foot in which a basal osteotomy was performed with fixation with a screw and a wire tension band. This technique allows for precise elevation of the affected metatarsal. (Reproduced with permission from Coughlin MJ, Mann RA (eds): *Surgery of the Foot and Ankle*. St. Louis, MO, Mosby, 1999, p 410.)

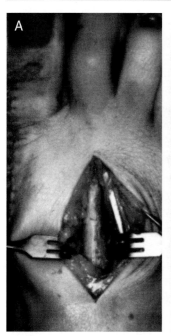 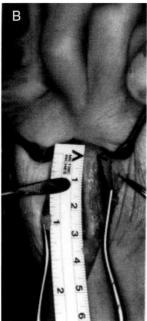 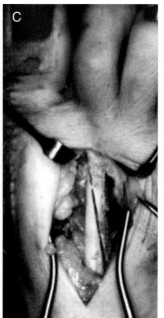 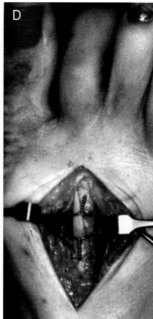

Figure 20 Surgical technique for the oblique metatarsal osteotomy. **A,** The metatarsal is exposed through a longitudinal incision. Care is taken to avoid the superficial nerves. The periosteum is incised, and the muscle is stripped from the metatarsal shaft. **B,** A mark is made on the metatarsal (*arrow*), and then a ruler is used to measure a fixed distance on the metatarsal shaft so that shortening can be performed accurately. **C,** A long oblique osteotomy has been performed. When it is performed on the second metatarsal, the osteotomy is performed in the direction shown, to avoid the artery in the first web space. **D,** The metatarsal is accurately shortened by using marks on the bone as a guide. A cerclage wire is passed through a drill hole after the metatarsal has been shortened. This helps to stabilize the metatarsal length. A second cerclage wire is then placed to increase the stability of the osteotomy site. (Reproduced with permission from Coughlin MJ, Mann RA (eds): *Surgery of the Foot and Ankle.* St. Louis, MO, Mosby, 1999, p 408.)

taken to identify and retract the cutaneous nerves.

2. The extensor tendons are moved aside, and the metatarsal is identified and is exposed subperiosteally (Figure 20, *A*).

3. If more than about 5 mm of shortening is required, the transverse metatarsal ligament is sectioned, particularly when the third and fourth metatarsals are involved. It is usually not necessary to do this when the second metatarsal is involved.

4. When the osteotomy is performed, a transverse mark is etched in the metatarsal at the midpoint of the osteotomy so that, as the osteotomy site is displaced, the surgeon can measure

precisely how much shortening is occurring (Figure 20, *B*).

5. A long oblique osteotomy is performed in the metatarsal shaft with a thin inline tooth saw blade. When the osteotomy is performed on the second metatarsal, the blade should be directed laterally to avoid bringing it into the interspace between the base of the first and second metatarsals, where the communicating artery passes (Figure 20, *C*).

6. Fixation of the osteotomy site can be performed with the use of a cerclage wire, small-fragment screws, or a plate. As a general rule, two cerclage wires produce satisfactory immobilization. One of the wires is passed through the

bone at its corrected length to control the length of the metatarsal, and the other is used to maintain apposition (Figure 20, *D*). A small-fragment screw can also be used, but technically it is somewhat difficult to place screws at the angle required to obtain good fixation without fracturing the bone. The use of a miniplate would seem ideal, but several nonunions after use of such a plate have been noted.

7. The intrinsic muscles that have been stripped to expose the metatarsal are sutured back over the top of the metatarsal shaft when possible, and the skin is closed in a routine manner (Figure 21,*A* and *B*).

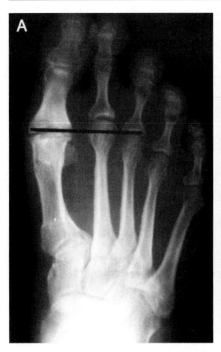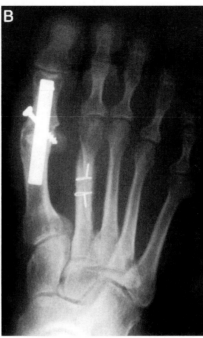

Figure 21 Preoperative **(A)** and postoperative **(B)** radiographs demonstrating shortening of the second metatarsal to create a smooth metatarsal arch. (Reproduced with permission from Coughlin MJ, Mann RA (eds): *Surgery of the Foot and Ankle*. St. Louis, MO, Mosby, 1999, p 409.)

8. A compression dressing is applied and is used for the initial 18 to 24 hours.

Postoperative Care The initial postoperative dressing is changed to a firm circumferential dressing in 18 to 24 hours. The patient is permitted to walk as tolerated while wearing a postoperative shoe. Usually, healing occurs in 8 to 10 weeks, although the radiograph is sometimes difficult to interpret from a healing standpoint.

Results We have not reviewed our experience with these operations because we carry out only one or two per year. The main complication is a transfer lesion, which occurs in about 10% of patients. Usually, this complication occurs not because the metatarsal was shortened excessively but because the distal fragment healed in a dorsiflexed position. With better internal fixation, this problem could probably be overcome.

Distal Metatarsal Osteotomy

The distal metatarsal osteotomy (Weil procedure) is used to shorten a metatarsal (LS Weil, Bordeaux, France, unpublished data, 1994). The procedure is most useful for the treatment of a subluxated or dislocated metatarsophalangeal joint, but it is also useful for the management of a diffuse intractable plantar keratosis resulting from a long metatarsal and occasionally for the management of a lesion that has been caused by dorsiflexion of an adjacent metatarsal. It can be performed on two or three metatarsals at the same time, and it has the advantage, compared with the other osteotomies, that the osteotomy site is stable and dorsiflexion deformity does not occur. Occasionally, metatarsalgia develops as patients get older and the fat pad becomes somewhat atrophied so that a long metatarsal (usually the second) becomes symptomatic; a distal metatarsal osteotomy

can often relieve this problem.

Surgical Technique

1. The skin incision begins in the web space and is then gently curved proximally over the metatarsal for a distance of about 3 cm. It is deepened to expose the extensor tendons.

2. The extensor tendons can be pulled aside or the raphe between the extensor digitorum longus and extensor digitorum brevis tendons can be split, exposing the joint. If there is hypertrophied synovial tissue, it should be excised.

3. Care is taken not to disrupt the collateral ligaments because one does not want to interfere with the blood supply to the metatarsal head.

4. The metatarsophalangeal joint is subluxated by plantar flexing the proximal phalanx, and a Weitlaner retractor is used to expose the metatarsal head.

5. With use of a fine-tooth saw blade and a sagittal saw, a longitudinal cut is made in the metatarsal head beginning about 1 to 2 mm plantar to the edge of the dorsal articulating surface. It is important that the saw blade be in the same plane as the metatarsal shaft and not rotated. As long a cut as possible is then created in the metatarsal (Figure 22, *A*).

6. As the saw blade is passed into the metatarsal, it is important that it be moved from side to side so that the medial and lateral aspects of the metatarsal are cut. The osteotomy site usually slides after approximately 70% to 80% of the length of the blade has been inserted. If it slides sooner, a sufficiently oblique angle has not been achieved.

7. The degree of shortening of the osteotomy depends on the overall

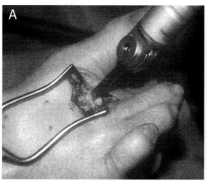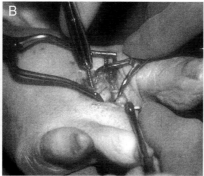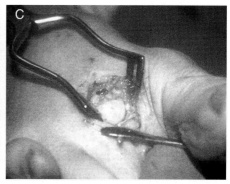

Figure 22 Surgical technique for the distal metatarsal osteotomy. **A,** After exposure, the osteotomy is performed with an oscillating saw. Note that the cut begins just beneath the dorsal aspect of the articular surface of the metatarsal head. The saw cut is made as obliquely as possible to create as large a bone contact area as possible. **B,** After shortening, the head fragment is stabilized with a small towel clip, and a 2.7-mm screw is inserted. The proximal cortex is overdrilled with a 2.7-mm drill bit. **C,** The dorsal overhanging bone has been "buffed" with a saw to create a smooth surface between the edge of the bone and the articular cartilage.

length of the metatarsal. The amount of shortening to be performed is determined by drawing a line that passes from the distal portion of the metatarsal head on either side of the long metatarsal. This sometimes involves a line from the first to the third metatarsal and, at the point at which the line intersects the second metatarsal, the degree of shortening to be performed is determined by measuring the distance from this line to the end of the second metatarsal head. If two metatarsals are long (usually the second and third metatarsals), then the initial line passes from the first to the fourth metatarsal, and the point at which it intersects the second and third metatarsal heads determines the degree of shortening to be achieved.

8. The osteotomy site is stabilized with use of a small towel clip.
9. A 2.7-mm lag screw is then inserted across the osteotomy site to stabilize it (Figure 22, *B*). The lag-screw method, with overdrilling of the proximal hole with a 2.7-mm drill bit, is preferred be-

cause self-tapping screws tend to slightly distract the osteotomy site.
10. Once the osteotomy site is stable, the overhanging portion of the remaining metatarsal head is buffed with the saw (Figure 22, *C*). A rongeur should not be used for this purpose as the bone might fracture, jeopardizing the screw fixation. Finally, it is imperative to check dorsiflexion of the joint to be sure that there is no impingement between the proximal phalanx and the dorsal aspect of the metatarsal head.
11. The skin is closed in a routine fashion, and a compression dressing is applied.

Postoperative Care The day after the operation, the circumferential dressing is changed and the patient is permitted to walk in a postoperative shoe. The sutures are removed at 10 days, and the dressings are removed in about 3 weeks. At that point, range-of-motion exercises should be begun. The foot is kept in a postoperative shoe for about 6 weeks, until the osteotomy site is completely healed radiographically.

The postoperative management does not differ if more than one osteotomy is performed.

Results The literature indicates that this procedure is most frequently used to treat a dislocated or subluxated metatarsophalangeal joint. In a series of 39 feet, only 7 without pathology of the metatarsophalangeal joint underwent this procedure.[11] In these 7 feet, 11 osteotomies were performed, with 4 of them performed on the second metatarsal; 5, on the third metatarsal; and 2, on the fourth metatarsal. A single osteotomy was performed in four feet; two osteotomies, in two; and three osteotomies, in one. There were three excellent results, three good results, and one poor result. Most patients had a reduced range of motion. The callus resolved in six of the seven patients.

Summary

An intractable plantar keratosis beneath a metatarsal head can be a mere annoyance or, in the worst case, a disabling condition for a patient. The clinician must make an accurate diagnosis of the etiology of the condition. Most patients with intractable plantar keratosis can be treated nonsurgically with proper shoe wear and adequate padding of the metatarsal area. If the keratotic lesion is refractory to nonsurgical treatment, surgical treatment offers a reasonable chance for success. It is imperative to choose the correct surgical procedure for the clinical condition because one operation will not resolve all keratotic lesions. In patients with hyperkeratotic skin, the lesion may not resolve despite adequate surgical treatment.

References

1. Mann RA, Poppen NK, O'Konski M: Amputation of the great toe: A clinical and biomechanical study. *Clin Orthop* 1988;226:192-205.

2. Hutton WC, Stott JRR, Stokes JAF, Klinerman L (eds): *The Foot and Its Allied Disorders.* Oxford, England, Blackwell Scientific, 1982, p 42.

3. Clarke TE: *The Pressure Distribution Under the Foot During Barefoot Walking* (doctoral dissertation). University Park, PA, Pennsylvania State University, 1980.

4. DuVries HL: *Surgery of the Foot,* ed 2. St. Louis, MO, Mosby, 1965, pp 456-462.

5. Mann RA, Coughlin MJ: Intractable plantar keratoses, in *The Video Textbook of Foot and Ankle Surgery.* St. Louis, MO, Medical Video Production, 1991, p 86.

6. Mann RA, DuVries HL: Intractable plantar keratosis. *Orthop Clin North Am* 1973;4:67-73.

7. Dreeben SM, Noble PC, Hammerman S, Bishop JO, Tullos HS: Metatarsal osteotomy for primary metatarsalgia: Radiographic and pedobarographic study. *Foot Ankle* 1989;9:214-218.

8. Kitaoka HB, Patzer GL: Chevron osteotomy of lesser metatarsals for intractable plantar callosities. *J Bone Joint Surg Br* 1998;80:516-518.

9. Mann RA, Wapner KL: Tibial sesamoid shaving for treatment of intractable plantar keratosis under tibial sesamoid. *Foot Ankle* 1992;13:196-198.

10. Giannestras NJ: Shortening of the metatarsal shaft in the treatment of plantar keratosis: An end-result study. *J Bone Joint Surg Am* 1958;49:61-71.

11. Vandeputte G, Dereymaeker G, Steenwerckx A, Peeraer L: The Weil osteotomy of the lesser metatarsals: A clinical and pedobarographic follow-up study. *Foot Ankle Int* 2000;21:370-374.

The Bunionette Deformity

Roger A. Mann, MD
Jeffrey A. Mann, MD

Abstract

The bunionette deformity results in pain about the lateral and/or the plantar aspect of the fifth metatarsal head. It is important to carefully assess the deformity anatomically in order to select the proper surgical procedure to correct this painful affliction. Knowledge of pathoanatomy and certain surgical procedures can be used to correct the deformity.

The bunionette deformity, or tailor's bunion, is a painful affliction of the fifth metatarsophalangeal (MTP) joint. It becomes symptomatic as a result of pressure against the fifth metatarsal head. The painful area may be on the lateral aspect of the metatarsal head because of pressure against a shoe, or on the plantar aspect of the metatarsal head where an intractable plantar keratosis may occur (Figure 1). Sometimes the fifth metatarsal head is prominent laterally and the metatarsal head is plantar flexed, giving rise to a lesion both laterally and plantarly. Occasionally, a painful lesion beneath the fifth metatarsal may be associated with a postural problem of the foot (for example, cavus foot, a malaligned fusion, or in a posttraumatic foot) (Figure 2). Regardless of the etiology, the symptom complex is aggravated by constricting shoe wear, which places pressure on the prominent fifth metatarsal head. In certain systemic diseases such as rheumatoid arthritis or psoriatic arthritis, there may be subluxation or dislocation of the fifth MTP joint, leading to abnormal pressure (Figure 3). In patients with impaired sensation, such as those with diabetes, an ulceration may occur beneath the fifth metatarsal head because of chronic pressure associated with an insensate foot.

Because the bunionette deformity has multiple causes, it is important to recognize the pathologic anatomy in order to correctly diagnose and, if necessary, surgically manage the deformity.

Anatomic Measurements

All radiographic measurements are made from weight-bearing AP, lateral, and oblique views. The following radiographic determinations are made: (1) Subluxation or dislocation of the MTP joint; (2) Evidence of systemic disorder such as rheumatoid arthritis; (3) Size of the metatarsal head; (4) The size of the MTP-5 angle, which calculates the magnitude of the medial deviation of the fifth toe in relation to the long axis of the metatarsal shaft. The MTP-5 angle has been reported as 10.2° in normal feet and 16° in patients with bunionettes[1,2] (Figure 4); (5) the size of the intermetatarsal angle between the fourth and fifth metatarsals, which normally averages 6.2° (range, 3° to 11°);[2] (6) degree of lateral deviation of the distal aspect of the fifth metatarsal shaft with a normal 4-5 intermetatarsal angle; (7) extent of the plantar flexion of the fifth metatarsal on the lateral radiograph.

Classification

Type 1

A type 1 deformity is caused by a prominent lateral condyle, which may be caused by hypertrophy of the lateral condyle or anatomically an enlarged metatarsal head. This type of deformity has been reported in 16% to 27% of cases in various series[1,3](Figure 5).

Type 2

A type 2 deformity is caused by a lateral bowing of the diaphysis of the fifth metatarsal shaft. In these cases, the intermetatarsal angle is normal and it is the lateral deviation of the

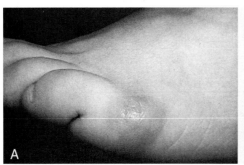
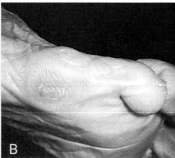

Figure 1 A, A keratotic lesion over a prominent fifth metatarsal head. **B,** A keratotic lesion involving the plantar lateral aspect of the foot caused by plantar flexion of the fifth metatarsal. (Reproduced with permission from Coughlin M, Mann R: Keratotic disorders of the plantar skin, in Coughlin M, Mann R (eds): *Surgery of the Foot and Ankle.* St. Louis, MO, Mosby, 1999, pp 394-441.)

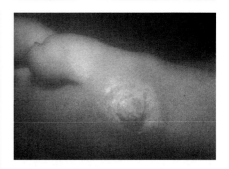

Figure 2 A large plantar lateral keratotic lesion secondary to a malaligned fifth metatarsal fracture.

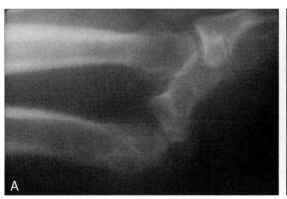
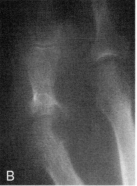

Figure 3 A and **B,** Subluxation of the fifth MTP joint as a result of rheumatoid arthritis.

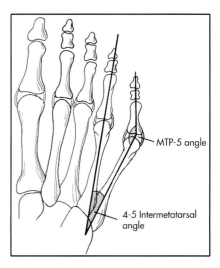

Figure 4 The degree of lateral deviation of the fifth metatarsal is determined by measuring the intermetatarsal angle between the fourth and fifth metatarsal shafts. The fifth toe angle represents the degree of medial deviation of the phalanx on the fifth metatarsal head. (Reproduced with permission from Coughlin M, Mann R: Keratotic disorders of the plantar skin, in Coughlin M, Mann R (eds): *Surgery of the Foot and Ankle.* St. Louis, MO, Mosby, 1999, pp 394-441.)

distal half of the fifth metatarsal that leads to the bunionette deformity. There may or may not be some degree of plantar flexion of the distal metatarsal. A type 2 deformity was noted in 23% of cases reported by Coughlin[1] (Figure 6).

Type 3
A type 3 deformity is characterized by an increased 4-5 intermetatarsal angle. The normal 4-5 angle is reported to be 6.2° (range, 3° to 11°).[2] In patients with a symptomatic bunionette deformity the 4-5 intermetatarsal angle averaged 9.6° (range, 5° to 14°) in one series[4] and 10.6° in another.[1] There may or may not be some degree of plantar flexion of the

metatarsal shaft. This type of deformity was reported by Coughlin[1] in 50% of his series of 28 patients (Figure 7).

Regardless of the type of bony deformity, the patient's clinical complaints are basically the same, namely that of lateral and/or plantar pain about the fifth metatarsal head.

Physical Evaluation
The patient with a symptomatic bunionette deformity may have an enlarged bursa over the lateral aspect of the fifth metatarsal head, or a painful callus along the lateral aspect of the metatarsal head and/or plantar aspect of the foot. In Coughlin's series[1] of 28 patients, 70% developed a

lateral keratotic lesion, 10% a plantar lesion, and 20% a combined lateral and plantar lesion. In patients with a rheumatologic disorder there may be significant synovitis of the MTP joint with or without dislocation of the joint. In all of these patients, however, the main problem is pain about the fifth metatarsal head area.

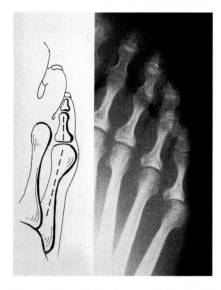

Figure 5 Type 1 bunionette deformity is characterized by an enlarged fifth metatarsal head. (Reproduced with permission from Coughlin M, Mann R: Keratotic disorders of the plantar skin, in Coughlin M, Mann R (eds): *Surgery of the Foot and Ankle*. St. Louis, MO, Mosby, 1999, pp 394-441.)

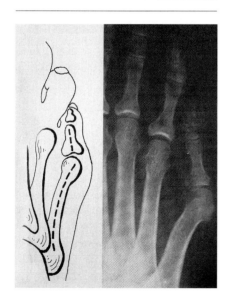

Figure 6 Type 2 bunionette deformity is characterized by lateral bowing of the fifth metatarsal head and neck. (Reproduced with permission from Coughlin M, Mann R: Keratotic disorders of the plantar skin, in Coughlin M, Mann R (eds): *Surgery of the Foot and Ankle*. St. Louis, MO, Mosby, 1999, pp 394-441.)

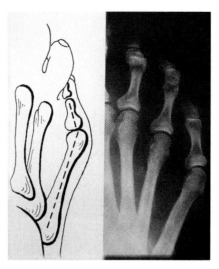

Figure 7 Type 3 bunionette deformity is characterized by lateral and plantar deviation, giving rise to an increased 4-5 intermetatarsal angle. (Reproduced with permission from Coughlin M, Mann R: Keratotic disorders of the plantar skin, in Coughlin M, Mann R (eds): *Surgery of the Foot and Ankle*. St. Louis, MO, Mosby, 1999, pp 394-441.)

The symptom complex is aggravated by constricting shoe wear. It is not uncommon for an asymptomatic patient wearing a tight shoe that cuts across the fifth metatarsal head area to develop painful bursitis. Usually, this type of bursal irritation will respond to conservative management and usually is an isolated incident. In patients who are more athletic and wear constricting and sometimes rigid shoe gear, the bursal irritation may be chronic.

The posture of the foot in the standing position should be noted during physical examination. A cavus type foot or a fixed forefoot varus both can place increased stress on the lateral aspect of the foot. The skin should be carefully evaluated because a patient will sometimes develop a small seed corn within a callus that is quite symptomatic, and if débrided alleviates the entire clinical problem.

The symptomatic patient is managed conservatively with a less constricting shoe and instructions to avoid pressure over the fifth metatarsal head. The seam pattern of the shoe should be evaluated. A small felt pad placed into the shoe just proximal to the plantar lesion may alleviate pressure on it. It is important that shoe wear be of adequate size because the addition of a pad to an already tight shoe will only lead to additional problems. If conservative management fails, then surgical intervention may be considered.

Surgical Management

The successful surgical treatment of a bunionette deformity is dependent upon selecting the correct surgical procedure for the patient's specific problem. For the patient with a type 1 deformity in which the main problem is brought about by the lateral prominence of the fifth metatarsal head, some type of distal metatarsal osteotomy, either a chevron or oblique type, is most useful. Careful evaluation of the fourth metatarsal head for flexibility is important if there is going to be any shortening of the fifth metatarsal, which occurs in an oblique sliding type of osteotomy. The fourth and fifth metatarsals are the most flexible of the metatarsals, with the fifth metatarsal tending to be more flexible than the fourth. In a situation in which the fourth metatarsal is rigid, significant shortening of the fifth metatarsal may lead to a transfer lesion, so a distal chevron procedure in which there is little or no shortening would be preferable. If the patient has plantar pain, elevation of the fifth metatarsal head is necessary.

A fifth metatarsal head resection to correct a bunionette deformity should only be used in the diabetic patient

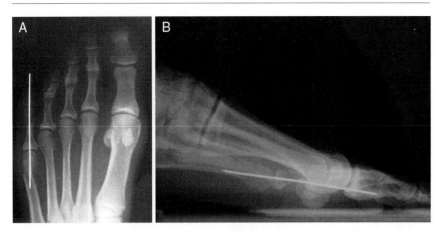

Figure 8 AP (**A**) and lateral (**B**) radiographs following a distal chevron osteotomy fixed with a longitudinal K-wire.

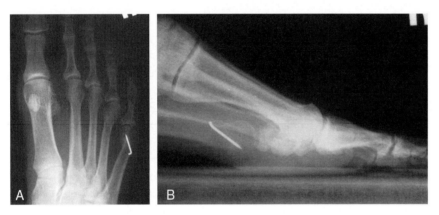

Figure 9 AP (**A**) and lateral (**B**) radiographs demonstrating fixation of the chevron osteotomy with a short K-wire drilled from proximal to distal.

with a plantar ulcer, or occasionally the patient with rheumatoid or psoriatic arthritis because of the chronic disability associated with these diseases. Resection of the fifth metatarsal head leads to a floppy fifth toe and a possible transfer lesion beneath the fourth metatarsal head.

Authors' Preferred Method of Treatment of Type 1 Deformity

For a type 1 deformity, a distal chevron procedure will usually produce a satisfactory result. The fifth metatarsal head is small and great care needs to be taken so it is not fractured.

A longitudinal incision starting over the lateral aspect of the proximal phalanx of the fifth toe is gently curved dorsally over the fifth metatarsal head and then slightly plantarward to the midline. As the incision is deepened through the subcutaneous tissue it is important that the dorsal nerve is identified and retracted dorsally. This curved incision avoids the possible complication of a painful callus developing within the scar over the lateral aspect of the joint. The capsule is released through a dorsal incision brought proximally, creating an inverted L-shaped flap. It is important that the flap is left attached to the

base of the proximal phalanx and the tendon of the abductor digiti quinti is not damaged. After the lateral capsular flap has been created, release of the medial joint capsule is important because it will prevent the fifth toe from subluxating in a medial direction. The metatarsal head is exposed and a wafer of bone is removed with a power saw from its lateral border. A 0.045-inch Kirschner wire (K-wire) is drilled through the center of the metatarsal head from lateral to medial to mark the apex of the chevron cut. A sagittal saw with a small blade with inline teeth is used to create the osteotomy at an angle of approximately 60°. The osteotomy site is freed up and displaced in a medial direction approximately 50% of the width of the shaft. Stabilization of the osteotomy by subluxating the fifth MTP joint and drilling a 0.045-inch K-wire starting in the middle of the base of the proximal phalanx out through the tip of the toe is preferred. This procedure is technically challenging. The osteotomy site is then displaced medially, the fifth MTP joint reduced, and the K-wire drilled into the metatarsal head and across the osteotomy site. This provides excellent alignment and fixation of the osteotomy. Another technique for stabilizing the osteotomy site is to place an oblique K-wire into the small capital fragment, leaving the end buried or protruding through the skin. The bony prominence created by the medially displaced metatarsal head is shaved off flush to the metatarsal. The capsule is closed and is sutured into the surrounding tissues. The skin is closed in a routine manner and the patient placed into a compression dressing.

In the occasional patient with a plantar lesion and a lateral lesion but no deviation of the metatarsal shaft, the chevron cut can be made slightly oblique to allow slight dorsiflexion of the metatarsal head as it is displaced medially (Figures 8 and 9).

Postoperative Care

The patient is permitted to ambulate in a postoperative shoe. The K-wire is removed in 4 weeks, but the postoperative shoe is worn an additional 2 to 4 weeks until there is radiographic evidence of healing.

The results following a chevron osteotomy reported by Kitaoka and associates,[4] at an average follow-up of 7.1 years, noted that 12 of 14 feet (63%) had a good or excellent result. The feet were narrowed an average of 3 mm. Complications included a postoperative keratosis over the bunionette in one patient and a transfer metatarsalgia in another. Osteonecrosis of the metatarsal head is a possible complication, although not encountered by the authors.

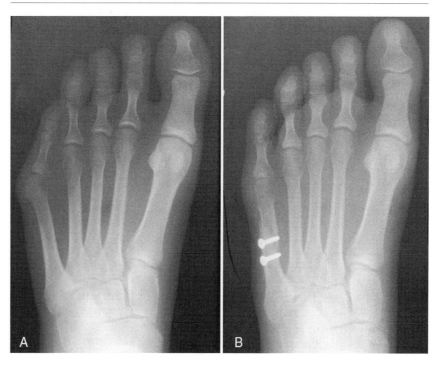

Figure 10 Preoperative **(A)** and postoperative **(B)** radiographs following repair of a type 3 bunionette deformity using an oblique metatarsal osteotomy.

Authors' Preferred Method of Treatment of Type 2 and Type 3 Deformity

The surgical procedure selected to correct the type 2 deformity is usually dependent upon the severity of the deformity and whether or not a plantar lesion is present. When the deformity is more severe, we prefer to manage the problem in the same way as a type 3 deformity with a long oblique osteotomy. The osteotomy is usually a little more distal, closer to the apex of the deformity. If, however, the deformity is quite distal, then a distal oblique osteotomy can be considered, although from a technical standpoint this is sometimes difficult because the bone in this region is quite small and fixation can be difficult. If there is a plantar flexion component to the deformity, the osteotomy is performed in an oblique plane.

The type 3 deformity is charac-

terized by a painful lesion laterally and a plantar keratotic lesion. The correction of this deformity, particularly if it is severe, cannot be carried out distally any more than a severe hallux valgus deformity can be corrected with a distal metatarsal osteotomy. The osteotomy must be placed more proximal in order to gain a greater degree of correction. For this reason, an oblique diaphyseal osteotomy is preferred to correct a deformity of this type.

A midlateral longitudinal incision is made starting from the middle of the proximal phalanx and extending proximally to the proximal aspect of the fifth metatarsal base. The incision is curved slightly as it passes over the metatarsal head to avoid making a direct lateral incision over the lateral eminence of the fifth metatarsal. As the incision is deepened, care is taken to avoid the dorsal nerve coursing over the fifth

metatarsal. The interval just above the abductor digiti minimi muscle is identified so the muscle belly can be reflected in a plantarward direction. In this manner, the entire distal two thirds of the metatarsal shaft is exposed. An inverted L-incision is made over the dorsal capsule with care being taken not to detach the capsule from the base of the proximal phalanx. The tendon of the abductor digiti minimi should not be detached. The fifth MTP joint is distracted and the capsule on the medial side of the joint is cut so that the fifth toe can be pulled into lateral deviation. With a power saw, a thin wafer of lateral eminence is removed and the edges buffed. If the patient's problem is only a prominent lateral eminence of the fifth metatarsal because of lateral deviation of the fifth metatarsal shaft, a horizontal osteotomy is performed. This enables the surgeon to displace

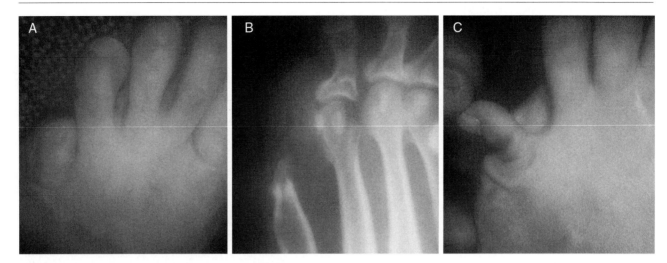

Figure 11 Problems associated with resecting the fifth metatarsal head for correction of bunionette deformity. **A,** The fifth toe is shortened and retracted. **B,** A radiograph demonstrating excised metatarsal head. **C,** The fifth toe becomes floppy, resulting in catching of the toe when putting on a sock. This can be corrected using a syndactyly between the fourth and fifth toes.

the distal shaft medially, therefore decreasing the intermetatarsal angle and, hence, the prominent metatarsal head. If, however, there is a lateral prominence as well as a plantar keratosis, an oblique metatarsal osteotomy is used, which displaces the metatarsal shaft medially and dorsally. The osteotomy site is created in such a way that it permits the distal fragment to move beneath the proximal fragment in a dorsal medial direction. The horizontal osteotomy is lined up by placing the saw along the dorsal aspect of the distal metatarsal in the metaphyseal area. The saw cut is angled proximally and plantarward to end at about the junction of the proximal third and distal two thirds of the bone. To produce the obliquity in the cut, the saw handle is dropped in a plantarward direction so the cut is angled slightly upward as it proceeds from medial to lateral. A cut in this plane as it is displaced medially will, therefore, dorsally angulate the distal metatarsal. Once the cut has been made, the osteotomy site is displaced so that the metatarsal head moves medially and/or medially and dorsally. The

osteotomy is stabilized with bone-holding forceps and fixed using one or two 2.7-mm or 3.5-mm cortical screws. When the screws are placed, the proximal cortex is over-drilled and the screw is slightly countersunk. If the bone happens to split, a cerclage wire can be used to stabilize the osteotomy site (Figure 10). The capsular flap of the fifth MTP joint is then repaired in such a way as to hold it in satisfactory alignment. The abductor digiti quinti muscle is closed over the fifth metatarsal shaft and the skin is closed with interrupted sutures.

Postoperative Care
The patient's foot is kept securely wrapped in a compression dressing for a period of 4 weeks, after which immobilization is continued until the osteotomy site has healed, usually 8 to 10 weeks. During the first 6 weeks the fifth toe is held in neutral to slight lateral deviation so as to prevent medial subluxation.

Results
Coughlin[1] reported on 20 patients (30 feet) undergoing this procedure

at an average of 31 months' follow-up. All osteotomies healed. The 4-5 intermetatarsal angle improved from 10.6° to 0.8° and the MTP-5 angle improved from 16° preoperatively to 0.5° postoperatively. There were no symptomatic transfer lesions noted and 93% of the patients were satisfied with the results. The width of the foot was reduced by 6 mm (range, 2 to 15 mm) and there was an average shortening of 0.5 mm.

Summary
Although there are more than 20 different surgical techniques recommended for the correction of a bunionette deformity, the ones presented here are designed to correct the specific pathologic anatomy. Although other osteotomies can give a satisfactory result, we believe these procedures correct the anatomic deformity.

Osteotomies that are carried out at the base of the fifth metatarsal in the area where a Jones fracture occurs should be avoided because the possibility of a nonunion is increased in this region. The fifth metatarsal head should not be ex-

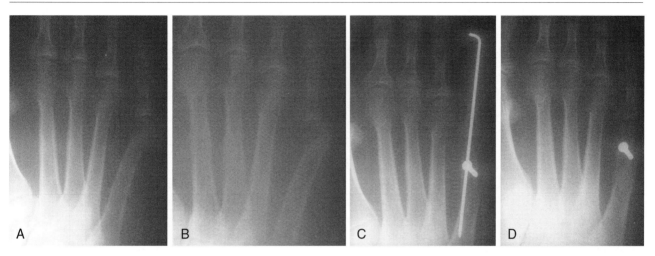

Figure 12 Complications following incomplete correction of bunionette deformity. **A,** A preoperative radiograph demonstrates a type 3 bunionette deformity. **B,** A radiograph demonstrating subluxation of the MTP joint following attempted correction using a lateral exostectomy. **C,** Correction using an oblique distal metatarsal osteotomy and capsulotomy. **D,** Maintenance of the postoperative correction following pin removal. When a bony deformity is present, a metatarsal osteotomy is essential to obtain a satisfactory long-term correction.

cised in the treatment of this condition because it leads to excessive shortening of the metatarsal and the possibility of a transfer lesion beneath the fourth metatarsal and cocking up and retraction of the fifth toe (Figure 11). The salvage procedure for this condition is usually a syndactyly of the fourth and fifth toes to correct the malalignment of the fifth toe and a plantar condylectomy of the fourth metatarsal if an intractable plantar keratosis is present.

The use of a lateral condylectomy to treat a bunionette deformity may give a satisfactory result, but only in the patient who only has a lateral lesion and no increase in the 4-5 intermetatarsal angle. If the patient has a plantar keratosis, a lateral condylectomy would be contraindicated.

Unfortunately, following the lateral condylectomy, medial subluxation of the MTP joint may occur and, as such, it is imperative that a strong capsular repair and medial capsular release be carried out to prevent this complication. A postoperative dressing should be worn for 6 weeks and the toe maintained in neutral to slight lateral deviation. For this reason, we rarely use this procedure and prefer the distal chevron osteotomy instead.

In patients in whom a lateral condylectomy has been performed and subluxation of the joint occurs, salvage of this problem can be achieved by carrying out a complete dorsal, medial, and lateral capsulotomy to release the soft-tissue contracture and a distal oblique osteotomy to shorten the metatarsal (Figure

12). The MTP joint is stabilized with a K-wire for a period of 6 weeks. Usually, this combination of release, shortening, and capsular repair will result in stabilization of the fifth MTP joint, although some joint motion may be lost.

References

1. Coughlin MJ: Treatment of bunionette deformity with longitudinal diaphyseal osteotomy with soft tissue repair. *Foot Ankle* 1991;11:195-203.

2. Fallat LM, Buckholz J: An analysis of the tailor's bunion by radiographic and anatomical display. *J Am Podiatry Assoc* 1980;70:597-603.

3. Konradsen L, Nielsen P: Distal metatarsal osteotomy for bunionette deformity. *J Foot Surg* 1988;27:493-496.

4. Kitaoka H, Holiday A, Campbell D: Distal chevron metatarsal osteotomy for bunionette. *Foot Ankle* 1991;12:80-85.

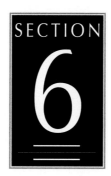

SECTION 6

Ankle Arthrosis

Ankle Arthrosis

Ankle arthrosis is one of the more challenging disorders affecting the ankle. The surgical treatment of ankle arthrosis poses a dilemma—whether to opt for ankle arthrodesis and sacrifice the residual motion of the ankle joint or to proceed with ankle replacement surgery, which has higher failure and complication rates than hip or knee arthroplasty. The chapters in this section review ankle arthrosis, including anatomy, pathophysiology, treatment options, and complications of surgical treatment.

The chapter by Buckwalter and Saltzman presents a review of the differences between ankle arthritis and arthritis affecting the hip and knee. A recent study confirmed that, in contrast with primary osteoarthritis of the hip and knee, ankle osteoarthritis most commonly occurs secondary to trauma.[1] The ankle is more vulnerable to injury than the hip or knee. The articular cartilage of the ankle is thinner and has a smaller contact area, and the high peak contact stresses make the ankle joint more susceptible to the development of posttraumatic secondary osteoarthritis.

Ankle articular cartilage can withstand greater tensile loads than hip articular cartilage; this may be a reason for the lower incidence of primary osteoarthritis of the ankle compared with the hip. Ankle cartilage has different biochemical and metabolic properties, such as greater proteoglycan and water content, decreased response to catabolic factors such as interleukin-1, and lower levels of prostaglandin E_2 and E_4 receptors than knee articular cartilage.[2,3]

Ankle arthrodesis, including the use of arthrodesis to treat rheumatoid arthritis, sepsis, osteonecrosis, bone deficit, malunion, Charcot ankle, and multiple joint disease, is discussed in the chapter

by Kitaoka. The importance of alignment, regardless of the fixation method, is emphasized. The recommended alignment is neutral dorsiflexion, 5° to 10° of hindfoot valgus, and 5° to 10° of external rotation of the foot. Posterior translation of the talus (0 to 1 cm) with respect to the tibia decreases the anterior lever arm and midfoot overloading.

Kitaoka reviews the technique of transfibular osteotomy and the use of the fibula as an onlay bone graft. More recently, some authors have reported that preservation of the fibula may decrease complications of future conversion of the arthrodesis to a total ankle replacement.[4] External ring fixation can achieve similar ankle fusion site stability as internal fixation screws,[5] and external ring fixation may be useful in achieving ankle fusion in patients with bone loss and infection.[6] Increased subtalar and medial column motion in the sagittal plane have been documented after ankle arthrodesis, and this may contribute to the progressive development of subtalar arthritis.[7]

The chapter by Gill discusses the history and design considerations for total ankle replacements. The anatomic and biomechanical properties of the ankle are compared and contrasted with those of the hip and knee, providing a conceptual understanding of the principles, pitfalls, and goals in designing ankle replacement implants. Gill concludes that successful ankle replacement is more challenging than hip or knee arthroplasty because of issues intrinsic to the ankle, including high forces, a small surface area, talar size and shape, poor bone quality, poor soft-tissue coverage, the high potential for injury, and the proximity of the neurovascular structures.

The chapter by DeOrio and Easley provides a comprehensive review of total ankle replacement arthroplasty including indications, contraindications, design features of available implants, surgical techniques, results, revision surgery, and conversion to arthrodesis. The authors discuss various ankle implants with respect to advantages, disadvantages, and clinical results (including complications). One of the major indications for total ankle replacement is end-stage ankle arthritis with prior subtalar or triple hindfoot arthrodesis; however, not all implants are suitable to treat this condition because of the potential subsidence associated with a compromised talar blood supply and bone stock. Key technical aspects include balancing the soft tissues and correcting varus or valgus malalignment.

A recent gait analysis study has shown that ankle arthrodesis is associated with faster gait and longer step length than ankle replacement, but ankle replacement is associated with better gait timing and ground reaction force pattern.[8] Gait analysis before and after total ankle replacement shows postoperative improvement of gait parameters including decreased energy expenditure.[9] After total ankle replacement, the ankle appears to have proprioception similar to the contralateral, unaffected side.[10]

Total ankle replacement has a steep surgical learning curve, with a markedly higher complication rate in earlier than later cases in a consecutive series.[11] A randomized, controlled trial of two ankle replacement implants confirmed that major varus or valgus ankle deformity is associated with a higher potential for failure of ankle replacements.[12] Nevertheless, major hindfoot deformity may be corrected during total ankle replacement surgery.[13] Ankle replacement also may be indicated for salvage of a painful ankle arthrodesis, but moderate pain may persist in most patients treated with this procedure.[14] Reoperation after primary total ankle replacement has been reported in almost one third of patients, and amputation is sometimes necessary after a failed arthroplasty.[15]

The chapter by Wapner reviews arthrodesis for the salvage of failed and infected total ankle replacements and discusses the challenges of limited bone stock, compromised soft tissues, and the large bony defect after implant removal. The lateral approach with fibular resection may minimize the potential for breakdown of the thin anterior soft tissues. A staged procedure is discussed for managing infection or questionable talar viability. Successful arthrodesis after failed ankle replacement has been report-ed with a tricortical iliac crest bone graft to preserve ankle height and the subtalar joint.[16] A large, bony defect associated with a nonviable talus or subtalar joint arthritis may be salvaged with a tibiotalo-calcaneal fusion or talar excision with tibiocalcaneal fusion using external fixation,[17] an intramedullary nail and femoral head allograft,[18] or a posterior blade plate and iliac crest bone graft.[19] Some aseptic failed ankle replacements may be salvaged with either arthrodesis or revision ankle replacement.[20]

The chapter by van Roermund and Lafeber presents a review of the background and early results of joint distraction, an emerging method for treating ankle arthritis. This procedure is based on the hypothesis that injured cartilage has reparative potential when the joint is unloaded and when intermittent synovial fluid flow and pressure are maintained. The ankle is treated with 5 mm of tibio-talar distraction for 3 months with an Ilizarov frame, with loading and unloading of the joint. This treatment may allow dedifferentiated chondrocytes to redifferentiate, stop proliferation, and create a reparative cartilage matrix. Since this chapter appeared, several additional studies have confirmed the potential clinical efficacy of ankle joint distraction for ankle arthritis, with 73% to 91% of patients having improvement of pain at follow-up evaluation 7 years or more after the procedure.[21-23] It is anticipated that further study will clarify the indications and potential long-term benefit of ankle distraction.

Aneel Nihal, MD, FRCS UK (Ortho), FRACS (Ortho)
Consulting Orthopaedic Surgeon
Department of Orthopaedics
Logan Hospital, Metro South District
Meadowbrook, South Brisbane,
Queensland, Australia

References

1. Valderrabano V, Horisberger M, Russell I, Dougall H, Hintermann B: Etiology of ankle osteoarthritis. *Clin Orthop Relat Res* 2009;467:1800-1806.

2. Kuettner KE, Cole AA: Cartilage degeneration in different human joints. *Osteoarthritis Cartilage* 2005;13:93-103.

3. Li X, Ellman M, Muddasani P, et al: Prostaglandin E2 and its cognate EP receptors control human adult articular cartilage homeostasis and are linked to the pathophysiology of osteoarthritis. *Arthritis Rheum* 2009;60:513-523.

4. Greisberg J, Assal M, Flueckiger G, Hansen ST: Takedown of ankle fusion and conversion to total ankle replacement. *Clin Orthop Relat Res* 2004;424:80-88.

5. Ogut T, Glisson RR, Chuckpaiwong B, Le IL, Easley ME: External ring fixation versus screw fixation for ankle arthrodesis: A biomechanical comparison. *Foot Ankle Int* 2009;30:353-360.

6. Kovoor CC, Padmanabhan V, Bhaskar D, George VV, Viswanath S: Ankle fusion for bone loss around the ankle joint using the Ilizarov technique. *J Bone Joint Surg Br* 2009;91:361-366.

7. Sealey RJ, Myerson MS, Molloy A, Gamba C, Jeng C, Kalesan B: Sagittal plane motion of the hindfoot following ankle arthrodesis: A prospective analysis. *Foot Ankle Int* 2009;30:187-196.

8. Piriou P, Culpan P, Mullins M, Cardon JN, Pozzi D, Judet T: Ankle replacement versus arthrodesis: A comparative gait analysis study. *Foot Ankle Int* 2008;29:3-9.

9. Detrembleur C, Leemrijse T: The effects of total ankle replacement on gait disability: Analysis of energetic and mechanical variables. *Gait Posture* 2009;29:270-274.

10. Conti SF, Dazen D, Stewart G, et al: Proprioception after total ankle arthroplasty. *Foot Ankle Int* 2008;29:1069-1073.

11. Lee KB, Cho SG, Hur CI, Yoon TR: Perioperative complications of HINTEGRA total ankle replacement: Our initial 50 cases. *Foot Ankle Int* 2008;29:978-984.

12. Wood PL, Sutton C, Mishra V, Suneja R: A randomised, controlled trial of two mobile-bearing total ankle replacements. *J Bone Joint Surg Br* 2009;91:69-74.

13. Hobson SA, Karantana A, Dhar S: Total ankle replacement in patients with significant preoperative deformity of the hindfoot. *J Bone Joint Surg Br* 2009;91:481-486.

14. Hintermann B, Barg A, Knupp M, Valderrabano V: Conversion of painful ankle arthrodesis to total ankle arthroplasty. *J Bone Joint Surg Am* 2009;91:850-858.

15. Spirt AA, Assal M, Hansen ST: Complications and failure after total ankle arthroplasty. *J Bone Joint Surg Am* 2004;86:1172-1178.

16. Culpan P, Le Strat V, Piriou P, Judet T: Arthrodesis after failed total ankle replacement. *J Bone Joint Surg Br* 2007;89:1178-1183.

17. Rochman R, Jackson Hutson J, Alade O: Tibiocalcaneal arthrodesis using the Ilizarov technique in the presence of bone loss and infection of the talus. *Foot Ankle Int* 2008;29:1001-1008.

18. Thomason K, Eyres KS: A technique of fusion for failed total replacement of the ankle: Tibio-allograft-calcaneal fusion with a locked retrograde intramedullary nail. *J Bone Joint Surg Br* 2008;90:885-888.

19. Ritter M, Nickisch F, DiGiovanni C: Technique tip: Posterior blade plate for salvage of failed total ankle arthroplasty. *Foot Ankle Int* 2006;27:303-304.

20. Kotnis R, Pasapula C, Anwar F, Cooke PH, Sharp RJ: The management of failed ankle replacement. *J Bone Joint Surg Br* 2006;88: 1039-1047.

21. Ploegmakers JJ, van Roermund PM, van Melkebeek J, et al: Prolonged clinical benefit from joint distraction in the treatment of ankle osteoarthritis. *Osteoarthritis Cartilage* 2005;13:582-588.

22. Paley D, Lamm BM, Purohit RM, Specht SC: Distraction arthroplasty of the ankle: How far can you stretch the indications? *Foot Ankle Clin* 2008;13:471-484.

23. Tellisi N, Fragomen AT, Kleinman D, O'Malley MJ, Rozbruch SR: Joint preservation of the osteoarthritic ankle using distraction arthroplasty. *Foot Ankle Int* 2009;30:318-325.

Aneel Nihal, MD or a member of his immediate family has received research or institutional support from Synthes.

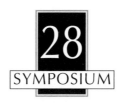

28
SYMPOSIUM

Ankle Osteoarthritis: Distinctive Characteristics

Joseph A. Buckwalter, MD
Charles L. Saltzman, MD

Because osteoarthritis causes similar symptoms of pain and loss of motion in different joints, few investigators have made an attempt to determine if osteoarthritis differs among joints in pathogenesis, clinical presentation, and response to treatment. The majority of clinical and basic scientific studies have focused on hip and knee osteoarthritis, and physicians have generally assumed that information developed from these studies applies equally well to other joints. Ankle osteoarthritis has received relatively little attention, making it difficult to identify and define differences between ankle osteoarthritis and osteoarthritis in other synovial joints. Nonetheless, review of available clinical and experimental studies shows that ankle osteoarthritis has characteristics that distinguish it from osteoarthritis occurring in other synovial joints, including the hip and knee, and that these distinctive characteristics result in differences in prevalence, clinical presentation, natural history, and, possibly, in results of treatment.

This chapter first reviews current understanding of the clinical syndrome of osteoarthritis and its relationship to joint degeneration. Subsequent sections consider the unique characteristics of the ankle joint, the prevalence and pathogenesis of ankle osteoarthritis, and the implications of the response of ankle osteoarthritis to

alterations in joint contact stress for understanding of the pathogenesis and treatment of ankle osteoarthritis.

Osteoarthritis

Osteoarthritis, also referred to as degenerative joint disease, degenerative arthritis, osteoarthrosis, or hypertrophic arthritis, is a clinical syndrome that results from degeneration of a synovial joint.[1,2] The critical feature of the joint degeneration responsible for osteoarthritis is a progressive loss of articular cartilage, accompanied by attempted repair of articular cartilage, remodeling, and sclerosis of subchondral bone.[1,2] In many instances, subchondral bone cysts and osteophytes form as part of the syndrome of osteoarthritis. However, subchondral bone cysts and osteophytes may form in the absence of clinically significant articular cartilage degeneration and, thus, in themselves are not diagnostic of osteoarthritis. Furthermore, in addition to degenerative changes in the synovial joint, the diagnosis of osteoarthritis requires the presence of symptoms that include joint pain and loss of joint function. Patients with osteoarthritis may also have restriction of joint motion, crepitus with joint motion, joint effusions, and deformity.

In most joints, osteoarthritis most commonly develops in the absence of a known cause, a condition referred to as primary or idiopathic osteoarthritis.

Less frequently, it develops as a result of joint injuries, infections, or a variety of hereditary, developmental, metabolic, and neurologic disorders, a group of conditions referred to as secondary osteoarthritis.[2] The age of onset of secondary osteoarthritis depends on the underlying cause. Thus, it may develop in young adults and even children as well as the elderly. In contrast, a strong association exists between the prevalence of primary osteoarthritis and age. The percentage of people with evidence of osteoarthritis in one or more joints increases from less than 5% of people between 15 and 44 years of age, to 25% to 30% of people 45 to 64 years of age, to more than 60% and in some populations as high as 90% of the people over 65 years of age.[3] Despite this strong association with age and the widespread view that primary osteoarthritis results from "wear and tear" of synovial joints, the relationships between age and osteoarthritis remain poorly defined. Furthermore, the changes observed in articular cartilage with aging differ from those observed in osteoarthritis, and normal lifelong joint use has not been shown to cause articular joint degeneration.[2,4–6] Thus, osteoarthritis is not simply the result of aging or of mechanical wear from normal joint use.

The joint degeneration responsible for osteoarthritis is not uniformly

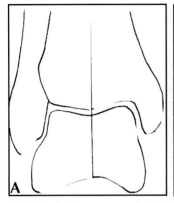
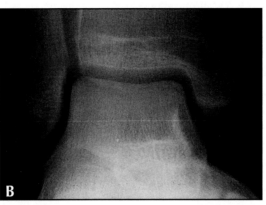

Fig. 1 Ankle joint structure. **A,** Drawing of the ankle joint showing how the talus fits in the mortise formed by the distal ends of the fibula and tibia. The medial malleolus and the medial surface of the talus form the opposing medial articular surfaces, the distal tibia and the superior talus form the opposing central articular surfaces, and the lateral malleolus and the lateral surface of the talus form the opposing lateral articular surfaces. Notice how the convexity of the distal tibial articular surface matches the concavity of the superior talar articular surface. The center of the matching convexity and concavity is used to divide the joint into medial and lateral compartments for study of joint loading and joint degeneration. **B,** Standing radiograph of the ankle joint showing the features outlined in the drawing.

progressive. Because repair and remodeling reactions can alter the rate of progression of the disorder, the rate of joint degeneration varies considerably among individuals and among joints. Occasionally it occurs rapidly, but in most instances it progresses slowly over many years, although it may stabilize or even improve spontaneously, with at least partial restoration of an articular surface and a decrease in symptoms. This phenomenon of stabilization and even regression of the degenerative changes has been observed in almost every synovial joint, including the ankle.

Unique Characteristics of the Ankle Joint

The differences in anatomy and motion between the ankle joint and the other major joints of the lower limb, the hip and the knee, are readily apparent. Other differences, including the area of contact between opposing articular surfaces and articular cartilage thickness, tensile properties, and metabolism, are less apparent. Taken

together, the unique mechanical and biologic characteristics of the ankle affect the development, clinical presentation, and course of osteoarthritis and the response to treatment of osteoarthritis in this joint.

Anatomy and Motion

The bony anatomy of the ankle joint determines the planes and ranges of joint motion and confers a high degree of stability and congruence when the joint is loaded. The 3 bones that form the ankle joint, the tibia, fibula, and talus, support 3 sets of opposing articular surfaces. The tibial medial malleolus and the medial facet of the talus form the medial articular surfaces, the fibular lateral malleolus and the talar lateral articular surface form the lateral articular surfaces, and the distal tibia and the superior dome of the talus form the central articular surfaces (Fig. 1). The distal tibial articular surface has a longitudinal convexity that matches a concavity on the surface of the talus. The center of the matching convexi-

ty and concavity of the distal tibial and superior talar articular surfaces is used to divide the tibiotalar articulation into the medial and lateral compartments for evaluation of ankle loading and degenerative changes (Fig. 1, *A*). The distal tibia, including the medial malleolus together with the lateral malleolus form the ankle mortise, which contains the talus. Firm anterior and posterior ligaments bind the distal tibia and fibula together, forming the distal tibiofibular syndesmosis. Medial and lateral ligamentous complexes and the ankle joint capsule stabilize the relationship between the talus and the mortise.

The bony anatomy, ligaments, and joint capsule guide and restrain movement between the talus and the mortise so that the talus has a continuously changing axis of rotation as it moves from maximum dorsiflexion to maximum plantarflexion relative to the mortise. The talus and mortise widen slightly from posterior to anterior. Thus when the talus is plantarflexed, the narrowest portion of the talus sits in the ankle mortise and allows rotatory movement between the talus and mortise. When the talus is maximally dorsiflexed, the tibiofibular syndesmosis spreads and the wider portion of the talar articular surface locks into the ankle mortise, allowing little or no rotation between the talus and the mortise. In most normal ankles, the soft-tissue structures, including joint capsule, ligaments, and muscle tendon units that cross the joint, prevent significant translation of the talus relative to the mortise.

Articular Surface Contact Area

When loaded, the human ankle joint has a smaller area of contact between the opposing articular surfaces than the knee or hip. At 500 N of load, the contact area of the ankle joint averages 350 mm^2,[7,8] compared with 1,120 mm^2 for the knee[9] and 1,100 mm^2 for the hip.[10] Although in vivo contact stress has not been measured in the ankle, the smaller contact area must make the normal peak contact stress higher in the ankle than in the knee or hip.

Articular Cartilage Thickness and Tensile Properties

Ankle joint articular cartilage differs from that of the knee and hip in thickness and tensile properties. The thickness of ankle articular cartilage ranges from less than 1 mm to slightly less than 2 mm.[11,12] In contrast, the knee and hip joints have regions of articular cartilage that may be more than 6 mm thick and in most load-bearing areas the articular cartilage of these joints is at least 3 mm thick.[13] Work by Kempson[14] shows that the tensile properties of ankle and hip articular cartilage differ and that these differences increase with age (Figs. 2 and 3). In particular, the tensile fracture stress and tensile stiffness of ankle articular cartilage deteriorate less rapidly with age than hip articular cartilage tensile properties.[14] Although the tensile fracture stress of hip femoral articular cartilage is initially greater than the tensile fracture stress of talar articular cartilage, hip cartilage tensile fracture stress declines exponentially with age while talar articular cartilage tensile fracture stress declines linearly (Fig. 2). As a result of these aging changes, beginning in middle age, ankle articular cartilage can withstand greater tensile loads than hip articular cartilage, and this difference increases with increasing age. Age-related changes in hip and ankle articular cartilage tensile stiffness follow a similar pattern (Fig. 3). Presumably, age-related declines in articular cartilage tensile properties result from

progressive weakening of the articular cartilage collagen fibril network. The cause or causes of the age-related weakening of the articular cartilage matrix have not been explained, but age-related changes in articular cartilage collagen fibril structure and collagen cross-linking have been identified that may contribute to changes in matrix tensile properties.[4,5] Kempson has suggested that the differences in articular cartilage tensile properties may explain the apparent vulnerability of the hip and knee for the development of degenerative changes with increasing age, and the relative resistance of the ankle to the development of primary osteoarthritis.[14]

Articular Cartilage Metabolism

Ankle articular cartilage may differ from articular cartilage from other joints in expression of an enzyme that can degrade articular cartilage and in response to the catabolic cytokine interleukin-1. Recently Chubinskaya and associates[15] detected messenger RNA for neutrophil collagenase (MMP-8) in human knee articular cartilage chondrocytes, but not in ankle articular cartilage chondrocytes. Häuselmann and associates[16] have reported that the catabolic cytokine interleukin-1 inhibited proteoglycan synthesis by knee articular cartilage chondrocytes more effectively than it inhibited proteoglycan synthesis by ankle articular cartilage chondrocytes.[16,17] The difference in the response to interleukin-1 between knee and ankle articular cartilage chondrocytes appears to be caused by the greater number of interleukin-1 receptors in knee articular cartilage chondrocytes. These observations will need further study, but they suggest that there are metabolic differences between knee and ankle articular cartilage that might help explain

the relative rarity of primary ankle osteoarthritis.

Prevalence of Ankle Osteoarthritis

Determining the prevalence of ankle osteoarthritis is more difficult than it might at first seem. As in other joints, the correlation between degenerative changes in the joint and the clinical syndrome of osteoarthritis is not consistent.[18,19] In addition, it is extremely expensive and difficult to obtain and study unbiased samples of populations to determine the prevalence of osteoarthritis. For these reasons, studies of the prevalence of osteoarthritis by examination of autopsy specimens, evaluation of radiographs of populations of patients, and evaluation of patients presenting with symptomatic osteoarthritis have significant limitations.

Autopsy Studies

Despite their limitations, including relatively small numbers of joints examined and lack of random or systematic sampling of populations, studies of joints at autopsy can provide useful information concerning differences in prevalence of degeneration among joints. Meachim and Emery[20–23] examined knee, shoulder, and ankle joints at autopsies performed on adults. They found full-thickness chondral defects in 1 of 20 ankle joints from people older than 70 years of age.[22] Cartilage fibrillation was much more frequent than full-thickness defects in all joints. Huch and associates[17] resected 36 knees and 78 ankles from both limbs of 39 organ donors to evaluate the prevalence of ankle osteoarthritis. Joints were evaluated using a scale described by Collins: grade 0–normal gross appearance of a joint, grade I–fraying or fibrillation of the articular cartilage, grade 2–fibrillation and fissuring of

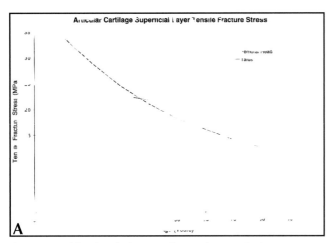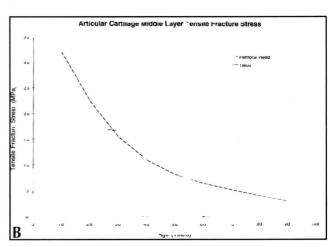

Fig. 2 Femoral head and talus articular cartilage tensile fracture stress versus age. **A,** Articular cartilage superficial layer tensile fracture stress versus age. **B,** Articular cartilage middle layer tensile fracture stress versus age. Notice that the tensile fracture stress of ankle articular cartilage is greater beginning in middle age than the tensile fracture stress of femoral head articular cartilage and that the difference increases with increasing age. These illustrations were developed from data reported by Kempson.[14]

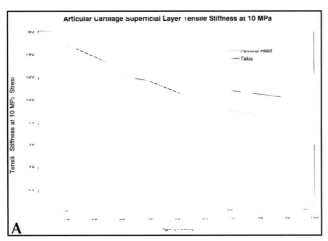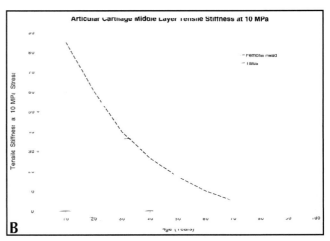

Fig. 3 Femoral head and talus articular cartilage tensile stiffness versus age. **A,** Articular cartilage superficial layer tensile stiffness versus age. **B,** Articular cartilage middle layer tensile stiffness versus age. Notice that the tensile stiffness of ankle articular cartilage is greater beginning in middle age than the tensile fracture stress of femoral head articular cartilage and that the difference increases with increasing age. These illustrations were developed from data reported by Kempson.[14]

the cartilage and osteophytes, grade 3–extensive fibrillation and fissuring with frequent osteophytes and 30% or less full-thickness chondral defects, grade 4–frequent osteophytes and greater than 30% full-thickness chondral defects.[17,24] In these studies, grades 3 and 4 were defined as osteoarthritis, and grade 2 was defined as early osteoarthritis.[17] However, the authors did not have information con-cerning possible symptoms associated with the joints studied, so it is not certain if the degenerative changes they identified were associated with clinical osteoarthritis. Using the Collins grading scale, Huch and associates[17] found grades 3 and 4 degenerative changes in 5 of 78 (6%) ankle joints and in 9 of 36 (25%) knee joints (Fig. 4). Degenerative changes were most commonly found on the medial aspect of the ankle. In another series of investigations Muehleman and associates[25] examined 7 joints, including the knee and ankle of both lower extremities in 50 cadavers.[17,25] The individuals studied ranged in age from 36 to 94 years, with a mean age of 76 years. Sixty-six percent of the knee joints had grades 3 and 4 degenerative changes, compared with 18% of the ankle joints (Fig. 4). Ninety-five percent of the knees had grade 2, 3, or 4 degenerative changes compared with 76% of the ankles. The authors also observed that the medial compartments of both the knees and the ankles were more frequently involved than the lateral compartments, and that radiographs often showed no evidence of degenerative changes when direct examination of the joint showed regions of full-thickness cartilage erosion. Overall, the autopsy studies demonstrate that advanced degenerative changes are at least 3 times more prevalent in the knee than in the ankle, and that the prevalence of degenerative changes in both joints increases with increasing age (Fig. 4).

Radiographic Evaluations

Although epidemiologic studies based on radiographic evaluations document a striking increase in the prevalence of degenerative changes of all joints, including those of the foot and ankle, with increasing age,[3] the reported studies have not focused on ankle osteoarthritis. Radiographic studies of ankle joint degeneration have important limitations because of the lack of a strong correlation between the formation of osteophytes and clinical osteoarthritis[19] (Fig. 5), and the difficulty in evaluating the thickness of ankle articular cartilage, particularly on radiographs that were not performed in a standardized fashion. Furthermore, ankle radiographs often do not show signs of joint degeneration even when the ankle joint has regions of full-thickness erosion of articular cartilage.[25] For these reasons, attempts to evaluate the prevalence of ankle degeneration and osteoarthritis by plain radiographs alone have limited value.

Clinical Studies

Very few studies of the prevalence of osteoarthritis have included patients

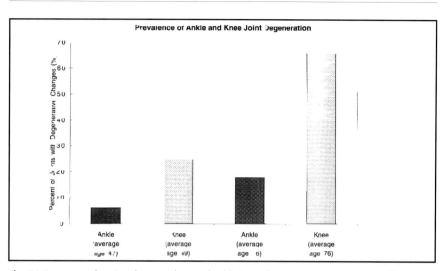

Fig. 4 Histograms showing the prevalence of ankle joint degeneration in autopsy studies reported by Huch and associates[17] and Muehleman and associates.[25] In these studies, the criteria for joint degeneration (osteoarthritis) were extensive articular cartilage fibrillation, osteophytes, and regions of full-thickness cartilage loss (Collins grades 3 and 4). Notice that joint degeneration was more than 3 times more common in the knee than in the ankle, and that the prevalence of joint degeneration in the knee and the ankle increased with age.

with ankle osteoarthritis. The available information suggests that knee osteoarthritis is 8 to 10 times more common than ankle osteoarthritis.[17,26–28] However, the best currently available estimates suggest that knee replacements are performed at least 25 times more frequently than ankle replacements and ankle fusions combined.[3] These observations, combined with the data from autopsy studies showing that advanced knee joint degeneration is about 3 to 5 times more common than advanced ankle joint degeneration, suggest that surgical procedures are performed less frequently for patients with advanced ankle osteoarthritis than for patients with advanced osteoarthritis of the knee. The reasons for this are unclear. It is possible that ankle joint degeneration and osteoarthritis cause less severe pain and functional limitation than knee degeneration and osteoarthritis. Lack of understanding of the evaluation and treatment of ankle osteoarthritis among physicians,

the efficacy of nonsurgical treatments for ankle osteoarthritis or the lack of effective and widely accepted surgical treatments for ankle osteoarthritis may also contribute to the apparent difference in the frequency of surgical treatment of ankle and knee osteoarthritis.

Pathogenesis of Ankle Osteoarthritis

Review of clinical experience and published reports of the treatment of ankle osteoarthritis indicates that primary ankle osteoarthritis is rare and that secondary ankle osteoarthritis that develops following ankle fractures or ligamentous injury is the most common cause of ankle osteoarthritis.[29–36] Patients with neuropathic degenerative disease of the ankle and degenerative disease following necrosis of the talus with collapse of the articular surface make up a small portion of the individuals with degenerative disease of the ankle.[32,37–39] Primary osteoarthritis is the most common diagnosis for patients treated with hip and knee

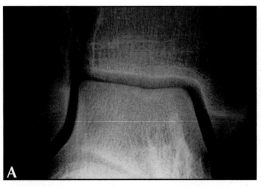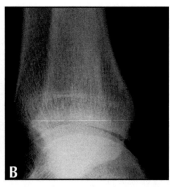

Fig. 5 Standing radiographs showing the ankle of a middle-age adult. **A,** Anteroposterior radiograph, and **B,** lateral radiograph. These studies were obtained to evaluate an acute ankle injury. The patient participated in a variety of athletic activities but she had no history of joint pain, swelling, crepitus or stiffness, and, therefore, she did not have osteoarthritis. The radiographs do not show a fracture or decreased articular cartilage thickness, but osteophytes are present at the tip of the medial malleolus (seen on the anteroposterior view) and the posterior edge of the tibia (seen on the lateral view).

Outline 1

Stages in development of posttraumatic ankle osteoarthritis

Stage I. Increased Contact Stress Damages Articular Cartilage
Disruption or alteration of the matrix macromolecular framework associated with an increase in water concentration may be caused by high levels of contact stress. At first, the type 11 collagen concentration remains unchanged, but the collagen meshwork may be damaged and the concentration of aggrecan and the degree of proteoglycan aggregation decrease.

Stage II. Chondrocyte Response to Matrix Disruption or Alteration
When chondrocytes detect a disruption or alteration of their matrix they respond by increasing matrix synthesis and degradation and by proliferating. Their response may restore the tissue, maintain the tissue in an altered state, or increase cartilage volume. They may sustain an increased level of activity for years.

Stage III. Decline in the Chondrocyte Response
Failure of the chondrocytic response to restore or maintain the tissue leads to loss of articular cartilage accompanied or preceded by a decline in the chondrocytic response. The causes for the decline in chondrocytic response remain poorly understood, but it may be partially the result of mechanical damage to the tissue with injury to chondrocytes and a down regulation of the chondrocytic response to anabolic cytokines.

---

replacements. In contrast, posttraumatic osteoarthritis is the most common diagnosis for patients treated with ankle arthrodesis or replacement. This observation raises the possibility that the ankle may be at least as vulnerable and perhaps more vulnerable than the hip and knee for the development of severe posttraumatic osteoarthritis. The relative rarity of primary osteoarthritis of the ankle may be the result of the congruency, stability, and restrained motion of the ankle joint, tensile properties of ankle articular cartilage, the metabolic characteristics of ankle joint articular cartilage, or a combination of these factors. The thinness of ankle articular cartilage and the small contact area leading to high peak-contact stresses may make the joint more susceptible to posttraumatic osteoarthritis. In particular, the thinner, stiffer articular cartilage of the ankle may be less able to adapt to articular surface incongruity and increased contact stresses than the thicker articular cartilage of the hip and knee, and the contact stresses may be higher in the ankle.

Joint injuries can cause articular cartilage and subchondral bone damage that is not repaired, create articular surface incongruencies, and decrease joint stability. Long-term incongruency or instability can increase localized contact stress. The ankle osteoarthritis that occurs following joint injuries appears to follow a pattern consistent with the hypothesis that posttraumatic ankle osteoarthritis is a result of elevated contact stress that exceeds the capacity of the joint to repair itself or adapt. According to this hypothesis, the development of posttraumatic ankle osteoarthritis progresses through 3 overlapping stages: (1) articular cartilage injury, (2) chondrocyte response to tissue injury, and (3) decline in the chondrocyte response (Outline 1).

Neuropathies and necrosis of the talus that cause incongruity of the articular surface also lead to secondary ankle osteoarthritis. Patients with neuropathies can develop rapidly progressive joint degeneration following minimal injury or in the absence of a history of an injury. This may occur because the loss of positional sense leads to undetected ligamentous or articular surface injuries that create localized regions of increased contact stress. Articular surface incongruency caused by necrosis of the talus may have the same effect.

Consistent with the hypothesis that excessive contact stress leads to degeneration of ankle articular cartilage, significant residual joint incongruity and severe disruption of the ankle joint articular surface predictably lead to joint degeneration, commonly within 2 years of injury

(Fig. 6); but advanced joint degeneration also can develop within 2 years of injuries that cause relatively little apparent damage to the articular surface (Fig. 7). In some of these latter cases the joint surface many have sustained damage that is not apparent by radiographic evaluation. In others, joint instability caused by alteration of the anatomy of the mortise, like spreading of the distal tibiofibular syndesmosis or shortening and rotation of the fibula or capsular and ligamentous laxity, may be responsible for degeneration of the joint. However, some patients develop progressive joint degeneration following ankle injuries in the absence of apparent articular surface damage, alteration of the joint anatomy, or instability, and other patients with articular surface incongruity or joint instability do not develop progressive joint degeneration. Thus, the pathogenesis of posttraumatic ankle osteoarthritis is more complex than it appears, and needs extensive further study.

Effects of Decreased Joint Contact Stress on Ankle Osteoarthritis

A variety of treatments of ankle osteoarthritis, including weight reduction, shoe modifications, orthoses, joint distraction, osteotomies, and procedures intended to restore ligamentous stability, have been based on the assumptions that these treatments redistribute or decrease articular surface contact stresses and that decreasing or redistributing stress will decrease symptoms. Some authors have also suggested that decreasing joint contact stress may slow the progression of articular cartilage degeneration and possibly stimulate restoration of some form of articular surface. Several sets of experimental and clinical observations support these assumptions.

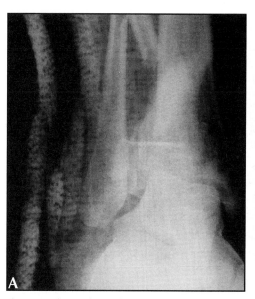
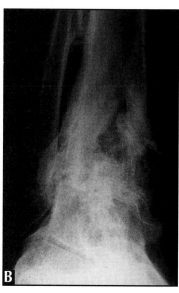

Fig. 6 Standing radiographs showing an ankle injury with extensive damage to the tibial articular surface. **A,** Anteroposterior radiograph showing almost complete disruption of the tibial articular surface and a fibula fracture immediately after the injury. **B,** Anteroposterior radiograph showing complete loss of articular cartilage less than 2 years after the injury.

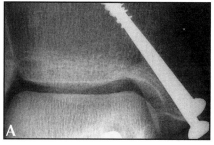
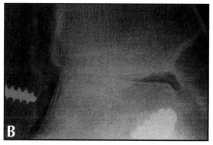

Fig. 7 Standing radiographs showing an ankle injury with relatively minor apparent damage to the tibial articular surface. **A,** Anteroposterior radiograph showing a medial malleolar fracture with minimal involvement of the tibial articular surface. The patient also had a fibula fracture and a talus fracture. The injuries were treated by internal fixation. **B,** Anteroposterior radiograph showing loss of articular cartilage less than 2 years after the injury.

Joint Distraction

Limited experimental studies indicate that joint distraction with external fixation devices promotes formation of a new articular surface.[40,41] Clinical studies of the effects of distraction of arthritic ankle joints using external fixators also suggest that decreasing joint contact stress can decrease symptoms and stimulate formation of a new articular surface.[42–44] In 1978, Judet and Judet[44] reported the results

of treating 16 patients with advanced ankle osteoarthritis by distraction and motion of the joint. They distracted the joints 4 to 8 mm while allowing motion for 6 to 12 weeks. Eight of their patients regained the ability to walk for unlimited distances and 13 of their patients had symptomatic improvement. More recently, van Valburg and associates[43] treated advanced posttraumatic osteoarthritis of the ankle with joint distraction in 11 patients. After application of an Ilizarov device, the authors distracted the joints 0.5 mm per day for 5 days and then maintained the distraction of the articular surfaces throughout the course of treatment. Patients were allowed to walk a few days after surgery, active joint motion was started between 6 and 12 weeks after surgery, and after 12 to 22 weeks the distraction device was removed. At an average of 20 months after treatment none of the patients had proceeded with an arthrodesis: all 11 patients had less pain, and 5 were pain free; 6 had more motion; and, 3 of 6 that had radiographic studies had increased joint space. The authors concluded that distraction of an osteoarthritic ankle joint delays arthrodesis, and that it may stimulate repair of osteoarthritic cartilage.

Osteotomies

Osteotomies of osteoarthritic hips and knees have been shown to decrease symptoms and stimulate formation of a new articular surface in some patients.[2] Osteotomies have not been widely used for the treatment of primary or posttraumatic ankle osteoarthritis, but in 1 study tibial osteotomies produced good or excellent results in 15 of 18 patients with primary ankle osteoarthritis.[45] Another report described significant improvement in ankle function and decreased pain in 8 patients with ankle osteoarthritis treated by tibial osteotomy.[46] The authors attributed the functional and symptomatic improvement to redistribution of pressure on the joint surface.

Ligament Reconstruction

Some patients with instability of the ankle due to laxity of the lateral ligaments develop osteoarthritis in the medial compartment of the joint,[31,33,35,47] possibly as a result of increased loading of the medial joint.[31,48] Harrington[31] studied 36 patients with a history of lateral ankle instability for more than 10 years. These patients had increasing ankle pain and radiographic evidence of degeneration of the medial joint compartment. In addition to demonstrating an association between chronic lateral ligamentous instability and development of medial compartment degeneration, he found that 14 of 22 ankles in patients with symptomatic ankle osteoarthritis had decreased symptoms and widening of the medial joint space following lateral ligament reconstruction. He concluded that restoration of lateral ligamentous stability has the potential to prevent progression of joint degeneration and, in selected patients, may reverse some of the degenerative changes.

Conclusion

The available evidence strongly suggests that ankle osteoarthritis has distinctive characteristics. This condition is less well understood and has been less thoroughly investigated than osteoarthritis of the knee, hip, and shoulder. Autopsy studies and clinical experience show that primary ankle degeneration and osteoarthritis occur less frequently than primary joint degeneration and osteoarthritis in other joints of the lower limb, including the knee. The reasons for this have not been clearly demonstrated, but relatively greater tensile strength of ankle articular cartilage in people of middle age and older may be partially responsible. Differences in articular cartilage metabolism may also contribute to the decreased susceptibility of the ankle for development of primary osteoarthritis. Perhaps because of the relative rarity of primary ankle osteoarthritis, a high proportion of the patients with ankle osteoarthritis have a history of ankle joint injuries including fractures, dislocations, or subluxations associated with fractures and capsular and ligamentous injuries. In these patients, the development of joint degeneration appears to result from increased joint contact stress that exceeds the capacity of the joint to repair itself or adapt to higher stress levels. The thinness of ankle articular cartilage and the small contact area of the ankle joint articular surfaces may increase the susceptibility of the joint to posttraumatic osteoarthritis. Other experimental and clinical evidence demonstrates that redistributing or decreasing joint contact stress has the potential to decrease symptoms of ankle osteoarthritis and, possibly, in some instances, restore a functional articular surface. These observations are necessarily speculative as a result of the lack of extensive study of ankle osteoarthritis. Nonetheless, they strongly suggest that ankle osteoarthritis has distinctive characteristics that need further investigation and that should guide treatment of this condition.

References

1. Buckwalter JA, Martin JA: Degenerative joint disease. *Clin Symp* 1995;47:1–32.

2. Buckwalter JA, Mankin HJ: Articular cartilage: Part II. Degeneration and osteoarthrosis, repair, regeneration, and transplantation. *J Bone Joint Surg* 1997;79A:612–632.

3. Praemer A, Furner S, Rice DP (eds): *Musculoskeletal Conditions in the United States.* Park Ridge, IL, American Academy of Orthopaedic Surgeons, 1992.

4. Buckwalter JA, Woo SL, Goldberg VM, et al: Soft-tissue aging and musculoskeletal function. *J Bone Joint Surg* 1993;75A:1533–1548.

5. Buckwalter JA, Mankin HJ: Articular cartilage: Part I. Tissue design and chondrocyte-matrix interactions. *J Bone Joint Surg* 1997;79A:600–611.

6. Newton PM, Mow VC, Gardner TR, Buckwalter JA, Albright JP: The effect of lifelong exercise on canine articular cartilage. *Am J Sports Med* 1997;25:282–287.

7. Beaudoin AJ, Fiore SM, Krause WR, Adelaar RS: Effect of isolated talocalcaneal fusion on contact in the ankle and talonavicular joints. *Foot Ankle* 1991;12:19–25.

8. Kimizuka M, Kurosawa H, Fukubayashi T: Load-bearing pattern of the ankle joint: Contact area and pressure distribution. *Arch Orthop Trauma Surg* 1980;96:45–49.

9. Ihn JC, Kim SJ, Park IH: In vitro study of contact area and pressure distribution in the human knee after partial and total meniscectomy. *Int Orthop* 1993;17:214–218.

10. Brown TD, Shaw DT: In vitro contact stress distributions in the natural human hip. *J Biomech* 1983;16:373–384.

11. Schenck RC Jr, Athanasiou KA: Biomechanical topography of human ankle cartilage. *Trans Ors* 1993;18:279.

12. Athanasiou KA, Niederauer GG, Schenck RC Jr: Biomechanical topography of human ankle cartilage. *Ann Biomed Eng* 1995;23:697–704.

13. Ateshian GA, Soslowsky U, Mow VC: Quantitation of articular surface topography and cartilage thickness in knee joints using stereophotogrammetry. *J Biomech* 1991;24: 761–776.

14. Kempson GE: Age-related changes in the tensile properties of human articular cartilage: A comparative study between the femoral head of the hip joint and the talus of the ankle joint. *Biochim Biophys Acta* 1991;1075:223–230.

15. Chubinskaya S, Huch K, Mikecz K, et al: Chondrocyte matrix metalloproteinase-8: Up-regulation of neutrophil collagenase by interleukin-I beta in human cartilage from knee and ankle joints. *Lab Invest* 1996;74:232–240.

16. Häuselmann HJ, Flechtenmacher J, Gitelis SH, Kuettner KE, Aydelotte MB: Chondrocytes from human knee and ankle joints show differences in response to IL-1 and IL-1 receptor inhibitor. *Orthop Trans* 1993;17:710.

17. Huch K, Kuettner KE, Dieppe P: Osteoarthritis in ankle and knee joints. *Semin Arthritis Rheum* 1997;26:667–674.

18. Dieppe PA, Cushnaghan J, Shepstone L: The Bristol "OA500" study: Progression of osteoarthritis (OA) over 3 years and the relationship between clinical and radiographic changes at the knee joint. *Osteoarthritis Cartilage* 1997;5:87–97.

19. van-der-Schoot DK, Den Outer AJ, Bode PJ, Obermann WR, van Vugt AB: Degenerative changes at the knee and ankle related to malunion of tibial fractures: 15-year follow-up of 88 patients. *J Bone Joint Surg* 1996;78B:722–725.

20. Meachim G, Emery IH: Cartilage fibrillation in shoulder and hip joints in Liverpool necropsies. *J Anat* 1973;116:161–179.

21. Meachim G, Emery IH: Quantitative aspects of patello-femoral cartilage fibrillation in Liverpool necropsies. *Ann Rheum Dis* 1974;33:39–47.

22. Meachim G: Cartilage fibrillation at the ankle joint in Liverpool necropsies. *J Anat* 1975; 119:601–610.

23. Meachim G: Cartilage fibrillation on the lateral tibial plateau in Liverpool necropsies. *J Anat* 1976;121:97–106.

24. Collins DH (ed): *Osteoarthritis: The Pathology of Articular and Spinal Diseases.* London, England, Edward Arnold, 1949, pp 74–115.

25. Muehleman C, Bareither D, Huch K, Cole AA, Kuettner KE: Prevalence of degenerative morphological changes in the joints of the lower extremity. *Osteoarthritis Cartilage* 1997;5:23–37.

26. Cushnaghan J, Dieppe P: Study of 500 patients with limb joint osteoarthritis: I. Analysis by age, sex, and distribution of symptomatic joint sites. *Ann Rheum Dis* 1991;50:8–13.

27. Peyron JG: The epidemiology of osteoarthritis, in Moskowitz RW, Howell DS, Goldberg VM, Mankin HJ (eds): *Osteoarthritis: Diagnosis and Management.* Philadelphia, PA, WB Saunders, 1984, pp 9–27.

28. Wilson MG, Michet CJ Jr, Ilstrup DM, Melton LJ III: Idiopathic symptomatic osteoarthritis of the hip and knee: A population-based incidence study. *Mayo Clin Proc* 1990;65:1214–1221.

29. Demetriades L, Strauss E, Gallina J: Osteoarthritis of the ankle. *Clin Orthop* 1998;349: 28–42.

30. Wyss C, Zollinger H: The causes of subsequent arthrodesis of the ankle joint. *Acta Orthop Belg* 1991;57(suppl 1):22–27.

31. Harrington KD: Degenerative arthritis of the ankle secondary to long-standing lateral ligament instability. *J Bone Joint Surg* 1979;61A: 354–361.

32. Inokuchi S, Ogawa K, Usami N, Hashimoto T: Long-term follow up of talus fractures. *Orthopedics* 1996;19:477–481.

33. Schafer D, Hintermann B: Arthroscopic assessment of the chronic unstable ankle joint. *Knee Surg Sports Traumatol Arthrosc* 1996;4:48–52.

34. Taga I, Shino K, Inoue M, Nakata K, Maeda A: Articular cartilage lesions in ankles with lateral ligament injury: An arthroscopic study. *Am J Sports Med* 1993;21:120–126.

35. Rieck B, Reiser M, Bernett P: Post-traumatic arthrosis of the upper ankle joint in chronic insufficiency of the fibular ligament [German]. *Orthopade* 1986;15:466–471.

36. Leeds HC, Ehrlich MG: Instability of the distal tibiofibular syndesmosis after bimalleolar and trimalleolar ankle fractures. *J Bone Joint Surg* 1984;66A:490–503.

37. Slowman-Kovacs SD, Braunstein EM, Brandt KD: Rapidly progressive Charcot arthropathy following minor joint trauma in patients with diabetic neuropathy. *Arthritis Rheum* 1990; 33:412–417.

38. Cheng YM, Lin SY, Tien YC, Wu HS: Ankle arthrodesis. *Kao Hsiung I Hsueh Ko Hsueh Tsa Chih* 1993;9:524–531.

39. Buechel FF, Pappas MJ, Lorio LJ: New Jersey low contact stress total ankle replacement: Biomechanical rationale and review of 23 cementless cases. *Foot Ankle* 1988;8:279–290.

40. Krogsgaard MR, Blyme P: Formation of joint surfaces by traction. *Acta Orthop Scand* 1997; (suppl 274):46.

41. Van Valburg AA, Van Roermund PM, Van Roy HLAM, Verbout AJ, Lafeber FPJG, Bijlsma JWJ: Repair of cartilage by Ilizarov joint distraction, tested in the Pond-Nuki model for osteoarthritis. *Trans Orthop Res Soc* 1997;22:494.

42. Van Valburg AA, Van Roermund PM, Larnmens J: Promising results of Ilizarov joint distraction in the treatment of ankle osteoarthritis. *Trans Orthop Res Soc* 1997;22:271.

43. Van Valburg AA, Van Roermund PM, Lammens J, et al: Can Ilizarov joint distraction delay the need for an arthrodesis of the ankle? A preliminary report. *J Bone Joint Surg* 1995; 77B:720–725.

44. Judet R, Judet T: The use of a hinge distraction apparatus after arthrolysis and arthroplasty. *Rev Chir Orthop* 1978;64:353–365.

45. Takakura Y, Tanaka Y, Kumai T, Tamai S: Low tibial osteotomy for osteoarthritis of the ankle: Results of a new operation in 18 patients. *J Bone Joint Surg* 1995;77B:50–54.

46. Cheng YM, Chang JK, Hsu CY, Huang SD, Lin SY: Lower tibial osteotomy for osteoarthritis of the ankle. *Kao Hsiung I Hsueh Ko Hsueh Tsa Chih* 1994;10:430–437.

47. Lofvenberg R, Karrholm J, Lund B: The outcome of nonoperated patients with chronic lateral instability of the ankle: A 20-year follow-up study. *Foot Ankle Int* 1994;15:165–169.

48. Noguchi K: Biomechanical analysis for osteoarthritis of the ankle. *Nippon Seikeigeka Gakkai Zasshi* 1985;59:215–222.

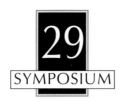

Arthrodesis of the Ankle: Technique, Complications, and Salvage Treatment

Harold B. Kitaoka, MD

Introduction

In recent years, advances have been made in the management of arthritis of the ankle. Clinical results with longer duration of follow-up of ankle reconstruction techniques such as arthrodesis and arthroplasty are now available. Techniques for managing limited arthritis such as cheilectomy and low tibial osteotomy are gaining favor. Other techniques, such as distraction arthroplasty, are promising alternatives that demand further investigation. Information regarding the efficacy of managing specific complex problems that affect the ankle is now available.

Ankle Arthritis and Treatment

Painful, disabling arthrosis of the ankle may occur following trauma or chronic instability, or it may be related to rheumatoid arthritis, degenerative joint disease, synovial osteochondromatosis, osteochondritis dissecans, talar osteonecrosis, tumors, hemophilia, infection, or neuropathy.

Evaluation of the painful or malaligned ankle joint begins with a thorough history and physical examination. Questions concerning a previous history of trauma, instability episodes, swelling, fever, night pain, or progressive sensory changes of the foot should all be addressed to the patient in an attempt to delineate an underlying disease process. In addition, the patient's response to previous forms of therapy should be assessed. Each joint of the lower extremity should be examined, documenting range of motion, painful motion, localized tenderness, swelling, stability, and alignment. Selective lidocaine injection into a specific joint may aid localization of the most symptomatic joint.

For assessment of ankle and hindfoot disorders, plain film radiography should be performed with standing anteroposterior and lateral views of the ankle as well as standing anteroposterior and oblique views of the foot. A mortise view is also useful for evaluating the ankle. Ankle and hindfoot alignment while weightbearing may be assessed with a standing tibiocalcaneal view (modified Cobey or Morrey view). Sometimes plain tomograms or computed tomography (CT) scans oriented parallel and perpendicular to the longitudinal axis of the foot are useful in delineating ankle and hindfoot pathology such as arthritis, tumors, and fractures. Technetium and indium bone scans are helpful in evaluating the likelihood of infection, stress fracture, bone tumor, or inflammatory disease, and for localizing an area of pathology that is not apparent on plain radiographs. Occasionally, a magnetic resonance imaging (MRI) scan is indicated to evaluate such painful ankle conditions as tendon disorders, osteonecrosis, stress fractures, infections, and soft-tissue tumors. In patients suspected of having inflammatory arthritis, testing may include blood count, blood chemistry group, rheumatoid factor, antinuclear antibody, sedimentation rate, and HLA-B27.

In general, most patients with ankle arthritis should initially receive nonsurgical treatment. Nonsurgical management of the ankle includes oral nonsteroidal anti-inflammatory medications, judicious use of intra-articular corticosteroid injections, footwear modifications, and bracing. Modifying the shoe with a rocker bottom sole and a solid ankle cushion heel may provide some relief for the stiff, arthritic ankle. This may not be adequate and immobilization with a laced ankle support or a polypropylene ankle foot orthosis should be considered. The ankle foot orthosis provides stability to ankle and hindfoot and therefore is applicable for patients with combined ankle and hindfoot arthrosis and for patients who are not candidates for surgery due to either local or general conditions.

Ankle cheilectomy is useful in selected patients who develop symptomatic anterior ankle osteophytes.

These osteophytes usually affect the distal tibia, but they may also occur on the talus and restrict ankle dorsiflexion. Patients may recognize the limitation of dorsiflexion with stair climbing and complain of anterior ankle pain. On examination, restriction of dorsiflexion, tenderness of the anterior joint line, pain with passive dorsiflexion of the ankle, and the presence of anterior osteophytes on the lateral radiograph of the ankle are consistent with this disorder. The osteophytes may be palpable. It is important to distinguish this condition from other disorders, as it is not unusual to observe anterior ankle osteophytes radiographically in patients who are asymptomatic. Nonsteroidal oral anti-inflammatory medications are useful, and if these do not provide adequate relief, surgery such as cheilectomy may be indicated. This is easily accomplished through an ankle arthrotomy and there are also advocates of the arthroscopic technique. While there are some potential advantages of arthroscopy for this condition, rare complications, such as dorsal foot numbness, have been reported.

For advanced arthrosis of the ankle, refractory to nonsurgical treatment efforts, ankle reconstruction operations may be considered. Several authors recently presented good results with total ankle replacement with limited (less than 5 year) follow-up, but nearly all reports of long-term results cited problems of recurrent pain, stiffness, component migration, loosening, and malalignment.[1-3] There are newer designs of total ankle replacement prostheses under investigation, which have the potential of addressing some of the deficiencies of previous designs. Until more critical analysis of these devices is available (such as long-term clinical and radiologic results,

gait analysis, mechanical testing) most would agree that the current standard treatment for advanced ankle arthrosis is arthrodesis. Distraction arthroplasty of the ankle and low tibial osteotomy have also been performed for ankle arthritis, with success in selected patients.

Ankle Arthrodesis

Posttraumatic arthritis is the most common indication for ankle fusion. Ankle fusion is also indicated in arthritis and in deformities resulting from rheumatoid arthritis, degenerative arthritis, osteonecrosis of the talus, neuromuscular conditions, and failed operations, such as total ankle arthroplasty. Arthrodesis of the ankle should rarely be performed in patients with neuropathic (Charcot) arthropathy secondary to a sensory neuropathy, because many of these patients have limited symptoms, and high complication and failure rates have been reported. With current methods of open reduction and internal fixation, acute ankle trauma is rarely treated by primary arthrodesis.

Each year new variations of ankle arthrodesis methods are reported and in general the results are good (approximately 90% union rate) when applied to patients with isolated ankle arthrosis uncomplicated by neuropathy, infection, multiple joint involvement, severe malalignment, severe bony deficiency, or major soft-tissue problems. In adults, rigid fixation is necessary. Internal fixation using compression screws has become a standard method in the past decade. There are variations in surgical approach, screw types, number of screws, and screw placement, but most authors recommend at least two screws for fixation, and some advocate adding an onlay fibular graft.

In recent years, there have been additional publications relating to

specific complex ankle problems such as salvage of ankle arthrodesis nonunion, management of infected nonunion, arthrodesis in patients with major bony deficit (eg, from failed total ankle replacement, infection, or tumor), arthrodesis in patients with sensory neuropathy, arthrodesis in patients with ongoing sepsis, severe osteopenia, and combined ankle and hindfoot arthrosis.[1,4-10] Because of the complexity of these disorders, it is suggested that a number of different arthrodesis methods be available in a surgeon's armamentarium, including external fixation techniques.

Regardless of the fixation methods, alignment is critical. Preferred alignment is neutral flexion-extension, hindfoot valgus of 5° to 10°, external rotation of 5° to 10°, neutral medial-lateral displacement, and posterior translation of the talus with respect to the tibia of between 0 and 1 cm. This posterior translation is designed to decrease the anterior lever arm of the foot, which reduces the overloading of the intact midfoot joints. The malleoli may need to be excised or shaved to prevent painful impingement against the upper margin of the counter of the shoe.

Approaches to the ankle include the anteromedial, anterolateral, posterior, and combined medial and lateral approaches. The combined medial and lateral transmalleolar approach consists of hockey stick-shaped incisions over the medial malleolus and anterior margin of the distal fibula respectively. Dissection is carried out over the malleoli, taking care to protect the superficial peroneal nerve laterally and the saphenous nerve medially. The fibula is transected obliquely 4 to 6 cm proximal to the tip with an oscillating saw and can be used as an onlay graft, preserving soft-tissue attachment to the malleolus. Dissection along the anterior ankle further exposes the joint for resection and realignment.

The anteromedial incision is longitudinally oriented medial to the anterior tibial tendon and centered over the ankle. The anterolateral approach is lateral to the extensor digitorum longus and peroneus tertius tendons and centered over the ankle. The posterior approach is generally along the lateral margin of the Achilles tendon, taking care to protect the sural nerve. The interval between the flexor hallucis longus and the peroneal tendons is developed. The Achilles tendon can be divided to maximize the exposure but should be repaired.

Methods of preparing the joint for arthrodesis include osteotomies of the distal tibia and talar dome perpendicular to the long axis of the tibia producing flat, parallel surfaces. This results in limited shortening (1 cm) of the extremity. Others prefer to remove the remaining articular cartilage while preserving the subchondral bone and bony contour or to use chevron-shaped osteotomies to maximize bony contact and stability. Simply removing the articular cartilage with or without the underlying subchondral bone minimizes shortening of the extremity and has the potential of improving stability (compared to flat parallel cuts), but this method is not applicable when there is substantial deformity to be corrected. Cartilage removal can be accomplished with the standard arthrotomy or arthroscopically.

Fusion may also be accomplished by bridging the ankle joint with an onlay or inlay graft. The inlay graft may be constructed from the distal anterior tibia, sliding the graft distally into the neck of the talus. This technique, popularized by Blair, is useful in ankle arthrosis with talar

osteonecrosis. The distal fibula may be used as an onlay graft. Combined intra-articular and extra-articular arthrodesis is another option, performed posteriorly by creating a trough in the distal tibia, talus, and calcaneus, which is then packed with morcellated iliac crest bone graft. With each of these methods some form of fixation is recommended.

Methods of ankle arthrodesis fixation include internal compression screws, external fixation devices, internal fixation with plates and screws or staples, percutaneous pins, and intramedullary nailing (Fig. 1). Large (6.5 mm or 7.0 mm) cancellous screws may be effective, but care must be taken not to violate the subtalar joint. Intraoperative radiographs are helpful to assess fixation placement, bony apposition, and alignment. Most authors agree that the internal compression arthrodesis technique with at least two screws is necessary for adequate fixation. Supplemental fibular onlay grafting has been shown to add stability to the screw fixation in cadaveric testing.[11]

External fixation devices, such as the Calandruccio triangular external fixation device or small wire ring fixators, may also be used. They play an important role in patients with open wounds or active infection or with a failed ankle arthrodesis. These devices are also useful in patients with severe talar bone deficiency or severe osteopenia, where adequate purchase with compression screws is not possible. Complications such as pin tract infections may occur and are normally successfully managed by oral antibiotics. Because neuromas can occur with external fixation, pins should be carefully placed.

Fixation with a plate and screws or a blade plate through a posterior approach has been described with

high union rates. Arthrodesis of the ankle with two longitudinally placed Steinmann pins in patients with rheumatoid arthritis has also been shown to be successful, as has fixation with a locked intramedullary nail passed from the plantar hindfoot and spanning the subtalar and ankle joints. The latter procedure should be reserved for the rare patient who has both ankle and subtalar arthritis.

Arthrodeses are usually united by 4 months postoperatively, and most patients obtain full clinical benefit of an ankle fusion by approximately 6 to 8 months postoperatively. Long-term studies of ankle fusion results report satisfactory clinical results in over 80% of patients. Following ankle fusion, gait is normal in the majority of patients, although it has been shown that walking speed is decreased because of a shortened stride length. Motion through Chopart's (talonavicular and calcaneocuboid) and Lisfranc's (tarsometatarsal) joints allows residual tibiopedal motion approximately 30% to 40% of normal. Subtalar motion following ankle fusion is often diminished, but many of these patients have some degree of subtalar joint stiffness before surgery. Some longer-term follow-up studies demonstrated degenerative changes at Chopart's and Lisfranc joints, but most of these radiologic abnormalities were asymptomatic.

Complications and Failures

Common reasons for failures of ankle arthrodesis are nonunion, malunion, infection, leg length discrepancy, painful hindfoot motion, and neurovascular injury. While nonunion was a frequent complication with older techniques, modern compression techniques commonly have union rates of approximately 90%. Ankle arthrodesis nonunion

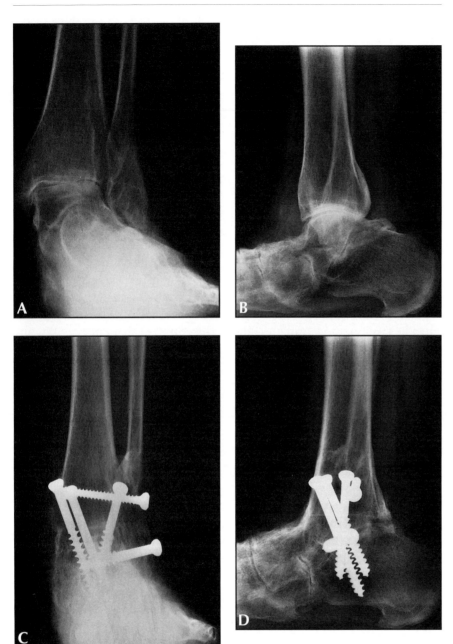

Fig. 1 Radiographs of a 40-year-old woman with rheumatoid arthritis of the ankle and hindfoot, valgus deformity at both the ankle and hindfoot levels, and ankylosed subtalar joint; anteroposterior (**A**) and lateral (**B**) radiographs. Patient underwent arthrodesis with internal fixation with screws, and lateral malleolar only graft. Valgus malalignment was improved by correction of ankle valgus, internal rotation of foot, and medial displacement of foot. Anteroposterior (**C**) and lateral (**D**) radiographs 2.7 years postoperatively with good clinical and radiologic results. (Reproduced with permission from Felix N, Kitaoka HB: Ankle arthrodesis in patients with rheumatoid arthritis. *Clin Orthop* 1998;349:58–64.)

surgeons advocated postponing arthrodesis until the patient has discontinued tobacco use.

Special Reconstruction Problems
Arthrodesis for Rheumatoid Arthritis
Rheumatoid arthritis may involve the ankle joint.[5,8] The early stage of the disease is characterized by painful synovitis, and treatment may include appropriate drug therapy, corticosteroid joint injection, immobilization in a splint, brace, or cast, and (rarely) synovectomy. Later stages of the disease are characterized by arthritis and deformity for which arthrodesis of the affected joints may be indicated.

Rheumatoid arthritis affecting the ankle may be a challenge to manage because of the frequency with which complicating factors occur, such as malalignment, hindfoot joint involvement, severe osteopenia, advanced joint erosive changes with loss of bone stock, and poor soft-tissue envelope about the ankle. The standard surgical treatment for the ankle is arthrodesis. A recently published series had a 96% union rate, and complications were comparable to other reports of arthrodesis in nonrheumatoid patients using either internal or external fixation.[5] Because of the osteopenia, some authors recommend the use of longitudinal Steinmann pins. Based on a laboratory study, the fixation stability of the internal compression arthrodesis technique with screws may be improved with the addition of a fibular onlay graft.

Arthrodesis in Patients with Ongoing Sepsis
Arthrodesis in patients with ongoing sepsis may be addressed by debridement, antibiotics, revision arthrodesis with external fixation, and soft-tissue coverage as needed.[4,6] It is important in these patients to define any local or

may be successfully salvaged by revision arthrodesis using external fixation and supplemental bone graft (Fig. 2).[7] In selected cases, internal fixation may be used. Arthrodesis of the ankle in patients who smoke is associated with a higher incidence of pseudoarthrosis; therefore, some

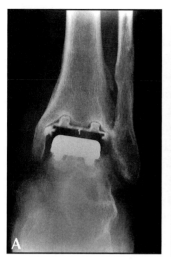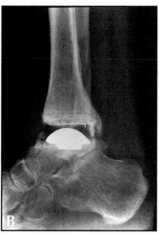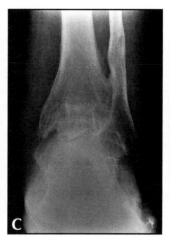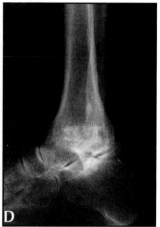

Fig. 2 Radiograph of a patient with a painful total ankle replacement. Anteroposterior (**A**) and lateral (**B**) radiographs demonstrate loosening of both tibial and talar components, subsidence, and malleolar impingement. Anteroposterior (**C**) and lateral (**D**) radiographs 14.5 years later, following modified Chuinard arthrodesis with intercalated iliac crest bone graft and external fixation. Patient had a good clinical and radiologic result, with preservation of ankle height and hindfoot joints. (Reproduced with permission from Kitaoka HB, Romness DW: Arthrodesis for failed ankle arthroplasty. *J Arthroplasty* 1992;7:277–284.)

systemic factors compromising the results, as well as the degree and distribution of bony involvement in order to predict the likelihood of success. Either locally or systemically compromised hosts with diffuse bony involvement (especially central column deficiency) have a much higher failure rate.

Arthrodesis in the Setting of Talar Osteonecrosis

Conventional ankle arthrodesis techniques for arthrosis associated with talar osteonecrosis may fail, as union to necrotic bone may not occur.[1] When osteonecrosis of the entire talar body leads to segmental collapse, arthrosis of both ankle and subtalar joints may occur, requiring arthrodesis with bone graft spanning both levels. In cases in which there is partial body necrosis and only ankle arthrosis (not subtalar), a conventional joint resection arthrodesis may be appropriate, bone grafting the defect.

If there is ankle arthrosis and talar body osteonecrosis without subtalar

arthrosis, other operations, such as the Blair anterior distal tibial sliding bone graft technique, are preferred. The sliding graft technique involves arthrodesis between the anterior tibia to the talar head and neck, which has more viable bone than the talar body. The ankle is approached anteriorly through the interval between the extensor digitorum longus and extensor hallucis longus tendons. The deep dissection requires careful retraction of neurovascular structures (deep peroneal nerve and anterior tibial artery) medially and is carried down to the ankle joint. A rectangular tibial graft measuring 2 to 2.5 cm in width and 3.5 to 5 cm in length is cut with an oscillating saw. A slot is cut into the talar neck about 2 cm in depth to accept the sliding tibial graft. A compression screw is used to fix the proximal graft to the tibia; a longitudinal Steinmann pin through the calcaneus into the tibia may be used for additional stabilization. It is usually not necessary to resect the entire talar body.

Arthrodesis in the Setting of Major Bony Deficit

Large defects resulting from debridement of infected bone, tumor resection, arthrodesis nonunion, or failed ankle replacement present a difficult reconstruction problem.[9] A massive residual defect may be addressed by achieving direct bony apposition, but this results in considerable shortening of the extremity. Intercalated tricortical iliac crest bone graft may be fashioned to fill the defect in order to preserve length. Union rates of up to 89% were reported in a large series of patients with failed ankle replacement. Vascularized fibula transfer and Ilizarov external fixation methods may also have application in selected cases of patients with large bony defects.

Ankle Arthrodesis Malunion

Malposition of the ankle in excessive equinus makes it difficult for the foot to clear the floor while walking. Patients may compensate by externally rotating the extremity. Genu recurvatum may occur resulting from the chronic "back-knee" gait or laxity of the medial collateral ligament from the repetitive valgus stress to the knee. Equinus alignment may cause metatarsalgia and excessive loading of the midfoot joints, with subsequent pain and/or arthrosis. Residual varus or excessive valgus can result in the formation of painful calluses under the fifth or first metatarsals, respectively, and may lead to subtalar arthrosis. Anterior translation of the talus relative to the tibia will cause excessive loading of the midtarsal joints as well. Revision arthrodesis with realignment may be successfully performed.

Arthrodesis of Neuropathic Ankle

Ankle arthrodesis in the neuropathic joint, as in patients with diabetes mellitus, could be considered for carefully selected patients. Neuropathic arthropathy can occur in patients with a subclinical disease without the loss of superficial and deep pain sensation. Typical radiologic features of neuropathic arthropathy may not present. Unfortunately, complications and failures are common following arthrodesis in these patients, with union rates much lower than normal. There may be a role for surgical treatment in patients who fail brace immobilization, or who have intractable ulcers or recurrent infection. Careful assessment of the vascular condition before surgery is essential.

Multiple Joint Disease

Patients with longstanding ankle disorders often develop stiffness of the subtalar joint, which may or may not be associated with pain.[7] It is tempting to extend the arthrodesis across both ankle and subtalar joints in order to eliminate the possibility of late symptoms at the subtalar level,

but it is generally advisable to limit the arthrodesis to the symptomatic joint or joints.

Tibiotalocalcaneal Arthrodesis In patients with arthrosis affecting the ankle and hindfoot, tibiotalar arthrodesis may not be appropriate if there is a high likelihood of residual hindfoot pain.[5,7,11,12] Differential joint injection of a local anesthetic agent may help clarify the contribution of a particular joint to a patient's symptoms and therefore may help the surgeon decide whether to extend the arthrodesis to include the hindfoot. Severe bony (talar) deficiency or selected cases of talar osteonecrosis may also necessitate extension of the arthrodesis due to the limited potential for union of the isolated tibiotalar arthrodesis in these patients. Tibiotalocalcaneal arthrodesis is indicated for symptomatic ankle and subtalar arthrosis unresponsive to bracing, injections, and nonsteroidal anti-inflammatory medications. This may be accomplished in one stage with fusion rates approximating those for primary tibiotalar arthrodesis. The operation may be accomplished through medial and lateral incisions with the patient supine on the operating table. As with the isolated ankle arthrodesis, the ankle joint is resected using an oscillating saw to make 2 parallel cuts, with care taken to minimize the degree of bony resection. Residual articular cartilage and subchondral bone are removed at the subtalar level and fixation applied across both ankle and subtalar levels. Different fixation methods have been used with success, but a commonly performed technique involves multiple cancellous screws placed from proximal to distal extending across both ankle and subtalar levels. A fibular onlay graft may be applied with screw fixation into the tibia and the calcaneus. As an alternative, ex-

ternal fixation may be used, with pins placed transversely in the tibia and the calcaneus. Some investigators use a posterior approach with the patient positioned prone, with fixation consisting of either a posterior plate or external fixator. Achieving appropriate alignment is critical with this operation, particularly with respect to varus-valgus position, as there is limited compensation from the adjacent unfused joints for even small degrees of malalignment. Malalignment in the varus-valgus plane will often result in a painful, intractable plantar keratosis under the medial or lateral plantar forefoot.

Tibiocalcaneal Arthrodesis When the talar body is either deficient, infected, or osteonecrotic, tibiocalcaneal arthrodesis could be considered.[12] If it is determined that the little remaining talar body is not salvageable, the remaining fragments of talar body may be removed and arthrodesis of the distal tibia directly to the calcaneus may be performed with internal or external fixation. As with the tibiotalocalcaneal arthrodesis, appropriate alignment is crucial. Although this procedure may have acceptable clinical results, the operation has the inherent disadvantage of creating considerable shortening of the extremity. The malleoli may be resected to prevent impingement from footwear.

Pantalar Arthrodesis The indications for pantalar arthrodesis are very limited, but its use has been reported to treat severe rheumatoid arthritis involving the ankle and hindfoot.[8] Occasionally, patients who undergo triple arthrodesis and develop subsequent ankle arthrosis require extension of the arthrodesis across the ankle, which results in a pantalar arthrodesis. The operation can be performed either in a one-stage or two-stage procedure.

References

1. Kitaoka HB, Johnson KA: Ankle replacement arthroplasty, in Morrey BF, An KN (eds): *Reconstructive Surgery of the Joints*, ed 2. New York, NY, Churchill Livingstone, 1996, pp 1757–1769.

2. Kitaoka HB, Patzer GL: Clinical results of the Mayo total ankle arthroplasty. *J Bone Joint Surg* 1996;78A:1658–1664.

3. Kitaoka HB, Patzer GL, Ilstrup DM, Wallrichs SL: Survivorship analysis of the Mayo total ankle arthroplasty. *J Bone Joint Surg* 1994;76A:974–979.

4. Cierny G III, Cook WG, Mader JT: Ankle arthrodesis in the presence of ongoing sepsis: Indications, methods, and results. *Orthop Clin North Am* 1989;20:709–721.

5. Felix NA, Kitaoka HB: Ankle arthrodesis in patients with rheumatoid arthritis. *Clin Orthop* 1998;349:58–64.

6. Johnson EE, Weltmer J, Lian GJ, Cracchiolo A III: Ilizarov ankle arthrodesis. *Clin Orthop* 1992;280:160–169.

7. Kitaoka HB, Anderson PJ, Morrey BF: Revision of ankle arthrodesis with external fixation for non-union. *J Bone Joint Surg* 1992;74A:1191–1200.

8. Kitaoka HB: Rheumatoid hindfoot. *Orthop Clin North Am* 1989;20:593–604.

9. Kitaoka HB, Romness DW: Arthrodesis for failed ankle arthroplasty. *J Arthroplasty* 1992;7:277–284.

10. Russotti GM, Johnson KA, Cass JR: Tibiotalocalcaneal arthrodesis for arthritis and deformity of the hind part of the foot. *J Bone Joint Surg* 1988;70A:1304–1307.

11. Thordarson DB, Markolf KL, Cracchiolo A III: Arthrodesis of the ankle with cancellous-bone screws and fibular strut graft: Biomechanical analysis. *J Bone Joint Surg* 1990;72A:1359–1363.

12. Kitaoka HB, Patzer GL: Arthrodesis for the treatment of arthrosis of the ankle and osteonecrosis of the talus. *J Bone Joint Surg* 1998;80A:370–379.

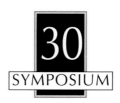

Principles of Joint Arthroplasty as Applied to the Ankle

Lowell H. Gill, MD

Introduction

During the past 30 years much has been learned about total joint arthroplasty. Past failures have often provided the direction for improvements. Proper recognition of design and material limitations is important, as is patient selection. Initial attempts at total ankle arthroplasty largely failed. Nevertheless, interest has recently renewed in the procedure.

The stimulus for total ankle arthroplasty derives from a partial dissatisfaction with ankle arthrodesis as well as the success of total hip and knee arthroplasties.[1] Although function after ankle arthrodesis is very good, it is not normal.[2] In addition to the loss of motion that results from ankle arthrodesis, patients have changes in gait. Lynch and associates[3] and Mazur and associates[2] have shown that patients with ankle arthrodesis walking barefoot have decreased stride length and gait velocity. There has also been the concern that ankle arthrodesis will place excessive stress on surrounding joints, leading to subsequent arthritis.[4-6] Patients with ankle arthritis and concomitant subtalar arthritis or arthrodesis could particularly benefit from a successful ankle arthroplasty.

Nonunion rates after ankle arthrodesis vary among different studies but are approximately 10% to 20% and are more common than after hindfoot arthrodeses.[1,7,8] Factors such as a previous history of high-energy ankle trauma and, particularly, smoking can contribute to considerably higher nonunion rates. The risk for nonunion of ankle arthrodesis among cigarette smokers can be 16 times that of nonsmokers.[7]

Despite these problems, ankle arthrodesis most commonly provides a reliable and durable solution for painful ankle arthritis.[2] Because total ankle arthroplasty has been associated with very high rates of complications and failures, present efforts for ankle arthroplasty need to provide results as least as good as, if not superior to, those of ankle arthrodesis. Whether newer designs in total ankle arthroplasties will provide results superior to those of ankle arthrodesis remains to be seen.

History of Total Ankle Arthroplasty

The first total ankle arthroplasty was performed by Lord, a French surgeon, in 1970.[9] Interestingly, the tibial component of his prosthesis had a long stem not unlike an upside-down femoral stem of a total hip prosthesis. After 10 years, Lord and Marotte published the results of 25 arthroplasties, of which 12 were failures and only 7 results could be considered satisfactory. They discontinued the procedure, believing that ankle arthrodesis was more reliable.[10]

The early reports of total ankle arthroplasty were actually quite good. In an initial review of 20 ankles treated with the Irvine total ankle arthroplasty (University of California, Irvine), Waugh and associates[11] reported that "the immediate results on 20 ankles are most encouraging." Stauffer,[12] at the Mayo Clinic, reported 52 excellent, 6 fair, and 5 poor results in 63 total ankles reviewed at an average of 6 months postoperatively. Subsequently, Stauffer[8] reported results in 102 ankle arthroplasties at a longer follow-up of 23 months: there were 43 excellent and 29 good results (72.5% of the series). More than 90% of patients were noted to have relief of most of their ankle pain, and results were noted to be better in patients with a diagnosis of rheumatoid arthritis. Lachiewicz and associates[13] reported 7 excellent and 8 good results with 15 ankle arthroplasties in patients with rheumatoid arthritis reviewed at an average of 39 months postoperatively. In a 1979 study of 50 arthroplasties, Newton[4] reported that "predictably good results" could be obtained in selected patients. He noted that 24 of 34 patients with osteoarthritis were "extremely happy" and that the patients with rheumatoid arthritis did well when they had not had long-term steroid use because of its secondary deleterious effects on bone quality.[4]

After this initial optimistic period, however, the reports of results of total ankle arthroplasty became more cautious. Such terms as "excellent" and "encouraging" were replaced with "successful," "acceptable," or "satisfactory." Satisfactory and successful results can cover a broad range; in fact, results counted as successful at times meant only that the prosthesis was still in place. Many of these patients actually had radiolucent lines or other evidence of loosening.

Unger and associates[14] reviewed 23 ankle replacements with an average follow-up of 5.6 years. Importantly, this study provided longer follow-up on the same 15 patients originally reported in the earlier study of Lachiewicz and associates,[13] as well as an additional 8 patients. Whereas the earlier report[13] found that all results were good or excellent at 39 months, the results in these same patients had deteriorated at the longer follow-up of 5.6 years. Although Unger and associates reported satisfactory results in 83% of the 17 patients available for review, clinical scores had diminished. Among this slightly larger group of 17 patients, only 2 ankles were rated as excellent, and 8 were rated as fair or poor. Furthermore, of the 15 patients with sufficient radiographs available for review, migration and settling had occurred in 14 of 15 talar components, and bone radiolucencies were found in 14 of 15 tibial components. Twelve of 15 tibial components had actually tilted. Therefore, many of the patients counted as satisfactory were actually impending failures.[14]

In 1982, Samuelson and associates[15] reported that the percentage of acceptable results in their series of 75 implanted Imperial College London Hospital (ICLH) prostheses was about 70%. The authors added that "the procedure should be approached with caution."[15] This same orthopaedic practice had published an earlier study[16] on total ankles in which their findings were noted to "encourage optimism." In another study, Helm and Stevens[17] noted in 19 total ankle arthroplasties that 3 had failed and that an additional 8 showed radiologic signs of loosening at an average of 4 years postoperatively.

Ultimately, as the number of failures continued to increase, total ankle arthroplasty was largely abandoned. Numerous authors recommended against ankle arthroplasty or recommended its use only with marked restrictions.[18-27] Jensen and Kroner[22] reviewed 23 ankles in 18 patients at an average of 59 months postoperatively. Twenty-one ankles were in patients with rheumatoid arthritis, which is often considered a favorable diagnosis for this procedure. Despite this, the authors reported poor results, with a lower percentage of pain relief— 30%— than in patients treated with arthrodesis, whose pain relief was greater than 60%. There were no significant increases in motion after the total ankle arthroplasties, and the overall results were judged to be "so poor that it should be indicated in only a few carefully selected cases."[22] Early advocates Bolton-Maggs and associates[18] reported on 62 total ankle arthroplasties with the ICLH prosthesis and recommended against the procedure. They noted that, "in view of the high complication rate and generally poor long term clinical results, we recommend arthrodesis as the treatment of choice for the painful, stiff arthritic ankle, regardless of the underlying pathologic process."[18] Newton, another early proponent of total ankle arthroplasty, subsequently also reported fusion as the procedure of choice.[26]

Variations in prosthetic designs seemed to make little difference. The Mayo Clinic total ankle was a relatively constrained design. Kitaoka and associates,[24] after a review of 204 primary Mayo Clinic total ankle arthroplasties, recommended against its use. Wynn and Wilde[27] reported on another relatively constrained design, the conaxial total ankle, at an average follow-up of 10 years and recommended against its use because of a 90% loosening rate. Kirkup[25] reviewed the results of a nonconstrained design, the Smith total ankle arthroplasty, and recommended abandoning that prosthesis, as well. In a 1982 review of 50 total ankle arthroplasties of another nonconstrained design, Newton noted that, "because of the high failure rate in this study, fusion remains the procedure of choice for most painful conditions of the ankle."[26] In summary, essentially all available prosthesis designs failed because of poor survivorship.

Demottaz and associates[20] noted that 88% of 21 total ankle arthroplasties of various designs had progressive radiolucent lines at an average of only 14.7 months postoperatively. Furthermore, the authors noted better pain relief in an ankle arthrodesis group, in which 9 of 12 patients (75%) remained pain free for up to 15 years, compared with the arthroplasty patients, only 4 of 21 (19%) of whom were relieved of pain after an average of just 15 months. Finally, and importantly, this study is one of the few to include gait analysis in the evaluation of total ankle arthroplasty patients. Demottaz and associates found abnormal gait patterns in speed, stride dimension, and temporal aspects of gait, as well as considerable muscle weakness about the ankle, in the arthroplasty patients. These results were compared with the gait analyses of patients with arthrodesis, whose gait performance was found to be superior. The authors concluded that arthrodesis is the procedure of choice.[20]

Support

Proper support is fundamental to the success of any construct, whether of a prosthetic joint or some other structure, such as a building. Prosthetic arthroplasty depends on bone for support. Conservation of as much bone as possible at the time of surgery not only helps ensure better support but also saves bone, which is valuable should revision become necessary. Total joint arthroplasties at the hip and knee have clearly demonstrated the fundamental importance of proper bone support, which is crucial for the long-term success of any arthroplasty.

The spherocentric knee introduced in the 1970s had a unique and advanced design concept for its time. This prosthesis allowed triaxial motion by incorporating a ball and socket within the linkage between the femoral and tibial components. This allowed some rotation, as well as varus-valgus tilt, in addition to flexion and extension. By allowing triaxial motion, this knee design should have diminished the rotatory and shear forces at bone-cement and bone-prosthesis interfaces, thereby reducing the high rate of loosening seen with earlier, more constrained hinged-knee designs. Despite the advance of triaxial motion over the earlier fixed-hinge designs, however, many spherocentric knees still failed because of loosening (Fig. 1, *A*). The reason was thought to be, in part, the excessive bone removal necessary during insertion of this bulky prosthesis. Furthermore, revision surgery after the removal of this prosthesis was complicated by the very large amount of bone loss at the time of the initial surgery. Fortunately, however, after a failed total knee arthroplasty, it often is possible to revise the arthroplasty with long-stemmed implants. The long stem allows bypass of the area of bone loss (Fig. 1, *B*).

It is important to note in comparison that, because of the size and shape of the talus, a long-stem talar prosthesis is not an option after a failed total ankle arthroplasty (Fig. 2). It is therefore critically important at the time of total ankle arthroplasty that the initial bone cuts be as conservative as possible.

Newton[4] recognized the importance of bone support very early in his work with total ankle arthroplasty. In his initial reports, he drew attention to the increased risks associated with osteonecrosis as well as bone depleted by long-term disease, inactivity, or steroid use.[4,26] Candidates for total joint arthroplasty frequently have these risks. Newton therefore recommended against ankle arthroplasty in patients with osteonecrosis and advised caution in patients on steroid therapy for rheumatoid arthritis.[4,26]

In one of the very few early laboratory studies, Kempson and associates[16] performed total ankle arthroplasties on cadaveric bone and subjected these arthroplasties to various tests using physiol-

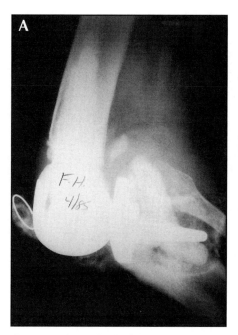
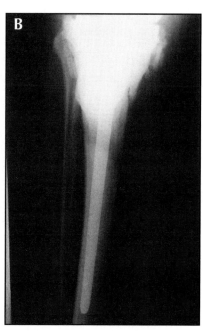

Fig. 1 A, Radiograph of a failed spherocentric total knee arthroplasty. **B**, The same patient as in panel *A*. Postoperative radiograph of a revision spherocentric total knee arthroplasty with long tibial stem component.

ogic forces. A force of 3,400 N (approximately 5.5 times body weight) was used for the compression testing. A force of 5.5 times body weight was chosen because this had recently been reported and later published by Stauffer[12] and Stauffer and associates[28] as the compressive force at the ankle during normal ambulation, based on their gait analysis studies. Stability, strength, and wear tests were also performed. The investigators found that after a total ankle arthroplasty, fractures occur-red in the ankle with 30% less force when a twisting motion was applied.[16] In the compression testing, the study documented rapid failure of the cadaveric bone supporting the prosthesis in just a few days of testing using these physiol-ogic forces. Despite this finding, the authors believed in 1979 that the results "encourage optimism," based on polyethylene wear studies and on the assumption that differences must occur between cadaveric bone and live bone, which is capable of repair.[16] Unintentionally, this article actually predicted

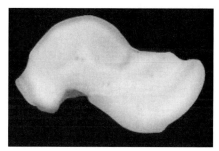

Fig. 2 The size and shape of the talus make stem and keel designs difficult.

the failures that subsequently became so evident.

Calderale and associates[29] studied three-dimensional models of the talar and tibial components of an implanted ankle prosthesis. A uniform vertical force was applied and a finite element analysis done. The researchers found that removing part of the cortical shell of the talus placed abnormal increased stress on the remaining talar cancellous bone.[29] Although logical, the confirmation of changed, abnormal, increased stress in remaining talar cancellous bone after

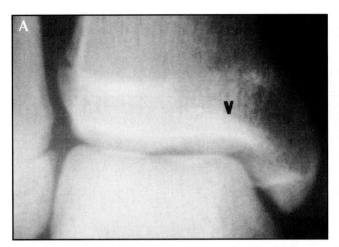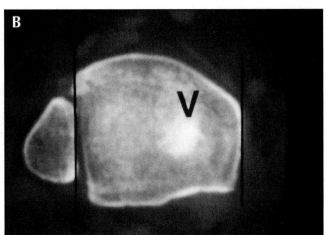

Fig. 3 A and **B**, The area of maximal bone strength at the distal tibia is often posteromedial (*arrowheads*).

bone cuts for prosthetic replacement is noteworthy. It means that when part of the cortical shell of the talus is removed at the time of arthroplasty, the remaining bone must support a greater load than it did before the arthroplasty. (An analogy would be the removal of some of the supports of a foundation; the remaining supports must then bear additional stress.) This study provided more evidence of the importance of saving talar bone.

Hvid and associates[30] studied bone strength at the ankle and documented marked reduction in the strength of bone as sections were taken farther from the articular surface. Although the talus was noted to be 40% stronger than tibial bone, the distal tibia was found to be dangerously close to or below the failure point for prosthetic replacement. Making several assumptions, including activity levels, the authors estimated that the tibial cancellous bone strength should equal 20 MPa; but they found that few of their cadaveric tibias reached this level. The authors summarized that "the resection surfaces—especially on the tibial side—might be too weak to support the loads imposed by current prosthetic designs."[30] The study also documents the eccentricity of the area of maximal bone strength of the distal tibia, which is posteromedial, not central (Fig. 3). This reflects the area of distal tibia receiving stress at the time of heel strike. Because relative bone strength is not uniform across the distal tibia, there can be a tendency for prosthetic settling in the weaker anterolateral aspects of the tibia, which could lead to micromotion and subsequent loosening.

The findings of these studies are not surprising considering the history of total ankle arthroplasty, because the failures of 20 years ago were most commonly caused by loosening and failure of bone support. The few basic laboratory studies that have been done regarding bone support should strongly caution those who attempt prosthetic replacement at the ankle.

Force

Forces at the joints of the lower extremity are great: they are estimated to be two to three times body weight at the hip, three to four times body weight at the knee, and even higher at the ankle.[12,31] These estimates are for normal ambulation only; forces are considerably higher with more vigorous activity.

The reason for the higher force at the ankle is that the forefoot acts like a lever arm to magnify forces across the ankle. Before the toe-off phase of the gait cycle, the body weight is borne on the forefoot. The length of the lever arm of the forefoot to the fulcrum at the ankle exceeds the much shorter length lever arm from the fulcrum at the ankle to the hindfoot. Therefore, while contracting, the Achilles tendon generates a force vector that is multiples of body weight to support body weight on the forefoot, as well as to help propel the body through space.

A familiar analogy is the common hammer with a claw nail extractor. Because of the longer lever arm of the hammer handle, an individual pushing down with 50 to 75 pounds of force on the hammer handle can create up to thousands of pounds of force on the nail extractor. It is because of this principle of leverage that nail extraction is possible. At the foot and ankle, the forefoot is analogous to the hammer handle and the hindfoot to the nail extractor. Because of the shorter lever arm at the hindfoot compared with that of the forefoot, the Achilles tendon must contract with a force of multiples of body weight, subjecting the ankle joint to high compressive loads.

Using mathematical models, Seirig and Arvikar[32] estimated the force at the ankle to be greater than five times body weight during ambulation. Stauffer and associates[28] performed force analyses on normal volunteers in a gait laboratory

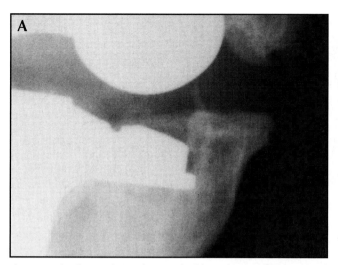 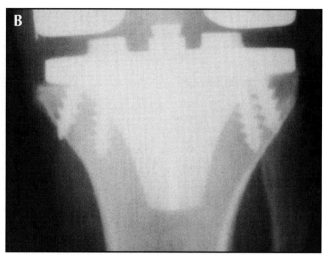

Fig. 4 A, Subsidence of a single-size tibial baseplate used before the development of a range of sizes. This baseplate has inadequate coverage. **B**, Newer baseplates improve bone coverage for better support.

using dynamic force plates. Compressive forces of the ankle were found to reach approximately 5.5 times body weight during normal ambulation.[12,28] Stauffer and associates therefore confirmed Seirig and Arvikar's mathematical prediction. Furthermore, significant tangential and shear forces are also found across the ankle joint.

Demottaz and associates[20] performed similar studies using force plate measurements on patients with total ankle arthroplasty. These authors found forces of approximately three times body weight in total ankle arthroplasty patients. Importantly, however, the study also documented considerable muscle weakness around the ankle in these patients, as well as changes in the normal gait pattern, such as a shortened stride length and decreased contact time. Because total ankle arthroplasty patients were documented to have significant muscle deficits, the finding of less force across the ankle in these patients, compared with normal individuals, is expected. The patients were effectively off-loading their total ankles by changing gait in such a way as to generate less force. If ankle arthroplasty patients are able to recover from the muscle strength deficits, then

more force would be generated during gait, and the values would be expected to rise toward the normal higher values. Significantly, despite the lower forces at the ankle in these arthroplasty patients, the results, in the view of Demottaz and associates,[20] were still poor. High loosening rates were observed despite the protective gait pattern. Whether the gait pattern and forces are normal or abnormal as documented by Demottaz and associates, it is apparent that an ankle arthroplasty must be able to withstand large forces that are multiples of body weight.

Force is always measured per unit area. In fact, surface area is a fundamental part of the definition of force. A newton, a unit of force, is one-quarter pound spread over 1 square meter (0.25 lb/m²). For a given load, expanding the surface area for support of that load decreases the load per unit area.

The earliest prostheses designed for total knee arthroplasties were available in only one size. With only one size, the prostheses were often undersized and therefore were prone to subsidence in the remaining soft cancellous bone (Fig. 4, A). Not only was the strongest bone removed at the time of the surgery, but also the remaining bone surface was not

fully utilized for support. Later, multiple sizes with more anatomic shapes were developed (Fig. 4, B). With these, the bone remaining after the surgical procedure is more fully utilized for support. By expanding the tibial baseplate to encompass all available bone, the load is diminished per unit area.

Stauffer[12] pointed out that the human ankle joint has a comparatively large surface area of about 12 cm², which is larger than that of the hip. However, much of the surface area of the ankle is in the medial and lateral gutters as well as in the anterior and posterior aspects of the curved dome of the talus and may not, in fact, be in areas used for prosthetic support. Depending on the specific design, the area utilized for prosthetic support is often approximately 6 to 7 cm², or about half the total surface area in the ankle. This is considerably less surface area for support than with the support surfaces of the knee, where the forces generated are less but the surface area for support is larger. Compared with the knee, therefore, the cut bone surface at the ankle must support larger forces over comparatively smaller surface areas for prosthetic support.

Force is not necessarily directly perpendicular to the baseplate of a prosthesis.

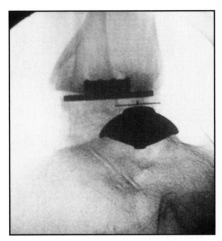

Fig. 5 Prostheses are often eccentrically loaded.

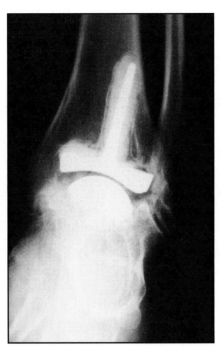

Fig. 6 Proper alignment in total ankle arthroplasty can be challenging because of the limitations of exposure at the ankle.

Instead, because of the variability of human activity, the direction of force may be angular. This introduces shear forces in addition to those of direct compression. Furthermore, a force vector on a prosthesis often is not central; instead, force is often placed "off center," that is, eccentrically (Fig. 5). Although proper alignment of a prosthesis helps minimize this, eccentric force can never be completely eliminated. Perfect alignment, if even possible, may be difficult to achieve surgically (Fig. 6). Even when alignment is perfect, the direction of forces will change with normal variability in human activity. In the human knee, Johnson and associates[33] have shown that forces are usually eccentric and greater on the medial side, even in a valgus knee.

Therefore, using the tibial baseplate in a total knee arthroplasty as an example, eccentric force placed on the medial side of a prosthesis will likely occur even in a well-aligned prosthesis. Malalignment can markedly aggravate this problem and has been associated with early failure. With an eccentric force placed on the medial side of the tibial prosthesis, there will be a downward force vector on this side and a corresponding lift-off force on the lateral side. The same phenomenon can occur in the anteroposterior direction, as well. The repeated direct compressive force on one side of the baseplate and the corresponding lift-off force on the other side leads to micromotion, which eventually can lead to loosening. Such micromotion can prevent bony ingrowth in a cementless prosthesis.[34] It is thought that micromotion in excess of 0.15 mm will prevent bony ingrowth into a prosthetic implant.[34]

The understructure of a tibial baseplate in a total knee arthroplasty is important in resisting such micromotion as well as in resisting shear, rotatory, and eccentric forces. Volz and associates[34] studied tibial baseplate micromotion in the laboratory using four tibial baseplates of different designs. They implanted the baseplates into paired cadaveric tibias, subjected them to eccentric loads, and measured the resulting micromotion. They found that four peripherally placed screws with a central peg best resisted micromotion. It should be noted that this study did not evaluate a keel or fin design.

Ewald and Walker[35] and Walker[36] studied the ability of tibial baseplates to resist shear and torque forces. Walker looked at several generic baseplate designs, which included a flat tray with no pegs, a tray with two pegs, a flat plate with four round pegs, a flat plate with a central stem, and a flat plate with a stem that included two fins or a keel. He showed that the keel design best resisted offset loading, that is, eccentrically applied loads. Furthermore, these same constructs were retested for resistance to shear and torque stresses and, again, the best design was the one with a keel or fin. The worst design in all tests was the baseplate without any understructure. The advantage of a keel makes sense because this design uses the same concept mentioned previously for tibial baseplate size: that is, by increasing the surface area for force dissipation, force per unit area is reduced. This means that a keel best prevents micromotion, given a certain strength of bone subjected to an applied load. Many of today's prosthetic designs for total knee arthroplasties have a keel on the undersurface of the tibial baseplate. At the ankle, however, because of the anatomy of the talus, use of a keel is difficult, if even possible, particularly on the lower side (Fig. 2). The talus is simply too small to allow a sizable keel or fin, which would require resection of more bone where little is available.

Finally, as noted, Hvid and associates[30] documented not only that forces are often eccentric but also that the strength of the bone support itself is eccentric. Instead of bone strength being evenly distributed, the strongest bone is likely posteromedial in the distal tibia (Fig. 3). This area of stiffer bone could act as a pivot point, with the risk of overloading the surrounding weaker anterolateral bone. A somewhat anterolaterally placed component could potentially aggravate this problem.

Limitations of Polyethylene

Understanding the materials used and

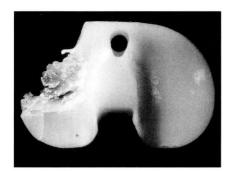

Fig. 7 Complete wear-through of a tibial polyethylene component.

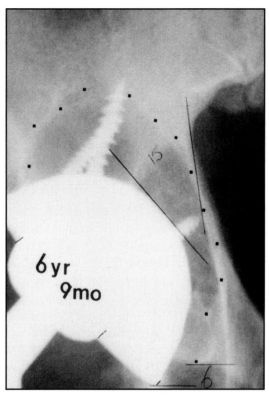

Fig. 8 Dots outline the borders of a large area of osteolysis caused by excessive polyethylene wear in less than 7 years.

their limitations is essential for success in arthroplasty. After initial failures using polytetrafluoroethylene (Fluon, often incorrectly confused with Teflon[37]), Sir John Charnley tried polyethylene in 1962. An advantage of a metal-polyethylene bearing surface is the low friction at the bearing surface, a feature that attracted Charnley and others to this bearing surface in the design of total hip arthroplasty. Wear particles from polyethylene were initially believed to be innocuous with this seemingly well-tolerated, biologically inert material.[16]

With its continued use, however, the disadvantages of polyethylene are now profoundly obvious. Numerous patterns of wear are seen in polyethylene, including pitting, delamination, and creep, with the loss of original contour.[38] Frank breakage can occur, and numerous retrievals show complete wear through the structure (Fig. 7). Finally, it is now known that the wear products often are neither innocuous nor biologically inert.[39]

The magnitude of the problem of polyethylene wear is greater than many surgeons recognize. Reports to the US Food and Drug Administration of medical device failures began in 1984. A study by the General Accounting Office in 1986 showed that fewer than 1% of medical device failures occurring at hospitals are actually reported.[40] Since then, the number of reported failures has

increased, although it is still estimated that fewer than 5% of such failures are actually reported. Despite this, 1,717 total hip and 2,769 total knee arthroplasty failures were recorded between 1984 and 1993. An analysis of these failures clearly shows the magnitude of the polyethylene problem. In an evaluation of the many different types of total joint failure, polyethylene failure was the most common complication category for total hip arthroplasty and accounted for 68% of failures in total knee arthroplasty.[40] In addition, other types of failure, such as loosening, can relate to polyethylene debris.

Polyethylene wear can be severe (Fig. 7). Wear is associated with many factors, but one of the primary factors is the activity level or number of cycles. Ambulation studies among adults with total joint arthroplasty show tremendous variability in activity levels, with up to a 45-fold difference among different patients.[41] An average of 0.9 million

cycles per year has been documented among total joint arthroplasty patients. Measurement of wear in the hip also shows tremendous variability, but the average of many studies is approximately 0.1 mm per year.[41] Based on the average amount of wear and the number of cycles per year, it has been calculated that wear particles can exceed 500,000 particles per step. Billions of polyethylene debris particles can therefore be generated in a single year. This particulate polyethylene debris appears to incite an inflammatory type of reaction that, through a cascade of events, leads to osteolysis and loss of support around the prosthesis[39,42] (Fig. 8). It is therefore essential that wear be minimized.

Previous laboratory tests did not predict the amount of wear observed clinically[37,42] (Fig. 8). This was partially because of the lack of crossing-path motion on earlier hip-wear simulators.[42] Furthermore, pin-on-disk experiments, which use a linear-track motion, led to

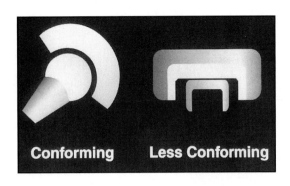

Fig. 9 The hip is a more conforming geometry than other potential design prostheses at the knee and ankle.

false conclusions regarding polyethylene wear in vivo because polyethylene can become resistant to a purely linear pattern of wear. Polyethylene wear is greater with a crossing-path or circular type of motion.

Backside wear of the polyethylene against the tibial metallic tray or acetabular liner has been documented and can be severe in both the hips and knees. This underscores the importance of secure locking mechanisms between the polyethylene and metal to minimize backside wear.[38] Locking mechanisms have been improved considerably in hips and knees but have been given scant attention in total ankle arthroplasty.

The polyethylene problem has led to the search for improved polyethylene as well as alternative bearing surfaces, such as ceramic on polyethylene or metal on metal. At present, most total ankle arthroplasty designs use the more traditional metal-on-polyethylene bearing surface.

Material transfer refers to the changed behavior of a material when it is transferred from one use to another or from one area to another. For example, polyethylene shows different and more severe wear patterns when it is used at the knee compared with the hip.[43] The ball-and-socket shape of total hip arthroplasty is a conforming geometry (Fig. 9). Polyethylene wear is minimized in this type of environment, where the contact stress is spread along a larger surface area. For some time, the geometry of total

knee prosthetic designs was flat on round rather than round on round, as seen in hip arthroplasties. The tibial polyethylene was designed flat to allow rollback of the femoral component in an effort to improve flexion and mimic more normal knee motion. The flatness of the tibial component, however, caused an increase in point-contact stress on the polyethylene, which then exceeded its yield strength in many designs.[43-46] It is for this reason that many of the newer total knee arthroplasties use a more "dished" tibial polyethylene surface.

The physical properties of polyethylene can vary according to the specific polyethylene used and because of a number of other variables. In general, however, the yield strength of polyethylene is relatively low compared with the forces generated in the lower extremity. Black[47] stated that the yield strength of polyethylene is approximately 13 MPa; Wright and Bartel[46] reported the yield strength as approximately 25 MPa. Wright and Bartel measured the contact stresses on five different total knee designs using Fuji pressure-sensitive film. These five different designs showed peak contact stresses of between 20 and 80 MPa. The contact stresses increased with knee flexion so that all designs studied exceeded the yield strength of polyethylene with flexion.[46] Ewald and Walker[35] showed that by rounding or dishing the polyethylene tray, the peak contact stress was reduced from 55 MPa for a round-on-flat design to 18 MPa for a design in which the poly-

ethylene is more conforming. Increasing the conformity reduces the peak contact stress on the polyethylene but also increases stresses that are transferred to the bone-prosthesis interface, which can contribute to loosening. Therefore, a proper balance is needed between reducing peak contact stress to protect the polyethylene and allowing enough freedom of movement to protect bone-prosthesis interfaces.

Polyethylene strength is improved with increased thickness.[43-45] Thin polyethylene wears faster. Because of this, it has been estimated that a minimum thickness of 4 to 6 mm is needed at the hip, where there is more conformity and the forces are smaller, and that a minimum thickness of 6 to 8 mm is needed at the knee, where there are larger forces and less conformity.[18]

Minimum polyethylene thickness standards for the ankle have not been determined at this time. Because of the behavioral differences observed with material transfer between the hip and knee, it would be reasonable to assume that the thickness at the ankle should be even greater. Furthermore, ankle prostheses that use a mobile bearing have no locking mechanism and, by design, are intended to wear on both sides.

Design

In his presidential address to the Knee Society, John N. Insall said in regard to the design of total knee arthroplasty: "Consider the analogy of automobiles: All have certain fundamental resemblances in that they possess an engine and four wheels. However, the engineers who design a racing car clearly have different priorities than those who design a mass-produced passenger car.... Similar compromises exist in the design of knee prostheses with one important difference: Whereas the designers of cars base their decisions on scientific knowledge and fact, the designers of knee prostheses rely to a much greater extent on opinion."[48]

These comments almost certainly pertain to the design of total ankle arthroplasty as well. There has been a relative paucity of basic scientific laboratory investigation on total ankle arthroplasty, and very little investigation into design criteria. Instead, most of the available literature consists of reviews of clinical use of a particular design.[4,6,8-15,17-20,22-28,49-54] There is, therefore, little scientific guidance available for the design criteria for total ankle arthroplasty. Undoubtedly, this situation is partly because the procedure was largely abandoned for many years. In view of the past failures, however, it would be prudent for basic laboratory investigation to be performed before another series of clinical trials is undertaken.

In one of the few laboratory investigations on total ankle arthroplasty design, Falsig and associates[55] evaluated stress transfer to the distal tibial trabecular bone. Aware of the critically low distal tibial bone strength about the ankle, as reported by Hvid and associates,[30] Falsig and associates[55] performed finite element stress analysis in the laboratory using three different generic distal tibial prostheses; (1) a polyethylene tibial component; (2) a metal-backed polyethylene tibial component; and (3) a long-stem metal-backed tibial component, using a much longer stem than is common with total ankle arthroplasty prostheses. An eccentric anterolateral load of 2,100 N (approximately three times body weight) was applied to the three different generic tibial prosthetic designs. The investigators found that the addition of metal backing reduced compressive stresses in the trabecular bone by 25%, from 20 N/mm^{-2} for an all-polyethylene tibial component to 15 N/mm^{-2} for a metal-backed component.[55] Shear stresses were also reduced. The long-stem implant resulted in almost complete reduction of compressive stresses in the metaphyseal trabecular bone because the stresses were transferred to the long stem, bypassing

---

Table 1
Goals for the Design of a Total Ankle Arthroplasty

Goal 1: Minimize bone removal on both sides of the joint
Goal 2: Maximize the surface area for support of the prosthesis
Goal 3: Maximize the surface area for stabilization of the prosthesis, but without excessive bone loss and without an excessively long stem
Goal 4: If polyethylene is used, allow sufficient thickness of polyethylene as well as a conforming geometry
Goal 5: Establish the proper balance between constraint and freedom
Goal 6: Use a bearing surface that minimizes wear
Goal 7: Use a firm, expanded surface-area locking mechanism for ankles that use a fixed, nonmobile polyethylene
Goal 8: Improve instrumentation to help ensure proper alignment to minimize shear, angular, and eccentric forces

---

the distal tibia.[55] This was considered undesirable because of the likelihood of stress shielding of distal tibial bone, which could potentially result in further weakening of bone at the ankle level.

Based on the studies that have been done in arthroplasty for the hip and knee, as well as the few studies done on bone strength at the ankle that have been cited,[16,29,30] and the study by Falsig and associates on tibial arthroplasty design, the goals at present for the design of a total ankle arthroplasty may be as outlined in Table 1.

It is obvious that compromises with the goals must be made. Achieving goal 4, for example, directly inhibits the ability to achieve goal 1. Furthermore, particularly because of the anatomic constraints of the relatively small amount of bone available at the ankle, goals 1, 2, and 3 are difficult to achieve.

Exposure at the ankle is very difficult because of the confines of ankle anatomy. This has a direct bearing on prosthesis design. Complete dislocation of the hip and marked subluxation at the knee are commonplace during total joint arthroplasty at these locations because they allow adequate exposure for the procedure and placement of the particular prosthesis, which may include a long stem or keel. By comparison, circulation to the talus would be jeopardized by such degrees of displacement at the ankle.[56]

Early laboratory wear studies of polyethylene at the ankle suggested a favorable longevity.[16] However, subsequent clinical observations (Fig. 8) and retrieval studies in total hip and knee arthroplasties have shown that such wear studies were very misleading. If the problems of long-term prosthesis fixation and maintenance of bone support are substantially improved or solved at the ankle, then the issue of polyethylene failure may become more apparent. In the earlier use of total ankle arthroplasties, the prostheses did not last long enough to make polyethylene failure apparent.

Thicker polyethylene components at the ankle may help prevent polyethylene failures, but at the expense of more generous bone cuts. Studies previously cited have already shown the fundamental importance of bone conservation, particularly at the ankle, where bone may be weak and surface areas for support small, yet forces very high. Polyethylene requirements of the ankle are therefore contradictory to what is necessary for conserving bone strength. Newer, more highly cross-linked polyethylenes may help this problem. However, other desirable qualities may be compromised in the manufacture of the highly cross-linked polyethylenes.[38] Whether the newer polyethylenes will solve the existing wear problems and allow greater conservation of bone is undetermined at this time.

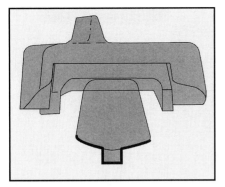

Fig. 10 The Agility Ankle prosthesis. The upper component includes a polyethylene insert.

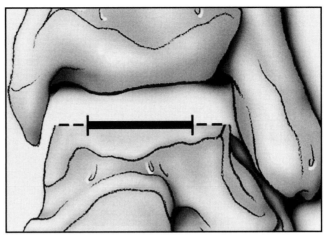

Fig. 11 Some total ankle designs do not use all available bone surface for support.

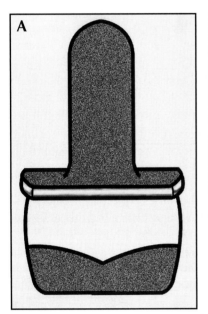

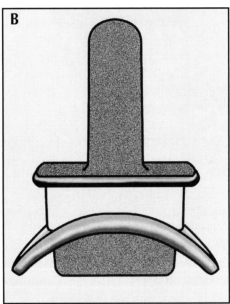

Fig. 12 Anterior (**A**) and lateral (**B**) view of the Buechel-Pappas Total Ankle replacement prosthesis.

There are currently three different total ankle arthroplasties being used in the United States: the Agility Ankle (DePuy, Warsaw, IN), the Buechel-Pappas Total Ankle Replacement (Endotec, South Orange, NJ), and the Scandinavian Total Ankle Replacement (STAR; Waldemar-Link, Hamburg, Germany). The STAR prosthesis was initially developed in Denmark and is presently in clinical trials in the United States.

The Agility Ankle (Fig. 10) has a metal-backed tibial component that is supported by both the tibia and fibula.[49] An arthrodesis is done between the tibia and fibula at the time of arthroplasty. This unique feature allows maximal expansion of the surface area for support on the upper side. The polyethylene component is dished or concave in the sagittal plane, much like the normal ankle, which helps anteroposterior stability. The tibial polyethylene component is larger in dimension than the talar component, which is free to seek its own position medially and laterally in the larger tibial polyethylene

component. This deliberate mismatch in articulation reduces constraint, helping to diminish rotatory and shear stresses.

The original talar component did not always cover the talar bone available for support (Fig. 11). A new modification helps improve this potential problem. The locking mechanism for the polyethylene on the top side does not have the expanded surface area for improved locking, as seen on the newer acetabular and tibial components of total hip and total knee arthroplasties. There is the potential for increased contact stress on the polyethylene, particularly if malalignment should occur. Finally, insertion of the prosthesis requires relatively aggressive bone cuts, although this is partially diminished by the use of a distractor at the time of surgery. Even using the distractor, the bone cuts are relatively substantial.

The Buechel-Pappas Total Ankle replacement (Fig. 12) has a medium-length stem on the tibial component which, according to the study by Falsig and associates,[16] will help protect the trabecular bone at the distal tibial metaphysis.[50,51] The metal components have a true metallic-ceramic bearing surface, which is different from alumina and zirconium ceramics. The polyethylene component is fully conforming with the metal tibial and talar components. These two features should help protect the polyethylene. The polyethylene component is a mobile bearing that is designed to articulate on both sides, thus reducing rotatory and shear stresses.[50,51] However, the flat upper surface of the polyethylene-metal articulation does not give the same degree of anteroposterior stability without the dishing or anteroposterior "capture" of the normal ankle on the tibial side.[57] The talar component is an onlay component with two fins to help increase surface area for fixation, although more bone removal is required to make two slots in the relatively small talus.

The STAR prosthesis (Fig. 13) also has a mobile-bearing polyethylene component.[52,53,58] The tibial component has two dowels or cylindrical bars used for fixation, and the component is designed to sit on cortical bone of the distal tibia. As with the Buechel-Pappas Total Ankle replacement, the mobile bearing reduces rotatory and shear stresses, thus avoiding excessive constraint, but also uses a flat upper surface, which diminishes anteroposterior stability.[57] Garde and Kofoed[58] have performed stabilometry studies on patients with meniscal bearing arthroplasty showing that, clinically, patients are able to maintain sufficient anteroposterior stability. The talar component maximizes surface area for force distribution and fixation by having a medial and lateral resurfacing in addition to the superior onlay resurfacing. In this way, the surface area for fixation and load distribution is maximized on the talar component.

All three total ankle arthroplasty designs have shown acceptable short-term and midterm results in clinical use.[49-54] Long-term follow-up is not yet available.

Summary

The challenges for the development of a successful total ankle prosthesis are formidable. The forces at the ankle are large and the surface area for bone support is

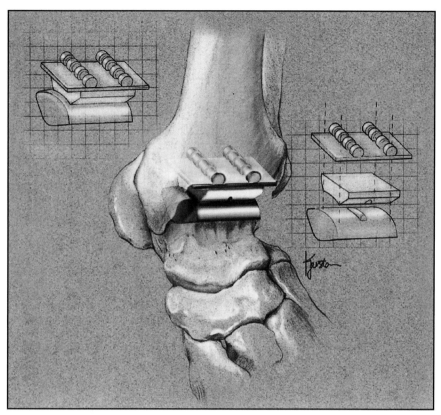

Fig. 13 The Scandinavian Total Ankle Replacement (STAR) prosthesis.

small. The size and shape of the talus make expansion of the surface area for fixation very difficult and greatly minimize options for prosthetic revision. The quality of bone in the distal tibia frequently may be questionable, and the bone strength is not uniform across the distal tibia.

Finally, the soft-tissue envelope at the ankle is poor. The distal location of the ankle magnifies the circulatory risk in any patient with peripheral vascular disease. Wound problems are more common and more dangerous than in more proximal sites. Fractures and other injuries are very common at the ankle and potentially can add to the frequency of complications. The proximity of the medial and anterior neurovascular structures also increases the likelihood of serious complication. Total ankle arthroplasty is much closer to the limit of what can be successfully accomplished with accept-

able risk to the patient. There is little room for error. This, coupled with the larger compressive forces generated at the ankle, makes successful ankle arthroplasty a bigger challenge than arthroplasty at the hip or knee.

References

1. Lewis G: The ankle joint prosthetic replacement: Clinical performance and research challenges. *Foot Ankle Int* 1994;15:471-476.

2. Mazur JM, Schwartz E, Simon SR: Ankle arthrodesis: Long-term follow-up with gait analysis. *J Bone Joint Surg Am* 1979;61:964-975.

3. Lynch AF, Bourne RB, Rorabeck CH: The long-term results of ankle arthrodesis. *J Bone Joint Surg Br* 1988;70:113-116.

4. Newton SE: An artificial ankle joint. *Clin Orthop* 1979;142:141-145.

5. Schaap EJ, Huy J, Tonino AJ: Long-term results of arthrodesis of the ankle. *Int Orthop* 1990;14:9-12.

6. Takakura Y, Tanaka Y, Sugimoto K, Tamai S, Masuhara K: Ankle arthroplasty: A comparative study of cemented metal and uncemented ceramic prostheses. *Clin Orthop* 1990;252:209-216.

7. Myerson MS: Revision foot and ankle surgery, in Myerson M (ed): *Foot and Ankle Disorders.* Philadelphia, PA, WB Saunders, 2000, vol 2, pp 1103-1134.

8. Stauffer RN: Total joint arthroplasty: The ankle. *Mayo Clin Proc* 1979;54:570-575.

9. Lord G, Gentaz R, Gagey PM, Baron JB: Pasturographic study of total prostheses in the leg: Apropos of 88 patients examined. *Rev Chir Orthop Reparatrice Appar Mot* 1976;62:363-374.

10. Lord G, Marotte JH: Total ankle replacement. *Rev Chir Orthop Reparatrice Appar Mot* 1980;66: 527-530.

11. Waugh TR, Evanski PM, McMaster WC: Irvine ankle arthroplasty: Prosthetic design and surgical technique. *Clin Orthop* 1976;114: 180-184.

12. Stauffer RN: Total ankle joint replacement. *Arch Surg* 1977;112:1105-1109.

13. Lachiewicz PF, Inglis AE, Ranawat CS: Total ankle replacement in rheumatoid arthritis. *J Bone Joint Surg Am* 1984;66:340-343.

14. Unger AS, Inglis AE, Mow CS, Figgie HE III: Total ankle arthroplasty in rheumatoid arthritis: A long-term follow-up study. *Foot Ankle* 1988;8:173-179.

15. Samuelson KM, Freeman MA, Tuke MA: Development and evolution of the ICLH ankle replacement. *Foot Ankle* 1982;3:32-36.

16. Kempson GE, Freeman MA, Tuke MA: Engineering considerations in the design of an ankle joint. *Biomed Eng* 1975;10:166-171.

17. Helm R, Stevens J: Long-term results of total ankle replacement. *J Arthroplasty* 1986;1: 271-277.

18. Bolton-Maggs BG, Sudlow RA, Freeman MA: Total ankle arthroplasty: A long-term review of the London hospital experience. *J Bone Joint Surg Br* 1985;67:785-790.

19. Das AK Jr: Total ankle arthroplasty: A review of 37 cases. *J Tenn Med Assoc* 1988;81:682-685.

20. Demottaz JD, Mazur JM, Thomas WH, Sledge CB, Simon SR: Clinical study of total ankle replacement with gait analysis: A preliminary report. *J Bone Joint Surg Am* 1979;61:976-988.

21. Hamblen DL: Editorial: Can the ankle joint be replaced? *J Bone Joint Surg Br* 1985;67:689-690.

22. Jensen NC, Kroner K: Total ankle joint replacement: A clinical follow up. *Orthopedics* 1992;15:236-239.

23. Kitaoka HB, Patzer GL: Clinical results of the Mayo total ankle arthroplasty. *J Bone Joint Surg Am* 1996;78:1658-1664.

24. Kitaoka HB, Patzer GL, Ilstrup DM, Wallrichs SL: Survivorship analysis of the Mayo total ankle arthroplasty. *J Bone Joint Surg Am* 1994; 76:974-979.

25. Kirkup J: Richard Smith ankle arthroplasty. *J Soc Med* 1985;78:301-304.

26. Newton SE: Total ankle arthroplasty: Clinical study of fifty cases. *J Bone Joint Surg Am* 1982; 64:104-111.

27. Wynn AH, Wilde AH: Long-term follow-up of the Conaxial (Beck-Steffee) total ankle arthroplasty. *Foot Ankle* 1992;13:303-306.

28. Stauffer RN, Chao EY, Brewster RC: Force and motion analysis of the normal, diseased, and prosthetic ankle joint. *Clin Orthop* 1977; 127:189-196.

29. Calderale PM, Garro A, Barbiero R, Fasolio G, Pipino F: Biomechanical design of the total ankle prosthesis. *Eng Med* 1983;12:69-80.

30. Hvid I, Rasmussen O, Jensen NC, Nielsen S: Trabecular bone strength profiles at the ankle joint. *Clin Orthop* 1985;199:306-312.

31. Andriacchi TP, Mikosz RP: Musculoskeletal dynamics, locomotion and clinical applications, in Mow VC, Hayes WC (eds): *Basic Orthopaedic Biomechanics.* New York, NY, Raven Press, 1991, pp 51-92.

32. Seirig A, Arvikar RJ: The prediction of muscular load sharing and joint-forces in the lower extremities during walking. *J Biomech* 1975;8: 89-102.

33. Johnson F, Leitl S, Waugh W: The distribution of load across the knee: A comparison of static and dynamic measurements. *J Bone Joint Surg Br* 1980;62:346-349.

34. Volz RG, Nisbet JK, Lee RW, McMurtry MG: The mechanical stability of various non-cemented tibial components. *Clin Orthop* 1988; 226:38-42.

35. Ewald FC, Walker PS: The current status of total knee replacement. *Rheum Dis Clin North Am* 1988;14:579-590.

36. Walker PS: Requirements for successful total knee replacements: Design considerations. *Orthop Clin North Am* 1989;20:15-29.

37. Li S, Burstein AH: Ultra-high molecular weight polyethylene: The material and its use in total joint implants. *J Bone Joint Surg Am* 1994;76:1080-1090.

38. Li S: Ultra-high-molecular-weight polyethylene: The weak link, in Lotke PA, Garino JP (eds): *Revision Total Knee Arthroplasty.* Philadelphia, PA, Lippincott-Raven, 1999, pp 43-65.

39. Kadoya Y, Kobayashi A, Ohashi H: Wear and osteolysis in total joint replacements. *Acta Orthop Scand Suppl* 1998;278:1-16.

40. Castro FP Jr, Chimento G, Munn BG, Levy RS, Timon S, Barrack RL: An analysis of Food and Drug administration medical device reports relating to total joint components. *J Arthroplasty* 1997;12:765-771.

41. Schmalzried TP, Dorey FJ, McKellop H: The multifactorial nature of polyethylene wear in vivo. *J Bone Joint Surg Am* 1998;80:1234-1242.

42. Poss R, Spector M: Discussion of commentary above. *J Bone Joint Surg Am* 1998;80:1242-1243.

43. Bartel DL, Rawlinson JJ, Burstein AH, Ranawat CS, Flynn WF Jr: Stresses in polyethylene components of contemporary total knee replacements. *Clin Orthop* 1995;317:76-82.

44. Bartel DL, Bicknell MS, Wright TM: The effect of conformity, thickness, and material on stresses in ultra-high molecular weight components for total joint replacement. *J Bone Joint Surg Am* 1986;68:1041-1051.

45. Bartel DL, Burstein AH, Toda MD, Edwards DL: The effect of conformity and plastic thickness on contact stresses in metal-backed plastic implants. *J Biomech Eng* 1985;107:193-199.

46. Wright TM, Bartel DL: The problem of surface damage in polyethylene total knee components. *Clin Orthop* 1986;205:67-74.

47. Black J: Requirements for successful total knee replacement: Material considerations. *Orthop Clin North Am* 1989;20:1-13.

48. Insall JN: Presidential address to The Knee Society: Choices and compromises in total knee arthroplasty. *Clin Orthop* 1988;226:43-48.

49. Alvine F: Total ankle arthroplasty, in Myerson M (ed): *Foot and Ankle Disorders.* Philadelphia, PA, WB Saunders, 2000, vol 2, pp 1085-1102.

50. Buechel FF, Pappas MJ, Iorio LJ: New Jersey low contact stress total ankle replacement: Biomechanical rationale and review of 23 cementless cases. *Foot Ankle* 1988;8:279-290.

51. Buechel FF, Pappas MJ: Survivorship and clinical evaluation of cementless, meniscal-bearing total ankle replacements. *Semin Arthroplasty* 1992;3:43-50.

52. Kofoed H: Cylindrical cemented ankle arthroplasty: A prospective series with long-term follow-up. *Foot Ankle Int* 1995;16:474-479.

53. Kofoed H, Sorensen TS: Ankle arthroplasty for rheumatoid arthritis and osteoarthritis: Prospective long-term study of cemented replacements. *J Bone Joint Surg Br* 1998;80: 328-332.

54. Pyevich MT, Saltzman CL, Callaghan JJ, Alvine FG: Total ankle arthroplasty: A unique design: Two to twelve-year follow-up. *J Bone Joint Surg Am* 1998;80:1410-1420.

55. Falsig J, Hvid I, Jensen N: Finite element stress analysis of some ankle joint prostheses. *Clin Biomech* 1986;1:71-76.

56. Gill LH: Avascular necrosis of the talus secondary to trauma, disease, drugs, and treatment. *Foot Ankle Clin* 1999;4:431-446.

57. Burge P, Evans M: Effect of surface replacement arthroplasty on stability of the ankle. *Foot Ankle* 1986;7:10-17.

58. Garde L, Kofoed H: Meniscal-bearing ankle arthroplasty is stable: In vivo analysis using stabilometry. *Foot Ankle Surg* 1996;2:137-143.

Total Ankle Arthroplasty

*James K. DeOrio, MD
Mark E. Easley, MD

Abstract

Recent investigations support the belief that ankle replacement represents an attractive surgical alternative to arthrodesis for patients with advanced ankle arthritis. Although longer follow-up is necessary for total ankle arthroplasty (TAA) to displace arthrodesis as the surgical "gold standard," intermediate-term results are encouraging. Indications for TAA include primarily posttraumatic and inflammatory arthritis. Contraindications to TAA include unresectable osteonecrotic bone, peripheral vascular disease, neuropathy, active and/or recent ankle infection, nonreconstructible ankle ligaments, loss of lower leg muscular control, and severe osteopenia or osteoporosis. Young, active, high-demand patients with ankle arthritis may be better candidates for arthrodesis than for TAA. Rigorous patient selection is essential in the success of TAA, more than in other joint arthroplasty procedures.

Total ankle prosthetic designs (Agility, Scandinavian Total Ankle Replacement, Hintegra, Salto, and Buechel-Pappas) with a minimum of published intermediate follow-up results, and several other innovative and biomechanically supported designs (the Mobility Total Ankle System, BOX, INBONE, and Salto-Talaris) are reviewed to demonstrate the recent evolution of TAA.

Some TAA designs feature a nonconstrained polyethylene meniscus (mobile bearing) that articulates between the porous-coated tibial and talar components. The concern for edge loading (when the polyethylene component comes in contact with a metal edge) has been addressed in more recent designs by reducing the superior polyethylene surface area, expanding the tibial component surface, and even offering a convex tibial component. More practical, effective, and safer instrumentation for implantation has also been developed and has been essential to the success of TAA. However, complications with TAA (such as inadequate wound healing and malleolar fractures) are more frequent when compared with total hip and knee arthroplasty, irrespective of the surgeon's training method. As an individual surgeon gains more experience, the chances of a favorable outcome are increased.

*James K. DeOrio, MD or the department with which he is affiliated has received research or institutional support from Link Orthopaedics; miscellaneous nonincome support, commercially derived honoraria, or other nonresearch-related funding from Tornier, INBONE, and Link Orthopaedics; and is a consultant or employee for Link Orthopaedics and INBONE.

Despite the failures of first-generation ankle prostheses implanted approximately 30 years ago, the interest in total ankle arthroplasty (TAA) has grown over the past decade. Currently, more than 20 different TAA designs are marketed worldwide, and several other designs are in development. This evolution of TAA from a procedure that was near extinction to a procedure with growing recognition can be attributed to four factors. (1) In the face of adversity, several pioneers designed ankle implants and techniques to perpetuate this procedure. Frank Alvine (Agility Ankle; DePuy, Warsaw, IN), Hakon Kofoed (Scandinavian Total Ankle Replacement [STAR]; W. Link GmbH and Co, Hamburg, Germany), and Fred Buechel (Low Contact Stress [LCS]/Buechel-Pappas Ankle; Endotec, South Orange, NJ) managed to develop and refine designs that are still currently in use; these designs have served as the foundations for current developments in TAA. Without the persistence of these individuals, the art of TAA may have ceased because of the original failures. (2) Several important studies have shown favorable outcomes with second-generation implants.[1-4]

(3) Several long-term outcome studies of ankle arthrodeses showed that although many patients do well initially with an ankle arthrodesis, some will ultimately suffer debilitating, secondary adjacent hindfoot arthritis in the subtalar and talonavicular joints.[5,6] This secondary hindfoot arthritis is so debilitating that it has prompted some surgeons to convert ankle arthrodeses to ankle replacements.[7] (4) TAA affords a nearly physiologic gait pattern in comparison with that of ankle arthrodesis using validated outcome measures.[8-10]

First-generation, cemented, constrained, two-component designs were replaced with first-generation, cementless, two-component designs, specifically the Agility Ankle[4] and the ceramic, polyethylene-lined TNK ankle (Kyocera, Kyoto, Japan).[11] Second-generation, three-component implants with minimal constraint are currently being used internationally. These implants include the STAR, Hintegra ankle replacement (New Deal SA, Lyon, France), the Salto prosthesis (Tornier SAS, Saint Ismier, France), the Buechel-Pappas ankle, Mobility (DePuy), and the Bologna Oxford (BOX) ankle (Finsbury, Leatherhead, Surrey, UK). Other three-component TAAs also have been developed, including the ESKA implant (GmbH and Co), the Ankle Evolution System (AES; Biomet, Dordrecht, Netherlands), the OSG ankle (Corin, Cirencester, England), the Albatross (Groupe Lepine, Lyon, France), and the Ramses (Fournitures Hospitaliers, Mulhouse, France). Three more designs in early trials are the CCI Evolution (van Straten Medical/Argomedical, Doets, Germany), the German Ankle System (ARGE Medizintechnik, Hannover, Germany), and the Al-

phamed ankle (Alphamed Medizintechnik Fischer GmbH, Lassnitzhöhe, Austria).

For the past decade, the Agility Ankle has been the only total ankle prosthetic design system approved by the US Food and Drug Administration (FDA). In 2006, the FDA approved three new two-component prostheses, the INBONE total ankle system (INBONE Orthopaedics, Boulder, CO), the Salto-Talaris (Tornier, Stafford, TX), and the Eclipse (Integra Life Sciences Holding Corporation, Plainsboro, NJ). To date, no three-component design has received full FDA approval; however, in April 2007 the STAR prosthesis was granted conditional FDA approval but with the need to fulfill several requirements before release to the US market.

This chapter focuses on total ankle replacement designs with FDA approval and/or available peer-reviewed outcome studies. The Agility is the only TAA system that has both FDA approval and intermediate to long-term peer-reviewed outcome data. The STAR, Buechel-Pappas, Hintegra, and Salto prostheses lack FDA approval but have more than 2 years of follow-up data in peer-reviewed outcome studies. The INBONE and Salto-Talaris prostheses also will be discussed because they are currently being used in the United States. Despite FDA approval, little information is available for the Eclipse, and it has had limited use to date. Although the Mobility and BOX implants lack both FDA approval and peer-reviewed outcomes data exceeding 2 years, these prostheses will be mentioned because these designs provide insight into recent developments in TAA.[12-14]

Whereas the hip is dislocated and the knee subluxated during arthro-

plasty procedures, TAA implants must be placed in situ.[15] The techniques to perform TAA vary with prosthetic design and the required implant-specific instrumentation. Although many complications in TAA surgery are common to all ankles, some are unique to a specific ankle replacement design. Few TAA outcome studies are available in the literature. A recent systematic meta-analysis of the three-component TAAs (1,086 patients) observed that only 18 of 1,830 citations fulfilled the eligibility criteria for a satisfactory, evidence-based study.[16] Using a standardized 100-point ankle and hindfoot score, formal data pooling was possible for only 10 trials and 497 patients. Nonetheless, many of these studies report on complications, providing knowledge about each ankle design.

Indications/Contraindications
Overview
Patient selection is critical in ankle arthroplasty for this relatively small but major weight-bearing joint. Good candidates for TAA have lower activity demands and are middle-aged or elderly patients with painful ankle arthritis (either traumatic or inflammatory), without osteopenia or osteoporosis. Ankle replacement is an end-stage procedure designed to relieve pain experienced with activities of daily living; it is not intended to enable patients to return to jobs requiring heavy labor or participate in impact athletics. Candidates for TAA must have satisfactory peripheral perfusion, intact sensation, and physiologic neuromuscular function. Patients with peripheral vascular disease, concomitant skin disorders, neuropathy, or Charcot joints are not suited to treatment with this procedure. Active and chronic ankle infections represent

absolute contraindications. Osteonecrosis, either of the tibial plafond or talus, is a relative contraindication (for example, patients with avascular bone segments that cannot be resected at surgery are poor candidates for TAA). However, if the avascular segment can be resected with adequate bone remaining to support an implant, TAA may be considered.

Prior Hindfoot Arthrodesis

End-stage ankle arthritis associated with prior subtalar or triple arthrodeses may represent an ideal indication for TAA because ankle arthrodesis would add further rigidity to an already stiff ankle-hindfoot complex. However, a previous hindfoot arthrodesis that compromises the primary talar blood supply (sinus tarsi artery) may lead to subsequent talar component subsidence. Talar implants that require resection of the medial and/or lateral talar dome surfaces (such as STAR, Hintegra, and Salto) or implants that do not use the entire prepared talar surface (such as the first-generation Agility talar component) may be particularly prone to subsidence. In contrast, the INBONE, Buechel-Pappas, Mobility, and BOX talar components preserve the medial and lateral talar dome cortices and are potentially more protective against subsidence. Currently, no evidence exists to determine whether preserving medial/lateral cortical support to the talar dome or creating greater surface area for bone ingrowth with medial/lateral talar dome resection confers a greater advantage in talar component survivorship.

Ligament Insufficiency

Similar to knee replacement, soft-tissue balancing is critical in TAA. Preoperative varus tilting in the ankle typically demands lateral ankle ligament reconstruction and potentially some deltoid ligament release. Although TAA in patients with medial (deltoid) ligament laxity is feasible, nonreconstructible ligament instability, particularly deltoid ligament absence, represents a contraindication to TAA because a satisfactory procedure for deltoid ligament reconstruction has not been perfected. Many preoperative deformities occur secondary to chronic ligament imbalance; resultant tibial plafond erosions secondary to long-standing talar tilt will create edge loading within the ankle mortise, which can result in asymmetric wear of the tibia and/or talus. Standard tibial and talar preparation with or without minor bone grafting normally addresses these bony deficiencies.

Malalignment

Varus or valgus talar tilt in the ankle mortise in patients with end-stage ankle arthritis can be corrected with TAA. Although no absolute degree of talar tilt has been established as a limit to correction with TAA, anecdotal experience suggests that talar tilt exceeding 10° to 20° may represent a contraindication for TAA. In patients with preoperative ligament instability and/or malalignment, the surgeon should obtain preoperative informed consent to intraoperatively abandon TAA in favor of arthrodesis when satisfactory alignment and balance cannot be established. Haskell and Mann[17] suggested that patients with incongruent ankle joints (talar tilt within ankle mortise) were at greater risk for progressive edge loading of a TAA. Extra-articular deformities are generally best addressed with periarticular (supramalleolar or calcaneal) osteotomies. Although these osteotomies can be performed simultaneously with TAA, staging these procedures separately before TAA may be safer and may occasionally alleviate the patient's symptoms adequately to delay the need for TAA, similar to periarticular osteotomies for arthritis of the knee.[18-21]

Preoperative Range of Motion

As for other joints being considered for joint arthroplasty, preoperative range of motion (ROM) of an arthritic joint typically predicts postoperative ROM. Patients with less than 10° of ankle ROM may function equally well after arthrodesis because even uncomplicated TAA in these patients may not reliably increase ROM.

Implant Design
Overview

The ideal ankle implant has yet to be developed. However, current expectations for TAA are (1) reproducible technique, (2) minimal bone resection, (3) rapid and adequate bone ingrowth, (4) minimal constraint, (5) replication of physiologic ankle motion (optimal soft-tissue tensioning throughout ambulation), (6) minimal complications and need for early revision, (7) long-term survivorship, and (8) predictable pain relief. In general, past experiences demonstrate that successful total hip and total knee arthroplasty designs closely mimic the anatomy of the joints they replace. Although it is logical that TAA designs and human ankle joint anatomy and function should converge, this is not necessarily the situation for all currently marketed implants. Some designs closely mimic human ankle joint morphology, whereas others differ considerably from normal anatomy. Of note, morphologic ankle joint measurements collected in 36 individuals with normal ankle anatomy show that the bones of the ankle are in direct proportion to each

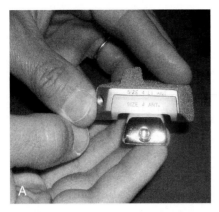 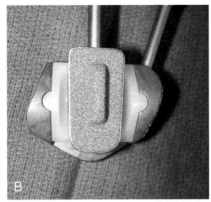 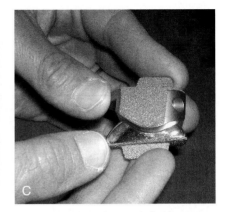

Figure 1   The Agility ankle prosthesis. **A,** Front view. **B,** Footprint of the talar component. **C,** View from the medial side.

other.[22] The implication with this finding is that developing an inventory of progressively larger, anatomically precise TAA component sizes is appropriate.

Currently, more than 20 different designs are either released for clinical use or are in development internationally. FDA approval for TAA implantation is currently restricted to two component designs, with the exception of the STAR, which was approved in March 2007 with some additional requirements before release. Specifically, the Agility, the INBONE, the Salto-Talaris, and the Eclipse prostheses are approved, with the Salto-Talaris being a fixed-bearing modification of the mobile-bearing Salto prosthesis. These designs are approved for use with cement only, and thus are all used "off-label." Outside the United States, the mobile-bearing, three-component prostheses have been favored over fixed-bearing, two-component designs. Implantation of three-component prostheses in the United States has been limited to select FDA-monitored clinical trials.

Specific Implant Designs
Agility Prosthesis
Overview/Primary Design
The Agility total ankle prosthesis was

designed in 1984 and is one of the few current TAA designs with FDA approval (Figure 1). Although approved for use with cement, it is routinely used off-label without cement, provided informed consent is obtained from the patient. The inventory of the Agility includes six sizes of matching tibial and talar components. Unique to this design is a titanium alloy tibial component with an ongrowth surface that rests simultaneously on the tibial plafond and inner aspects of the medial and lateral malleoli. Proper tibial component positioning requires resection of the residual tibial plafond articular surface and the articular surfaces of both malleoli. To facilitate this combined tibial/fibular support, a syndesmotic fusion is necessary for a successful outcome; a requirement unique to the Agility system.[2,4,23] This fixed-bearing implant has a size-matched, separate, high-density polyethylene insert that slides into the tibial component. This articular surface is rotated 22° externally to mimic ankle anatomy. The most recent designs afford greater tibial plafond and talar dome coverage than the original models, and a front-loading polyethylene component insert helps to facilitate polyethylene exchange. The talar

component is an onlay cobalt-chromium replacement of the talar dome, with a bone ingrowth surface facing the residual talar dome. A concern for talar component subsidence has prompted revamping of the original posteriorly tapered design to a nearly rectangular flared base (originally, the posterior taper was intended to limit posterior impingement). Currently available tibial and talar components have single fins, also with bone ingrowth surfaces, to provide greater stability. In an attempt to further limit subsidence, a broader, multifinned talar component also has been designed.

Revision Components
Revision components are available for the talar and polyethylene implants. With the tibial and talar components implanted, the original polyethylene insert was difficult to exchange in revision surgery because it inserted vertically. Now, the revision polyethylene component has half columns that allow it to be inserted from the front, and it is 2 mm thicker than the standard polyethylene component. The revision talar component has a completely rectangular base and a 2-mm increase in vertical thickness relative to the primary implant. These op-

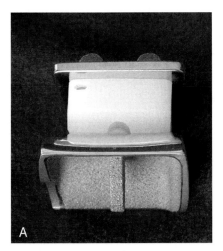 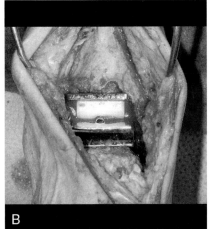 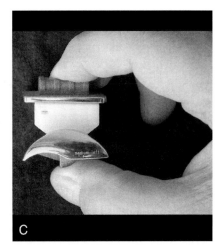

Figure 2 STAR prosthesis. **A,** Front view. **B,** Implanted at the time of surgery. **C,** Side view.

tions afford the potential to increase the total height of the revision prosthesis by 4 mm. Custom revision implants feature stemmed talar and tibial components.

Biomechanics

Motion in the Agility ankle prosthesis is constrained by the implant's articulating surfaces and the ankle ligaments.[24-26] In a cadaver model simulating physiologic motion and loading during a walking cycle, the anterior talofibular and tibiocalcaneal ligaments proved to be reasonable guides for tibial component positioning. The anterior talofibular and tibiocalcaneal ligaments were shown to be sensitive to transverse plane and coronal plane displacements, respectively.

In another study, 10 cadaveric specimens were implanted with the Agility ankle prosthesis and axially loaded to 700 N.[27] The average contact pressure of the system was 5.6 MPa with mean peak pressures of 21.2 MPa. When physiologic ankle forces are considered for routine patient activity, peak pressures may exceed recommended contact pressures (10 MPa) and the compressive yield point (13 to 22 MPa) for poly-

ethylene. Based on the contact pressure data, the investigators suggested that a heavy patient with a larger ankle may be a better candidate for this procedure than a heavy patient with a small ankle.

STAR Prosthesis
Overview

The STAR Prosthesis, designed in 1981, is the prototypical three-component TAA (Figure 2). The original two-piece cemented prosthesis evolved into the current three-piece, meniscal-bearing, ongrowth design. The symmetrically trapezoidal tibial component is wider in the front and has two cylinders or barrels that provide an interference fit with the prepared tibial surface.

The symmetrically convex, bone ingrowth, talar component resurfaces the talar dome (including the medial and lateral aspects) so that the talar implant articulates with the polyethylene meniscus and the ankle's natural malleolar articular surfaces. To accomplish this, the medial and lateral articular surfaces of the talus are resected. Support for the talar cap is enhanced by a single bone ingrowth fin. A criticism of this talar component design is a fail-

ure to respect the relatively smaller medial curvature and larger lateral radius of curvature of the natural talus, which may occasionally lead to relatively loose lateral ligaments and relatively tight medial ligaments after implantation. The high density polyethylene implant is concave on its inferior surface and articulates with the domed talar component. The congruent talar convexity and polyethylene concavity maintain anteroposterior polyethylene stability. The articulating dorsal talar component surface has a smooth, central, longitudinally oriented ridge that congruently articulates with a groove in the inferior polyethylene surface to maintain proper mediolateral polyethylene position. The increased constraint created by these features at the polyethylene-talar component interface is offset by the nonconstrained tibial component polyethylene interface; the flat superior polyethylene surface freely glides on the flat, polished, tibial component. The bony interfaces of the cobalt-chromium metal implants have a titanium spray coating to promote bony ingrowth; alternatively, outside the United States, a hydroxyapatite coating is available.

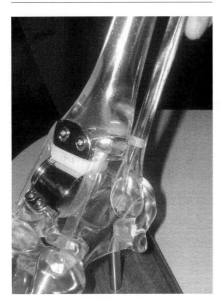

Figure 3 Hintegra ankle prosthesis.

Talar component inventory includes five sizes. The tibial component is available in anteroposterior dimensions of 30, 35, 40, and 45 mm, with widths only varying from 30 to 32.5 mm. The polyethylene component increases in 1-mm increments between 6 and 10 mm. Polyethylene revision components are manufactured in 1-mm increments from 11 mm to 15 mm. A revision tibial-stemmed component is available; however, to date no revision talar component is available without custom specifications.

Biomechanics

Testing in cadavers demonstrates that optimal polyethylene thickness and sagittal plane talar component positioning maximize ankle ROM and limit polyethylene lift-off.[28] Six cadaver ankles with STAR prostheses were tested under weight-bearing conditions to determine ROM, while the strain in the ankle ligaments was monitored. Each specimen was tested with the talar component positions in neutral, 3 mm, and 6 mm of anterior and pos-

terior displacement. The sequence was repeated with an anatomic bearing thickness, as well as at 2 mm reduced and increased thicknesses. Both anterior talar component displacement and bearing thickness reduction caused a decrease in plantar flexion, associated with polyethylene lift-off. With increased bearing thickness, posterior displacement of the talar component decreased plantar flexion, whereas anterior displacement decreased dorsiflexion.

Another study evaluated the function of the ankle joint during walking before and after STAR implantation. Nine patients were evaluated both preoperatively and postoperatively in a gait analysis laboratory. Arthroplasty patients showed reduced ankle ROM compared with normal control subjects. However, postoperative arthroplasty patients had significantly improved external ankle dorsiflexion moment when compared with their preoperative status, suggesting improved function of the ankle joint.[9]

Hintegra Prosthesis
Overview

The Hintegra total ankle prosthesis was designed in 2000 (Figure 3). Much like the STAR prosthesis, the Hintegra is a nonconstrained, three-component system that provides inversion/eversion stability. Axial rotation and normal flexion/extension mobility are provided by a mobile-bearing element with limits to motion imposed only by natural soft-tissue constraints. No more than 2 to 3 mm of bone removal on each side of the joint is necessary to insert the tibial and talar components.

Flat-cut tibial preparation affords apposition of the tibial component with structurally sound subchondral bone. To eliminate coronal plane micromotion in the immediate

postoperative period, two screws may be inserted through the anterior phalange of the tibial component. These screws do not lock into the oval holes of the tibial component; instead, they are inserted into the superior aspect of these holes so the benefit of axial loading is not limited in optimizing apposition between resected tibial plafond and tibial component.

The talar component caps the entire talar dome, necessitating not only superior surface resection but also medial and lateral dome subchondral bone removal for the talar implant to articulate with the natural malleolar articular surfaces. The talar component has an asymmetric dual-radius curvature, with a smaller radius of curvature on the medial rather than the lateral sides. The sides of the talar component hemiprosthetically replace medial and lateral talar facets, mimicking the morphology of the physiologic talus. An anterior extension from the talar component to the talar neck features two holes that permit screw fixation if desired. The talar component has two pegs that create greater stability, and the slightly curved medial and lateral component surfaces afford press-fit fixation, making screw fixation optional. The curved superior articular surface of the talar component is congruent with the polyethylene insert and controls sagittal plane position of the polyethylene. Medial and lateral rails on the borders of the dorsal talar surface control the coronal plane position of the polyethylene. Theoretically, the increased constraint created by these features at the polyethylene-talar component interface is offset by the nonconstrained tibial component polyethylene interface; the flat superior polyethylene surface freely glides on the flat, polished, tibial component.

Biomechanics

In biomechanical testing, Valderrabano and associates[24-26] compared cadaver ankles that were normal, had been treated with arthrodesis, or had been implanted with either the Agility, STAR, or Hintegra prostheses, with the Hintegra most closely reproducing physiologic ankle ROM in their cadaver model. The investigation showed that the three-component ankles (Hintegra, STAR) afforded motion that approached that of the unoperated cadaver ankle.[24] In contrast, the study suggested that the fixed-bearing, two-component design (Agility) restricted talar motion within the ankle mortise, thereby increasing stress/constraint at the bone-implant interface.[24] The authors concluded that successful TAA relies on how effectively designs can mimic physiologic human ankle movement transfer, while simultaneously dissipating rotational forces and maintaining joint stability.[24-26] In particular, these investigators noted that an anatomic talar component design conferred a biomechanical advantage over nonanatomic designs.

Another study suggested that establishing physiologic hindfoot alignment is essential for optimal foot and ankle function, and preoperative malalignment should be corrected. Using the Heidelberg Foot Model, Muller and associates[29] analyzed 11 patients with the unilateral Hintegra ankle prosthesis. Although the timing of the kinematics between the physiologically normal and operated extremities appeared similar, diminished ROM was found in all operated foot segments. A limitation in hindfoot mobility, as experienced after ankle arthrodesis, was not observed. Concerning kinetics, the replaced ankle showed a decrease in power generation compensated by an increase in power in the ipsilateral knee.

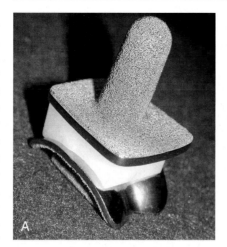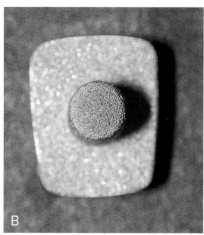

Figure 4 Buechal-Pappas implant. **A,** Ankle components. **B,** View from top stem.

Buechel-Pappas Implant
Overview
The original LCS TAA implant designed by Buechel and Pappas evolved into the current Buechel-Pappas implant[30,31] (Figure 4). The first-generation device (Mark I) was first implanted in 1978 and was modified into the second-generation device (Mark II) in 1989.[1,30-32] The Buechel-Pappas design has three components. The tibial component has a flat, polished platform that articulates with the flat superior polyethylene surface, and a central stem requires that a window be cut into the anterior tibial cortex for its implantation into the tibial metaphysis. The convex talar component has a single radius and a central sulcus that is congruent with the inferior polyethylene surface. This configuration controls coronal plane polyethylene translation and permits a mild degree of inversion/eversion while maintaining full conformity and limiting the risk of edge loading. The constraint created by the polyethylene talar implant is offset by the flat interface between the tibial component and polyethylene articulations. Modifications that have led

to the currently available design include a thicker tibial component, a second talar component backside fin for improved fixation, a titanium nitride porous coating to enhance bone ingrowth, and a deeper talar sulcus for improved polyethylene stability. A nitride ceramic film on the titanium articulating surfaces may afford improved wear characteristics with the polyethylene insert. The talar component only resurfaces the superior aspect of the talar dome; the medial and lateral cartilage is left intact to continue physiologic articulation with the malleolar articular surfaces.

Biomechanics
A fluoroscopic evaluation of 10 patients with unilateral Buechel-Pappas implants showed an average ROM of 37.4° for normal ankles and 32.3° for implanted ankles. Implanted ankles showed rotational and translational motion but had relatively more posterior talar contact, particularly with plantar flexion, when compared with the nonoperated ankles. The authors suggested that the increased posterior contact was related to surgical technique or alterations of ligamentous tension.[33]

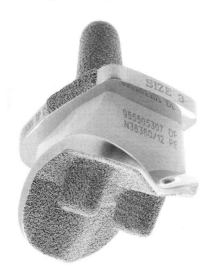

Figure 5 Mobility ankle prosthesis.

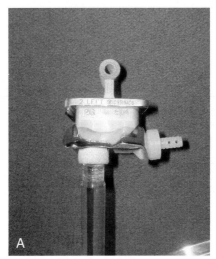
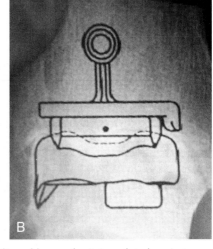

Figure 6 **A,** Salto ankle prosthesis. **B,** Salto ankle prosthesis templated against a radiograph.

Mobility Total Ankle System
Overview
The Mobility Total Ankle System was developed by a surgeon design team in collaboration with DePuy and became commercially available in October 2004 (Figure 5). The device was first implanted in September 2003 and has been released for general use in Europe, Australia, New Zealand, South Africa, and Canada. In the United States, a multicenter FDA trial comparing the Agility and Mobility prostheses has been initiated.

The Mobility unconstrained, three-component, mobile-bearing prosthesis resembles the Buechel-Pappas total ankle system. The short, conical stem, set on the central nonarticulating aspect of the tibial component, is similar to the Buechel-Pappas implant. However, the sagittal plane dimensions of the tibial component exceed those of the Buechel-Pappas implant to optimize tibial plafond coverage while being tapered posteriorly to avoid overhang and soft-tissue impingement. The talar component resurfaces only the superior dome of the talus without violating the native medial and lateral aspects of the talar dome like the Buechel-Pappas implant. The talar component also features a central, longitudinal sulcus. Talar component stability is enhanced by two fins on the nonarticulating aspect of the implant. The constraint imparted by the conforming, congruent interface of the talar component and polyethylene insert is dissipated by the flat tibial component-polyethylene articulation. The porous coated, nonarticulating metal surfaces are covered with a titanium spray.

Comparison
In simulated mechanical testing by the manufacturer, the Mobility total ankle prosthesis compares favorably with the Buechel-Pappas implant. Similar shear loads were required to dislocate the Mobility and Buechel-Pappas bearing inserts in both the sagittal and coronal planes. However, under similar circumstances, the Mobility talar component was less likely to subside when compared with the Buechel-Pappas talar component. In a comparative study of stability testing performed at Leeds University and sponsored by DePuy, researchers noted (in an internal company document) that the Mobility prosthesis demonstrated significantly higher average peak loads to failure in the coronal and sagittal planes compared with the Buechel-Pappas implant.[34] Similarly, in a simulator test, the wear rate for the Mobility ankle prosthesis was less than that of the Buechel-Pappas implant.[35]

Salto and Salto-Talaris Prostheses
Overview
The three-component Salto TAA prosthesis was designed in 1998 and offers a unique and optional polyethylene fibular implant to articulate with the lateral talar component (Figure 6); however, the fibular component is now rarely used. Tibial component stability is enhanced by a central pedestal-like stem that necessitates a keyhole-shaped anterior tibial cortical window for insertion. Medially, a low-profile medial rail extends vertically from the horizontal tibial surface that protects the medial malleolus and limits medial

translation of the polyethylene insert.

Because of the restrictions imposed by the FDA on three-component TAA devices implanted in the United States, the two-component Salto-Talaris prosthesis (Figure 7) was recently introduced and is essentially the fixed-bearing version of the Salto prosthesis. The polyethylene component is secured to the tibial component via a locking mechanism and no fibular component is available. The Salto-Talaris prosthesis was approved for use in the United States in November 2006. The manufacturer introduced the concept of "mobile-bearing instruments." Although the tibia and talus are prepared separately, the orientation of the bony cuts are at least in part interrelated to facilitate the symmetrical articulation of the talar and fixed-bearing tibial components. With the talar component seated, an instrument unique to the Salto-Talaris system allows the surgeon to determine the ideal tibial component position relative to tracking of the talus within the ankle mortise. The tibial component is then fixed in that position. However, with larger component sizes, this "auto-alignment" feature may be limited by the ankle's coronal dimensions because the tibial component may not have sufficient space to rotate.

The concave talar component resurfaces the talar dome and mimics physiologic talar morphology, with the medial radius being shorter than the lateral radius. Although the lateral aspect of the talar component fully resurfaces the lateral talar dome, the medial side does not. Medially, the natural talar dome is not violated. The superior surface of the talar component has a central, sagittal sulcus that conforms to the

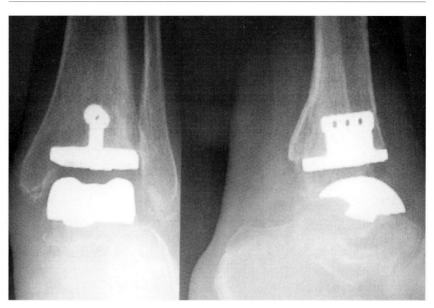

Figure 7 AP (left) and lateral (right) radiographic views of the Salto-Talaris ankle prosthesis.

central ridge on the inferior polyethylene surface. This configuration affords coronal plane stability and limits the risks for polyethylene dislocation while reducing edge loading. The conformity of the polyethylene to the talar component combined with the medial stop mechanism of the tibial component creates some degree of constraint. The tibial and talar components are made of cobalt-chromium and feature a titanium spray ingrowth surface; only the Salto prosthesis (not the Salto-Talaris) has a hydroxyapatite coating.

BOX Prosthesis
Overview
The name BOX is derived from the joint efforts of the prostheses designers from the Istituti Ortopedici Rizzoli, Bologna, Italy, and the laboratory in Oxford, England. Like the Buechel-Pappas and Mobility prostheses, the BOX does not resurface the sides of the talus, only the superior dome. Similar to the STAR prosthesis, the BOX has ingrowth

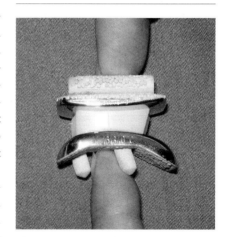

Figure 8 BOX ankle prosthesis.

cylinders on its tibial base plate. It has an anatomic talar component with the radius of curvature longer than that of the natural talus in the sagittal plane, and a fully conforming meniscal component. It is made of cobalt-chromium with a titanium spray coating on its surface. The BOX has a unique design with a convex tibial component that articulates with a biconcave polyethylene spacer (Figure 8).

Biomechanics

Several researchers described how the unique BOX prosthetic design maintains optimal biomechanical behavior of coupled human ankle-hindfoot physiologic motion, while allowing complete congruence over the entire range of ankle motion. Claiming the first realistic representation of the biomechanical behavior of a prosthetic joint replacing a human ankle, researchers noted that the meniscal bearing of the BOX ankle prosthesis was observed to move 5.6 mm posteriorly during the simulated stance, and the corresponding anteroposterior displacement of the talar component was 8.3 mm.[13,14] The predicted pattern and the amount (10.6°) of internal-external rotation of the ankle complex were found to be in agreement with corresponding in vivo measurements on normal ankles. A peak contact pressure of 16.8 MPa was observed, with most of the contact pressures below 10 MPa. For most ligaments, reaction forces remain within corresponding physiologic ranges.[14] Preliminary observations in trial implantation in a few patients suggest that while reproducing physiologic ankle mobility, the new design is capable of maintaining complete congruence at the two articulating surfaces of the meniscal bearing over the entire motion arc, with the prospect of minimizing wear of this component.[12]

In another study, one of the designers of the BOX prosthesis found that rolling as well as sliding motion occurs in the natural ankle, governed by a ligamentous linkage.[36] Elongation of the tibiocalcaneal and calcaneofibular ligaments was 1.5% and 4.8%, respectively. A 13% change in lever arm length occurred for both the tibialis anterior and gastrocnemius muscles during ankle flexion. Unlike the currently available three-component designs, the newly proposed convex, tibial ligament-compatible prosthesis was found to restore the original mobility and physiologic function of the ligaments. The authors believe that the BOX prosthesis combines freedom from restraint with congruity of the components throughout the range of flexion. The designers also evaluated the kinematics of the ankle when replaced by nonconforming two-component designs and by fully conforming three-component designs with flat, concave, or convex tibial surfaces; these designs were assessed by their dynamic ankle joint simulation model. A ligament-compatible, convex-tibia, fully congruent three-component prosthesis showed the best features. The three-component prosthesis allows complete congruence over the entire ROM.[36] A convex shape for the tibial arc was preferred because of the improved degree of entrapment of the meniscal bearing. A 5-cm, convex-tibia arc radius provided 2 mm of entrapment together with 9.8 mm of tibial bone cut. Ligament elongation imposed by full congruence of the articular surfaces was less than 0.03% of the original length. The original patterns of joint kinematics and ligament tensioning were closely restored in the joint replaced by the proposed prosthesis.[37]

INBONE Prosthesis
Overview

The INBONE total ankle system is a fixed-bearing, two-component design with a modular stem system for both tibia and talar components (Figure 9). Multiple modular segments may be added to the tibial stem, depending on the surgeon's determination of how much stability is needed or the distance the stem should pass beyond a simultaneous supramalleolar osteotomy performed for tibial malunion. The tibia is inset into the tibial metaphysis but, unlike the Agility, does not resurface the malleoli. The talar component entirely replaces the superiormost aspect of the natural talus, after a flat dome resection. The stem of the talar component may be limited to the body of the talus or can be extended across the subtalar joint into the calcaneus if greater support for the talar component is required, or when a simultaneous subtalar arthrodesis is warranted. The longer talar component calcaneal stem is not currently FDA approved.

Unique to the INBONE total ankle system is the alignment guide placed after the ankle is exposed via an anterior approach. The device demands simultaneous alignment of the talus with the tibia in both the coronal and sagittal planes. Once that is achieved, a drill is passed from the plantar foot through the calcaneus, just anterior to the posterior facet of the subtalar joint, through the center of the talar body into the center of the tibial metaphysis; much like the guide pin for a retrograde ankle arthrodesis nail. Although many surgeons believe that it is undesirable to violate the subtalar joint when performing TAA, the designers of this alignment guide maintain that appropriate application of the device permits the 6-mm drill to safely negotiate the subtalar joint between the arterial anastomosis on the inferior talar neck and the articulation of the posterior facet with the inferior talus.

Biomechanics

No reports are yet available documenting the kinematics of the INBONE ankle prosthesis in biomechanical testing. More information is needed to define the biome-

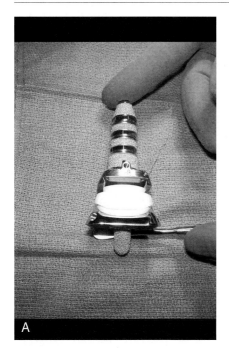
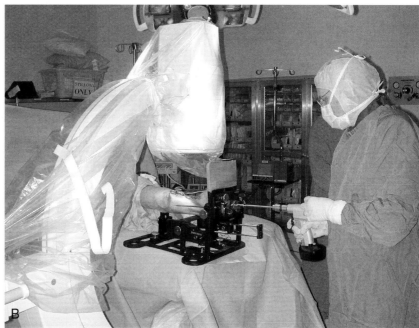

Figure 9   **A,** INBONE ankle prosthesis with the polyethylene component not yet inserted. **B,** Leg holder used to insert INBONE ankle prosthesis.

chanical characteristics of the INBONE total ankle system.

Surgical Technique
Overview
Relative to arthroplasties of other joints, the surgical technique for TAA is demanding because the soft tissue envelope is relatively vulnerable, vital neurovascular structures are in close proximity to the joint, and the ankle cannot be dislocated to improve exposure. Implant alignment determined intraoperatively under non–weight-bearing conditions is subject to tibiotalar joint distortions, the affected limb's mechanical axis, and the multiplanar function of the ankle-hindfoot complex. Similar to total knee arthroplasty in concept, bone resection alone in TAA does not determine alignment; optimal polyethylene articulation with the tibial and talar components requires proper soft-tissue balance. Soft-tissue balancing about the ankle and hindfoot for

TAA may necessitate lateral ligament reconstruction and/or a medial deltoid release and/or lengthening of the Achilles tendon either with a percutaneous triple hemisection or a gastrocnemius release. Unlike total knee arthroplasty, soft-tissue balancing techniques for TAA lack standardization but are evolving.

Exposure and Closure
Although most TAA prostheses are implanted via an anterior approach, several implants are inserted via a transfibular approach. All prostheses mentioned in this chapter are implanted via the more conventional anterior approach except the ESKA, which is inserted laterally, and the Eclipse (Figure 10), which can be inserted medially or laterally. The other designs use a longitudinal anterior skin incision to expose the extensor retinaculum, which is divided directly medial to the extensor hallucis longus (EHL) tendon. Dis-

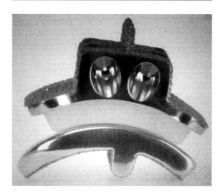

Figure 10   Eclipse ankle prosthesis.

tally, the superficial peroneal nerve is at risk for injury during this approach. The interval to the anterior ankle is between the tibialis anterior and EHL. By avoiding an incision directly over the tibialis anterior tendon and shifting the division of the extensor retinaculum toward the EHL tendon, less tension will be placed on the fibrous retinaculum by the tibialis anterior after closure. However, located immediately deep to the EHL is the anterior tibial

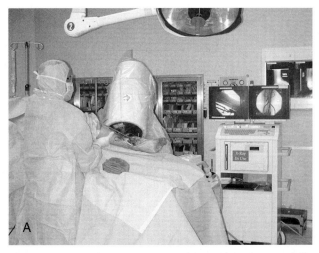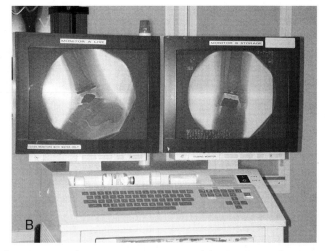

Figure 11 **A,** Fluoroscopy is used to confirm extramedullary alignment. **B,** Fluoroscopic inspection of the STAR prosthesis at the end of the arthroplasty procedure.

artery and deep peroneal nerve. With the neurovascular structures and tendons protected, an anterior capsulotomy is performed.

A layered closure of the anterior ankle capsule, extensor retinaculum, subcutaneous tissue, and skin affords the joint more than one barrier in the event of wound dehiscence. Also, by maintaining the extensor retinaculum over the tibialis anterior, wound suction appliances and split-thickness skin grafts, in lieu of free-tissue transfer, may be feasible in situations involving wound breakdown. To minimize the risk for skin necrosis, direct skin retraction should be avoided throughout the procedure; however, deep retractors (Adson-Beckman, Langenbeck, or Gelpi) are recommended to avoid repetitive trauma or excessive tension to the skin with subsequent creation of vascular channel blockers.

Tibial and Talar Preparation

Most surgeons familiar with TAA agree that the tibial cut must be perpendicular to the tibial shaft axis in the coronal plane, with slight dorsi-flexion in the sagittal plane for success of the procedure. This concept is no different than that of tibial preparation in total knee arthroplasty—perpendicular in the coronal plane with a slight posterior slope in the sagittal plane. For TAA the trend is similar to findings of outcomes studies for total knee arthroplasty—a tibial cut made in varus produces a higher failure rate than neutral-symmetric tibial cuts. External tibial alignment guides align the tibial cutting block for tibial preparation. Except for a few select experts (who may even perform freehand cuts), most surgeons confirm proper tibial cutting block alignment with intraoperative fluoroscopy. The use of a large fluoroscopic C-arm to assess alignment intraoperatively facilitates instant assessment of the alignment relative to the tibia (Figure 11, *A*); a mini C-arm limits the surgeon's ability to evaluate proper alignment and is not recommended. Only a few degrees of malalignment negatively influence ligamentous tensioning and/or the compressive effect of the prosthesis on adjacent bone. Once proper

alignment is established, it is particularly important to orient the saw directly centrally and posteriorly, carefully avoiding saw blade excursion into the malleoli.

Initial talar dome preparation is typically performed by a cutting guide suspended or aligned from the same base that supported the tibial cutting block. The initial talar cut has the chance of creating a relatively serious and perhaps irreversible complication. Nowhere is the "ship in the bottle" analogy to TAA more relevant than with the initial talar preparation because the cutting guide obscures most of the joint, and visualization is further compromised by the saw that must be held directly over the joint. With minor saw blade deviation or overpenetration, the malleoli and posterior soft-tissue and/or neurovascular structures are at risk. Because the talus is not symmetrically hinged to the tibia, an assistant must maintain proper dorsiflexion and coronal plane position when applying the jigs or cutting the talus to ensure the desired talar cut. Cutting the talus in a plantar-flexed position can lead to excessive posterior talar dome resection, which is particularly true in a patient with an equinus contracture. Overresection of the posterior talus may lead to talar component subsidence. Similarly, holding the foot in excessive dorsiflexion while the talar cutting guide is secured into position or when the talus is cut can lead to anterior overresection and a plantar-flexed talar component, although this resection error is far less likely than overresection of the posterior talus. Poor coronal plane talar position during talar preparation leads to difficulties in proper varus/valgus position or tension on the collateral ligaments.

Component Positioning

Several universal recommendations exist for TAA component positioning. After completing tibial and talar preparation, the talar component should be centered directly beneath the tibia; poorly centered components often result in polyethylene edge loading. Oversizing the prosthesis may lead to friction between the bone and components, a painful ankle, and early polyethylene wear. This is the most commonly reported complication, which is not initially recognized, following TAA. Based on anecdotal experience, the general rule is that in situations of in-between sizing, downsizing is appropriate. Although in most systems the tibial component's coronal dimensions rather than sagittal dimensions determine tibial component size, this is usually a unique feature of the chosen prosthesis. For example, the STAR prosthesis has very similar coronal dimensions and a 15-mm variance in the sagittal plane dimensions of the tibial component. The talar component, aligned with the long axis of the talus, typically parallels the second or third metatarsal.

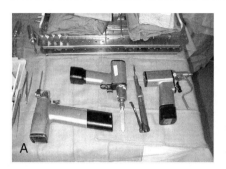 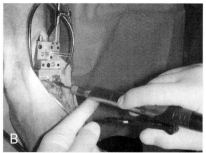

Figure 12   **A,** A variety of saws are used to make surgery safer and easier. **B,** The small reciprocating saw can be used to cut small corners out of bone.

Ideal rotational orientation of the tibial component may be challenging, given the oblique slope of the anterior distal tibia. Placement of an osteotome in the medial gutter of the ankle joint, between the medial malleolus and the medial talar dome, will assist in determining the angle to cut the tibia. However, this technique is prosthesis dependent. For example, the Salto-Talaris instrumentation recommends "splitting" the sagittal alignment angle of the malleolar walls to find the true axis of the talus longitudinally. Because the polyethylene in mobile-bearing prostheses without stop mechanisms (STAR, Hintegra, Buechel-Pappas, and Mobility) is afforded full freedom, some minor degree of malrotation is typically tolerated, or the risk of impingement or edge loading will increase with greater malrotation. The potential for malrotation is probably greatest with the Agility prosthesis. Because the implant requires partial resections of the malleoli, errors in rotation may lead to compromise of the posterior malleolus and, in extreme circumstances, the posteromedial neurovascular bundle. If the cutting block is oriented into external rotation relative to the sagittal plane, the resultant external rotation may be dramatic because the polyethylene is designed with 22° of

external rotation within the tibial component housing. Using the C-arm to confirm trial and final component positioning before leaving the operating room is currently advised (Figure 11, B).

Tools

Three saws are recommended for TAA: a 1-inch nonbending 0.5-inch oscillating saw for flat tibial and talar cuts, a 0.5-inch wide × 3-cm thin reciprocating saw with circumferential and end-cutting ability, and a 0.25-inch × 1-inch reciprocating saw to remove minor bony irregularities with minimal pressure against the bone (Figure 12). A thin oscillating saw is often valuable for trimming flat areas with a ridge of bone. Osteotomes, if levered inappropriately, may lead to intraoperative malleolar fractures, some of which are not detected until postoperative radiographic evaluation. Several TAA surgeons recommend placing prophylactic malleolar guidewire; in the event an intraoperative malleolar fracture occurs, a cannulated screw may be placed over the guidewire.

Soft-Tissue Balancing and Deformity Correction

Bone resection is critical to alignment. However, if ligamentous imbalance is not corrected at the time of surgery, varus or valgus deformity will ensue despite perfect bone cuts. Even though techniques for TAA soft-tissue balancing and corrective osteotomies about the ankle and hindfoot have not been standardized, anecdotal experience is gradually evolving into general guidelines. Simply changing the polyethylene thickness alone is not appropriate in establishing soft-tissue balance for TAA.

Equinus Contracture

Whereas some surgeons routinely perform Achilles tendon lengthening for ankle arthritis associated with equinus, others maintain that the gastrocnemius-soleus complex will gradually stretch out if a posterior capsular release is performed at the time of surgery and proper component implantation is achieved. Typically, increased tibial resection will provide greater motion in TAA; however, there is a fine balance between appropriate and excessive resection.[38] Resecting too much bone from the tibial plafond may result in implant subsidence into the weaker proximal bone, whereas underresection may lead to inadequate dorsiflexion and increased stress on the anterior tibial cortex with weight bearing.

In patients with limited preoperative dorsiflexion, anterior osteophytes are removed and a gastrocnemius recession may be performed. Performing this procedure early in the operation avoids having to stress the "cut bone" with dorsiflexion when the prosthesis is in place and potentially damaging the newly cut surface or fracturing a malleolus. After tibial and talar resections, a posterior capsular release is performed, typically through the anterior incision. Some authors maintain a high threshold for

triple hemisection Achilles tendon lengthening, relying on the posterior capsular release and gradual Achilles tendon accommodation postoperatively. However, if at least 5° of dorsiflexion is not achieved intraoperatively during TAA, the patient will vault over their plantar-flexed forefoot when walking in shoes without heels. Bone resection performed before Achilles tendon lengthening may result in excessive resection of the posterior talus, which (based on anecdotal reports) can lead to talar component subsidence as previously described. When 5° of ankle dorsiflexion cannot be achieved despite adequate bone resection, and a posterior Achilles tendon lengthening has not already been performed, a gastrocnemius recession through a medial approach at the musculotendinous junction of the gastrocnemius-soleus complex is performed; care should be taken to avoid the sural nerve. If gastrocnemius-soleus recession fails to achieve a least 5° of ankle dorsiflexion and tibial resection is appropriate, a percutaneous triple hemisection of the Achilles tendon may be added to further lengthen the Achilles tendon.

Varus Malalignment

Typically, a graduated deltoid ligament release and proper component positioning with appropriate sizing of the polyethylene permits satisfactory soft-tissue balance. Deltoid ligament release can be performed through the anterior approach; occasionally, a small separate incision over the posterior medial malleolus may be required to lengthen otherwise inaccessible tight deltoid fibers. Overrelease can be avoided by limiting the release to the deep deltoid fibers and preserving the superficial fibers. If it is decided that an entire deltoid ligament release is needed, taking the periosteum off the tibia in continuity with the

deltoid ligament can avoid late-term gross medial instability. Lateral ligament attenuation generally warrants lateral ligament stabilization with a modified Broström repair, Evans procedure (augmentation with the anterior third of the peroneus brevis), or a free tendon autograft or allograft reconstruction. Deltoid tightness may not always require deltoid fiber release; instead, appropriate coronal plane positioning of TAA components influences deltoid tension. Additionally, cavus or varus foot positioning may warrant osteotomies and/or arthrodeses of the foot to maintain proper ankle balance; these procedures may either be staged or performed simultaneously with TAA. Commonly performed osteotomies include a lateral closing wedge and/or lateralizing calcaneal osteotomies for valgus deformity, or dorsiflexion, first metatarsal osteotomies for forefoot-driven hindfoot varus. Tibia vara deformity proximal to the ankle may require staged or simultaneous supramalleolar medial opening or lateral closing wedge osteotomies to achieve optimal ankle alignment. Often the fibula is also cut to obtain greater correction.

Valgus Malalignment

Unlike varus deformity, the logical approach of lateral release and medial capsular plication is not reliable or even feasible in most patients. Several techniques for deltoid ligament reconstruction have been proposed but lack objective clinical validation or even adequate anecdotal experience to recommend their use in soft-tissue balancing for TAA.[39] An intraoperative decision to convert to arthrodesis may be prudent when the deltoid ligament is incompetent. Medial displacement calcaneal osteotomies, plantar flexion osteotomies and/or arthrodeses of the medial column, or even supramalleolar medial closing wedge osteotomies may be required to appropriately treat valgus deformities that cannot be corrected with proper bone cuts for TAA and soft-tissue rebalancing alone.

Postoperative Care

Variations in postoperative protocols are used by surgeons performing TAA. Although a surgeon confident in initial implant stability and wound resilience may recommend ROM activities and weight bearing within the first 2 weeks, a more conservative approach may involve 6 weeks of immobilization and protected weight bearing. Generally, most surgeons follow the more conservative approach of allowing patients with uncomplicated, isolated TAA to progress to regular shoe wear by 6 weeks after surgery. Routine, supervised physical therapy is not always warranted, although some patients will require such therapy to achieve maximum ROM. Usually, patients ambulate reasonably well by 3 months and return to full activities (such as golf, walking, and skiing) at 6 months. Further functional improvement is typically observed up to 24 months following successful TAA.

Bone ingrowth requires approximately 6 weeks of protected weight bearing to avoid component micromotion and associated fibrous ingrowth. Initial implant stability varies; therefore, the treating surgeon must determine when to initiate weight bearing and ROM. Enthusiasm for early ankle motion must be tempered by the potential for early manipulation of the wound resulting in delayed healing. Other factors to consider are adjunctive procedures (corrective osteotomies and ligament reconstructions), intraoperative fractures, and time to syndesmotic union (specific to the Agility prosthesis).

Implant-Specific Aspects of Surgical Technique
Agility Prosthesis
Unique Features
Intraoperative medial external fixation, syndesmotic arthrodesis, using a monoblock cutting guide for both the tibia and talus, and resurfacing the medial and lateral malleolar articular surfaces are unique features of the Agility prosthesis. Many surgeons who use other systems view the external fixator as an unnecessary and cumbersome extra step in TAA. However, for surgeons who routinely implant the Agility prosthesis, this extra step adds no more than 10 minutes to the procedure and can be applied (at least the pins) before tourniquet inflation. The advantage of the external fixator is that distraction reduces the amount of bone resection when using the recommended cutting monoblock for both tibial and talar resection. The external fixator also maintains the proper alignment for the bone cuts; if properly applied, no change in ankle position is needed between fluoroscopic confirmation and execution of the bone resections. A disadvantage is that surgeons less experienced with the Agility system may have a false sense of proper alignment with the external fixator in place. The external fixator can easily overpower or mask ankle ligamentous imbalance. Therefore, proper assessment requires release of the external fixator. Overtensioning of the external fixator may lead to an intraoperative malleolar fracture.

Component Positioning
For coronal plane tibial component positioning, the Agility prosthesis is subject to errors related to the resultant effects of deltoid ligament tension. The Agility is the only TAA prosthesis reviewed in this chapter that requires resection of a sizable portion of the medial malleolar articular surface. The Agility prosthesis creates a conflict for the surgeon less experienced with its recommended technique. In an attempt to avoid medial malleolar fracture (a goal in all TAA procedures) a careful surgeon may resect too little medial malleolus. The resultant tibial component lateralization forces the talus and talar component more laterally, thereby overtensioning the deltoid ligament, particularly a deltoid ligament with a preoperative contracture. The clinical effect is a varus talar tilt, edge loading, potential for talar component loosening and/or subsidence, and early polyethylene wear. Fortunately, when potential varus malalignment is observed intraoperatively, more medial malleolus can be resected, the tibial fin cut can be adjusted, and the tibial component properly positioned.

The talus must be positioned properly relative to the monoblock cutting guide of the Agility prosthesis. Direct visualization is often obscured by the instrumentation; therefore, fluoroscopic confirmation in the sagittal plane is desirable. The sagittal axis of the talar component is aligned with the second or third metatarsals. The Agility talar component has been redesigned with a wider base to avoid subsidence. Ideally, the bone interface of the talar component should be sized to cover the maximum resected talar surface without overhang, and the talar component should rest on the posterior cortex of the talar body.

Syndesmotic Fusion
The Agility is the only prosthesis discussed in this chapter that requires syndesmotic débridement

and arthrodesis.[2,4] Although these procedures were originally performed through a separate extensile lateral incision, they may be performed via the single anterior approach. The risk of tibial component migration has been reported to increase 8.5 times if a solid syndesmotic fusion is absent.[4] Use of platelet-rich product mixed with autograft bone from the ankle, autologous concentrated growth factors, and a lateral plate has been reported to improve the syndesmotic fusion rates.[40-42]

STAR Prosthesis

The STAR prosthesis represents the prototypical unconstrained three-component design. The surgical technique used to implant the STAR prosthesis has been described by Anderson and associates.[43]

Tibial Preparation

Tibial preparation is not unique to the STAR design. The cutting block must be properly aligned in the coronal, sagittal, and rotational orientations and may be confirmed using fluoroscopy. The recommended resection level is 5 mm proximal to the anterior tibia, measured after osteophyte removal. Taking into consideration the sagittal plane concavity of the tibial plafond, this generally leads to a 2-mm resection at the midtibial plafond level, similar to recommended resection levels for the most involved tibial hemiplateau in total knee arthroplasty. Proper rotation of the external tibial alignment guide cannot be assessed via fluoroscopy, but a thin osteotome inserted into the medial ankle gutter usually adequately defines rotation. The cutting block has capture guides, but divergence of the saw blade from the true sagittal plane may still result in malleolar injury.

Talar Preparation

Because the talar cutting guide is suspended from the tibial cutting block, it is not a monoblock as described for the Agility prosthesis. Like the surgical technique used for the Agility prosthesis, however, the talus must be positioned in the desired position for ideal resection relative to the fixed cutting guide. Osteophytes may need to be removed from the gutters to ensure that the talus can be placed in its anatomic position for dome resection (avoiding varus). Because the talar block lacks capture guides, it is advisable to place metal ribbon retractors in the gutters to protect the malleoli. Unlike the Agility prosthesis, talar preparation dictates talar component positioning because the talar component is a "talar cap," fully resurfacing the talar dome. The following observations have been made (several of which are applicable to most TAA talar components): oversizing leads to symptomatic malleolar impingement; anterior positioning increases the potential risk of untoward contact stresses, edge loading, and anterior tibial component subsidence; and inadequate posterior talar preparation leads to talar component flexion. Final talar preparation for the STAR prosthesis involves creation of a slot for the talar component fin.

A 4-mm talar resection level is desirable for the STAR prosthesis. In combination with the 5-mm tibial resection, a 9-mm space is created, which is adequate to accommodate the implants with a 6-mm or preferably 7- to 8-mm polyethylene insert. (The 6-mm polyethylene insert has been known to crack in the groove.) Next, the medial and lateral sides of the talar dome are prepared with the lateral cut 5 mm more distal than the medial cut to accommodate the longer lateral aspect of the talar component that articulates with the fibula. A tapered orientation of the medial and lateral cuts (wider anteriorly) dictates sagittal plane position of the talar component. Performed properly, the error of placing the talar component too anteriorly can be avoided.

The STAR system lacks true trial tibial and talar components, but several instruments and steps provide confirmation of appropriate joint preparation. One of these instruments serves to cap the talus to determine ideal polyethylene component thickness. In the authors' experience, the 8-mm spacer should easily fit between the trial talar cap and the tibial cut, simulating the 2-mm thickness of the tibial component, and ensuring that at least a 6-mm polyethylene component can be inserted with both the tibial and talar component implanted. If not, the tibia can be easily recut, as done in total knee arthroplasty.

Final Component Positioning

The tibial component must be centered under the tibial shaft axis. This necessitates proper positioning of the channels for the fixation barrels on the nonarticulating aspect of the tibial component while simultaneously ensuring appropriate tibial component balance in the coronal plane to avoid medial malleolar fracture during tibial component impaction. Because most of the stresses tend to focus on the anterior aspect of the ankle following TAA, the anterior aspect of the tibial implant should rest on the anterior tibial cortex and not be recessed beyond the cortex. Fluoroscopic confirmation of proper component position is recommended. A trial spacer is then used to determine the thickness necessary to achieve ligamentous stability. Residual coronal plane ankle instability can be corrected with lateral ligament reconstruction and/or deltoid ligament release. The trial polyethylene spacer is removed, and the true polyethylene component inserted.

Hintegra Prosthesis

Although Hintegra cutting guides are distinct, tibial and talar preparations resemble those for the STAR prosthesis. As is common with mobile-bearing prostheses, a spacer block is available to evaluate appropriate ligamentous balance. Once proper talar preparation is confirmed, peg holes are created in the talus to accommodate pegs on the nonarticulating talar component surface. The tibial component is centered on the cut surface of the tibial plafond, and its position is clinically confirmed with an anterior phalange contacting the anterior tibial cortex. Optional screw fixation is available for both components.

Buechel-Pappas Implant

Tibial preparation for the Buechel-Pappas implant is similar to that of the STAR and Hintegra, except that an anterior cortical window to accommodate the tibial stem must be created. Ideal tibial component positioning over the talar component (over the polyethylene bearing) avoids edge loading and contact wear. Although not ideal, the cortical window can be recut to allow adjustments in the coronal plane. Because the tibial stem is centered on the tibial component, rotation may easily be altered. Talar preparation preserves physiologic talar subchondral architecture, except that the talar trochlea is deepened to create a 5-mm, central, longitudinal sulcus and two slots to accommodate the fins on the underside of the talar component. Unlike the STAR

and Hintegra, but similar to the Mobility, the medial and lateral talar walls are left intact. Balanced talar component impaction is facilitated with the anterior tibial cortical window. Next, the tibial component is properly seated and the resected tibial window is replaced with added bone graft as needed; this prevents joint fluid from migrating to the tibial stem and backside of the tibial component, which may cause loosening. The polyethylene component of the proper thickness is then inserted.

Mobility Total Ankle System

The instrumentation for the Mobility ankle has been refined from past experience with three-piece designs and allows for AP and lateral-medial centering of tibial and talar components. Combined with a superior tapering of the polyethylene component, optimal centering of the components is believed to result in favorable balancing with less likelihood of polyethylene component overhang. The system also allows for a visual "double check" before every important resection, thus allowing the surgeon to estimate the sufficiency of the initial tibial resection. The general technique for insertion is similar to that used for the Buechel-Pappas implant.

Salto-Talaris Prosthesis

For the Salto-Talaris ankle prosthesis, the tibial alignment guide is stabilized to the tibia with one pin in the tibial tubercle and a second pin in the distal medial tibia. Adjustments to the tibial alignment guide are made to ensure the guide is parallel to the sagittal and coronal axis of the tibia. Optimal sagittal and coronal alignment can be confirmed fluoroscopically. Rotation of the tibial resection guide is determined vi-

sually. Rotation of the tibial component is based on the sagittal axis of the talus. Sizing of the tibial component is determined simultaneously with confirmation of talar rotation. The guide is set to allow 9-mm tibial resection from the apex of the tibial plafond. To determine this resection level, anterior tibial osteophytes must be removed beforehand. Following tibial preparation and removal of most of the cut tibial bone, the foot is held at a 90° angle to the tibia. A talar alignment pin is then placed into the talus through the guide. Next, a posterior chamfer talar dome cutting guide is placed over this pin, secured with three to four additional pins, and the posterior superior talus is cut and the bone removed. An anterior chamfer guide is then positioned, and the anterior superior portion of the talus is planed down with a milling device. Final talar preparation is performed with a third talar cutting guide that allows drilling of both a cylindrical hole to accommodate the talar stem and the cutting of lateral chamfer off the talus. The trial implants are then placed in position. The ankle is dorsiflexed and plantarflexed to allow the tibial component drill guide to rotate into the ideal position relative to the talar implant. Residual lateral tibial bone adjacent to the fibula must be removed to permit this automatic adjustment of the tibial trial implant. Trial polyethylene thicknesses allow for final adjustment of the tension. If adequate dorsiflexion is not possible, additional resection of the tibia or gastrocnemius resection is performed. Final preparation of the tibial component is achieved through pedestal drilling and pedestal strut preparation. The final implants are then inserted and the pedestal area bone grafted to avoid ingress of joint fluid.

INBONE Prosthesis

The approach used with the INBONE prosthesis is identical to that of the other ankles between the tibialis anterior and the EHL. The leg is then placed in the leg holder, and the rotation of the ankle determined by aligning the holder parallel to a 0.25-inch osteotome in the medial mortise. The calcaneus is fixed with two pins, and the foot and lower leg secured to the leg holder with elastic bandaging. The large fluoroscopic C-arm is guided into place, and the anteroposterior rotation sites are aligned by rotating the C-arm or operating room table. This rotation confirms the center location of the guide over the talus and the tibia. Then, using a similar procedure, the lateral rotation site centering is accomplished with the C-arm in the lateral view. The AP view is then reobtained with proper centering and the cutting guide applied. Selection of the ideal cutting guide is determined using preoperative templating, intraoperative fluoroscopy, and direct visualization. The plantar calcaneal heel pad is carefully incised, a cannula is inserted through the soft tissue and locked into position, and the talus and tibia are drilled. Alignment of the monoblock cutting guide is accomplished under fluoroscopy, and the guide is pinned into position. Tibia and talus are cut through the monoblock saw guide. The saw guide is removed and the bone extracted. The tibia is reamed by applying the reamer tip into the ankle and onto the reaming rod inserted up through the calcaneus and talus. The ankle is then plantar flexed, talar component positioning is fine-tuned, and the hole for the talar stem is drilled. The tibial screw is assembled within the prepared ankle and advanced into the reamed tibia. The Morse taper tibial component is then tamped into the modular stem's lowest cylinder and fully seated on the resected tibial surface. Next, the talar component with the 10-mm stem attached is positioned and impacted into the prepared tibia. Alternatively, a longer 14-mm stem or a not yet FDA-approved calcaneal stem is inserted first and then the talar component is inserted and locked onto this stem. Finally, the polyethylene component is inserted via a screw-pushing mechanism and then tamped into place.

Results

Overview

The levels of evidence and grades of recommendation remain limited to retrospective and intermediate prospective data. In the published studies, it is often difficult to determine the level of the surgeon's experience with TAA and/or the recommended surgical technique for the particular implant. The ideal study would be a prospective, randomized trial comparing TAA and ankle arthrodesis; however, expecting informed patients to accept randomized surgical options of arthrodesis versus ankle replacement is unrealistic. Currently, TAA outcomes are based on prospective, comparative studies and retrospective, case-controlled studies—some intermediate, but others have only short-term results. It is hoped that registries of TAAs will become available to provide useful data regarding particular design features, surgeon experience, institutional data, and carefully selected outcomes measures.

One concern is that currently available intermediate-term results will drive enthusiasm for TAA. Consistent long-term follow-up for current TAA implants is needed but not yet available. Most concerning is the reported survivorship analysis. Although many implanted TAAs may maintain excellent function with long-term follow-up, there are probably an equal number that are surviving but not functioning perfectly. Reviewing the current literature with a critical eye reveals many instances of persistent malalignment, radiolucencies, osteolysis, and bone overgrowth at intermediate-term (5- to 7-year) follow-up. Nonetheless, many patients have good to excellent results in these follow-up studies. Although these patients may be functioning well at intermediate-term follow-up, it is important to remember that such positive results may not be experienced at long-term (10- to 15-year) follow-up.

Revision surgery for TAA does not necessarily mean failure of a TAA implant; if this was the situation, good to excellent results would drop to approximately 50%, rendering TAA obsolete. Many of the current studies report on successful revision surgeries. These "touch-up" surgeries include fixation of malleolar fractures not noted at the time of surgery, replacing the mobile polyethylene component with a thicker component to gain better ligamentous stability, resection of bony overgrowth causing impingement in well-fixed components, and periarticular osteotomy. The number of patients needing revision surgery may decrease as the techniques of TAA become more defined.[44,45]

Meta-Analysis

In the meta-analysis previously mentioned, data pooling was only possible for 10 studies of three-component TAA designs (n = 497).[16] These trials showed a mean improvement of 45.2 points on the American Orthopaedic Foot and

Ankle Society (AOFAS) ankle-hindfoot scoring system (95% confidence interval [CI] 39.3 to 51.1). Average ROM improved slightly (6.3°, 95% CI 2.2° to 10.5°). Weighted complication rates ranged from 1.6% (deep infections) to 14.7% (impingement). The prevalence of secondary surgery was 12.5% and secondary arthrodesis was 6.3%. The weighted 5-year prosthesis survival rate averaged 90.6%. This meta-analysis concluded that TAA improves pain and joint mobility in end-stage ankle arthritis but cautioned that its performance in comparison to ankle arthrodesis remains to be defined in a properly designed randomized trial.

Implant-Specific Results
Agility Prosthesis
Mean follow-up of published studies for the Agility prosthesis ranges from nearly 3 years to 9 years.[2,4,23,45] In most of these studies, patient satisfaction ranged from 90% to 97% for patients who did not have conversion to arthrodesis and were available for follow-up. One study showed an improvement in AOFAS ankle-hindfoot score from 34 to 83 points, with 49 points on the Medical Outcomes Study 36-Item Short Form physical component and 56 points on the mental component at a mean follow-up of 44 months.[23] Despite these apparently favorable results, progressive radiolucency rates (76% to 85%) have been reported.[2,23] Although it has been suggested that not all peri-implant lucency is related to failure but instead to stress shielding, high rates (24% to 45%) of component migration and subsidence have been reported.[2,4,23] One study noted a high correlation of tibial component migration with syndesmotic delayed union and particularly nonunion,

with syndesmotic nonunions occurring in 8% to 10% of Agility TAAs.[4]

One investigation suggested that not all revision surgeries represent failures.[45] In a study of 306 ankles with Agility prostheses, the authors reported a 28% revision rate, with the procedures ranging from osteophyte removal to amputation. With revision as the end point, the 5-year survival was 54%; with implant survival as the end point, the 5-year survival was 80%. If the patient cohort is limited to patients older than 54 years, the 5-year survival increased to 89%. In the study with the longest mean follow-up (9 years),[2] 11% conversion to arthrodesis was observed; in the study with the shortest mean follow-up (33 months), the amputation rate approached 3%.[45] TAA is also believed to be protective of the hindfoot articulations, particularly in comparison with ankle arthrodesis. However, despite TAA, one study noted radiographic evidence of progressive arthritis of the subtalar joint in 19% of ankles and 15% in the talonavicular joint.[2]

STAR Prosthesis
Mean follow-up for published series for the currently available STAR prosthesis ranges from 3 to 5 years.[3,43,44,46-50] Two of the studies, with some of the same patients in their cohorts, show an AOFAS ankle-hindfoot score improvement from 25 to 84 points with 98% good to excellent results.[48] Best implant survival rates (ranging from 93% to 98%) were observed with double-coated (hydroxyapatite and titanium) cementless prostheses with optimal component fit at the implant-bone interface.[46,49] Life table survivorship analysis estimated cementless implant survival at 95% at 12 years.[3] In contrast, 5-year sur-

vival rates for single-coating components and 12-year survivorship rates for cemented components have been reported at 70%.[3,50] Some of these less favorable outcomes may be attributable to a learning curve for surgeons and possibly by limitations in prosthetic design (a design that has remained virtually unchanged since inception of the implant more than 15 years ago).[44,46,48,50,51]

Revision rates for cementless prostheses range from 7% to 37%.[48-50] Not all revisions are indicative of prosthesis failure. In one study, no revisions involved component removal; all revision procedures were "touch-ups," again suggesting limitations of prosthetic design, characteristics common to TAA, or a learning curve for surgeons.[44] However, the rate of revision surgery for component exchange or conversion to arthrodesis is not negligible, ranging from 7% to 29% in some studies.[46,49,50]

Hintegra Prosthesis
Only two reports of outcomes for the Hintegra prosthesis have been published, both by one of the inventors of the prosthesis.[52,53] One study of 271 Hintegra TAAs, with a mean follow-up of 3 years, reported an increase in the AOFAS ankle-hindfoot score from 40 to 85 points.[53] Revisions were performed in 14% of ankles, with 2% of TAAs being converted to arthrodesis. The revisions that did not require conversion to arthrodesis had outcomes that matched those of the residual cohort that did not undergo repeat surgery. Radiographic evaluation showed proper position without migration in 266 TAAs that were not converted to arthrodesis. Talar component positioning was deemed too posterior in 4% of the implants. The investigators, who had extensive prior clinical experience with the STAR

prosthesis, reported a short, steep learning curve with the Hintegra prosthesis and noted that many revisions were not failures but instead "touch-up" procedures.

Salto Prosthesis

The only published report on the Salto TAA is by the inventors of the prosthesis.[54] In a study of 98 consecutive Salto TAAs, with a mean follow-up of almost 3 years (minimum follow-up, 2 years), clinical and radiographic evaluation was possible for 91 patients (93 implants). Results showed an increase in the AOFAS ankle-hindfoot score from 32 to 83 points. Seventy-two patients were pain free, 54 patients could walk unlimited distances, and 25 patients had limitations but could walk more than 1 km. Sixty-seven patients had no limp but seven needed walking aids. Fifty-eight patients could walk on tiptoe, 49 patients could walk on uneven ground, 14 patients could run, 76 patients could ascend stairs normally, and 63 patients could descend stairs normally. ROM as measured on stress radiographs improved from 15.2° preoperatively to 28.3° at follow-up. Survivorship analysis (calculated at 68 months, the longest follow-up period available in the study cohort), with the end point set at implant removal, was 98% and 95% for best- and worse-case scenarios, respectively.[54]

Buechel-Pappas Prosthesis

Mean follow-up for the currently available Buechel-Pappas prosthesis (deep sulcus design) ranges from 5 to 12 years. Two studies by the inventors of the prosthesis showed 88% good to excellent results and a 10- and 12-year survivorship rate (with revision of any component) of 93.5 and 92%, respectively.[1,32] Most patients (82% to 84%) in these stud-

ies had osteoarthritis. Results of earlier-generation Buechel-Pappas prostheses (shallow sulcus design) from these same authors showed only 70% good to excellent results and a 12-year survivorship rate of 74%.[34]

Other studies of Buechel-Pappas prostheses, either using the shallow or deep sulcus designs, report on cohorts composed solely of patients with inflammatory arthritis.[55,56] At a mean follow-up of 8 years for these studies, clinical outcome scores improved significantly, and a patient satisfaction rate of 89% was reported for those patients who underwent clinical and radiographic follow-up.[55] The outcomes did not include patients who had died or those who had undergone reoperation. In one cohort, 6% of revision surgeries were performed for aseptic loosening and another 6% for axial deformity;[55] in another study, 6% of revision surgeries were converted to ankle arthrodesis.[56] One study showed 82% acceptable radiographic alignment and ingrowth of the Buechel-Pappas prosthesis, and another study showed 18% of implants had marked component subsidence, suggestive of impending failure.[55,56] The authors reported that subsidence did not appear to correlate with radiolucent lines noted on postoperative radiographs.

INBONE, Mobility Total Ankle, and Salto-Talaris Prostheses

At this time, published results with at least 2-year follow-up were not available for the INBONE, Mobility total ankle or Salto-Talaris prostheses.

Complications
Overview/Learning Curve

Despite advances in techniques, instrumentation, and implant design,

the complication rate for TAA continues to exceed that of total knee and total hip arthroplasty. Some complications require revision, with most of these revision surgeries being relatively minor procedures that are not indicative of TAA failure. In a recent investigation of complications in initial TAAs, surgeons were categorized based on their training in TAA.[57] Surgeons were classed as observers of the surgeon inventor; participants in a structured, hands-on surgical training course; and those who had completed a 1-year foot and ankle fellowship with a mentor who performed TAA. Review of surgical outcomes of these three groups was statistically indistinguishable with respect to rates of complications, revisions, or malalignment. However, experience in TAA appears to lower complication rates as shown by the experience of one surgeon who had a lower complication rate for his second 25 Agility TAAs compared with his first 25 procedures (two versus five intraoperative fractures, and zero versus five tendon/nerve lacerations, respectively). Component malalignment also decreased 9% from the first group to the second group of precedures.[15] Improved results with more experience also were found for other surgeons performing STAR TAAs.[49] However, no registry analysis has been published that shows improved outcomes and diminished complication rates based on an individual surgeon's experience and the volume of TAAs performed at an institution.

Specific Complications and Proposed Management
Wound Healing

For TAAs implanted via an anterior approach, postoperative wound complications are cited along with malleolar fractures as the most common complication in TAA.[49,50,55,56]

Although wound complication rates no longer approach 40% as in early reports of TAA, some recent studies cite an incidence of postoperative wound healing complications of approximately 10%.[49,50,55,56,58] Most of these wounds involve less than 1 cm of skin necrosis and often resolve with simple immobilization and local wound care. With more extensive wound dehiscence, a negative pressure wound system may prove effective, provided the extensor retinaculum remains intact. Communication with the ankle joint typically necessitates implant removal, irrigation, débridement, and possible free-tissue transfer, with eventual conversion to arthrodesis as the prudent treatment.

Anecdotal experience has introduced four recommendations that appear to limit wound complications but do not have proven scientific support. (1) Direct skin tension should be avoided and only deep retractors (for example, Adson-Beckman or deep Gelpis) should be used. (2) Adequate exposure should be provided by making an incision long enough to avoid undue tension on the wound edges (currently precluding the use of a minimally invasive technique). (3) Four-layer closure (capsule, extensor retinaculum, subcutaneous layer, and skin) should be used. (4) A brief period of immobilization is recommended following TAA, until the wound is stable.

For the Agility prosthesis, an adequate skin bridge between the anterior and lateral incisions must be maintained. Some surgeons suggest that nasal oxygen in the immediate postoperative period may have a positive effect on wound healing. There is no current clinically proven support for perioperatively interrupting the administration of immunosuppressive medications for a patient with rheumatoid arthritis.

Malleolar Fractures

Malleolar fractures are a relatively common complication in TAA, with the incidence significantly decreasing for surgeons with more TAA experience.[15,42,49,55,57,59] In several recent studies, the prevalence of malleolar fractures approached and sometimes exceeded 20%.[42,49,55,56,59] Such fractures can be attributed to the difficulty of performing TAA, with instrumentation that obscures already limited visualization, and a joint that narrows slightly posteriorly, making violation of the malleoli even more likely.

Malleolar fractures result from inadvertent excursion of the oscillating saw blade, levering with instrumentation, or malpositioning and improper sizing of the porous-coated tibial component.[15,42,55-57,59] Malleolar fractures may not be detected until postoperative radiographic evaluation; some are occult fractures occurring intraoperatively, and others represent postoperative stress fractures.[15,42,55-57]

Some authors suggest prophylactically pinning the malleoli before making the bone cuts.[59] This simple adjunct adds little surgical time. In the event of an intraoperative medial malleolar fracture, cannulated screw fixation and/or buttress plating is typically feasible but must be performed judiciously to avoid wound complications. A lateral malleolar fracture is generally managed with a small fragment plate, placed through a limited lateral incision with an adequate skin bridge from the anterior approach.[42]

Malalignment

Malalignment following TAA has been reported in 4% to 45% of patients.[1,4,55,56] All prostheses with published results use extramedullary alignment instrumentation. Most techniques recommend intraoperative imaging in the coronal and sagittal planes to confirm appropriate alignment of cutting guides. Occasionally, extra-articular corrections or tendon transfers may be required to attain desired alignment, performed either simultaneously with the TAA or in a staged fashion. In select patients, residual postoperative malalignment may be effectively corrected with second-stage extra-articular osteotomies. Proper talar component alignment demands appropriate hindfoot/talar positioning when the talar cut is made.

Preexisting malalignment must be corrected with TAA. One study reported the greatest number of failures when preoperative coronal plane deformity exceeded 10°.[56] Another study reported that in patients with preoperative incongruent joints (for example, varus talar tilt within the ankle mortise in patients with end-stage arthrosis) progressive edge loading is 10 times more likely to develop than in patients with congruent joints.[17]

Infection

Infection with TAA is a relatively uncommon complication, with an incidence similar to that of other major weight-bearing joint arthroplasties, and a reported prevalence ranging from 0% to 2%.[1,2,4,23,42,45,48-50,54-56] Management of infections associated with TAA empirically follow protocols established for infections occurring in total hip or total knee arthroplasties. Cellulitis or superficial wound infections typically respond well to irrigation, débridement, and antibiotic management, provided that an effective multilayer closure is maintained to avoid contamination of the joint. Acute joint sepsis, if detected immediately, often can be managed with irrigation and débridement, exchange of the polyethylene insert, and antibiotic therapy. Subacute or chronic infections necessitate treatment with irrigation and débridement, implant removal, a temporary antibiotic spacer, antibiotic therapy, and staged reimplantation or ankle arthrodesis. Standardized techniques for managing the infected TAA based on evidence-based outcomes have not been defined.

Subsidence and Component Migration

Subsidence and component migration is generally a result of inadequate bone ingrowth or inadequate component support with weight bearing. A mild amount of early migration of current cementless TAA implants is anticipated, with stabilization of most components by 6 months following implantation.[60] In one study of the Buechel-Pappas tibial components, the authors suggested that the method of fixation and surgical technique (an anterior cortical window) was responsible for component settling.[60]

Progressive component migration has been associated with tibial component undersizing and preoperative deformity exceeding 10° and osteonecrosis (both specific to the Buechel-Pappas implant); and failure of syndesmotic fusion (specific to Agility prosthesis).[1,2,4,56] Occasionally, component collapse into osteopenic bone or large subchondral cysts is observed. Large subchondral cysts detected on preoperative radiographs should prompt more detailed evaluation with CT to plan bone grafting at the time of TAA.

Optimal component bone ingrowth is facilitated by congruent

matching between components and prepared bony surfaces.[49] Hydroxyapatite coating, double coatings, and covering the backsides of components with platelet growth factors or mesenchymal stem cells have been studied to promote ingrowth.[3,40,46,48-50,61] With the STAR prosthesis, adding a titanium coating appears to promote more successful bony ingrowth than hydroxyapatite alone.[46,49] Initial component stability must be adequate but not excessive. Although supplemental screw fixation may limit initial micromotion at the bone-prosthesis interface, it may also restrict early component settling, which may be important for optimal bone ingrowth. If screw fixation is considered, nonlocking screws, which allow desirable minor component settling, are recommended. Even with congruent matching of component and prepared bony surfaces, stress shielding may lead to bone resorption and eventual component subsidence. For talar components that cap the prepared talar surfaces, ideal contact cannot be determined; this is another factor that may lead to inadequate bone ingrowth and/or stress shielding.

Most TAA outcome studies show a high prevalence (up to 85%) of peri-implant radiolucent lines on follow-up radiographs.[2,4,23,55] One study observed that component migration did not correlate with the presence of radiolucent lines, suggesting that progressive migration may not be solely caused by lack of bone ingrowth.[55] It is recommended that progressive peri-implant radiolucencies be followed closely for associated component migration beyond that observed with anticipated early settling. It is important to differentiate true lucency representing osteolysis from

movement from gaps inherent in inserting the prosthesis (for example, asymmetric drilled holes and cylindrical barrel replacements to fill the holes in the STAR prosthesis). Many of these surgical deficiencies will be physiologically replaced with bone over time.

Aseptic Loosening and Osteolysis

Whereas component subsidence is associated with a failure of initial component stabilization, osteolysis is caused by polyethylene particulate wear debris that stimulates an osteolytic or "bone cyst" response. Poor component alignment and incongruent polyethylene articulation with the talar and/or tibial components, including edge loading, is the primary cause leading to osteolysis (Figures 13 and 14). Two studies, one of the later-generation Buechel-Pappas implants and another of a single-coated version of the Hintegra prosthesis, show a 6% prevalence of aseptic loosening.[53,56] Conventional osteolysis should be distinguished from ballooning osteolysis that is believed to occur with component abutment against the malleoli, resulting in a loss of bone adjacent to the prosthesis (for example, the lateral malleolus in the Agility or STAR prosthesis in which one study reported a 4% prevalence of ballooning osteolysis).[48]

Newer TAA prostheses (Mobility and BOX) use a relatively small polyethylene tibial surface contact area and a larger talar articulating surface in an attempt to limit edge loading and component abutment. It may be acceptable to observe minor defects without surgical intervention; however, close follow-up is warranted to avoid missing the opportunity to salvage an ankle before gross loosening occurs. Provided component stability is maintained, larger defects (in par-

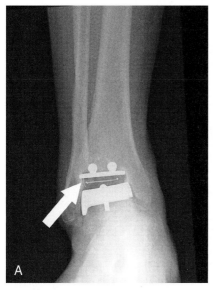
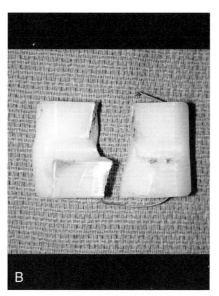

Figure 13 **A,** A STAR prosthesis placed in varus position in a 71-year-old man caused polyethylene wear and a cyst above the tibial component. Note the wire marker in the prosthesis is broken with small vertical piece of wire (*arrow*) in the joint of the lateral portion of ankle. **B,** Unilateral wear caused fracture of the polyethylene component.

ticular those with progression evident on serial radiographs) should be addressed with repeat surgery. Unless the cause for polyethylene wear (such as edge loading or malalignment) is rectified, recurrence of osteolysis can be expected. Although cyst débridement, bone grafting, and polyethylene exchange are appropriate, osteotomies to realign the joint may be necessary (Figure 15). Extensive osteolysis with component loosening may require revision TAA with custom implants or different designs or conversion to arthrodesis (Figure 16).

Impingement and Bone Overgrowth and Proliferation

A high prevalence of bone overgrowth and impingement has been reported in outcome studies for TAA, with one investigation showing impingement in 63% of patients.[45,48] Based on the available literature, bone overgrowth with symptomatic impingement has

prompted most revision surgeries in TAA.[45,48,53] Exposed cancellous surfaces are believed to promote bone overgrowth. This overgrowth, combined with the anticipated early settling of components, may be responsible for impingement that was not evident at the time of the index procedure. Empirically, many surgeons recommend comprehensive débridement of the gutters. In the Agility prosthesis, exposed cancellous talar surfaces are chamfered after talar component implantation. Although some surgeons recommend bone wax on the exposed bone surfaces and/or pulsed irrigation to remove loose bone fragments, others accept bone overgrowth as a matter of course and inform their patients that repeat surgery may become necessary to address symptomatic impingement.

The risk for postoperative impingement can be minimized by proper component sizing and osteo-

phyte removal. Occasionally, removal of osteophytes may expose instability and the surgeon should be prepared to perform a ligament balancing/reconstruction. Downsizing the talar component in three-component designs is recommended if there is concern for impingement. Although leaving as much bone as possible is preferable, leaving metal in too close proximity to bone may create pain as the metal abuts the bone. Also, bone overgrowth can block a meniscal bearing from moving and effectively converts a mobile-bearing TAA into a fixed-bearing TAA.

ROM and Postoperative Ankle Stiffness

Clinical assessment of ankle sagittal plane motion shows contributions from both the ankle and hindfoot. One study of the Agility TAA prosthesis used lateral ankle weight-bearing radiographs to determine ankle ROM before and after TAA.[62] Tibiotalar, midfoot, and combined ROM were measured preoperatively and 1 year postoperatively in a standardized, reproducible fashion. The preoperative tibiotalar ROM was 18.5° and combined ankle and midfoot motion was 25.1°. Isolated tibiotalar motion after an Agility TAA was 23.4°, and the combined ankle and midfoot motion was 31.3°. The average improvement in ROM in the tibiotalar joint was approximately 5°, and combined improvement in ROM was 6.1°. The authors concluded that preoperative ROM was the main determinant of eventual postoperative ROM and that TAA resulted in some, but less than expected, increase in ROM.[63] Other authors have used fluoroscopy or stress radiographs to document isolated ankle ROM after TAA with similar findings.[44,48,52-54] Although TAA rarely (if ever) restores physio-

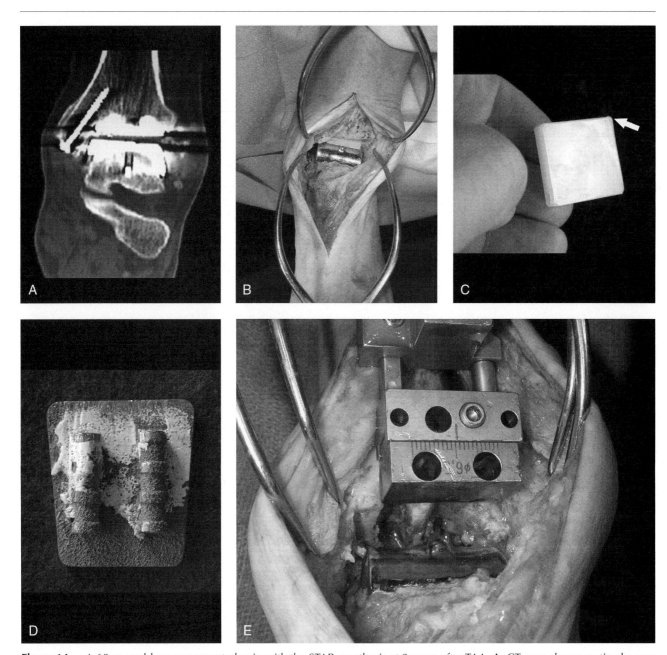

Figure 14   A 68-year-old woman reported pain with the STAR prosthesis at 2 years after TAA. **A,** CT scan shows cystic changes from polyethylene wear particles that migrated to the medial malleolar screw inserted during previous open reduction and internal fixation. **B,** The opened ankle shows that the polyethylene component is protruding from the leading edge of the tibial component. **C,** Slight wear is seen at the anterior edge of the polyethylene component (*arrow*). **D,** The removed tibial base plate shows bony ingrowth over the anterior two thirds of component. **E,** The ankle was revised secondary to excessive dorsiflexion of the tibial component in addition to polyethylene wear. For the revision, the tibia was cut superiorly and a 12-mm revision polyethylene component was used.

logic ankle ROM, several authors have reported an improvement in ankle ROM following TAA.[44,52-54] These authors reported mean postoperative ankle ROM with TAA to be 28° to 37° (based on imaging studies of the ankle).

There is debate concerning whether to perform gastrocnemius-soleus recession or Achilles tendon lengthening for TAA in patients with an intraoperatively confirmed equinus contracture. Some surgeons believe that the gastrocnemius-soleus complex will gradually adapt after removal of anterior ankle osteophytes, comprehensive posterior capsular release, and appropriate bone resection and component sizing. If the ankle fails to achieve adequate dorsiflexion postoperatively, greater physiologic compressive forces may lead to anterior tibial cortical impaction with tibial component subsidence into extension. Therefore, at least 5° of intraoperative dorsiflexion is recommended. If this degree of dorsiflexion is not achieved, more tibial bone must be resected and/or a gastrocnemius recession and/or a percutaneous triple hemisection of the Achilles tendon should be performed.

Instability

Ligament balancing for TAA must be achieved at the time of surgery. Although modular polyethylene inserts can enhance appropriate ligament tension, ligament repair or reconstruction may be required to establish satisfactory ankle stability with TAA. The varus ankle may require a deltoid ligament release combined with a modified Broström procedure (for mild instability), a modified Evans procedure (for mild to moderate instability), or complete or partial peroneus brevis or hamstring autograft or allograft reconstruction (for moderate instability). Because severe instability or deformity may not be reconstructible, preoperative consent should be obtained from a patient to perform arthrodesis when TAA is not appropriate based on intraoperative findings. Correction of valgus instability in conjunction with TAA remains challenging because a predictable deltoid ligament reconstruction has yet to be devised. Although several techniques of deltoid ligament reconstruction have been described, a study of their effectiveness for rebalancing valgus instability with TAA has not been published in a peer-reviewed journal. Ankle or tibiotalocalcaneal arthrodesis is currently recommended for medial ligament

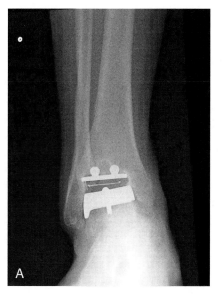
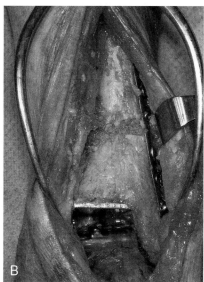

Figure 15   **A,** Varus malposition of STAR tibial component led to central osteolysis and fracture of the polyethylene bearing. **B,** Intraoperative view showing osteotomy used to correct malposition (polyethylene not yet implanted).

incompetence. When proper ligament balance can be achieved in conjunction with TAA, selective foot osteotomies and/or arthrodeses or supramalleolar osteotomies also ay be needed to maintain ankle balance. Fortunately, in most valgus ankles, there is lateral collapse as opposed to medial incompetence and correct alignment of the ankle, occasionally accompanied by a sliding medial calcaneal osteotomy, will effectively balance the ankle.

Adjacent Joint Arthritis

Adjacent joint pain occurs in some patients treated with TAA. Unless the pain is symptomatic preoperatively, many of these patients will gain relief with TAA alone. However, if CT scanning or preoperative differential anesthetic blocks confirm hindfoot arthritis as a contributor to the ankle pain, arthrodeses should be performed simultaneously with TAA, or in a staged manner, particularly if associated with hindfoot malalignment. TAA does not ensure that hindfoot arthri-

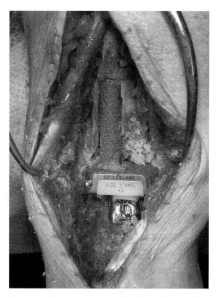

Figure 16   Custom tibial Agility ankle prosthesis component with stem.

tis will not develop. At an average follow-up of 9 years, hindfoot arthritis was reported in 15% of talonavicular and 19% of subtalar joints after TAA using the Agility prosthesis.[2] This finding suggests that TAA cannot completely protect hindfoot articulations from developing arthritis; however, the prevalence of hindfoot arthritis following TAA should prove to be less than that reported following ankle arthrodesis.[5,6]

Prosthetic Breakage

As previously mentioned, malalignment may lead to eccentric, narrow, contact stresses on the components. Although component failure is uncommon, the polyethylene component is most likely to fail, and rarely, the metal or metal-backed components may fracture. Although polyethylene exchange is possible for an isolated failure of the polyethylene component, malalignment, if present, must be corrected to reduce the risk of recurrent component failure.

Revision Surgery for Failed TAA

Few (if any) standardized techniques have been described for revision TAA. Because a full complement of revision components is not yet available, many revision surgeries require conversion to arthrodesis.[63-65] The surgeon performing revision TAA must be prepared for a full range of possible salvage options, which often requires a considerable collection of equipment, including revision and custom components, equipment for ankle arthrodesis, and structural bone graft material.

Revision TAA, even with careful removal of the primary components and judicious repeated preparation of the tibial and talar surfaces, creates a gap consistently larger than with primary TAA. Thus, the most commonly used components in revision TAA are thicker polyethylene inserts. Some systems offer augmented revision metal components to facilitate reestablishing proper joint line position and ligament function. Full complements of revision TAA components are gradually becoming more available. Occasionally, custom prostheses must be produced, often at great expense, or consideration needs to be given to the selection of another system that can better address the larger residual gap following removal of the primary implants. One modification to available tibial and talar components is implant stem extensions. In the event only one component needs to be revised, either the tibial or talar component may be replaced, while maintaining the same articulations with a polyethylene insert of revised or increased width. The INBONE prosthesis has a patented bone-ingrowth talar-calcaneal stem extension that is placed across the subtalar joint into the calcaneus to provide talar implant support when residual talar bone stock is limited. That stem, although initially implanted as a "custom" device, is not FDA approved and is unavailable in the United States. When the residual talar bone is insufficient for a primary or an augmented talar implant, a subtalar arthrodesis may prove effective in supporting the talar prosthesis, irrespective of implant design.

Some surgeons have suggested that given the Agility prosthesis' relatively large design dimensions, it may also be used in revision situations for failed implants.[66] Recutting the tibial surface in revision TAA often rests the tibial component in weaker subchondral bone; however, adequate support can generally be achieved with syndesmotic arthrodesis. In the talus, even if the medial and lateral talar dome surfaces have been removed as part of talar preparation for other designs, the residual recut talar bone may be adequate for the Agility augmented or revision talar components. As a custom implant, the talar component of the Agility prosthesis may be fitted with a stem extension for situations that warrant simultaneous subtalar arthrodesis. However, recognizing the difficulties of using an Agility prosthesis in ideal conditions makes surgery with the Agility as a revision prosthesis a challenging procedure. The INBONE prosthesis with its modular tibial stem design and its ingrowth calcaneal stem may be more suited for use in revision situations.

One study of revision TAA using the Hintegra prosthesis for 28 failed TAAs (STAR, 25; Buechel-Pappas, 2; Agility, 1) showed that at a mean follow-up of approximately 3 years, 23 patients (82%) were satisfied with their outcome.[67] The AOFAS hindfoot score improved from 41 points preoperatively to 86 points at follow-up. Radiographic evaluation suggested a single instance of revision tibial component loosening. However, in the absence of further symptoms, re-revision surgery was deemed unnecessary.

Conversion of TAA to Arthrodesis

The surgical challenge of converting TAA to arthrodesis is fusing surfaces separated by a large gap that have been subjected to implants (and potentially an antibiotic spacer) while attempting to retain near-physiologic limb length, occasionally in the presence of previous infection.[49,63-65,68,69] Proponents of several three-component designs claim that in the event of implant failure, the minimal bone resection (9 mm) at the index procedure makes conversion to arthrodesis relatively straightforward. However, experience indicates that regardless of design, despite minimal initial bone resection and careful removal of bone ingrowth implants (using thin power saws to avoid damaging too much bone), a considerable gap is created. Although some patients may accept an in situ fusion with the potential need for shoe modification, many patients request that the surgeon attempt to maintain equal limb length. To do so, the surgeon is faced with the challenge of interposing a bulk allograft (often a portion of a femoral head). Occasionally, the subtalar joint can be preserved; however, this salvage procedure usually warrants a tibiotalocalcaneal arthrodesis performed with a combination plate and screws (possible through the same anterior approach), blade plate fixation (typically requiring a second lateral or posterior approach) or a retrograde intramedullary arthrodesis nail (also through a lateral or posterior approach). A midline posterior Achilles tendon-splitting approach can be used to remove the ankle components. The fibula is left in place, the ankle and subtalar surfaces are prepared, and a bulk femoral head allograft is inserted to maintain length. The structural allograft is then held with a retrograde intramedullary rod supplemented by additional bone graft in any defects (Figure 17). If infection is present, a two-stage procedure is favored, with implant removal, irrigation/débridement, antibiotic bead or spacer placement, and delayed arthrodesis. External fixation is an alternative in the presence of infection. The residual bone surfaces can be acutely opposed and compressed (after débridement), while a simultaneous proximal tibial corticotomy is performed to initiate gradual distraction to restore limb length. Regardless of the technique used, the basic principles of arthrodesis must

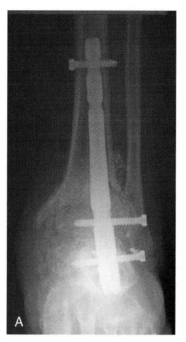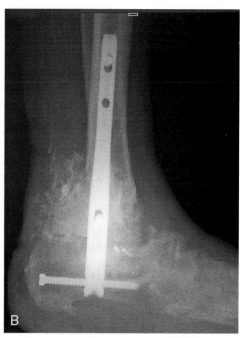

Figure 17 AP (**A**) and lateral (**B**) views of an intramedullary rod through femoral head used to fill the gap left by TAA prosthesis that had been removed.

be followed. All infected, nonviable tissue must be removed and bleeding surfaces established on both sides of the fusion site even if a considerable amount of bone needs to be resected.

Comprehensive studies of one institution's experience with arthrodesis and revision arthrodesis following failed TAA and failed arthrodesis after failed TAA have been published.[63-65] Using external fixation and autologous bone graft in virtually all patients, the authors reported an 89% fusion rate and little or no pain in 80% of patients at a mean follow-up of 8 years.[65] For patients undergoing revision ankle arthrodesis for nonunion following attempted conversion of failed TAA to ankle arthrodesis, outcomes were less favorable, despite successful union in most patients.[64] In another study (at a separate institution) using iliac crest bone, arthrodesis after failed TAA achieved successful fu-

sion in only two of four patients.[69] Although one of the two patients with a failed TAA had a successful union after repeat arthrodesis with an intramedullary rod, a persistent nonunion developed in the other patient. In a similar study of eight patients with failed TAA, the authors reported an 87% fusion rate and recommended an anterior plate fixation technique, reserving external fixation for patients with infection.[70]

Future Directions
Implant Design and Technique
The ideal TAA design has yet to be created. Despite the challenges in trying to restore physiologic, pain-free ankle function in patients with end-stage ankle arthritis, the evolution of TAA over the past decade has been extraordinary. Over the next decade several more designs currently in development will be introduced. Building on past experiences,

new designs will potentially achieve the goal of TAA results that are comparable to those achieved in total hip and total knee arthroplasty. As demonstrated with the BOX prosthesis, designs may not need to mimic human ankle anatomy to restore ankle-hindfoot function. Published results of TAA using a lateral rather than an anterior approach may confer advantages over implant designs inserted with the anterior approach. The Eclipse and ESKA are examples of such a concept, and another company is currently working on developing such a TAA. Outcomes of TAAs such as the INBONE will determine if intramedullary alignment guides confer advantages over more traditional methods using extramedullary alignment. Additionally, computer-assisted surgery with robotics and intraoperative pedobarography with TAA may improve the surgeon's ability to properly align TAA components and use a less invasive approach. Navigation systems for TAA may lag behind those for total knee and total hip arthroplasty because of industry's lack of financial incentives to develop ankle-specific software and the lower prevalence of ankle arthritis compared with that of the hip and knee.

Cost Effectiveness

A cost-effectiveness analysis of TAA using a model that assumed a 10-year prosthetic survival suggested an incremental TAA cost-effectiveness ratio of $18,419 per quality-adjusted life year gained, and a gain of 0.52 quality-adjusted life years at a cost of $9,578 when TAA is chosen instead of fusion.[71] This ratio compares favorably when compared with other medical and surgical interventions. If the prosthesis is assumed to fail before 7 years, sensitivity analysis suggested that the cost

per quality-adjusted life year gained with TAA is more than $50,000, a figure generally associated with limited cost-effectiveness. If the theoretic functional advantages of TAA over ankle fusion are proven in future long-term clinical trials, TAA has the potential to be a cost-effective alternative to ankle fusion.

Conversion of Ankle Fusion to TAA

In select patients with pain following ankle arthrodesis, conversion to TAA may confer advantages over correcting a malposition or adding fusions for adjacent areas of arthritis. Although no comparative studies exist, early reports of conversion of ankle arthrodesis to TAA have been published, with two studies showing similar increases in mean AOFAS ankle-hindfoot scores at short-term follow-up.[7,67] One prospective study of 19 consecutive conversions of ankle arthrodesis to Hintegra TAAs reported an improvement of the AOFAS score from 33.6 to 66.5 points.[67] The authors documented average ankle ROM (confirmed fluoroscopically) of 24°, roughly 52% of the motion of the healthy contralateral ankle. The results of the study were slightly inferior to those of studies with primary arthroplasty; however, the authors believed that ankle arthroplasty represents a valuable alternative to the current treatment for painful ankle arthrodesis. Similarly, a retrospective analysis of 16 symptomatic ankle arthrodeses converted to Agility TAAs showed an improvement of mean AOFAS hindfoot-ankle scores from a preoperative value of 42 points to 68 points at follow-up.[7] These authors observed that patients with a definitive source of pain following ankle arthrodesis, such as secondary hindfoot arthrosis,

tended to have a better outcome than patients without a distinct source of pain.[7] They also reported that patients who had the lateral malleolus resected as part of their ankle arthrodesis tended to have more complications following conversion to TAA.

Revision TAA

As previously mentioned, the techniques for revision TAA have not been standardized and many of the available revision systems are limited, often prompting surgeons to salvage a failed primary TAA with custom implants, conversion to another TAA system, or complex arthrodesis. The challenges in revising the current generation of primary TAAs, either necessitated by complications or anticipated polyethylene wear, will bring obligatory refinements in revision TAA techniques, components, and instrumentation. Also, though less desirable, revision TAA may also include standardized recommended techniques, implants, and instrumentation to convert failed TAAs to arthrodesis.

Summary

Adequate long-term follow-up and high levels of evidence are not available to support universal TAA over arthrodesis in the management of end-stage ankle arthritis. Although developments in TAA have been extraordinary since the procedure's inception, outcomes of TAA fall short of those reported for total hip and total ankle arthroplasty. However, the combined improvements in implants, instrumentation, patient selection, and surgical technique make 10-year implant survival of more than 90% a realistic goal. The incidence of malalignment, neurovascular injury, and material failure of

TAA implants is diminishing. Despite these improvements, impingement from bony proliferation, osteolysis/loosening, component subsidence, and failure to resolve preoperative ankle stiffness remain concerns. Further investigation will determine the cost-effectiveness of TAA and if conversion of ankle arthrodesis to arthroplasty is advisable. The future promises a full complement of revision and custom prostheses and incorporation of state-of-the-art adjuncts such as computer navigation to facilitate ideal alignment. Improved techniques, implants, and instrumentation, coupled with promising midterm results of newer prosthetic designs, make TAA a viable alternative for properly selected patients.

References

1. Buechel FF Sr, Buechel FF Jr, Pappas MJ: Ten-year evaluation of cementless Buechel-Pappas meniscal bearing total ankle replacement. *Foot Ankle Int* 2003;24:462-472.

2. Knecht SI, Estin M, Callaghan JJ, et al: The Agility total ankle arthroplasty: Seven to sixteen-year follow-up. *J Bone Joint Surg Am* 2004;86: 1161-1171.

3. Kofoed H: Scandinavian Total Ankle Replacement (STAR). *Clin Orthop Relat Res* 2004;424:73-79.

4. Pyevich MT, Saltzman CL, Callaghan JJ, Alvine FG: Total ankle arthroplasty: A unique design: Two to twelve-year follow-up. *J Bone Joint Surg Am* 1998;80:1410-1420.

5. Coester LM, Saltzman CL, Leupold J, Pontarelli W: Long-term results following ankle arthrodesis for post-traumatic arthritis. *J Bone Joint Surg Am* 2001;83:219-228.

6. Fuchs S, Sandmann C, Skwara A, Chylarecki C: Quality of life 20 years after arthrodesis of the ankle: A study of adjacent joints. *J Bone Joint Surg Br* 2003;85:994-998.

7. Greisberg J, Assal M., Flueckiger G, Hansen ST Jr: Takedown of ankle fusion and conversion to total ankle replacement. *Clin Orthop Relat Res* 2004; 424:80-88.

8. Conti S, Lalonde KA, Martin R: Kinematic analysis of the agility total ankle during gait. *Foot Ankle Int* 2006; 27:980-984.

9. Dyrby C, Chou LB, Andriacchi TP, Mann RA: Functional evaluation of the Scandinavian Total Ankle Replacement. *Foot Ankle Int* 2004;25: 377-381.

10. Thomas R, Daniels TR, Parker K: Gait analysis and functional outcomes following ankle arthrodesis for isolated ankle arthritis. *J Bone Joint Surg Am* 2006;88:526-535.

11. Tanaka Y, Takakura Y: The TNK ankle: Short- and mid-term results. *Orthopade* 2006;35:546-551.

12. Affatato S, Leardini A, Leardini W, Giannini S, Viceconti M: Meniscal wear at a three-component total ankle prosthesis by a knee joint simulator. *J Biomech* 2007;40:1871-1876.

13. Leardini A, O'Connor JJ, Catani F, Giannini S: Mobility of the human ankle and the design of total ankle replacement. *Clin Orthop Relat Res* 2004; 424:39-46.

14. Reggiani B, Leardini A, Corazza F, Taylor M: Finite element analysis of a total ankle replacement during the stance phase of gait. *J Biomech* 2006; 39:1435-1443.

15. Myerson MS, Mroczek K: Perioperative complications of total ankle arthroplasty. *Foot Ankle Int* 2003; 24:17-21.

16. Stengel D, Bauwens K, Ekkernkamp A, Cramer J: Efficacy of total ankle replacement with meniscal-bearing devices: A systematic review and meta-analysis. *Arch Orthop Trauma Surg* 2005;125:109-119.

17. Haskell A, Mann RA: Ankle arthroplasty with preoperative coronal plane deformity: Short-term results. *Clin Orthop Relat Res* 2004;424:98-103.

18. Stamatis ED, Cooper PS, Myerson MS: Supramalleolar osteotomy for the treatment of distal tibial angular deformities and arthritis of the ankle joint. *Foot Ankle Int* 2003;24: 754-764.

19. Takakura Y, Takaoka T, Tanaka Y, Yajima H, Tamai S: Results of opening-wedge osteotomy for the treatment of a post-traumatic varus deformity of the ankle. *J Bone Joint Surg Am* 1998; 80:213-218.

20. Takakura Y, Tanaka Y, Kumai T, Tamai S: Low tibial osteotomy for osteoarthritis of the ankle: Results of a new operation in 18 patients. *J Bone Joint Surg Br* 1995;77:50-54.

21. Tanaka Y, Takakura Y, Hayashi K, Taniguchi A, Kumai T, Sugimoto K: Low tibial osteotomy for varus-type osteoarthritis of the ankle. *J Bone Joint Surg Br* 2006;88:909-913.

22. Stagni R, Leardini A, Ensini A, Cappello A: Ankle morphometry evaluated using a new semi-automated technique based on X-ray pictures. *Clin Biomech (Bristol, Avon)* 2005;20: 307-311.

23. Kopp FJ, Patel MM, Deland JT, O'Malley MJ: Total ankle arthroplasty with the Agility prosthesis: Clinical and radiographic evaluation. *Foot Ankle Int* 2006;27:97-103.

24. Valderrabano V, Hintermann B, Nigg BM, Stefanyshyn D, Stergiou P: Kinematic changes after fusion and total replacement of the ankle: Part 1. Range of motion. *Foot Ankle Int* 2003; 24:881-887.

25. Valderrabano V, Hintermann B, Nigg BM, Stefanyshyn D, Stergiou P: Kinematic changes after fusion and total replacement of the ankle: Part 2. Movement transfer. *Foot Ankle Int* 2003;24:888-896.

26. Valderrabano V, Hintermann B, Nigg BM, Stefanyshyn D, Stergiou P: Kinematic changes after fusion and total replacement of the ankle: Part 3. Talar movement. *Foot Ankle Int* 2003;24: 897-900.

27. Nicholson JJ, Parks BG, Stroud CC, Myerson MS: Joint contact character-

istics in Agility total ankle arthroplasty. *Clin Orthop Relat Res* 2004;424: 125-129.

28. Tochigi Y, Rudert MJ, Brown TD, McIff TE, Saltzman CL: The effect of accuracy of implantation on range of movement of the Scandinavian Total Ankle Replacement. *J Bone Joint Surg Br* 2005;87:736-740.

29. Muller S, Wolf S, Doderlein L: Three-dimensional analysis of the foot following implantation of a HINTEGRA ankle prosthesis: Evaluation with the Heidelberg Foot Model. *Orthopade* 2006;35:506-512.

30. Buechel FF, Pappas MJ, Iorio LJ: New Jersey low contact stress total ankle replacement: Biomechanical rationale and review of 23 cementless cases. *Foot Ankle* 1988;8:279-290.

31. Pappas M, Buechel FF, DePalma AF: Cylindrical total ankle joint replacement: Surgical and biomechanical rationale. *Clin Orthop Relat Res* 1976; 118:82-92.

32. Buechel FF Sr, Buechel FF Jr, Pappas MJ: Twenty-year evaluation of cementless mobile-bearing total ankle replacements. *Clin Orthop Relat Res* 2004;424:19-26.

33. Komistek RD, Stiehl JB, Buechel FF, Northcut EJ, Hajner ME: A determination of ankle kinematics using fluoroscopy. *Foot Ankle Int* 2000;21: 343-350.

34. Parsons P, Leslie I, Kennard E, Barker M: *Comparative Mechanical Testing of the Mobility Total Ankle Joint Replacement Prosthesis: Talar Component Subsidence, Bearing Insert Push-Out, and Prosthesis Stability*. Leeds, UK, DePuy International, 2003.

35. Bell CJ, Fisher J: Simulation of polyethylene wear in ankle joint prostheses. *J Biomed Mater Res B Appl Biomater* 2007;81:162-167.

36. Leardini A, Moschella D: Dynamic simulation of the natural and replaced human ankle joint. *Med Biol Eng Comput* 2002;40:193-199.

37. Leardini A, Catani F, Giannini S, O'Connor JJ: Computer-assisted design of the sagittal shapes of a

ligament-compatible total ankle replacement. *Med Biol Eng Comput* 2001;39:168-175.

38. Hvid I, Rasmussen O, Jensen NC, Nielsen S: Trabecular bone strength profiles at the ankle joint. *Clin Orthop Relat Res* 1985;199:306-312.

39. Deland JT, de Asla RJ, Segal A: Reconstruction of the chronically failed deltoid ligament: A new technique. *Foot Ankle Int* 2004;25:795-799.

40. Coetzee JC, Pomeroy GC, Watts JD, Barrow C: The use of autologous concentrated growth factors to promote syndesmosis fusion in the Agility total ankle replacement: A preliminary study. *Foot Ankle Int* 2005;26: 840-846.

41. Jung HG, Nicholson JJ, Parks B, Myerson MS: Radiographic and biomechanical support for fibular plating of the agility total ankle. *Clin Orthop Relat Res* 2004;424:118-124.

42. Raikin SM, Myerson MS: Avoiding and managing complications of the Agility total ankle replacement system. *Orthopedics* 2006;29:930-938.

43. Anderson T, Montgomery F, Carlsson A: Uncemented STAR total ankle prostheses. *J Bone Joint Surg Am* 2004; 86-A(suppl 1):103-111.

44. Hintermann B, Valderrabano V: Total ankle joint replacement. *Z Arztl Fortbild Qualitatssich* 2001;95:187-194.

45. Spirt AA, Assal M, Hansen ST Jr: Complications and failure after total ankle arthroplasty. *J Bone Joint Surg Am* 2004;86:1172-1178.

46. Carlsson A: Single- and double-coated star total ankle replacements: A clinical and radiographic follow-up study of 109 cases. *Orthopade* 2006;35: 527-532.

47. Carlsson A, Markusson P, Sundberg M: Radiostereometric analysis of the double-coated STAR total ankle prosthesis: A 3-5 year follow-up of 5 cases with rheumatoid arthritis and 5 cases with osteoarthrosis. *Acta Orthop* 2005;76:573-579.

48. Valderrabano V, Hintermann B, Dick W: Scandinavian total ankle replace-

ment: A 3.7-year average followup of 65 patients. *Clin Orthop Relat Res* 2004;424:47-56.

49. Wood PL, Deakin S: Total ankle replacement: The results in 200 ankles. *J Bone Joint Surg Br* 2003;85:334-341.

50. Anderson T, Montgomery F, Carlsson A: Uncemented STAR total ankle prostheses. Three to eight-year follow-up of fifty-one consecutive ankles. *J Bone Joint Surg Am* 2003;85-A:1321-1329.

51. Haskell A, Mann RA: Perioperative complication rate of total ankle replacement is reduced by surgeon experience. *Foot Ankle Int* 2004;25: 283-289.

52. Hintermann B, Valderrabano V, Dereymaeker G, Dick W: The HINTEGRA ankle: Rationale and short-term results of 122 consecutive ankles. *Clin Orthop Relat Res* 2004;424: 57-68.

53. Hintermann B, Valderrabano V, Knupp M, Horisberger M: The HINTEGRA ankle: Short- and mid-term results. *Orthopade* 2006;35:533-545.

54. Bonnin M, Judet T, Colombier JA, Buscayret F, Graveleau N, Piriou P: Midterm results of the Salto Total Ankle Prosthesis. *Clin Orthop Relat Res* 2004;424:6-18.

55. San Giovanni TP, Keblish DJ, Thomas WH, Wilson MG: Eight-year results of a minimally constrained total ankle arthroplasty. *Foot Ankle Int* 2006;27:418-426.

56. Doets HC, Brand R, Nelissen RG: Total ankle arthroplasty in inflammatory joint disease with use of two mobile-bearing designs. *J Bone Joint Surg Am* 2006;88:1272-1284.

57. Saltzman CL, Amendola A, Anderson R, et al: Surgeon training and complications in total ankle arthroplasty. *Foot Ankle Int* 2003;24:514-518.

58. Bolton-Maggs BG, Sudlow RA, Freeman MA: Total ankle arthroplasty: A long-term review of the London Hospital experience. *J Bone Joint Surg Br* 1985;67:785-790.

59. McGarvey WC, Clanton TO, Lunz

D: Malleolar fracture after total ankle arthroplasty: A comparison of two designs. *Clin Orthop Relat Res* 2004;424: 104-110.

60. Nelissen RG, Doets HC, Valstar ER: Early migration of the tibial component of the Buechel-Pappas total ankle prosthesis. *Clin Orthop Relat Res* 2006;448:146-151.

61. Ohgushi H, Kitamura S, Kotobuki N, et al: Clinical application of marrow mesenchymal stem cells for hard tissue repair. *Yonsei Med J* 2004;45: 61-67.

62. Coetzee JC, Castro MD: Accurate measurement of ankle range of motion after total ankle arthroplasty. *Clin Orthop Relat Res* 2004;424:27-31.

63. Kitaoka HB: Fusion techniques for failed total ankle arthroplasty. *Semin*

Arthroplasty 1992;3:51-57.

64. Kitaoka HB: Salvage of nonunion following ankle arthrodesis for failed total ankle arthroplasty. *Clin Orthop Relat Res* 1991;268:37-43.

65. Kitaoka HB, Romness DW: Arthrodesis for failed ankle arthroplasty. *J Arthroplasty* 1992;7:277-284.

66. Assal M, Greisberg J, Hansen ST Jr: Revision total ankle arthroplasty: Conversion of New Jersey Low Contact Stress to Agility: Surgical technique and case report. *Foot Ankle Int* 2004;25:922-925.

67. Knupp M, Hintermann B: Abstract: Conversion of ankle arthrodesis into total ankle arthroplasty. *74th Annual Meeting Proceedings*, Rosemont, IL, American Academy of Orthopaedic

Surgeons, 2007, p 491.

68. Gabrion A, Jarde O, Havet E, Mertl P, Olory B, de Lestang M: Ankle arthrodesis after failure of a total ankle prosthesis: Eight cases. *Rev Chir Orthop Reparatrice Appar Mot* 2004;90:353-359.

69. Zwipp H, Grass R: Ankle arthrodesis after failed joint replacement. *Oper Orthop Traumatol* 2005;17:518-533.

70. Lodhi Y, McKenna J, Herron M, Stephens MM: Total ankle replacement. *Ir Med J* 2004;97:104-105.

71. SooHoo NF, Kominski G: Cost-effectiveness analysis of total ankle arthroplasty. *J Bone Joint Surg Am* 2004; 86:2446-2455.

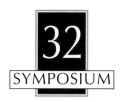

Salvage of Failed and Infected Total Ankle Replacements With Fusion

Keith L. Wapner, MD

Problems of Failed Arthroplasty

The salvage of failed and infected total ankle replacements presents challenges similar to those posed by the failure of other joint arthroplasties. However, the advantage of an array of adequate revision prostheses is lacking, the remaining bone stock is often limited on the talar side, and the soft-tissue envelope may be compromised. Therefore, removal of the prosthesis may be indicated. This leaves a large bony defect that must be dealt with unless the patient and physician are willing to accept significant shortening of the affected extremity.

Multiple problems can occur in conjunction with failed arthroplasty, including loss of bone stock, fracture and erosion of the malleoli, malleolar impingement, compromise of the soft-tissue envelope, wound dehiscence, talar avascular necrosis, and subtalar arthritis[1-8] (Fig. 1).

Loss of bone stock occurs in both the tibia and the talus and is often quite great. Defects in the tibial plafond may be reconstructed with either allograft or autograft. When significant malalignment is present, realignment may require corrective osteotomy and graft. Loss of bone in the body of the talus presents a greater challenge. There may not be enough viable body of the talus remaining to reconstruct it with structural bone graft and excision of the remaining talar body may be required.

Fracture and erosion of both the medial and lateral malleoli may lead to further shifting of the position of the prosthesis. This can increase either varus or valgus malalignment, causing further bony erosion on the tibial plafond or talar dome. This malalignment also may create skin breakdown from the increased pressure on the skin.

The soft-tissue envelope of the ankle is less forgiving than that of the hip or the knee. Most prostheses are placed through an anterior incision; the skin at this level can be easily compromised if meticulous technique is not used. Skin breakdown can lead to catastrophic infection with osteomyelitis. When skin slough occurs, a free flap may be required to obtain wound closure. In the aging patient, however, the distal vessels may not be adequate to perform a free flap; amputation may be the only option.[3,6,7,9]

As in other joint arthroplasties, infection may develop without skin breakdown. Infection complicates any attempt at salvage. Eradication of the soft-tissue infection and osteomyelitis must be accomplished to complete salvage of the limb.

Evaluation

In the evaluation of a patient with failed ankle arthroplasty, infection must be ruled out as either a primary cause of failure or as a secondary complication from failure. The use of MRI is not helpful

because of the degree of scatter that occurs from the implant. Bone scans will be positive but will not distinguish between infection and the consequences of loosening. A labeled white blood cell scan (indium In 111) combined with a bone scan (technetium Tc 99m) may be helpful. The labeled white cell scan may indicate an area of infection. Evaluation of the patient's erythrocyte sedimentation rate and C-reactive protein level also is helpful in ascertaining the presence of infection. In addition, joint aspiration can be used; although helpful if positive, a negative result is not conclusive.

Radiographic evaluation should be done with weight-bearing radiographs. Assessment of the degree of lucency surrounding the implant is important in planning the reconstruction. In addition, the degree and direction of subsidence need to be evaluated. These indicate the need for bone grafting and corrective osteotomy. These factors help in evaluating the options for methods of fixation.

The overall healing potential of the patient should be assessed. Pedal pulses should be evaluated to determine adequate circulation. If pulses cannot be palpated, an ischemic index study should be done. An ankle brachial index of 0.45 at both the tibialis posterior and dorsalis pedis arterial pulses is indicative of adequate healing potential. Evaluation of the condition of the skin surrounding the implant also is necessary and is helpful in

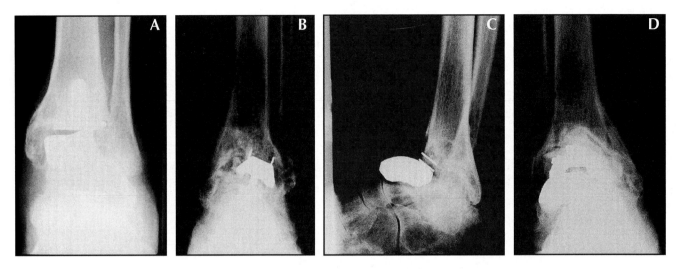

Fig. 1 A, AP radiograph demonstrating erosion of the medial malleolus with valgus malalignment of the prosthesis. **B,** AP radiograph demonstrating lateral subsidence of the prosthesis with significant bony erosion. **C,** Lateral radiograph demonstrating anterior extrusion of the talar component. **D,** AP radiograph demonstrating subsidence, bony erosions, and lucency around the prosthesis.

planning appropriate placement of the incision. Overall nutritional status of the patient should be assessed. If the patient is a smoker, he or she should be informed that smoking could impede the healing of any type of salvage procedure.

Surgery

In planning the surgical approach, the overall condition of the skin is assessed. Most ankle replacements are inserted through an anterior incision. The skin in this area is often thin and may not withstand vigorous manipulation. In general, a lateral incision is preferable in most salvage situations. The lateral fibula can be resected when converting to a fusion. Removal of the fibula allows access for removal of the loose joint components.

At the time of surgery, cultures should be taken of the synovium, joint fluid, and bone of both the talus and tibia. Often there is a severe reactive synovitis that requires a synovectomy. The implants are then removed. If cement has been used for placement of the implant, it must also be removed completely. Complete débridement down to the level of healthy cancellous bone is necessary to obtain healing. Opening of the tibial

canal may be required if sclerotic margins have developed. The viability of the talus and the amount of remaining bone must be determined. A decision must be made to try to achieve tibiotalar fusion, interposition bone graft fusion, or tibiocalcaneal fusion with excision of the talar body.

When infection is suspected, a staged procedure is advised.[10] After removal of the implant and complete synovectomy, cultures are sent for identification. An external fixator or an antibiotic-impregnated cement spacer can be used to maintain length. When infection is found, adequate antibiotic treatment is necessary.

When viability of the talus cannot be determined intraoperatively, staging the procedure and obtaining an MRI study to evaluate the talus can be considered. Once the tibial plafond and talar body remaining are determined, the options for fusion can be explored. The amount of shortening to be accepted can be discussed with the patient preoperatively. The need for and type of bone graft can be assessed once the size of the gap has been determined. Often the gap is too large to allow the use of an anterior iliac crest graft; it

may require a posterior iliac crest graft or an allograft. If enough viable talus remains, interposition bone grafting with salvage of the subtalar joint is preferable. If the talus is nonviable or if there is secondary degeneration of the subtalar joint, then excision of the body of the talus is indicated. Options at this time are either tibiocalcaneal fusion or interposition bone graft fusion to try to maintain length.

Salvage

The goals of salvage are to restore and maintain the length of the extremity. Loss of length comes from the initial resection of bone at the time of placement of the total ankle replacement, secondary loss of height from subsidence of the implant, and débridement back to viable bone at the time of salvage surgery.

Malalignment must be corrected. Malalignment can occur with subsidence or malposition of the implant. The ultimate goal is to achieve a stable arthrodesis with neutral dorsiflexion and plantar flexion of the ankle, 5° of residual hindfoot valgus, and external rotation equal to that of the contralateral limb.[11]

If the talar body is viable, an isolated ankle fusion can be done. If there are secondary changes in the subtalar joint, combined ankle and subtalar joint fusion may be required. If the talar body is not viable, a talectomy with interposition bone graft or tibiocalcaneal fusion can be used.

When large defects are present, the options are either posterior iliac crest graft or allograft. For smaller defects, anterior iliac crest, use of the resected distal fibula, or allograft can be considered. The technique of fixation is determined once the type of fusion has been decided on. When an isolated ankle fusion is to be done, multiple screws often are adequate. Cannulated screws are preferable because they allow evaluation of the overall alignment of the limb before final screw placement. This is most easily done through a lateral incision with fibulectomy. Fixation with 7.3-mm screws generally provides adequate compression if the residual bone stock is satisfactory. Additional fixation for either allograft or autograft may be required in the final construct.

When talectomy is necessary, fixation with an intramedullary rod is an option. This technique has the advantage of being familiar to the general orthopaedic surgeon. It does not provide excellent compression, however. Fixation with locking screws will provide a rigid construct, but it is difficult to secure bone grafts with this technique. An intramedullary rod is most easily used when talectomy and tibiocalcaneal fusion are done (Fig. 2).

An Ilizarov or other type of external fixator can secure fusion. If significant length discrepancy is present, the fixator can be used to try to lengthen the tibia in carefully selected patients. Most patients undergoing ankle replacements are older, however, and lengthening techniques may not have a place in this patient population. Another approach is to obtain fusion first and lengthen secondarily. As mentioned previously, fixation of bone grafting with external fixation alone may

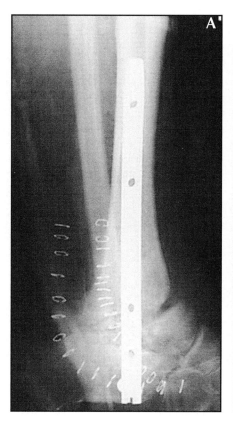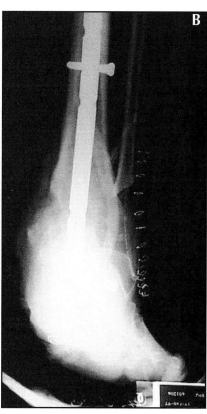

Fig. 2 Lateral (**A**) and AP (**B**) radiographs demonstrating partial talectomy and fusion with intramedullary rod fixation.

be difficult. Hybrid internal and external fixation may be required.

Another technique that provides rigid fixation and allows for secure fixation of bone grafts is the use of a pediatric blade plate. This was first described for the treatment of Charcot arthropathy. A pediatric blade plate can be used with talectomy or for combined ankle and subtalar joint fusion (Fig. 3).

With each of these fixation techniques, bone grafting is required unless shortening is to be accepted. Malleolar resection with removal of the margins of the tibia, fibula, and talus is the simplest technique but causes the most significant shortening.[5] Internal or external fixation can be used for fixation of the bones.

Chuinard and Peterson[12] described a technique for interposition iliac crest grafting for ankle fusion, which Stauffer[8] modified to apply to the salvage of failed

ankle prostheses. After removal of the prosthesis, a tricortical block of iliac crest is placed horizontally to fill the defect. Additional cancellous graft is used to fill any remaining voids. Campbell and associates[13] described a technique using a vertically oriented tricortical iliac crest graft augmented with cancellous graft. This technique has the advantage of filling a larger defect (Fig. 4). Both of these techniques can be augmented by using the resected fibula as either a vascularized graft or interposition graft. Initial alignment can be obtained by placing a percutaneous Steinmann pin retrograde through the heel. Fixation can be achieved with internal or external fixation.

Russotti and associates[9] described a posterolateral approach with transection of the Achilles tendon to expose the ankle and subtalar joints between the flexor hallucis longus muscle medially and the

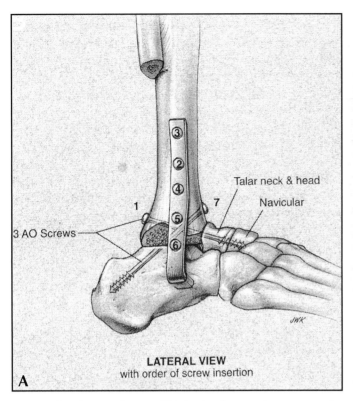
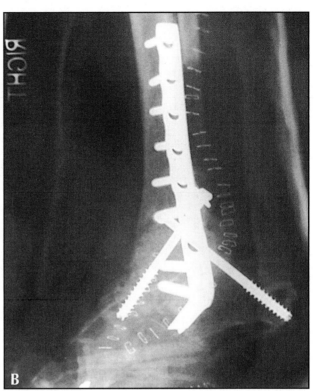

Fig. 3 A, The Alvarez technique of blade plate fixation, demonstrating the recommended order of screw replacement. **B,** Lateral radiograph of patient treated with blade plate fixation. (Reproduced with permission from Alvarez RG, McKibbin W: Tibiocalcaneal arthrodesis using pediatric blade plate. *Oper Tech Orthop* 1996;6:217-221.)

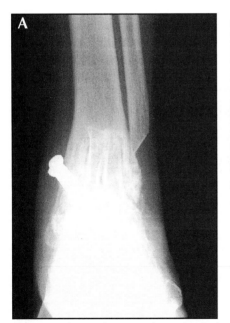
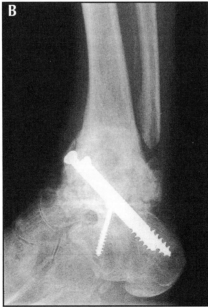

Fig. 4 Lateral (**A**) and AP (**B**) radiographs of salvage performed with a modified Campbell technique.

peroneus brevis muscle laterally. After removal of the implant, a trough is created in the posterior tibia, talus, and calcaneus and is packed with bone graft. The authors used an external fixator to secure the construct.

Newer prosthetic designs require less bony resection, and revision to another prosthesis, rather than resection and fusion, is becoming a more viable option. However, the long-term survivorship of this type of revision is unknown at this time. Ultimately, resection and fusion, or amputation, may be the only remaining options.

All of these techniques are demanding and require both good preoperative planning and meticulous surgical technique. The patient should be advised that these are salvage techniques and that, if unsuccessful, complications ranging from infection to nonunion can occur and below-knee amputation may be required.

References

1. Bolton-Maggs BG, Sudlow RA, Freeman MA: Total ankle arthroplasty: A long-term review of the London hospital experience. *J Bone Joint Surg Br* 1985;67:785-790.

2. Groth HE, Fitch HF: Salvage procedures for complications of total ankle arthroplasty. *Clin Orthop* 1987;224:244-250.

3. Kitaoka HB: Salvage of nonunion following ankle arthrodesis for failed total ankle arthroplasty. *Clin Orthop* 1991;268:37-43.

4. Kitaoka HB, Romness DW: Arthrodesis for failed ankle arthroplasty. *J Arthroplasty* 1992; 7:277-284.

5. Kitaoka HB: Fusion techniques for failed total ankle arthroplasty. *Semin Arthroplasty* 1992;3: 51-57.

6. McGuire MR, Kyle RF, Gustilo RB, Premer RF: Comparative analysis of ankle arthroplasty versus ankle arthrodesis. *Clin Orthop* 1988; 226:174-181.

7. Newton SE III: Total ankle arthroplasty: Clinical study of fifty cases. *J Bone Joint Surg Am* 1982;64:104-111.

8. Stauffer RN: Salvage of failed total ankle arthroplasty. *Clin Orthop* 1982;170:184-188.

9. Russotti GM, Johnson KA, Cass JR: Tibiotalocalcaneal arthrodesis for arthritis and deformity of the hind part of the foot. *J Bone Joint Surg Am* 1988;70:1304-1307.

10. Cierny G III, Cook WG, Mader JT: Ankle arthrodesis in the presence of ongoing sepsis: Indications, methods, and results. *Orthop Clin North Am* 1989;20:709-721.

11. Buck P, Morrey BF, Chao EY: The optimum position of arthrodesis of the ankle: A gait study of the knee and ankle. *J Bone Joint Surg Am* 1987;69:1052-1062.

12. Chuinard EG, Peterson RE: Distraction-compression bone-graft arthrodesis of the ankle: A method especially applicable in children. *J Bone Joint Surg Am* 1963;45:481-490.

13. Campbell CJ, Reinhart WT, Kalenak A: Arthrodesis of the ankle: Deep autogenous inlay grafts with maximum cancellous-bone apposition. *J Bone Joint Surg Am* 1974;56:63-70.

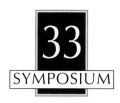

33
SYMPOSIUM

Joint Distraction as Treatment for Ankle Osteoarthritis

Peter M. van Roermund, PhD
Floris P.J.G. Lafeber, PhD

Osteoarthritis

The patient with ankle osteoarthritis has to cope with progressive pain, stiffness, and functional impairment. There is an ongoing deterioration of the joint cartilage due to rupture of the collagen network, loss of matrix molecules, mostly proteoglycans and collagen fragments, and, as a result, loss of the mechanical properties of the cartilage.[1] As a consequence of these mechanical and biochemical changes of the cartilage matrix, normal joint use will further increase cartilage damage. Chondrocytes sense these changes in the damaged matrix and will attempt to repair the matrix.[2] Finally, these chondrocytes lose their phenotype and dedifferentiate. They start to proliferate and produce inappropriate types of matrix molecules,[3] catabolic cytokines, and matrix proteases, damaging the cartilage further.[4] Bone is characteristically altered by sclerosis, and osteophytes are formed, possibly in an attempt to stabilize the joint, minimizing mechanical impact on the cartilage. Both for patient and physician the main question to be answered is: how can this process of progressive cartilage damage be stopped? How can a complete destruction of the joint be prevented? At present, severe osteoarthritis cannot be stopped. The only really effective procedures in treatment of

severely painful osteoarthritic ankle joints are ankle arthrodesis or arthroplasty. However, both of these procedures cause the patient to lose the joint. So the basic problem is that no proven effective remedy for osteoarthritis exists.

Attempts to treat osteoarthritis are numerous. Pain may be effectively treated with medication, possibly by suppression of mild secondary inflammation, which partly might delay destruction of articular cartilage.[5] Alternative nonmedicinal and noninvasive treatments, such as electromagnetic stimulation, acupuncture, diathermy, or yoga, may relieve pain but have never been proven to be effective in repair of joint destruction.[6,7] Much effort is put into the development of new modalities to treat moderate to severe cases of osteoarthritis. Only a limited number of reports on clinical application of these new approaches are available at present. In autologous chondrocyte transplantation,[8] healthy cartilage is taken from uninvolved areas of an injured joint during arthroscopy. Chondrocytes are isolated, cultured ex vivo, and then injected in the area of the defect. Results are not yet conclusive.[9] Further advances in the procedures of cell isolation, multiplication, and retransplantation will be required to improve the technique.

This technique may be specifically useful in repair of deep isolated cartilage defects, which are a precursor of osteoarthritis. Results of arthroscopic debridement of osteoarthritic joints, especially in the late stages of osteoarthritis, are reported to be unpredictable, and, if beneficial, lasting for an uncertain period of time. Laser-assisted arthroscopic debridement[10] is used to remove osteophytes, to reshape cartilage surface, and to remove inflamed synovial tissue. It has been suggested that this method offers an advantage over conventional debridement. However, further research is required to investigate possible adverse effects on articular chondrocytes, which may counteract the positive effects of laser debridement. Several clinical studies have evaluated the use of intra-articular injections of hyaluron,[11] a viscous substance important in joint lubrication. It may be questioned whether the minor effects justify serial intra-articular injections. Although this treatment is gaining acceptance for treatment of osteoarthritis, further evidence of efficacy and utility is required to determine whether hyaluron will become an established form of treatment. Osteochondral retransplantation[12] of intact tissue taken from nonweight-bearing areas to chondral defects seems promising judging from animal

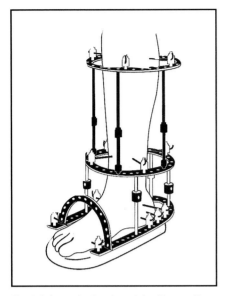

Fig. 1 Schematic drawing of the Ilizarov fixation used for ankle distraction.

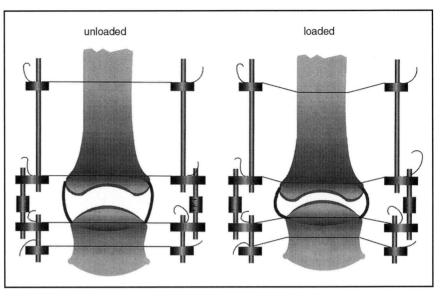

Fig. 2 Schematic depiction of the intra-articular intermittent fluid pressures during walking due to the axial flexibility in the Ilizarov external fixation.

studies, but clinical studies have still to be reported on.

Joint Distraction: A Relatively New Approach in the Treatment of Osteoarthritis

This technique is based on the hypothesis that osteoarthritic cartilage has some reparative activity if it is mechanically unloaded and if the intermittent synovial fluid flow and fluid pressure, essential for the nutrition of cartilage, is maintained. The aim is to achieve a temporary (about 3 months) release of mechanical stress on articular cartilage by a distraction of the articular surfaces combined with continuation of intra-articular intermittent fluid flow/fluid pressure (Fig. 1). This strategy was the basis for a study on the effects of joint distraction in treatment of severe ankle osteoarthritis, including the repair capacity of cartilage under these conditions, as reported by van Valburg.[13]

Apart from unloading the osteoarthritic cartilage, another characteristic of joint distraction is the maintenance of intra-articular intermittent fluid flow. Absence of mechanical contact between both degenerative articular surfaces is achieved by distraction of the joint by means of an external fixation frame. Intermittent fluid flow/fluid pressure can be maintained by the use of hinges in the distraction frame. Such an articulating distraction has been used for the osteoarthritic hip.[13] Intermittent intra-articular fluid flow can also be obtained by the use of an Ilizarov frame with thin (1.5 mm) Kirschner wires (K-wires), tensioned to external rings (Fig. 1). Loading and unloading of the joint in such a distraction frame will result in intermittent intra-articular fluid pressure/fluid flow due to the flexibility of the K-wires[14] (Fig. 2).

The Technique of Distraction

Distraction of the ankle joint is done by using Ilizarov ring fixation consisting of 2 rings around the leg, 1 half ring around the heel, and 2 long plates at both sides of the foot at the front connected by a half ring (Fig. 1). Two K-wires are drilled through the proximal and distal part of the tibia and fixed under 12 N to 2 external rings, both connected by screw-threaded rods. Two wires with olives are drilled through the calcaneus and fixed under 5 N tension to a half ring, 1 wire without tension through the talus and 1 wire under 9 N with an olive wire medial through the forefoot (Fig. 1). It is important to drill a pin through the talus, otherwise the subtalar joint is distracted as well, which is not preferred. Distraction is subsequently carried out for 0.5 mm twice daily until a total distraction of 5 mm is achieved. The absence of mechanical loading of both degenerative articular surfaces of tibia and talus, checked by radiograph under joint loading, is maintained for about 3 months, during which time full weightbearing is allowed. Intermittent changes in ankle joint fluid pressure during loading and unloading under distraction were measured in patients by the use of a pressure sensitive catheter placed intra-articularly. On average it appeared that intra-articular fluid pressure changed from 3 to 10 kPa during loading and unloading, with a frequency of around 0.5 Hz during walking.[14] A representative measurement is shown in Figure 3.

Clinical Experiences
A Retrospective Study

Eleven relatively young (35 ± 15 years) patients with severe posttraumatic ankle osteoarthritis had been treated with Ilizarov joint distraction for 3 months. The osteoarthritis was so painful that an arthrodesis was indicated but refused. Mean follow-up of these patients at the time of evaluation was 20 ± 6 month (ranging from 1 to 5 years). The retrospective data, collected from charts before and after treatment, were surprisingly good and revealed a prolonged relief of pain and unchanged or increased joint mobility. The radiographic joint space, initially narrowed because of osteoarthritis, was unchanged or had remained widened after distraction in 50% of the cases. Such data are inspiring and strongly suggest that joint distraction is a promising approach in treatment of severe ankle osteoarthritis. The observed prolonged clinical improvement and the joint space widening suggest that joint distraction has a beneficial effect on cartilage metabolism.

A Prospective Uncontrolled Study

Between 1993 and 1997, 26 patients were treated. In 16 cases the follow-up was 1 year, in 12 cases, 2 years, in 4 cases there was a follow-up of 3 years, and in a single case there was a follow-up of 4 years. Five had a follow-up of less than 1 year and 5 were failures in the first year and were treated with an arthrodesis. As in the retrospective evaluation, patients were relatively young, 39 years (range, 17 to 53 years), and mostly male. In most cases, the osteoarthritis was posttraumatic. Inclusion criterion was a severely painful ankle for

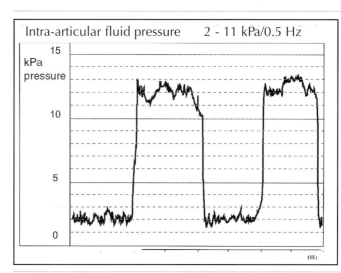

Fig. 3 Representation of an intra-articular pressure measurement in an ankle joint during Ilizarov distraction. During loading intra-articular fluid pressure increases, and there is a subsequent decrease during unloading.

which an arthrodesis was considered. If needed, osteophytes were removed arthroscopically to place and fix the foot into a plantigrade position. The 5-mm distraction for 3 months was carried out as described above. The clinical status, evaluated by measurement of pain, crepitus, and swelling, was expressed as a percentage of the maximum score. After removal of the external fixation frame, the scores remained initially high because of persisting swelling and crepitus, but they improved after 1 year and in the following years (Fig. 4). Functional loss was assessed by a questionnaire, a modification of the functional index for hip and knee osteoarthritis.[15] Function improved significantly after 1 year and this improvement continued (Fig. 4). Pain was measured by use of a box-scale, ranging from 10 (unbearable pain) to 0 (pain free). After 1 year there was a significant relief of pain, with a further improvement in the following years. Ankle mobility was measured by the range of motion. Joint mobility was maintained during the entire follow-up, showing a small improvement in the years after joint distraction. Moreover, radiographic measurements demonstrated an increase in joint space width (Fig. 5). All data

were comparable to the data from the retrospective study. Our conclusion is that Ilizarov joint distraction of a painful osteoarthritic ankle joint can result in clinical improvement after a year, and that this improvement continues for a significant period of time. Although we do not know at present how long these effects may last, in most patients, an arthrodesis could at least be delayed for several years.

Possible Underlying Mechanisms

A 3-month distraction period might be just enough to give the dedifferentiated chondrocytes in the osteoarthritic cartilage the opportunity to redifferentiate, to stop proliferation, and to create an appropriate matrix around them. In the follow-up after distraction, matrix repair might be continued, as is suggested by the slow but progressive increase in joint space widening in the years after distraction. Matrix repair may be facilitated by diminished mechanical impact on the cartilage during revalidation in the first months after distraction, a period of walking with crutches and low impact joint loading. We found a reduction of subchondral sclerosis and bone density in the tibial shaft as a result of the distraction. Bone den-

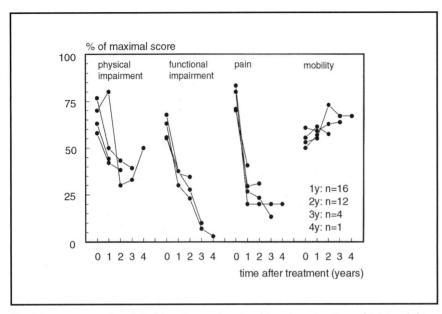

Fig. 4 Average scores for clinical impairment, functional impairment, pain, and joint mobility before Ilizarov joint distraction and after 1, 2, 3, and 4 years of follow-up. Data are presented as a percentage of the maximum score being: 10 points for clinical impairment; 30 points for functional impairment, and 10 points for pain. Mobility is presented as percentage from the contralateral control joint.

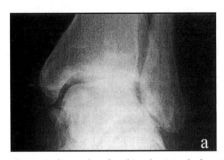
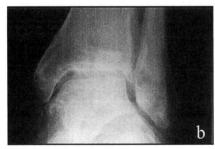

Fig. 5 Radiographs of a tibiotalar joint before (**A**) and 3 years after (**B**) joint distraction. Joint space was widened compared to the condition before distraction.

sity was restored within 1 year after distraction, but subchondral sclerosis remained reduced for more than 2 years (personal communication, AC Marÿnissen, 1998). This result of the distraction may improve shock absorption by the bone, diminishing the impact on the cartilage. The idea of actual repair of cartilage, however, remains difficult to prove in patients. Magnetic resonance imaging (MRI) and radiographs will not provide us with the proper data. More funda-

mental approaches, such as cultures of human articular cartilage and animal models for osteoarthritis, are needed to unravel the actual mechanisms behind possible cartilage repair as a result of joint distraction.

Does Joint Distraction Result in Cartilage Repair?
An Experimental In Vitro Study
Mild to moderate human preclinical osteoarthritic knee cartilage was subjected to the characteristics of joint

distraction: absence of mechanical loading and the presence of intermittent fluid pressure. This type of cartilage shows histologic changes of osteoarthritis comparable to clinically defined osteoarthritis.[16] In general, all changes observed in osteoarthritic joints are, to a lesser extent, observed in the joints with preclinical osteoarthritic cartilage and are significantly different from joints with normal cartilage. This type of osteoarthritic cartilage, normal healthy knee cartilage, and inflammatory cells (mononuclear cells) from the osteoarthritic synovial fluid were used to investigate the in vitro effects on articular cartilage of intermittent fluid pressures (0 to 13 kPa; 0. 33 Hz) as measured in the patients, in absence of mechanical stress. Cartilage and mononuclear cells were cultured both separately and together (coculture). Intermittent fluid pressure was applied via a pressure chamber to which a computer-controlled pressure system was connected (Fig. 6). Controls were placed in an identical chamber at ambient pressure. Cartilage matrix (proteoglycan) synthesis was stimulated by about 50% by intermittent fluid pressure in osteoarthritic cartilage; normal cartilage was not affected.[17] No effects on proteoglycan release were detected. Inhibition of proteoglycan synthesis, induced by osteoarthritic synovial fluid mononuclear cells in coculture, was reduced when cultures had been exposed to intermittent fluid pressure. Analysis of conditioned media of osteoarthritic synovial fluid cells revealed that the beneficial effect of intermittent fluid pressure was accompanied by a decrease in production of the catabolic cytokines interleukin-1 (IL-1) and tumor necrosis factor-alpha (TNFα), cytokines involved in upregulation of matrix-destructive metalloproteinase activity. Thus, low levels of intermittent fluid pressure as occurring in vivo during joint distraction may have beneficial effects on joint tissue in osteoarthritis, indicating that this factor could be involved in actual repair of cartilage.

A Canine In Vivo Model

Intermittent fluid pressure in absence of mechanical stresses in vitro strongly suggests that joint distraction can provide structural beneficial changes in osteoarthritic cartilage. Unfortunately, actual repair of osteoarthritic cartilage in patients is difficult to study. Evaluation of cartilage by MRI or histologic evaluation of cartilage biopsies after arthroscopy have their restrictions (not representative or too little material, no quantitative measures).[18,19] For this reason, an animal model was used to study the effects of joint distraction on the early changes in articular cartilage and on secondary inflammation in osteoarthritis. In beagle dogs, experimental osteoarthritis was induced by anterior cruciate ligament transection (ACLT) in 1 knee joint, with subsequent instability. The other knee served as internal control. Eleven weeks later, the ACLT dogs were randomly divided into 2 groups. One group was treated with articulating joint distraction (Fig. 7); the other dogs received no treatment after ACLT (osteoarthritic controls). The aim of distraction was to achieve the absence of mechanical stresses on the articular cartilage in combination with intra-articular intermittent fluid pressure, as observed during clinical treatment. Because the dogs did not load their treated joint significantly, changes in intra-articular fluid pressure were generated by motion of the joint. These changes in intra-articular fluid pressure, measured by means of a pressure transducer connected to an intra-articularly positioned catheter, revealed that flex-

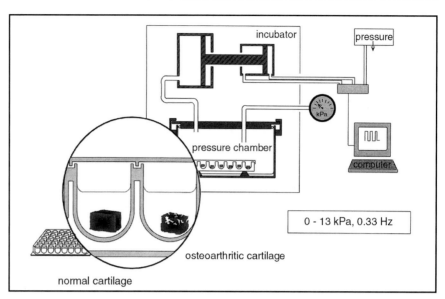

Fig. 6 Schematic drawing of the in vitro pressure device. Microtiter plates (96-well) with normal and osteoarthritic cartilage are placed in a pressure chamber to which a computer controlled pressure system is connected. Control cultures are carried out in an identical chamber under ambient pressure.

ion and extension of the canine knee joint, under distraction without joint loading, resulted in pressure levels from 3 ± 2 to 12 ± 5 kPa. The absence of mechanical contact between both articulating surfaces was demonstrated radiographically (Fig. 7). Dogs were exercised in a group twice a day for half an hour on a patio. Twenty-five weeks after ACLT all dogs were killed, and both cartilage and synovium of all knee joints were analyzed according to standard procedures.

Histologic gradation of inflammation of the synovial tissue revealed a mild degree of inflammation in the osteoarthritic control group which was significantly reduced by joint distraction. This corroborates the in vitro findings, showing that the absence of mechanical stress combined with intermittent fluid pressure decreases the secondary inflammatory features present in human osteoarthritis. In addition, joint distraction results in normalization of

cartilage matrix turnover. Changes in proteoglycan synthesis and release, characteristic for early osteoarthritis, were completely normalized in the osteoarthritic joints treated with distraction. Effects were observed in femoral as well as tibial cartilage. The decreased proteoglycan content, as a characteristic of osteoarthritis, was not improved by joint distraction. It is likely that a subsequent follow-up period is needed after removal of the fixation frame. In patients, clinical improvement, including joint space widening, was experienced gradually after removal of the distraction frame. In the presently used animal model, such a follow-up is impossible, because joint instability caused by ACLT remains a trigger for osteoarthritis. In conclusion, joint distraction, a combination of unloading of degenerative cartilage in the presence of intermittent fluid pressures, induces reduction of inflammation and normalization of matrix turnover. Both in vivo and in vitro experiments

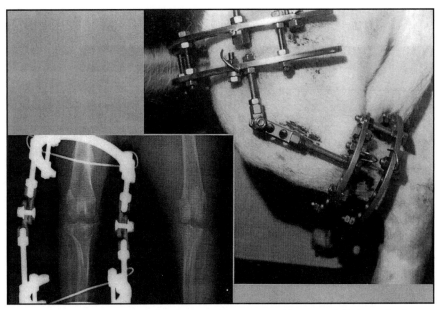

Fig. 7 Illustration of joint distraction of the dog knee joint. Half pins are drilled into the femur and connected with half oval rings around the upper limb. Kirschner wires are drilled through the tibia and connected to rings around the lower limb. Distraction of the femoral and tibial fixations is carried out by use of screw-threaded rods with hinges. The radiograph shows joint space widening as a control for the absence of mechanical stress during distraction.

suggest that the promising clinical results of ankle distraction are accompanied by actual changes in cartilage.

What is the Future for Joint Distraction as a Treatment for Osteoarthritis?

Evidence that ankle distraction results in cartilage repair and may be advocated as a remedy for osteoarthritis is still circumstantial. Nevertheless, the results of clinical, in vitro, and animal studies as described are hopeful. The clinical study has to be controlled, although such a set-up will be difficult. Animal studies that allow a prolonged follow-up after temporary joint distraction must be initiated to evaluate if there is real cartilage repair. The importance of the transient reduction of bone density in the tibial shaft after ankle distraction and the prolonged diminished subchondral sclerosis should also be investigated. Although the reported distraction

technique can be applied to many other joints,[20] its effect on osteoarthritis in particular joints must be studied separately. In other words, many more studies are needed before we can conclude that joint distraction is a remedy for osteoarthritis.

References

1. Buckwalter JA, Mankin HJ: Articular cartilage: Part I. Tissue design and chondrocyte-matrix interactions. *J Bone Joint Surg* 1997;79A:600–611.

2. Lafeber FP, van Roy H, Wilbrink B, Huber-Bruning O, Bijlsma JW: Human osteoarthritic cartilage is synthetically more active but in culture less vital than normal cartilage. *J Rheumatol* 1992;19:123–129.

3. Lafeber FP, van der Kraan PM, van Roy HL, et al: Local changes in proteoglycan synthesis during culture are different for normal and osteoarthritic cartilage. *Am J Pathol* 1992;140:1421–1429.

4. Buckwalter JA, Mankin HJ: Articular cartilage: Part II. Degeneration and osteoarthrosis, repair, regeneration, and transplantation. *J Bone Joint Surg* 1997;79A:612–632.

5. March LM, Brooks PM: Clinical trials in osteoarthritis. *Ann Rheum Dis* 1996;55:491–493.

6. Puett DW, Griffin MR: Published trials of nonmedicinal and noninvasive therapies for hip and knee osteoarthritis. *Ann Intern Med* 1994;121:133–140.

7. Takeda W, Wessel J: Acupuncture for the treatment of pain of osteoarthritic knees. *Arthritis Care Res* 1994;7:118–122.

8. Buckwalter JA, Lohmander S: Operative treatment of osteoarthrosis: Current practice and future development. *J Bone Joint Surg* 1994;76A:1405–1418.

9. Breinan HA, Minas T, Hsu HP, Nehrer S, Sledge CB, Spector M: Effect of cultured autologous chondrocytes on repair of chondral defects in a canine model. *J Bone Joint Surg* 1997;79A:1439–1451.

10. Zangger P, Gerber BE: Use of laser in arthroscopy of the ankle: Indications, method, first results [German]. *Orthopade* 1996;25:73–78.

11. Lohmander LS, Dalen N, Englund G, et al: Intra-articular hyaluronan injections in the treatment of osteoarthritis of the knee: A randomised, double blind, placebo controlled multicentre trial. Hyaluronan Multicentre Trial Group. *Ann Rheum Dis* 1996;55:424–431.

12. Bobic V: Arthroscopic osteochondral autograft transplantation in anterior cruciate ligament reconstruction: A preliminary clinical study. *Knee Surg Sports Traumatol Arthrosc* 1996;3:262–264.

13. van Valburg AA: *Ilizarov Joint Distraction in Treatment of Osteoarthritis.* Elinkwijk, Utrecht, University Medical Centre of Utrecht, The Netherlands. Thesis.

14. van Valburg AA, van Roermund PM, Lammens J, et al: Can Ilizarov joint distraction delay the need for an arthrodesis of the ankle? A preliminary report. *J Bone Joint Surg* 1995;77B:720–725.

15. Lequesne MG, Mery C, Samson M, Gerard P: Indexes of severity for osteoarthritis of the hip and knee: Validation. Value in comparison with other assessment tests. *Scand J Rheumatol* 1987;65(suppl):85–89.

16. van Valburg AA, Wenting MJ, Beekman B, Te Koppele JM, Lafeber FP, Bijlsma JW: Degenerated human articular cartilage at autopsy represents preclinical osteoarthritic cartilage: Comparison with clinically defined osteoarthritic cartilage. *J Rheumatol* 1997;24:358–364.

17. Lafeber F, Veldhuijzen JP, Vanroy JL, Huber-Bruning O, Bijlsma JW: Intermittent hydrostatic compressive force stimulates exclusively the proteoglycan synthesis of osteoarthritic human cartilage. *Br J Rheumatol* 1992;31:437–442.

18. Brandt KD, Fife RS, Braunstein EM, Katz B: Radiographic grading of the severity of knee osteoarthritis: Relation of the Kellgren and Lawrence grade to a grade based on joint space narrowing, and correlation with arthroscopic evidence of articular cartilage degeneration. *Arthritis Rheum* 1991;34:1381–1386.

19. Martel W, Adler RS, Chan K, Niklason L, Helvie MA, Jonsson K: Overview: New methods in imaging osteoarthritis. *J Rheumatol* 1991;27(suppl):32–37.

20. van Roermund PM, van Valburg AA, Duivemann E, et al: Function of stiff joints may be restored by Ilizarov joint distraction: Three case reports. *Clin Orthop* 1998;348:220–227.

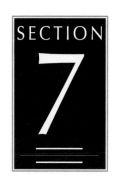

SECTION 7

Reconstruction of Foot and Ankle Deformity

Reconstruction of Foot and Ankle Deformity

Foot and ankle deformity can be attributed to malalignment of bones or joints caused by trauma, asymmetric cartilage wear, or ligament instability. The goals of deformity reconstruction include achieving a comfortable, stable, plantigrade foot. Successful reconstruction requires an understanding of the hindfoot, midfoot, and forefoot deformity and careful selection of the surgical procedures (arthrodesis, osteotomy, soft-tissue release, and tendon transfer) needed to correct the deformity.

Accurate measurements of the deformity are important for selecting the optimal reconstructive procedures; however, measuring angles is difficult because of the complex foot and ankle anatomy and short bone segments. Hindfoot varus deformity may be difficult to measure despite the availability of specific hindfoot radiographs. Secondary, compensatory foot deformities commonly develop to keep the foot plantigrade. For example, distal tibial varus deformity may be associated with hindfoot eversion and forefoot valgus deformity. If the secondary deformities become rigid, correction of the primary deformity may aggravate the compensatory deformity unless it also is reconstructed.

Other considerations in deformity reconstruction include the patient's age and skin condition, the location of previous surgical wounds at risk for poor healing, the vascular supply, the magnitude of the deformity, and the severity of arthrosis. Deformity correction requires an accurate diagnosis, including growth potential or progressive neurologic disease, because of the associated potential for deformity recurrence. For example, correction of an adult tibial varus mal-

union deformity may have a low incidence of recurrence, but equinovarus deformity in congenital clubfoot may recur after reconstruction. In a diagnosis associated with recurrence, the surgeon may select a more extensive reconstruction, and long-term bracing may be indicated. Technical factors to consider include the type of fixation, prophylactic tarsal tunnel release when correcting equinovarus deformity, and tendon transfer to prevent recurrence of deformity.

The chapter by Crawford and Amendola reviews the etiology of ankle osteoarthritis, the importance of correct limb and tibial mechanical axis alignment for normal ankle joint contact forces, and the evaluation of limb alignment. Further definitions and diagrams of angle measurements are available elsewhere.[1] The authors discuss staging of ankle osteoarthritis, preoperative planning, and the surgical technique of distal tibial osteotomy. In patients with valgus or varus ankle osteoarthritis, recent studies have confirmed that realignment surgery, including distal tibial osteotomy, can preserve the ankle joint and improve ankle pain and function in some patients.[2-5] If the ankle joint cannot be preserved and a total ankle replacement is considered, varus deformity may be corrected with a medial malleolar lengthening osteotomy.[6]

In their chapter, Joseph and Myerson review the correction of multiplanar hindfoot deformities, such as rigid cavovarus or planovalgus deformity, with arthrodesis, osteotomies, and soft-tissue or tendon releases. Cavovarus foot deformity may increase the anteromedial ankle joint pressure and contribute to ankle arthrosis.[7] Joseph and Myerson also discuss corrective osteotomy techniques for

reconstruction of foot deformity created by malunion of a previous triple arthrodesis. Preoperative evaluation of the foot and ankle, including the clinical and radiographic assessment of alignment, is reviewed. The authors emphasize the importance of defining the apex of the deformity for planning the corrective osteotomy or arthrodesis at the apex, if possible. Sequential correction of complex deformity is done from the hindfoot to the forefoot.

Johnson and Yu review the treatment of stage II and III adult acquired flatfoot deformity with arthrodesis, osteotomy, and tendon transfer. Arthrodesis options may include talonavicular, subtalar, double (talonavicular and calcaneocuboid), and triple (talonavicular, calcaneocuboid, and subtalar) arthrodesis. Adjunctive procedures are discussed including medial displacement calcaneal osteotomy, lateral column lengthening, medial cuneiform plantar-flexion osteotomy, gastrocnemius-soleus lengthening, and flexor digitorum longus tendon transfer. It is important to evaluate the entire medial column for instability and arthrosis that contribute to the flatfoot deformity.

There is controversy concerning the optimal procedure for reconstructing adult acquired flatfoot deformity. The appropriate procedure may vary, depending on the specific features of the deformity such as heel valgus, forefoot varus, and ankle equinus deformities. Biomechanical studies of posterior tibial tendon dysfunction showed that increased load on the medial arch contributes to flatfoot, and both medial displacement calcaneal osteotomy and lateral column lengthening may decrease this load.[8,9] A recent, small study of patients with adult acquired flatfoot (in whom arthrodesis was not included in the reconstruction) concluded that patients who were treated with lateral column lengthening had greater realignment and maintenance of correction, but an increased frequency of degenerative arthritis and nonunion, compared with those treated with medial displacement calcaneal osteotomy.[10] Another study of patients younger than 50 years with posterior tibial tendon dysfunction showed improved function after reconstruction with medial displacement calcaneal osteotomy with a flexor digitorum longus tendon transfer, with lateral column lengthening added to treat patients with greater deformity.[11]

For arthrodesis, recent studies have described correction of severe planovalgus deformity with a double (subtalar and talonavicular) arthrodesis through a medial approach, decreasing the potential risk of lateral wound complications.[12,13] The medial approach also may be used for triple arthrodesis for fixed hindfoot valgus deformity.[14,15] Furthermore, a posterior, Achilles tendon-splitting approach has been used for subtalar arthrodesis to correct a varus or valgus deformity.[16] Severe planovalgus foot deformity may be corrected with hindfoot arthrodesis using a tricortical allograft.[17]

The chapters by Cummings and associates and Dietz review congenital clubfoot deformity, including etiology, evaluation, nonsurgical management (for example, the Kite and Lovell, Ponseti, Denis Browne, and other methods), surgical correction, and the treatment of residual or recurrent deformity. The etiology and management of congenital clubfoot is the subject of much current research, evidenced in a recent symposium.[18] A recent comparative study of nonsurgical treatments showed that the Ponseti method may result in faster correction and greater ankle dorsiflexion with fewer casts than the Kite and Lovell method.[19] The Ponseti method also may be effective in older infants (age 4 to 13 months) with idiopathic, congenital clubfoot.[20]

Recurrent clubfoot deformity after nonsurgical treatment with the Ponseti method may result from inadequate bracing, and a recently described flexible abduction brace may be associated with improved compliance and a decreased risk of recurrent deformity.[21] Surgical treatment of congenital clubfoot with extensive subtalar ligament release may result in long-term correction without recurrence.[22] Newer treatments for residual or recurrent congenital clubfoot include Ilizarov correction with or without calcaneal osteotomy.[23-25]

Richard Evan Gellman, MD
Clinical Assistant Professor
Department of Orthopaedics
Oregon Health and Science University
Summit Orthopaedics
Portland, Oregon

References

1. Paley D, ed: *Principles of Deformity Correction.* New York, NY, Springer-Verlag, 2002.

2. Tanaka Y, Takakura Y, Hayashi K, Taniguchi A, Kumai T, Sugimoto K: Low tibial osteotomy for varus-type osteoarthritis of the ankle. *J Bone Joint Surg Br* 2006;88:909-913.

3. Pagenstert GI, Hintermann B, Barg A, Leumann A, Valderrabano V: Realignment surgery as alternative treatment of varus and valgus ankle osteoarthritis. *Clin Orthop Relat Res* 2007;462:156-168.

4. Pagenstert G, Leumann A, Hintermann B, Valderrabano V: Sports and recreation activity of varus and valgus ankle osteoarthritis before and after realignment surgery. *Foot Ankle Int* 2008;29:985-993.

5. Pagenstert G, Knupp M, Valderrabano V, Hintermann B: Realignment surgery for valgus ankle osteoarthritis. *Oper Orthop Traumatol* 2009;21:77-87.

6. Doets HC, van der Plaat LW, Klein JP: Medial malleolar osteotomy for the correction of varus deformity during total ankle arthroplasty: Results in 15 ankles. *Foot Ankle Int* 2008;29:171-177.

7. Krause F, Windolf M, Schwieger K, Weber M: Ankle joint pressure in pes cavovarus. *J Bone Joint Surg Br* 2007;89:1660-1665.

8. Arangio GA, Chopra V, Voloshin A, Salathe EP: A biomechanical analysis of the effect of lateral column lengthening calcaneal osteotomy on the flat foot. *Clin Biomech (Bristol, Avon)* 2007;22:472-477.

9. Arangio GA, Salathe EP: A biomechanical analysis of posterior tibial tendon dysfunction, medial displacement calcaneal osteotomy and flexor digitorum longus transfer in adult acquired flat foot. *Clin Biomech (Bristol, Avon)* 2009;24:385-390.

10. Bolt PM, Coy S, Toolan BC: A comparison of lateral column lengthening and medial translational osteotomy of the calcaneus for the reconstruction of adult acquired flatfoot. *Foot Ankle Int* 2007;28:1115-1123.

11. Tellisi N, Lobo M, O'Malley M, Kennedy JG, Elliott AJ, Deland JT: Functional outcome after surgical reconstruction of posterior tibial tendon insufficiency in patients under 50 years. *Foot Ankle Int* 2008;29:1179-1183.

12. Brilhault J: Single medial approach to modified double arthrodesis in rigid flatfoot with lateral deficient skin. *Foot Ankle Int* 2009;30:21-26.

13. Knupp M, Schuh R, Stufkens SA, Bolliger L, Hintermann B: Subtalar and talonavicular arthrodesis through a single medial approach for the correction of severe planovalgus deformity. *J Bone Joint Surg Br* 2009;91:612-615.

14. Jeng CL, Tankson CJ, Myerson MS: The single medial approach to triple arthrodesis: A cadaver study. *Foot Ankle Int* 2006;27:1122-1125.

15. Jackson WF, Tryfonidis M, Cooke PH, Sharp RJ: Arthrodesis of the hindfoot for valgus

deformity: An entirely medial approach. *J Bone Joint Surg Br* 2007;89:925-927.

16. DeOrio JK, Leaseburg JT, Shapiro SA: Subtalar distraction arthrodesis through a posterior approach. *Foot Ankle Int* 2008;29:1189-1194.

17. Chou LB, Halligan BW: Treatment of severe, painful pes planovalgus deformity with hindfoot arthrodesis and wedge-shaped tricortical allograft. *Foot Ankle Int* 2007;28:569-574.

18. Dobbs MB, Gurnett CA: Update on clubfoot: Etiology and treatment. *Clin Orthop Relat Res* 2009;467:1146-1153.

19. Sanghvi AV, Mittal VK: Conservative management of idiopathic clubfoot: Kite versus Ponseti method. *J Orthop Surg (Hong Kong)* 2009;17: 67-71.

20. Hegazy M, Nasef NM, Abdel-Ghani H: Results of treatment of idiopathic clubfoot in older infants using the Ponseti method: A preliminary report. *J Pediatr Orthop B* 2009;18: 76-78.

21. Kessler JI: A new flexible brace used in the Ponseti treatment of talipes equinovarus. *J Pediatr Orthop B* 2008;17:247-250.

22. Henn RF, Crawford DC, Eberson CP, Ehrlich MG: Subtalar release in clubfeet: A retrospective study of 10-year outcomes. *Foot Ankle Int* 2008;29:390-395.

23. Ferreira RC, Costa MT, Frizzo GG, Santin RA: Correction of severe recurrent clubfoot using a simplified setting of the Ilizarov device. *Foot Ankle Int* 2007;28:557-568.

24. Malizos KN, Gougoulias NE, Dailiana ZH, Rigopoulos N, Moraitis T: Relapsed clubfoot correction with soft-tissue release and selective application of Ilizarov technique. *Strategies Trauma Limb Reconstr* 2008;3:109-117.

25. El-Mowafi H, El-Alfy B, Refai M: Functional outcome of salvage of residual and recurrent deformities of clubfoot with Ilizarov technique. *Foot Ankle Surg* 2009;15:3-6.

Richard Evan Gellman, MD or a member of his immediate family is a member of a speakers' bureau or has made paid presentations on behalf of Smith & Nephew.

Periarticular Osteotomies: The Importance of Limb Alignment

Haemish A. Crawford, MBChB, FRACS
Annunziato Amendola, MD, FRCSC

Introduction

The role of the periarticular osteotomy in the ankle is to restore the mechanical alignment of the lower limb and to normalize the joint contact forces across the ankle joint as much as possible. In the lower limb, the planning, surgical techniques, and clinical outcomes of periarticular osteotomies of the hip and knee have been reported extensively. However, few papers have addressed the role of osteotomy in the treatment of osteoarthritis of the ankle,[1-3] perhaps because of the very low incidence of primary osteoarthritis in the ankle compared with the other joints.[1] Malalignment can lead to increased point contact forces across the joint and result in osteoarthritis in the affected "compartment" of the joint[4-6] (Fig. 1). Chronic compensation of a joint to adjacent malalignment can lead to joint overload and secondary osteoarthritis. Not only can malalignment of a long bone lead to osteoarthritis as in Figure 1, but, fusing a joint in a malreduced position can lead to premature osteoarthritis in adjacent joints of the same limb. In malunited ankle fractures, often correction of the malunion is all that is necessary. However, axial alignment must be assessed and corrected to prevent failure of the reconstructive procedure (Fig. 2).

Etiology of Osteoarthritis

Trueta[7] showed that osteoarthritis was a result of biochemical changes in the deep chondral layers of the cartilage and in the subchondral bone. With malalignment of the limb, the uneven contact pressures cause a vascular change in this area, leading to poor nutrition and subsequent death in the deep chondral cells, which results in fibrillation and subsequent degeneration of the cartilage. In addition to the increased point contact stress with malalignment, there is also an increased shear force on the cartilage if the joint surface is no longer perpendicular to the long axis of the bone.[8] An assumption often made in realigning a deformed limb is that in the new position "normal" cartilage will be loaded; however, this cartilage may have an underlying biologic derangement as in primary osteoarthritis or have been damaged in the same preceding trauma.

Both the proximity of the angular deformity to the joint and the position the joint is in contribute to the contact area and subsequent forces across the joint. In cadaver studies, it has been shown that a substantial decrease in tibiotalar contact area occurs when there is a distal tibial fracture angulated in recurvatum or antecurvatum.[4,5,9] An even smaller area of contact is present when the foot is placed in plantarflexion or dorsiflexion as well. A more proximal tibial fracture has its greatest effect on the knee, while middle third angulations in the tibia cause a minimal change in contact pressures in the knee or ankle. The subtalar joint may protect the ankle joint from premature osteoarthritis due to limb malalignment.[6] The ankle joint is most congruent in the neutral position, and the orientation of the subtalar joint axis helps maintain this congruency during the gait cycle. Inman[10] was the first to show that the subtalar joint compensates for tibial varus and valgus deformities and, more recently, cadaver studies have shown that the greatest decreases in contact area in the tibiotalar joint occur when the angulated tibia is loaded in the presence of a fixed subtalar joint.[6] The downside of these compensatory changes in the subtalar joint is that premature arthritis may occur in this joint as a result of altered forces across the joint.

Staging

The optimum time for intervention in the osteoarthritic ankle is difficult to ascertain, because the natural history of early changes in the tibiotalar

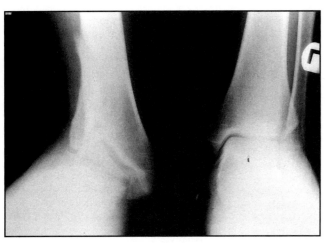
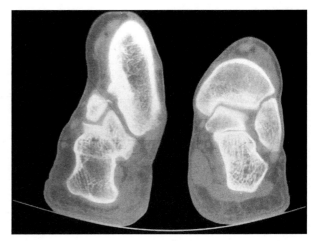

Fig. 1 Residual valgus deformity of the ankle joint and congenital tibial pseudoarthrosis. Although the hindfoot is in neutral through the subtalar joint, the obliquity of the ankle joint precludes long-term success.

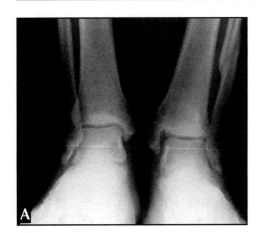
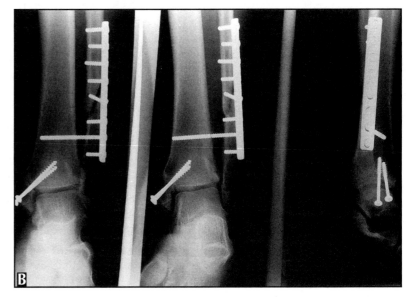
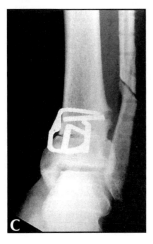

Fig. 2 A, A malunited AO Type C fibular fracture and medial malleolar fracture. **B,** A corrective osteotomy to realign the fracture fails due to failure to address the mechanical axis. **C,** Mechanical axis correction through distal tibial osteotomy using staples for fixation.

joint associated with malalignment is not clearly determined. The classification system produced by Takakura and associates[1] (Table 1) for primary osteoarthritis is useful in considering the surgical options for a patient with an arthritic ankle.[1] Stage 4 can usually be treated by arthrodesis and stage 1 by nonsurgical means. However, stages 2 and 3 present the most challenging decision making to the orthopaedic surgeon. It is in these lower

Table 1
Classification of ankle arthritis from weightbearing radiographs

Stage 1	No joint space narrowing; early sclerosis and osteophyte formation
Stage 2	Medial joint space narrowing
Stage 3	Joint space obliterated with sub-chondral bone contact medially
Stage 4	Whole joint space obliterated with complete bone contact

stages that periarticular osteotomy of the ankle may have some role in trying to prevent progression of the arthritis. More frequent use of ankle arthroscopy and magnetic resonance imaging (MRI) may help provide a more accurate assessment of the articular surface and influence the indications for osteotomy (Fig. 3).

Assessment of Limb Alignment

The assessment of limb alignment is difficult, because mechanical axis deviation accounts for all types of deformity: rotation, angulation, and translation. Not only is the overall limb alignment important (the mechanical axis) but the orientation of each joint to the anatomic axis of the individual bones also needs to be assessed. The most common way of assessing overall limb alignment is a standing long leg radiograph of both legs with the X-ray beam centered on the knee (Fig. 4). This examination is useful as it allows comparison of one limb to the other. However, it does not address the mechanical axis during the single leg stance phase of gait; which a single standing radiograph of each individual limb achieves. These radiographs should be taken with the patella facing directly forward equally centered between the femoral condyles, which characteristically results in a mortise view of the ankle joint.[11] These radiographs have been developed primarily for assessing the mechanical axis of the limb to assist

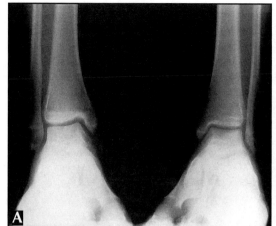
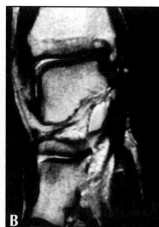
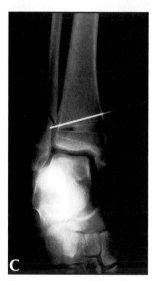
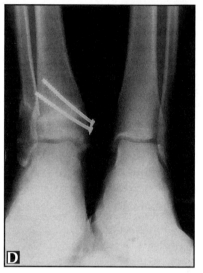

Fig. 3 A, Malunited bimalleolar fracture. **B,** MRI evaluation can be valuable to confirm medial overload. **C,** Intraoperative technique using fluoroscopic guidance for the fibular osteotomy and the opening wedge osteotomy of the tibia. **D,** Fixation is necessary on the tibial side.

in the preoperative planning of knee surgery.[12–14] The ankle joint is usually found right at the bottom edge of the radiograph, often with the subtalar joint missing and with the X-ray beam centered on the knee, which makes it difficult to calculate the tibiotalar angle. Any deformity distal to the ankle joint must also be recorded with the radiograph.

There is variation in the literature as to which bony landmark should be used to measure the tibiotalar angle. Either a line at a tangent to the dome of the talus or a line at a tangent to

the tibial diaphysis has been used.[1,13,15–17] Despite these variations, a number of authors have calculated the lateral distal tibial angle (LDTA) in representative samples of the normal population (Table 2).

In assessing deformity, the routine procedure is to take anteroposterior (AP) and lateral radiographs of the affected limb. However, these projections do not always lie in the plane of maximum deformity, and therefore may underestimate the degree of malalignment. In order to assess the deformity in more detail, further

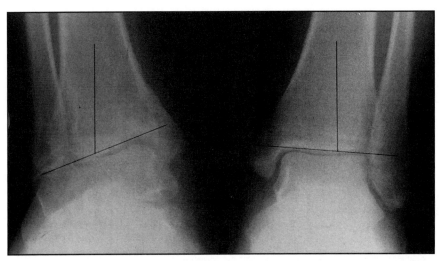

Fig. 4 The importance of standing anteroposterior radiographs of both ankles to measure the weightbearing deformity in the ankle joint.

Table 2 The variation in the lateral distal tibial angle (LDTA)	
Moreland[13]	89.8° + / -2.7° valgus
McKie[15]	91.4° +/ -3.8° varus
Chao[16]	92.9° +/ -3.3° varus
Takakura[2]	91° varus

radiographs can be taken at different angles, or else sophisticated algebraic equations can be used to determine the exact deformity.[18–20] As well as the angulation and translation deformity seen on plane radiographs, consideration must also be given to any rotational deformity that may co-exist.[21] Computed tomography (CT) scanning is an accurate way of measuring rotation.[22] If the patient does not move while being scanned, the resultant scan is not limb position dependent or technician dependent (Fig. 5). The published results of tibial rotation measured by CT scanning vary because of the definition of the reference axis chosen by the authors.[22–24] Eckhoff and Johnson[24] showed in a cadaver model that significant variation and tibial version existed between their 5 specimens, with a range of 15° to 30°. They used a reference axis of the proximal tibia as a line joining the posterior bony prominences of the tibia at least 2 mm distal to the articular surface but no more than 20 mm distal to the joint line. The reference axis of the distal tibia was a line joining the 2 most distal points of the malleoli.

Preoperative Planning

Before discussing the actual techniques for periarticular osteotomies of the ankle joint, it is necessary to consider the principles of correcting lower limb malalignment.[23] Before any surgical correction, there must be an adequate soft-tissue envelope, ankle joint stability, and sufficient joint motion to allow a functional range of motion after the osteotomy. The general medical condition of the patient must also be considered, especially any underlying vascular disease or diabetes mellitus. Once surgery has been decided on, the deformity has to be defined as part of the preoperative planning so that the appropriate procedure will be carried out. In most cases in the ankle joint, the deformity is a result of trauma to the distal tibia, physeal arrest in the growth plate at some time in childhood, or, rarely, because of idiopathic osteoarthritis. Consideration must be given to the whole limb alignment, as there may be a multilevel deformity, requiring a 2-level correction. Paley and associates[25] defined the center of rotation and angulation (CORA) as being the intersection point of the

proximal and distal mechanical or anatomic axis in the tibia. If there is a single level deformity, these 2 axes will intersect at the apex of the deformity. If they do not intersect here, then a multiplanar deformity or translation component must also be present. The orientation of the ankle joint to the mechanical or anatomic axis is calculated so that any rotational malalignment can also be corrected. One deformity often overlooked is leg-length inequality secondary to trauma or growth arrest. If this coexists with the malalignment, it can be corrected with an opening wedge osteotomy, if it is a small deformity, or by distraction osteogenesis, if greater length is required. If 2-level deformity is present, ie, varus gonarthrosis of the knee and ankle, then the proximal deformity should be addressed first. The reasons for this approach are twofold. First, it is difficult to assess the effect of proximal tibial osteotomy on the ankle alignment, and second, the proximal realignment may resolve some or most of the symptoms. If an arthrodesis of the ankle or foot is planned, proximal alignment correction should be carried out before any arthrodesis to avoid malposition of the fixed arthrodesis.

Because the mechanical axis is drawn from a point in the center of the femoral head to the center of the ankle joint, deformities in the femoral neck or tibial plafond may result in very little overall limb malalignment but marked joint malorientation. In these cases, it is necessary to calculate

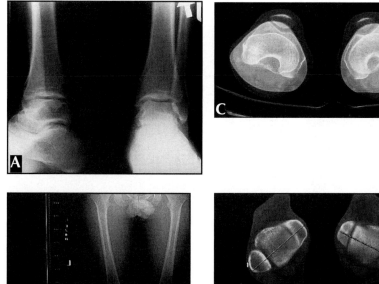

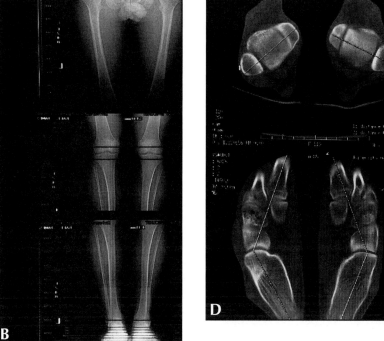

Fig. 5 A case of idiopathic tibial rotation deformity. **A,** Standing anteroposterior radiograph demonstrates the abnormal rotation in the right ankle. **B,** To assess the degree of rotation superimposed computed tomography (CT) at the hip, knee, ankle, and foot are used. **C,** No rotational deformity at the level of the knee. **D,** The rotational deformity can be seen at the ankle and foot levels.

is used for a valgus ankle. The medial side is much easier to approach and less destructive. The advantages of a closing wedge osteotomy are that it offers more inherent stability and does not require a bone graft. However, it does shorten the limb. An opening wedge osteotomy, on the other hand, usually requires internal fixation and structural bone graft, which results in lengthening of the shortened limb (Fig. 6). The opening wedge valgus osteotomy is performed at the level of the deformity or, if this is not possible, 4 cm proximal to the ankle joint line. If the distal tibial growth plate is still open, the osteotomy should be performed at least 3 cm proximal to the epiphyseal plate. An oblique osteotomy of the fibula is performed first at the same level as the site of the tibial osteotomy to allow angulation of the fibula. The tibial malalignment is corrected, which prevents deformation of the tibiofibular syndesmosis. An incomplete horizontal osteotomy is made through the tibia parallel to the distal tibial joint line, using the lateral tibial cortex as a fulcrum for the correction. The preplanned correction can then be performed and checked with the image intensifier before tricortical bone graft from the iliac crest is impacted into the bony defect. The use of rigid internal fixation, as shown in Figure 7, allows early weightbearing and movement of the ankle joint, which may avoid the postoperative stiffness that can occur when Kirschner wires alone are used.

Primary osteoarthritis of the ankle is a rare condition in which the deformity is characteristically in varus, with increased anterior opening of the tibiotalar joint. The condition has its highest incidence in Japanese women and is thought to be caused by the way they sit cross-legged. If the varus

the lateral distal tibial angle (LDTA) from the contralateral normal limb to help plan the amount of correction necessary.[25] The above has only outlined malalignment and malorientation in the sagittal plane. Malalignment in the coronal (lateral plane) is also calculated so that it can be corrected at the time of the osteotomy. Takakura and associates[2] found that the angle of the tibial joint surface on the lateral view (TLS) indicated the amount of anterior opening of the joint, and they were able to correct this approximately 6° in the posttraumatic cases by doing an appropriate opening wedge osteotomy.

Technique

An opening medial wedge osteotomy is used to correct a varus ankle joint, and a closing medial wedge osteotomy

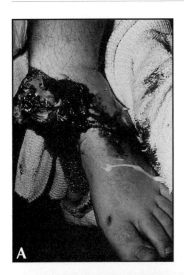
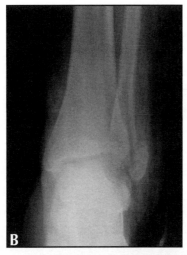
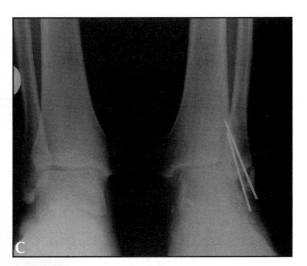

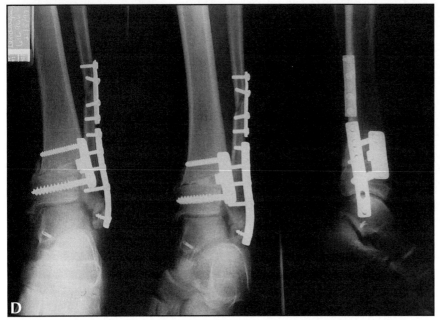

Fig. 6 A, Open fracture dislocation of the left ankle. **B,** Shearing of the lateral malleolus is likely related to underlying valgus angulation of the tibia. **C,** Malunion secondary to valgus tilt. **D,** The corrective osteotomy.

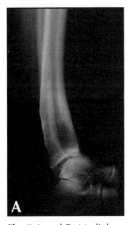
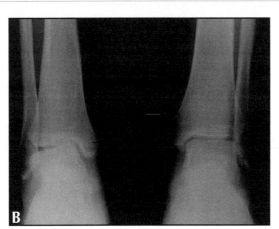
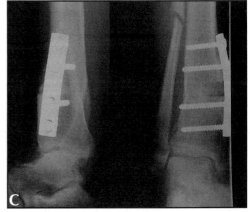

Fig. 7 A and **B,** Medial compartment osteoarthritis secondary to tibial malunion in the AP and lateral planes. **C,** Correction of distal tibial deformity in 2 planes.

deformity of the ankle is so great that the subtalar joint cannot compensate for it, osteoarthritis may develop on the medial side of the joint. After arthroscopic evaluation, Takakura and associates[1] performed distal tibial opening wedge osteotomies on 18 patients, with an excellent result in 6 cases, good in 9, fair in 3, and poor in none after an average follow-up of 6 years, 9 months.

The timing of the surgery is one of the crucial decisions in all osteotomies. The natural history of osteoarthritis of the ankle is not well defined, as it is in the hip or the knee, which makes the decision of when to operate difficult. A high risk patient, as outlined earlier, who has a coronal deformity close to the joint and a stiff subtalar joint but no symptoms or radiographic changes may benefit from a prophylactic osteotomy. On the other hand, the patient with pain, varus alignment and radiographic and arthroscopic changes on the medial side of the joint may benefit from an opening wedge osteotomy, to unload this area and transfer the forces through the lateral compartment. Advanced osteoarthritis that requires arthrodesis, in which varus and valgus coexist, usually requires an osteotomy at the time of the arthrodesis to correct the alignment appropriately rather than attempt to correct the alignment through the ankle arthrodesis alone (Fig. 6).

Achieving correct limb alignment is most important in the success of any reconstructive procedure. Corrective osteotomy has a definite place in the treatment of ankle osteoarthritis.

References

1. Takakura Y, Tanaka Y, Kumai T, Tamai S: Low tibial osteotomy for osteoarthritis of the ankle: Results of a new operation in 18 patients. *J Bone Joint Surg* 1995;77B:50–54.

2. Takakura Y, Takaoka T, Tanaka Y, Yajima H, Tamai S: Results of opening wedge osteotomy for the treatment of a post-traumatic varus deformity of the ankle. *J Bone Joint Surg* 1998; 80A:213–218.

3. Graehl PM, Hersh MR, Heckman JD: Supramalleolar osteotomy for the treatment of symptomatic tibial malunion. *J Orthop Trauma* 1987; 1:281–292.

4. Tarr RR, Resnick CT, Wagner KS, Sarmiento A: Changes in tibiotalar joint contact areas following experimentally induced tibial angular deformities. *Clin Orthop* 1985;199:72–80.

5. Wagner KS, Tarr RR, Resnick C, Sarmiento A: The effect of simulated tibial deformities on the ankle joint during the gait cycle. *Foot Ankle* 1984;5:131–141.

6. Ting AJ, Tarr RR, Sarmiento A, Wagner K, Resnick C: The role of subtalar motion and ankle contact pressure changes from angular deformities of the tibia. *Foot Ankle* 1987;7: 290–299.

7. Trueta J: Studies on the etiopathology of osteoarthritis of the hip. *Clin Orthop* 1963;31:7–19.

8. Radin EL, Burr DB, Caterson B, Fyhrie D, Brown TD, Boyd RD: Mechanical determinants of osteoarthrosis. *Semin Arthritis Rheum* 1991;21(3 suppl 2):12–21.

9. McKellop HA, Llinas A, Sarmiento A: Effects of tibial malalignment on the knee and ankle. *Orthop Clin North Am* 1994;25:415–423.

10. Inman VT (ed): *The Joints of the Ankle.* Baltimore, MD, Williams & Wilkins, 1976.

11. Wright JG, Treble N, Feinstein AR: Measurement of lower limb alignment using long radiographs. *J Bone Joint Surg* 1991;73B:- 721–723.

12. Bauer M, Bergstrom B, Hemborg A: Arthrosis of the ankle evaluated on films in weight-bearing position. *Acta Radiol (Stockh)* 1979;20:88–92.

13. Moreland JR, Bassett LW, Hanker GJ: Radiographic analysis of the axial alignment of the lower extremity. *J Bone Joint Surg* 1987;69A: 745–749.

14. Hsu RW, Himeno S, Coventry MB, Chao EY: Normal axial alignment of the lower extremity and load-bearing distribution at the knee. *Clin Orthop* 1990;255:215–227.

15. Tetsworth K, Paley D: Malalignment and degenerative arthropathy. *Orthop Clin North Am* 1994;25:367–377.

16. Chao EY, Neluheni EV, Hsu RW, Paley D: Biomechanics of malalignment. *Orthop Clin North Am* 1994;25:379–386.

17. Paley D, Tetsworth K: Mechanical axis deviation of the lower limbs: Preoperative planning of uniapical angular deformities of the tibia or femur. *Clin Orthop* 1992;280:48–64.

18. Green SA, Green HD: The influence of radiographic projection on the appearance of deformities. *Orthop Clin North Am* 1994;25:467–475.

19. Bar HF, Breitfuss H: Analysis of angular deformities on radiographs. *J Bone Joint Surg* 1989; 71B:710–711.

20. Ries M, O'Neill D: A method to determine the true angulation of long bone deformity. *Clin Orthop* 1987;218:191–194.

21. Eckhoff DG: Effect of limb malrotation on malalignment and osteoarthritis. *Orthop Clin North Am* 1994;25:405–414.

22. Jakob RP, Haertel M, Stussi E: Tibial torsion calculated by computerized tomography and compared to other methods of measurement. *J Bone Joint Surg* 1980;62B:238–242.

23. Jend HH, Heller M, Dallek M, Schoettle H: Measurement of tibial torsion by computer tomography. *Acta Radiol (Stockh)* 1981;22: 271–276.

24. Eckhoff DG, Johnson KK: Three-dimensional computed tomography reconstruction of tibial torsion. *Clin Orthop* 1994;302:42–46.

25. Paley D, Herzenberg JE, Tetsworth K, McKie J, Bhave A: Deformity planning for frontal and sagittal plane corrective osteotomies. *Orthop Clin North Am* 1994;25:425–465.

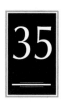

Correction of Multiplanar Hindfoot Deformity With Osteotomy, Arthrodesis, and Internal Fixation

Thomas N. Joseph, MD
Mark S. Myerson, MD

Abstract

Multiplanar deformity of the hindfoot is among the most daunting deformities of the foot and ankle to correct. Deformity correction must attempt to fix the overall orientation of the foot, and prior surgical procedures, arthritic conditions, neurologic abnormalities, musculotendinous insufficiency, and patient goals must be considered. The procedure must relieve pain, arthritis, or instability of the hindfoot and ankle, as well as pressure overload of the lateral foot, midfoot, and/or forefoot. The foot should achieve a plantigrade position that allows for easier shoe fitting and provide a stable platform for weight bearing. When multiple deformities are present, a staged approach to surgical correction is needed. The goal is to create a plantigrade and stable hindfoot first, and then focus on the forefoot. Multiplanar and severe deformities require a variation of basic arthrodesis and osteotomy techniques. Properly placed wedge excisions and soft-tissue releases will enable a plantigrade correction. In some situations, even arthrodesis is insufficient to correct deformity, and residual hindfoot varus or valgus must be corrected with various types of osteotomy of the calcaneus. Osteotomies of the midtarsal region can be considered for residual pes cavus, forefoot supination, adduction, or abduction. An algorithmic approach is used in which the hindfoot is corrected first, followed by the midfoot and forefoot. Correction using multiplanar cuts and internal fixation to establish a plantigrade foot provides the best opportunity for a successful result.

Multiplanar deformity of the hindfoot can be the most daunting deformity of the foot and ankle to correct. With this deformity, equinus, valgus, or varus are not addressed in a "pure" form, but in varying combinations of positions. The correction is of course not uniplanar but multiplanar, with wedges removed; this correction is often combined with derotation and translation. Unique challenges are presented in the decision making during execution of the surgery as to the combination of procedures, and the anticipation of correction on the hindfoot by creating an additional forefoot deformity.

The surgeries performed are generally either primary, or secondary following failed hindfoot correction. The goal of any of these surgeries is to create a plantigrade foot that is stable. Many of these failures seem to have a common cause, for example correcting the skeletal alignment while ignoring the potential for muscular imbalance. This is an important principle, because the hindfoot will always deform despite arthrodesis if remaining muscular imbalance is present. A triple arthrodesis may initially correct a cavovarus deformity associated with hereditary sensorimotor neuropathy (for example, Charcot-Marie-Tooth). However, if the posterior tibial muscle remains a deforming force, subsequent recurrence of deformity with worsening hindfoot varus will occur. This deformity can be multiplanar, and much more difficult to correct than the primary deformity. The surgical correction of the complex hindfoot deformity involves a combination of osteotomy or arthrodesis. As a rule, it is the authors' preference to use arthrodesis of the hindfoot sparingly, but there is no choice when a prior arthrodesis has already been performed. From a technical standpoint, the deformity is corrected with a multiplanar osteotomy through a prior arthrodesis. Frequently this osteotomy is performed in addition to tendon transfers to maintain the final balance of the foot. Although external fixation can be used in correcting deformity, especially in severe cases, most can be stabilized primarily using standard internal fixation techniques that will be the highlighted in this chapter.

Goals of Surgery

A successful outcome must accomplish several important goals. Deformity correction must attempt to fix the overall orientation of the foot; at the same time, prior surgical procedures, arthritic conditions, neurologic abnormalities, musculotendinous insufficiency, and patient goals must be taken into consideration. The procedure must relieve pain, arthritis, or instability of the hindfoot and ankle, as well as pressure overload of the lateral foot, midfoot, and/or forefoot. The foot should achieve a plantigrade position that allows for easier shoe fitting and provides a stable, painless platform for weight bearing without excessive muscular effort.

The foot must absorb shock during ambulation as well as become a rigid lever to propel the body forward during the push-off stage of gait. At heel strike, the heel is slightly inverted (foot supination). Anatomically, this places the long axis of the talus and calcaneus perpendicular to the floor, making the foot more rigid and stable to receive the weight-bearing load. As the body weight progresses forward onto the foot during foot-flat stance, the heel everts (foot pronation). The long axis of the talus and calcaneus become more parallel to the floor, allowing the foot to be more flexible. As this motion occurs, the tibia internally rotates, absorbing shock and allowing the foot to better accommodate and adjust to uneven surfaces. As the body weight continues forward, the foot prepares for push-off by becoming more rigid. The tibia and leg externally rotate and the foot supinates to allow a more rigid foot for mechanical advantage in push-off. To some extent, many of these physiologic needs cannot be met once the foot is rigid, either as a result of deformity or the surgery performed. This is precisely why the primary surgery must attempt to maintain flexibility, generally with osteotomy and tendon transfer rather than arthrodesis.

Evaluation of the Foot and Ankle
Basic evaluation may seem mundane, yet it is absolutely fundamental to a satisfactory outcome. The skin should be inspected for scars from previous injuries or surgery. Surprisingly, the foot is quite forgiving with respect to skin flaps; provided a reasonable time period has elapsed since the previous surgery (on the order of 6 months), skin flap necrosis is unlikely. This concept is important, because the procedure is complex enough without the need for worry about compromising the approach with unorthodox skin incisions. Occasionally a free flap or skin graft is present precisely where the skin incision needs to be made. Avoiding either the free flaps or graft is difficult, and if they have been viable for more than 6 months it is the authors' preference to cut right through them. Clearly, an incision immediately adjacent to the flap or graft is preferable, which can be lifted during the surgical approach. The skin incision must be made boldly to maintain viability, and full-thickness flaps should be used when possible to avoid potential for necrosis.

Vascular status should be assessed with clinical palpation of pulses or measurement of the ankle-brachial index (ABI). An ABI of 0.75 is associated with an excellent likelihood of healing, whereas an ABI less than 0.5 is considered borderline. Toe pressures greater than 45 mm Hg indicate a good chance of healing. Patients should be encouraged to stop smoking before surgery is performed. The combination of nicotine, carbon monoxide, and hydrogen cyanide in cigarette smoke has a toxic effect that is deleterious to skin and bone healing. Various suppressant aids should be considered to encourage the patient to discontinue smoking. Sensation should be carefully plotted out. Sensory testing is particularly important; sensory compromise following these reconstructive procedures is not unusual, and patients must understand the likelihood of sensory loss following surgery. Skin and bone healing are key; however; although loss of sural or superficial peroneal sensation is clearly not desirable, it is preferable if it ensures adequate skin healing. Although some patients are more likely to develop neuromata, again this can be dealt with on an as-needed basis. A discussion of Charcot neuropathic arthropathy is beyond the scope of this chapter. This condition often leads to bizarre and complex hindfoot deformity; patients with neuropathic arthropathy should be treated surgically only under specific circumstances.

Evaluation of Alignment
Examination of alignment is critical in planning surgical treatment, and should be judged by looking at the patient posteriorly when standing, and from as many angles as possible to get a true "feel" of the foot. One technique is to place the patient prone and with the knee flexed to examine the rotation in the limb as well as the position of the hindfoot. Determining whether the heel as well as the hindfoot is in varus, for example, can be difficult. Another useful technique is to cover up the heel and subsequently the midfoot with a towel, and then look at the alignment. Surprisingly, the location of the apex of the deformity is often apparent. The angle made by the Achilles tendon and the vertical axis of the calcaneus is normally 5° to 7° of valgus. Pes planus or cavus is best observed by viewing the foot medially during weight bearing. Forefoot abduction or adduction should be observed from above. Rotation of the forefoot can be evaluated with the patient seated. The examiner holds the hindfoot in neutral or slight valgus and notes the forefoot from the front. Forefoot varus (supination) occurs when the first metatarsal head is higher than the fifth; valgus (pronation) occurs when the first is lower than the fifth.

The flexibility of various deformities should be assessed while the patient is standing and walking, and then the motion in each joint segment examined. Any equinus contracture merits attention, whether in the Achilles tendon or the gastrocnemius soleus complex. The transverse tarsal joints can compensate for limited plantar flexion/dorsiflexion. Although the Coleman block test has been described as an objective measure of the stiffness of the hindfoot and its ability to compensate for forefoot deformity, this test has not been found to be very reliable in the adult.[1] This test attempts to note the predominant focus of deformity in a varus foot, and whether the hindfoot is flexible enough to compensate for a fixed forefoot valgus (when the first metatarsal is fixed in equinus). Although this test provides an overall appreciation of the hindfoot flexibility, it is not accurate enough in the adult to predict the need for osteotomy, tendon transfer, or arthrodesis.

Radiographic evaluation with weight-bearing AP, lateral, and oblique views should be routinely obtained. Patients with severe deformities of the hindfoot should also have weight-bearing AP and mortise radiographs of the ankle. If instability is suspected, varus and valgus stress views must be performed. The ankle, subtalar, and transverse talar joints are evaluated for degeneration, deformity, osteophytes, and instability. The normal lateral talocalcaneal angle is 25° to 50°, and the lateral talus-first metatarsal angle is 0°. On the AP view, the talocalcaneal angle is 15° to 50°, and the talus-first metatarsal angle is 0°. Careful evaluation of the talus in the concavity of the navicular normally shows uncovering of the talar head less than 7°.[2] Additional views are not commonly used to examine the hindfoot.[3]

General Concepts of Correction

To properly address severe deformity or residual deformity of the hindfoot and midfoot, the key is understanding exactly where the apex of the deformity is located. This will of course determine the direction of surgery, because the osteotomy must be located at the apex of the deformity. When multiple deformities are present, a staged approach to surgical cor-

rection is needed. Because the "driving" deformity is in the hindfoot, the hindfoot varus/valgus is addressed before correcting any forefoot supination/pronation. With multiple components of deformity, maximum correction often requires a correction proximal to the apex of the deformity. Whether correcting a varus or valgus deformity, a calcaneus osteotomy will need to be performed in addition to the rotation, angulation, and translation performed in the hindfoot and midfoot.

Although arthrodesis is not the authors' preferred method of correction, it must be incorporated into the correction for a painful deformity that is fixed and associated with painful arthritis. The magnitude of the deformity is not what dictates the need for arthrodesis. Very often with careful tendon releases or transfers, a severe deformity can be corrected by adding osteotomy instead of arthrodesis. In general, the hindfoot should be positioned to place the forefoot plantigrade to the floor. This is a good concept, but inevitably with correction of severe multiplanar deformity, the correction of the hindfoot will either create or aggravate forefoot deformity. Therefore, the goal is to create a plantigrade and stable hindfoot first, and then focus on the forefoot. Again, the objectives are to allow for maximum flexibility and absorption of impact during stance phase of gait, the least stress across adjacent joints, and the most normal-appearing gait possible. A subtalar fusion is placed in slight valgus, taking care to place the foot in a plantigrade position to allow the transverse tarsal joints to be in a parallel position and thus more flexible. This principle is adhered to provided there is no tibia vara, or internal rotation of the tibia that creates a severe torque on the hindfoot, which throws it into varus. What may appear to have been a perfectly positioned hindfoot fusion on the table becomes meaningless once the patient bears weight if tibia vara is present. The forefoot must not be forgotten, especially

in severe or revision cases, because the ankle cannot compensate for forefoot malalignment. Although preoperative evaluation is certainly important, consideration of forefoot realignment after hindfoot correction is best done intraoperatively.

Multiplanar and severe deformities require a variation of basic arthrodesis and osteotomy techniques. Severe cavovarus and pes planovalgus deformities can be addressed surgically with modifications to the triple arthrodesis. Although an attempt to correct deformity without resection of bone wedges is a good idea, in reality this is not easily done. Ideally, the correction should be obtained by rotation and translation rather than wedge resection that shortens the foot. However, properly placed wedge excisions and soft-tissue releases will allow for a plantigrade correction. There are times when even arthrodesis is insufficient to correct deformity, and residual hindfoot varus or valgus must be corrected with various types of osteotomy of the calcaneus. Osteotomies of the midtarsal region can be considered for residual pes cavus, forefoot supination, adduction, or abduction. Ideally the osteotomy should be at the level of the apex of the deformity. Although external fixation can be used for osteotomy fixation, especially in severe cases of deformity, most patients can be treated with modern internal fixation techniques. Moeckel and associates[4] and Thordarson and associates[5] have demonstrated that internal fixation provides a rate of union greater than that of external fixation in routinely used hindfoot and ankle arthrodeses. Certainly, this is not to say that external fixation is not indicated in certain situations. On the contrary, there are some deformities that defy imagination, for which gradual multiplanar correction with an external fixator is necessary. Caution should be exercised against a hasty decision to embrace external fixation in this situation. Although the foot is ultimately plantigrade, it is as stiff if not stiffer than would be obtained by the techniques described herein. Open reduction and internal fixation is preferred unless a severe deformity requires gradual correction (a rare situation). The type of internal fixation used merits consideration, because screw positioning can be a challenge. Using cannulated screws over guide pins is ideal, but even then, the screw may have to cross an open joint not included in the osteotomy or arthrodesis. This scenario is not serious, however; in the unlikely event that the screw eventually irritates the joint, it may be removed. This is important because the plane of the hindfoot does not always facilitate insertion of screws after correction. It can be helpful to perform the osteotomy, position the hindfoot, and then hold it with guide pins to check (and recheck) the position of the foot. The location of the guide pins at this time is not that important.

Revision after a triple arthrodesis leaves little margin for error. Recurrence rates for deformity range from 9% to 20%[6-9] and nonunion rates from 6% to 33%.[8-11] There is little capacity for biomechanical adaptation and a slight amount of hindfoot varus is poorly tolerated. Adjacent joints experience increased stresses in an attempt to compensate for the rigidity and residual deformity. Arthritic changes often result. Wetmore and Drennan[12] evaluated 16 patients with Charcot-Marie-Tooth disease who had 30 triple arthrodeses. Degenerative changes in the ankle and midfoot were noted in 23 of the 30 feet (77%). The procedure results were rated good or excellent in only seven feet (23%). Six limbs (20%) had arthrodesis of the ankle for degenerative disease.[12] Graves and associates[13] studied 17 older adults after triple arthrodesis. Three patients (18%) experienced a nonunion and seven patients (41%) had ankle arthritis at long-term follow-up.[13] Pell and associates[14] studied 132 feet (111 patients) after triple arthrodesis. They found nonunion in 3 feet (2%) and ankle arthritis in 79 feet

(60%). The authors found a correlation between patient satisfaction and postoperative alignment, but no correlation between patient satisfaction and arthritis.[14]

Correction of Varus (Malunion)

Varus malunion after triple arthrodesis may initially be managed with orthotic devices and/or custom orthopaedic shoes. However, many patients do not experience relief of symptoms and require surgical intervention. To some extent, correction of varus malunion must not be delayed because of unnecessary added stress on the ankle; over time, arthritis and instability of the ankle may worsen. Whenever possible, the hindfoot deformity should be revised, preserving as much motion as possible in the remaining joints of the foot and in the ankle in particular. In general, it is easier to correct a varus deformity because the bone wedges can be removed from the apex of the deformity on the lateral side of the foot. Opening wedges on the medial aspect of the foot should rarely if ever be used. In addition to the increased risk of nonunion, the risk of soft-tissue wound problems is increased because of the inelasticity of the tissue on the medial aspect of the foot and ankle. Accordingly, the deformity should be addressed through a lateral approach with resection of a biplanar or triplanar wedge, accepting the slight shortening of the length of the foot.

With a varus-based deformity (whether varus, equinovarus, or cavovarus), the principle is the same—using a lateral incision. The only time a medial incision is warranted is when additional soft-tissue release, including that of the posterior tibial tendon or spring ligament, is necessary. A medial incision is also used when a posterior tibial tendon transfer is performed. These patients should be approached with particular caution, because any incision on the medial foot is precarious when correcting a fixed varus hindfoot. The incision

should be watched closely, using minimal retraction and ensuring that adequate closure is possible. If it does not appear that the skin is closing without tension, it may be preferable to leave the incision open rather than risk necrosis, which is harder to treat. For severe varus deformity, tension on the medial skin should be anticipated as the foot is rotated into a plantigrade position; at times a Z-plasty of the medial skin may be necessary. Skin problems and wound compromise occur more commonly with fixed valgus deformity or malunion. Correction of severe valgus malunion requires a medial shift as well as a medial rotation of the lateral skin. These incisions need to be made according to the longitudinal axis of the foot and not based on the deformity to be corrected. Full-thickness flaps are made, including periosteum. Preservation of the sural and superficial peroneal nerves may not be possible in scarred feet, but an attempt should be made to do so. The entire dorsal and plantar surfaces of the foot should be protected after periosteal elevation. Large malleable retractors are placed on either side of the foot before the osteotomies are performed. Any saw blade that is used for correction has an excursion that may be harmful to the plantar or dorsal soft tissues; thus, the plane and excursion of the saw blade should be watched carefully. Despite the apparent potential for problems with a saw, in the authors' experience, laceration of a tendon or nerve has never been caused with the saw. Although some surgeons may prefer to use an osteotome to cut through the bone, the saw provides a much greater "feel".

In correction of the varus hindfoot, it is essential to determine where the apex of the deformity is located. Deformity may be isolated to the hindfoot, or there may be elements of midfoot varus with adduction and forefoot supination. In addition to the varus, equinus of the ankle or hindfoot may be present, associated with dorsiflexion of the midfoot or forefoot distal to the transverse tarsal joints, creating a rocker-bottom deformity. This deformity may be located centrally under the midfoot or more commonly under the lateral column of the foot.

With surgical correction, each component of the deformity is corrected sequentially. The hindfoot should be addressed first. As noted previously, the various components of the deformity must be identified. For example, a component of heel varus may exist, which is in addition to a second deformity with the apex at the lateral aspect of the transverse tarsal joint. If a "double" deformity is present, then the heel must be corrected in addition to the wedge correction at the transverse tarsal joint. For heel varus, a wedge is removed from the calcaneus and then a biplanar or triplanar correctional osteotomy is performed. In a triplanar osteotomy of the calcaneus, after the wedge is resected, the heel is not only closed down but is overcorrected by translating the calcaneus further laterally. In patients with an increase in the calcaneal pitch angle, the third component of the osteotomy correction is to translate the calcaneus cephalad. In the standard osteotomy, the calcaneal tuberosity is translated laterally and closed into valgus. If necessary in a cavus foot, the calcaneal pitch can be improved by allowing the calcaneus to slide slightly cephalad. For hindfoot valgus, the same lateral incision is used and the calcaneal tuberosity is translated medially. An opening wedge bone graft is not inserted, and furthermore is not to be recommended, because of tension on the lateral soft tissues. Also, removal of a wedge of bone medially is not necessary; translation alone is adequate. A partially threaded cannulated compression screw is used unless the bone is osteopenic, in which case a fully threaded screw is used.

To address midfoot varus, adductus, or supination, a derotational osteotomy across the transverse tarsal joint can concurrently correct forefoot supination and first metatarsus elevatus as well as forefoot adductus. If the problem is solely supination, for example with pain under the base of the fifth metatarsal, a derotational osteotomy is sufficient, and the osteotomy must be performed just proximal to the apex of the deformity. The position of the osteotomy is critical, and guide pins or Kirschner wires should be inserted transversely across the hindfoot to determine the ideal location for the rotational osteotomy. The cut is made on either side of the guide pin, and once the cut has gone in 1 cm the guide pin can then be removed. For combined supination and adductus, a wedge is removed with the base dorsal and slightly lateral. The apex of this wedge must be adjusted to the specifics of the deformity; sometimes it is more superior, sometimes directly lateral, depending on the adductus and varus components of the deformity. In some patients with severe deformity, a calcaneal osteotomy is not sufficient to correct the varus of the heel. When the apex of the heel varus is superior to the axis of the body of the calcaneus, the joint must be opened, and a wedge removed from the subtalar fusion mass as well as from the transverse tarsal joint. A second medial incision is generally not necessary, provided that the exposure is adequate through the extensile lateral incision.

Salvage of the Ankle Joint Associated With Hindfoot Deformity

Frequently, the ankle joint will take up the load after hindfoot malalignment with the development of worsening arthritis. The options for ankle salvage include an ankle or pantalar arthrodesis or a total ankle replacement. However, the joint arthroplasty cannot be performed in the presence of hindfoot deformity. An ankle replacement can only be considered once the hindfoot alignment is corrected. The same applies to severe deformity of the hindfoot and ankle, where attempts at hindfoot correction have not yet been performed. The ankle replacement thus must be staged. The effort is usually merited, because some ankle motion is invariably present and a pantalar arthrodesis causes significantly more severe motion restriction than a triple arthrodesis.[15]

Correction of Valgus Malunion

Although valgus malunion is usually caused by excessive bone removal from the calcaneal cuboid joint, there are times when the deformity was not adequately corrected, with fusion of the talonavicular joint left in abduction. This simultaneously abducts the midfoot and forefoot and pulls the heel into valgus. As the heel remains in valgus, the Achilles tendon drifts laterally and a contracture develops, further perpetuating the deformity. For valgus malunion, either a lengthening of the lateral column or a shortening of the medial column must be performed. For severe deformities, both procedures can be done. The decision as to when to use lateral lengthening or medial shortening depends on the severity of the deformity and the status of the soft tissues. If the lateral skin is tenuous, then it is preferable to avoid a lateral incision and to perform a medial column shortening. This decision must also be viewed in light of the potential for nonunion when a structural graft is used as an interposition, as opposed to a medial shortening with primary bone-to-bone healing. The problem with lateral column lengthening in some patients is not only the tension on the soft tissues and potential for wound complications, but also the inability to correct the deformity if ankle arthritis and deformity are present as well. If this problem is anticipated, a talectomy and tibiocalcaneal arthrodesis should be considered, because the wound will not close after such a severe correction. Performing a medial closing wedge osteotomy across the transverse tarsal joint is safer, combined with slight adduction of the mid-

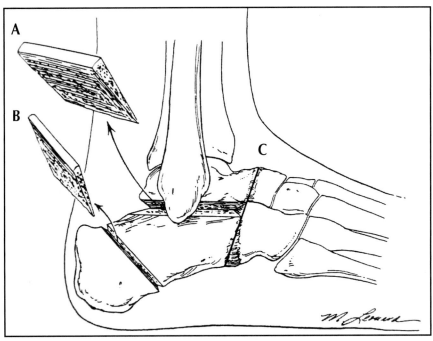

Figure 1 Correction of hindfoot varus by closing wedge osteotomy through the talocalcaneal fusion mass (A) or by closing wedge osteotomy through the calcaneal tuberosity (B). A transverse tarsal osteotomy (C) is necessary when correcting varus by an osteotomy through the fusion mass (B). (Reproduced with permission from Haddad SL, Myerson MS, Pell RF IV, Schon LC: Clinical and radiographic outcome of revision surgery for failed triple arthrodesis. *Foot Ankle Int* 1997;8:489-499.)

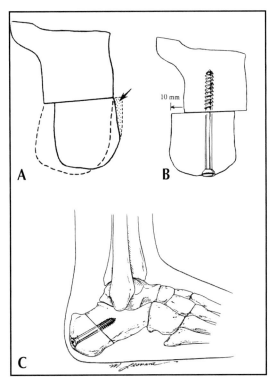

Figure 2 A, Axial view of a closing wedge osteotomy with lateral translation of the calcaneal tuberosity for varus hindfoot. **B,** Medial sliding osteotomy with screw fixation for a valgus hindfoot. **C,** Lateral view of screw placement across the osteotomy after either osteotomy through the calcaneal tuberosity. (Reproduced with permission from Haddad SL, Myerson MS, Pell RF IV, Schon LC: Clinical and radiographic outcome of revision surgery for failed triple arthrodesis. *Foot Ankle Int* 1997;8:489-499.)

foot. If there is sufficient tissue to work with or laxity is present, correction through rotation of the midfoot rather than bone resection may be possible. Although this method is clearly preferable and feasible for primary triple arthrodeses, it cannot always be accomplished in revision of malunion or nonunion. The incision is planned; usually a single incision is sufficient. Medially, the incision is located in the interval between the anterior and posterior tibialis tendons. Laterally, the incision begins at the tip of the fibula, crosses the dorsal lateral aspect of the calcaneocuboid joint, and ends over the cuboid. A periosteal elevator is used to strip the soft tissues off the bone across the dorsal and plantar surfaces of the transverse tarsal joint fusion mass. An oscillating saw with a long blade is then used to make a transverse cut across the foot at the level of the previous calcaneocuboid and talonavicular joints. Care is taken to preserve as much cuboid and navicular bone as possible to facilitate fixation. Cannulated screws can be used. The surfaces of the bones are flat after rotation of the osteotomy, and if the plane of deformity does not facilitate screw fixation, then staples can be used to stabilize the joints. In most cases of osteotomy for correction of hindfoot malunion, bone graft is not necessary. This is not the case, however, when treating patients with deformity as well as nonunion. One should then consider the use of bone graft. In the presence of avascular bone, bone sclerosis, or in a smoking patient, bone graft as well as an electrical bone stimulator (implantable or external) should be considered.

Results Reported in the Literature

Haddad and associates[16] established an algorithm for addressing complex deformity in surgical revision of failed triple arthrodesis. Hindfoot varus was corrected by two methods—a closing wedge osteotomy through the subtalar joint or a lateral closing wedge osteotomy with lat-

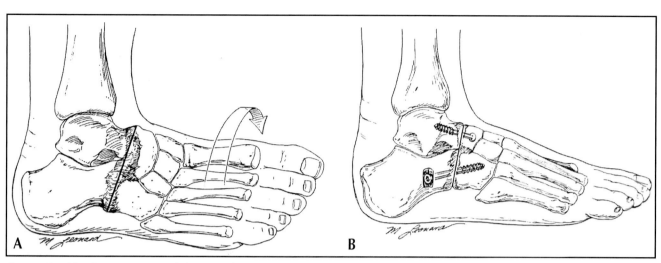

Figure 3 Fixed forefoot supination with location of transverse osteotomy through the fusion mass. **A,** Derotation of the forefoot. **B,** Fixation across the osteotomy after forefoot derotation. (Reproduced with permission from Haddad SL, Myerson MS, Pell RF IV, Schon LC: Clinical and radiographic outcome of revision surgery for failed triple arthrodesis. *Foot Ankle Int* 1997;8:489-499.)

eral translation through the tuberosity of the calcaneus (Figure 1). The presence of a callus under the fifth metatarsal head or base indicated a fixed forefoot supination; thus, a calcaneal osteotomy alone would not be sufficient. Correction through the midfoot would be addressed subsequently. Hindfoot valgus deformity was corrected with a medial displacement osteotomy through the tuberosity of the calcaneus. A lateral incision was made for both varus and valgus correction. A medially based wedge was never used. An oblique incision was used, beginning two fingerbreadths anterior to the insertion of the Achilles tendon and 1 cm inferior to the tip of the fibula. Cuts and bone wedges were made with an oscillating saw. The calcaneal tuberosity was translated 1.0 to 1.5 cm in the appropriate direction and secured with a cannulated cancellous lag screw (Figure 2). To correct an abducted or adducted forefoot, a biplanar closing wedge osteotomy was performed through the fusion mass. The wedge was medial for abduction and lateral for an adduction deformity. Derotation of the osteotomy alone was not sufficient to correct the midfoot deformity (Figure 3). To determine the angle of

the wedge, a proximal guide pin was placed perpendicular to the plane of the hindfoot. A second distal guide pin was placed perpendicular to the plane of the forefoot. Saw cuts were made parallel to the two pins. The cuts were planned to meet on the lateral or medial border of the foot, creating the apex of the wedge. The cuboid and navicular were preserved as much as possible to provide bone for distal fixation. Cannulated screws or power staples were used for fixation (Figure 4). Multiple deformities were addressed simultaneously by placing guide pins to establish angles for the

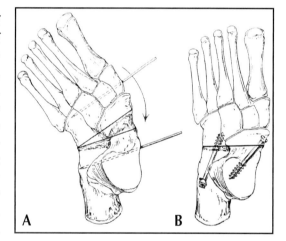

Figure 4 A, Guide pin placement for the closing wedge osteotomy through the talonavicular and calcaneocuboid fusion mass for excessive abduction of the forefoot. **B,** Fixation across the osteotomy site after correction of the abduction deformity. (Reproduced with permission from Haddad SL, Myerson MS, Pell RF IV, Schon LC: Clinical and radiographic outcome of revision surgery for failed triple arthrodesis. *Foot Ankle Int* 1997;8: 489-499.)

wedges of bone to be removed. Multiplanar wedge cuts could then be made. Similarly, a rocker-bottom deformity was corrected with a plantar-based closing wedge osteotomy.

For correction of a rocker-bottom deformity, an incision is made medially along the preaxial border. Subperiosteal dissection is performed, with care taken to avoid neurovascular damage. If the ankle is in equinus, a percutaneus tenotomy or gastrocnemius lengthening can be performed. If the ankle remains in a fixed equinus position, a posterior capsulotomy through a medial approach is per-

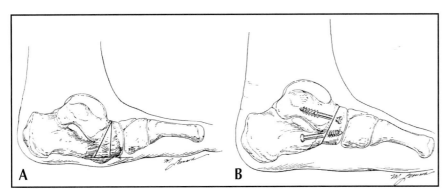

Figure 5 A, Plantar-based closing wedge osteotomy for correction of a rocker-bottom deformity. **B,** Fixation across the osteotomy site after removal of the plantar osteophytes and apposition of bone. (Reproduced with permission from Haddad SL, Myerson MS, Pell RF IV, Schon LC: Clinical and radiographic outcome of revision surgery for failed triple arthrodesis. *Foot Ankle Int* 1997;8:489-499.)

formed. A lengthening of the flexor hallucis longus, flexor digitorum longus, and posterior tibial tendon may be added if resistance is still felt after the capsulotomy. The planned wedge excision is templated with Kirschner wires placed under fluoroscopic guidance. The wedge is resected using a microsagittal saw and completed with osteotomies. The osteotomy is usually biplanar, with apices based laterally and dorsally (Figure 5). The forefoot is temporarily stabilized to the hindfoot with threaded Kirschner wires. The lateral column screw is placed from the calcaneus into the cuboid. The medial column screw may be placed retrograde from the medial cuneiform into the talus, or axially from the posterior talus into the medial cuneiform or first metatarsal base.[17]

Summary

To achieve a successful outcome in multiplanar deformity correction of the hindfoot, the surgeon must address several important objectives. The goal of achieving a plantigrade, functional, painless foot that can fit into regular shoe wear is not easy to accomplish. Careful evaluation of each separate deformity, prior incisions, and fusion location are valuable aids in formulating a treatment plan. An algorithmic approach is used, in which the hindfoot is corrected first, followed by the midfoot and forefoot. Correction using multiplanar cuts and internal fixation to establish a plantigrade foot provides the best chance of a successful result.

References

1. Coleman SS, Chesnut WJ: A simple test for hindfoot flexibility in the cavovarus foot. *Clin Orthop* 1977;123:60-62.

2. Mann RA, Baumgarten M: Subtalar fusion for isolated subtalar disorders: Preliminary report. *Clin Orthop* 1988;226:260-265.

3. Saltzman CL, el-Khoury GY: The hindfoot alignment view. *Foot Ankle Int* 1995;16:572-576.

4. Moeckel BH, Patterson BM, Inglis AE, Sculco TP: Ankle arthrodesis: A comparison of internal and external fixation. *Clin Orthop* 1991;268:78-83.

5. Thordarson DB, Markolf KL, Cracchiolo A III: External fixation in arthrodesis of the ankle: A biomechanical study comparing a unilateral frame with a modified transfixion frame. *J Bone Joint Surg Am* 1994;76:1541-1544.

6. Figgie MP, O'Malley MJ, Ranawat C, Inglis AE, Sculco TP: Triple arthrodesis in rheumatoid arthritis. *Clin Orthop* 1993;292:250-254.

7. Haritidis JH, Kirkos JM, Provellegios SM, Zachos AD: Long-term results of triple arthrodesis: 42 cases followed for 25 years. *Foot Ankle Int* 1994;15:548-551.

8. Sangeorzan BJ, Smith D, Veith R, Hansen ST Jr: Triple arthrodesis using internal fixation in treatment of adult foot disorders. *Clin Orthop* 1993;294:299-307.

9. Wukich DK, Bowen JR: A long-term study of triple arthrodesis for correction of pes cavovarus in Charcot-Marie-Tooth disease. *J Pediatr Orthop* 1989;9:433-437.

10. Galindo MJ Jr, Siff SJ, Butler JE, Cain TE: Triple arthrodesis in young children: A salvage procedure after failed releases in severely affected feet. *Foot Ankle* 1987;7:319-325.

11. Mulier E, De Rijcke J, Fabry G, Mulier JC: Triple arthrodesis in neuromuscular disorders. *Acta Orthop Belg* 1990;56:557-561.

12. Wetmore RS, Drennan JC: Long-term results of triple arthrodesis in Charcot-Marie-Tooth disease. *J Bone Joint Surg Am* 1989;71:417-422.

13. Graves SC, Mann RA, Graves KO: Triple arthrodesis in older adults: Results after long-term follow-up. *J Bone Joint Surg Am* 1993;75:355-362.

14. Pell RF IV, Myerson MS, Schon LC: Clinical outcome after primary triple arthrodesis. *J Bone Joint Surg Am* 2000;82:47-57.

15. Gellman H, Lenihan M, Halikis N, Botte MJ, Giordani M, Perry J: Selective tarsal arthrodesis: An in vitro analysis of the effect on foot motion. *Foot Ankle* 1987;8:127-133.

16. Haddad SL, Myerson MS, Pell RF IV, Schon LC: Clinical and radiographic outcome of revision surgery for failed triple arthrodesis. *Foot Ankle Int* 1997;18:489-499.

17. Cooper PS: Application of external fixators for management of Charcot deformities of the foot and ankle. *Foot Ankle Clin* 2002;7:207-254.

Arthrodesis Techniques in the Management of Stage II and III Acquired Adult Flatfoot Deformity

Jeffrey E. Johnson, MD
James R. Yu, MD

Abstract

The proper management of acquired flatfoot deformity requires obtaining a careful patient history and physical examination of the foot, ankle, and lower extremity. Accurate assessment of foot flexibility and localization of pain will aid in decision making. Nonsurgical management may not be successful in patients with advanced disease, particularly with the development of degenerative changes. Surgical management of advanced acquired adult flatfoot deformity (stages III and IV) is indicated with failure of nonsurgical management and consists primarily of arthrodesis for the foot component of the deformity. The foot component may include the subtalar, talonavicular, calcaneocuboid, or tibiotalar joints, or a combination of these joints. Adjunctive procedures, such as Achilles tendon lengthening, medial displacement calcaneal osteotomy, lateral column lengthening, and plantar flexion osteotomy of the first ray are useful in correcting residual deformities after hindfoot realignment. Proper selection of surgical procedures will maximize the potential for a good outcome. It is critical to correct all components of the deformity simultaneously in order to minimize recurrence of the deformity.

Arthrodesis is indicated for the management of an acquired adult flatfoot disorder with a fixed deformity or degenerative joint disease. In general, limited fusions of the hindfoot and midfoot preserve more motion than do extensive fusion procedures such as triple arthrodesis. However, full correction of the deformity is important for a durable outcome, and this may require a more extensive fusion procedure or the inclusion of adjunctive procedures.

Triple arthrodesis provides the most reliable and predictable correction of a fixed deformity. Careful preoperative and intraoperative physical examination and radiographic evaluation are critical to developing a surgical plan that will address all of the components of this complex deformity and to minimizing the chance of its recurrence.

Posterior tibial tendon dysfunction is the most common etiology of adult acquired flatfoot deformity. The pathologic process by which

this dysfunction occurs varies and may be inflammatory, degenerative, or traumatic in nature. Acquired adult flatfoot deformity can occur in younger patients (30 to 40 years old) with inflammatory arthropathy, but it is more common in older women (50 to 60 years old) with degenerative tears.[1] Posterior tibial tendon dysfunction with loss of the dynamic stabilizer of the medial aspect of the hindfoot can lead to a progressive valgus deformity of the hindfoot. Once the posterior tibial tendon ruptures or becomes elongated, the dynamic forces of weight bearing contribute to attritional rupture or laxity of the static hindfoot stabilizers and collapse of the medial longitudinal arch. There is sagging of the medial column of the foot with eversion and external rotation of the calcaneus in relation to the talus. With longer-standing deformity, compensatory forefoot varus often develops (Figure 1).

Stages of Deformity

Johnson and Strom[2] described three clinical stages of posterior tibial tendon dysfunction (stages I, II, and III). This staging system was subsequently modified to include stage

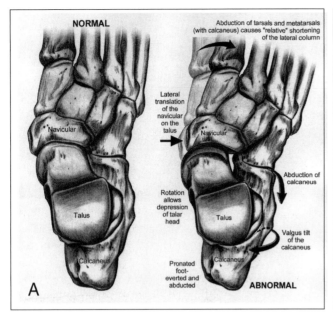
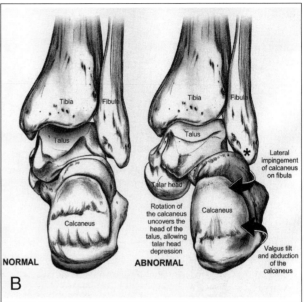

Figure 1 A typical flatfoot deformity. **A,** Dorsoplantar view. Note the lateral translation of the navicular on the talus, relative shortening of the lateral column causing forefoot abduction, and valgus (and abduction) of the calcaneus. **B,** Posteroanterior view. (Adapted with permission from Romas MM: Triple arthrodesis for treatment of painful flatfoot, grade III posterior tribal tendon disfunction. *Tech Foot Ankle Surg* 2003;2:109.)

IV, or the so-called tilted-ankle deformity, which indicates valgus tilt of the talus in the ankle mortise.[1]

Surgical intervention is indicated following failure of nonsurgical treatment. The surgical management of a flexible flatfoot without degenerative changes has been reviewed in detail elsewhere[1,3-5] (RG Alvarez, MD, AL Marini, MD, Boston, MA, unpublished data presented at the American Orthopaedic Foot and Ankle Society annual meeting, 1998). Every attempt should be made to fully correct the deformity with hindfoot osteotomies, midfoot osteotomies, soft-tissue balancing, and tendon transfers to fuse as few joints as possible; however, full correction of the deformity may necessitate fusion of one or more joints. Although there is controversy about whether full correction of the deformity is absolutely necessary for a good outcome,[6] residual hindfoot valgus de-

formity following hindfoot fusion with only partial correction will lead to substantially increased valgus stresses at the ankle and may result in late valgus deformity of the tibiotalar joint. Stage II disease with degenerative changes, stage III disease, and stage IV disease generally require an arthrodesis of some type. The management of a stage IV foot deformity is similar to that of a stage II or III deformity, depending on the degree of arthritis and the flexibility of the hindfoot. The valgus ankle component of a stage IV disorder has been managed with a variety of techniques, including reconstruction of the deltoid ligament, ankle fusion, total ankle replacement, and bracing. Management of this component is not the focus of this chapter.

Painful joints with modest to severe degenerative changes must be treated with arthrodesis to minimize residual postoperative pain. Arthro-

desis can be avoided when painful joints have minimal degenerative changes because such joints often become painless after repositional osteotomies and tendon transfers alone. Arthrodeses for acquired adult flatfoot deformity include subtalar, double, triple, tibiotalocalcaneal, and pantalar procedures. Limited arthrodesis, involving the talonavicular and calcaneocuboid joints, or isolated subtalar fusion allows more residual motion than does triple arthrodesis.[7]

Severe, fixed deformities of the hindfoot and forefoot (stage III) require triple arthrodesis. Occasionally, triple arthrodesis alone may not fully correct the deformity; adjunctive procedures may be necessary to correct residual forefoot varus, forefoot abduction, or hindfoot valgus deformities after the repositional triple arthrodesis. Adjunctive procedures include medial displacement calcaneal osteotomy to address residual hindfoot valgus; medial column procedures such as a plantar flexion osteotomy of the medial cuneiform, fusion of the first tarsometatarsal joint, or naviculocuneiform fusion to address residual forefoot varus deformity; and lateral column lengthening to address forefoot abduction. These procedures are best performed simultaneously with the triple arthrodesis, but they may be used later to correct a malunited or incompletely corrected planovalgus foot.

Arthrodesis Procedures for Acquired Adult Flatfoot Deformity

In general, the proper selection of surgical procedures depends on the severity and flexibility of the deformity as well as the presence and location of degenerative changes about the foot and ankle. Activity level, age, body habitus, and medical comorbidities need to be considered as well. Surgical goals include relief of pain, establishment of a stable plantigrade foot without the need for bracing, and maintenance of the integrity of adjacent unfused joints, especially the ankle joint. This chapter will focus on the indications, surgical techniques, and complications of the various arthrodesis procedures used for the management of stage II disease with degenerative changes and stage III disease.

In stage II disease, the deformity is flexible, and hindfoot osteotomies are usually performed because they spare the important hindfoot joints and are a powerful means with which to correct a wide range of deformities. Limited arthrodesis may be indicated, especially when there is a moderate deformity that cannot be fully corrected with reconstruction of the posterior tibial tendon and joint-sparing osteotomy alone.

Limited fusions are especially useful when the deformity is flexible and there is evidence of arthrosis in the hindfoot. According to Mann and Beaman,[8] talonavicular arthrodesis is indicated for management of an unstable talonavicular joint associated with a flexible subtalar joint in patients who are older than 50 years, whereas double arthrodesis is preferred for an unstable talonavicular joint associated with a flexible subtalar joint in a younger patient. Isolated arthrodesis of the subtalar joint is indicated for a fixed deformity of the subtalar joint associated with a flexible forefoot as well as for a flexible hindfoot deformity in the presence of degenerative changes in the subtalar joint. Subtalar fusion is also indicated for salvage of a failed reconstruction of a foot with acquired adult flatfoot deformity when there is residual subluxation, degenerative changes, or pain at the subtalar joint. The addition of a flexor digitorum longus tendon transfer to the navicular or the first cuneiform has been advocated to improve function and stabilize the talonavicular joint even when an isolated subtalar joint fusion is being performed.[9]

Patients with stage III disease require a more extensive repositional arthrodesis to fully correct the fixed deformity. Triple arthrodesis is indicated for a rigid subtalar joint and a fixed varus deformity of the forefoot. It may be necessary to include adjunctive procedures to fully correct all components of the deformity. The decision to use these adjunctive procedures is highly dependent on the degree of deformity and the intraoperative assessment of the correction obtained with the initial realignment. After reducing the subtalar, calcaneocuboid, and talonavicular joints, the surgeon should determine

whether the foot will be plantigrade. The heel should be evaluated for excessive residual hindfoot valgus, which, if present, may require additional correction with a medial displacement calcaneal osteotomy. The position of the forefoot relative to the hindfoot should be evaluated as well. Additional surgery, such as a lateral column lengthening with a bone block placed in the calcaneocuboid joint, may be indicated to fully correct the abducted forefoot to a neutral position. Any residual varus deformity of the forefoot needs to be corrected (Figure 2). This may require an osteotomy of the medial column, such as a plantar flexion osteotomy of the medial cuneiform, or an extended arthrodesis of the medial column.

At our institution, most of these procedures are performed with the patient under general anesthesia and with preemptive ankle block regional anesthesia. Antibiotic prophylaxis, a pneumatic tourniquet, and fluoroscopy are used routinely. Patients are initially cared for in the hospital and then are discharged on the day following the surgery. Splints and sutures are removed and a cast is applied in the clinic at approximately 2 weeks postoperatively.

Medial Column Arthrodesis

Loss of the medial longitudinal arch may be caused by pathologic changes in the talonavicular, naviculocuneiform, and/or metatarsocuneiform joints. Instability or hypermobility, degenerative changes, or residual forefoot varus at these joints are the primary indications for medial column fusion.[10] Isolated arthrodesis of the talonavicular joint essentially eliminates motion in the rest of the hindfoot.[7] A patient with a flexible hindfoot deformity who has no arthrosis in adjacent joints

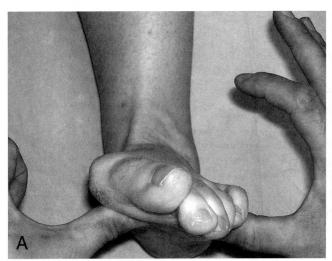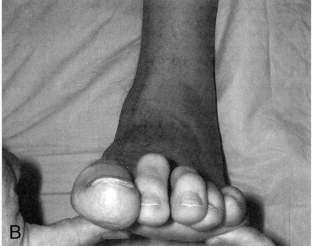

Figure 2 Evaluation for varus forefoot deformity. **A,** Forefoot varus with the subtalar joint corrected to neutral. **B,** Neutral forefoot alignment.

may be a candidate for isolated talonavicular arthrodesis; however, the specific indications remain controversial, and nonunion rates are higher than those following other hindfoot fusions.[11] Patients with residual hindfoot valgus, instability at multiple midfoot joints, or ankle arthrosis may require additional procedures such as a calcaneal osteotomy, midfoot fusions, ankle fusion, or ankle arthroplasty.[12] Arthrodesis of the naviculocuneiform joint is usually performed in conjunction with other procedures to correct hindfoot deformity and is done when there is residual forefoot varus secondary to severe instability or arthritis at this joint.

Surgical Technique for Talonavicular Arthrodesis A dorsomedial longitudinal incision is made over the talonavicular joint, along the lateral edge of the anterior tibial tendon to the tibialis anterior tendon. The talonavicular joint capsule is identified and is incised longitudinally. Subperiosteal dissection exposes the remainder of the talonavicular joint. A small lamina spreader can help distract and expose the joint. The talo-

navicular articular surfaces are then débrided. The forefoot is then reduced to the talus by adducting, plantar flexing, and pronating it. Lateral counter pressure is applied to the medial aspect of the talar head. Provisional fixation can be obtained with use of Kirschner wires or the guide pins for the cannulated screw system. The hindfoot should be in 5° to 10° of valgus. It is imperative that the hindfoot not be fused in varus and that the forefoot not be left in varus relative to the hindfoot. The reduction should be confirmed fluoroscopically as well as clinically. Once the reduction is deemed to be satisfactory, two 4.5-mm cannulated screws are placed across the talonavicular joint in a retrograde fashion. Occasionally, a third cannulated screw can be placed percutaneously from the lateral aspect of the navicular into the talus or a staple may be placed across the dorsal joint line. In severely sclerotic bone, a tricortical iliac bone allograft or autograft can be placed as a slot graft across the joint to augment the fusion. A saw is used to cut a rectangular trough perpendicular to the joint line. The slot

graft is then impacted into the trough, spanning the joint line. The wound is closed in the usual manner. It is important to assess the foot for excessive heel valgus, forefoot varus, or heel cord contracture preoperatively. The presence of these problems signifies the need for additional or different surgery to address them.

Postoperatively, a bulky compressive Robert Jones dressing and splint are applied. Sutures are removed at 2 weeks. A short leg non-weight-bearing cast is applied and worn for 4 weeks. The patient then wears a short leg weight-bearing cast for another 4 to 6 weeks.

Outcomes and Complications The outcomes of isolated talonavicular arthrodeses have varied in studies reported in the literature. Harper[13] reported that 24 of 27 patients treated with talonavicular arthrodesis to correct acquired adult flatfoot deformity had a good or excellent result with no pain or pain only with strenuous activity. The correction was maintained in all patients at an average of 27 months postoperatively. Progressive arthrosis was noted in one ankle, one calcaneocuboid joint, and three naviculocuneiform joints. In four of these joints, the arthrosis had been present preoperatively and had progressed after the talonavicular arthrodesis. There was one nonunion requiring revision and one major wound problem.

Below and McCluskey (Traverse City, MI, unpublished data presented at the American Orthopaedic Foot and Ankle Society annual meeting, 2002) reported the outcomes for 15 of 21 patients who had undergone isolated talonavicular arthrodesis for the treatment of acquired adult flatfoot deformity. Twelve patients had stage II posterior tibial tendon dysfunction, and nine patients had stage III disease with talonavicular degenerative joint disease. Most of the patients experienced daily pain postoperatively. Radiographic evidence of subtalar arthrosis developed in 8 patients, and 12 patients had pain at the subtalar joint on examination. Six patients had a nonunion.

Complications of talonavicular arthrodesis include residual lateral midfoot pain, malunion, nonunion, and the development of arthrosis at adjacent joints. For these reasons, talonavicular fusion alone is not commonly performed for stage II acquired adult flatfoot deformity.

Lateral Column Lengthening

Calcaneocuboid distraction arthrodesis or lateral column lengthening arthrodesis has been advocated for the treatment of stage II posterior tibial tendon dysfunction with dorsolateral peritalar subluxation.[14] Lengthening of the lateral column has been shown to restore the medial arch and correct hindfoot valgus and forefoot abduction.[15,16] The decision whether to perform a lengthening osteotomy through the distal

part of the calcaneus or with distraction arthrodesis of the calcaneocuboid joint is controversial.[6,17] Proponents of distraction arthrodesis of the calcaneocuboid joint cite the potential for the development of degenerative changes at the calcaneocuboid joint following osteotomy of the calcaneus as a result of increased contact pressures at the calcaneocuboid joint;[4,14-19] however, the nonunion rate following distraction arthrodesis of the calcaneocuboid joint is approximately 20%. Typically, if lateral column lengthening is required as a component of the correction of a flexible stage II acquired adult flatfoot deformity, a lengthening osteotomy of the calcaneal neck with interposition of bone graft is performed. When lateral column lengthening is needed for a stage III acquired adult flatfoot deformity, distraction arthrodesis of the calcaneocuboid joint is performed with interposition of bone graft as part of a triple arthrodesis.

Surgical Technique A lateral longitudinal incision is made over the anterolateral aspect of the calcaneus from just anterior to the tip of the fibula toward the base of the fourth metatarsal. Dissection through the soft tissues is performed to expose the extensor digitorum brevis, with care taken to avoid injury to the anterior branch of the sural nerve. Other cutaneous nerves, such as the intermediate branch of the superficial peroneal nerve, can occasionally enter the surgical field, and they need to be protected. The peroneal tendons and sural nerve are retracted inferiorly. The extensor digitorum brevis is retracted superiorly; the extensor digitorum brevis origin and the plantar aspect of the muscle may be elevated to facilitate exposure of the calcaneocuboid joint.

The articular surfaces of the

calcaneocuboid joint are then débrided. A lamina spreader without teeth is used to distract the joint.

Care must be taken to avoid overcorrecting the heel into varus or pushing the forefoot into varus. A tricortical iliac crest bone allograft or autograft is then fashioned to fit into the distracted calcaneocuboid joint. This graft usually measures between 8 and 12 mm in width.[14] Fixation is obtained with a 4.0- or 4.5-mm cannulated screw inserted in a retrograde direction. However, an isolated distraction arthrodesis of the calcaneocuboid joint usually requires additional fixation to help prevent a nonunion, and a lateral plate is often added. The extensor digitorum brevis is reapproximated, and the skin is closed in the usual manner. Postoperative care is similar to that described above.

Outcomes and Complications Complications of calcaneocuboid arthrodesis include cutaneous neuroma of the sural or superficial peroneal nerve, residual lateral midfoot pain, malunion, nonunion, and the development of arthrosis at adjacent joints. Symptomatic nonunion is treated with bone grafting and plate, screw, or staple fixation. Chi and associates[16] reported that 8 of 41 attempted distraction arthrodeses of the calcaneocuboid joint in 36 patients did not result in healing. Distraction arthrodesis of the calcaneocuboid joint causes some loss of motion in the foot, but less than that seen after subtalar or talonavicular arthrodesis.[19]

Isolated Subtalar Arthrodesis With Flexor Digitorum Longus Transfer

There is support in the literature for the use of isolated subtalar arthrodesis to treat acquired adult flatfoot deformity when the patient has a fixed

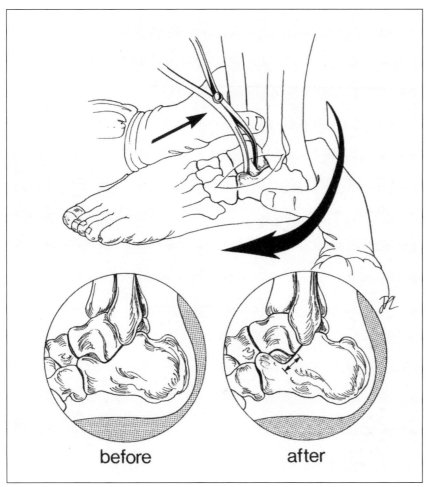

before   after

Figure 3 Manual reduction of the subtalar joint is accomplished by internally derotating the calcaneus underneath the talus. (Reproduced with permission from Schon LC: Derotational triple arthrodesis for severe pes plano valgus correction. *Tech Orthop* 1996;11:294-295.)

deformity of the subtalar joint and a flexible forefoot.[20,21] Mann and associates[9] stated that 10° to 15° of forefoot varus or joint hypermobility is a contraindication to isolated subtalar joint fusion. In such a situation, isolated subtalar joint arthrodesis will overload the lateral border during gait as a result of the fixed forefoot varus. Other indications for isolated subtalar joint arthrodesis include degenerative changes in the subtalar joint and salvage of a failed hindfoot reconstruction. The procedure allows residual motion at the talonavicular and calcaneocuboid joints (26% and 56% residual mo-

tion, respectively[7]). This may have a protective effect on the development of ankle arthritis when compared with triple arthrodesis.[21] However, the authors of an in vitro biomechanical study concluded that isolated subtalar or calcaneocuboid fusion cannot achieve full correction of a moderate flatfoot deformity with substantial transverse tarsal joint laxity; in contrast, a talonavicular, double, or triple arthrodesis completely corrected the deformity.[22] We believe that, when an isolated subtalar fusion is performed to treat acquired adult flatfoot deformity, the addition of a flexor digi-

torum longus transfer helps to support the talonavicular joint and balances the pull of the peroneus brevis.[20]

Surgical Technique An oblique longitudinal skin incision is made from the tip of the lateral malleolus toward the base of the fourth metatarsal, centered over the sinus tarsi. Alternatively, an oblique Ollier-type incision can be used, but this may limit the placement of a calcaneal osteotomy incision if one is needed during the procedure. Care is taken to preserve full-thickness skin flaps as well as the sural nerve at the inferior and distal aspect of the incision.

The origin of the extensor digitorum brevis muscle and the peroneal tendon sheath are identified. The origin of the extensor digitorum brevis is split in line with the muscle fibers and is retracted superiorly. The fat in the sinus tarsi is either excised or reflected to improve exposure. The calcaneocuboid joint capsule is not violated. The peroneal tendons are retracted posteriorly to expose the posterior facet of the subtalar joint. A small lamina spreader can be inserted into the sinus tarsi to distract the subtalar joint and improve visualization. Any obvious osteophytes should be resected, and any removed bone should be morcellized for bone graft. The talocalcaneal interosseous ligament is resected to allow greater distraction of the joint. The medial aspect of the subtalar joint capsule may be excised carefully with a rongeur if necessary to improve hindfoot mobility to allow reduction.

The articular surfaces of the subtalar joint are débrided. Care should be taken to preserve the subchondral contour of the joint surfaces to maximize the surface area of bone contact. The calcaneocuboid articulation, talonavicular articulation, and tibiotalar capsules should be preserved.

The posterior tibial tendon is then exposed through a medial incision and is débrided as needed. The flexor digitorum longus tendon is dissected distal to the knot of Henry and is divided just proximal to its decussation with the flexor hallucis longus tendon. A 4.5-mm drill hole is placed in the navicular tuberosity, and the flexor digitorum longus tendon is pulled up from plantar to dorsal through the drill hole with use of a grasping suture placed in the end of the tendon. Tensioning of the flexor digitorum longus is delayed until the subtalar joint is fused.

The subtalar joint is then reduced; this usually requires internal rotation and inversion of the calcaneus back under the talus (Figure 3) as well as elevation of the lateral column and depression of the medial column of the forefoot. The reduction can be aided by placing a lamina spreader between the lateral process of the talus and the anterior process of the calcaneus as described by Hansen[23] (Figures 4 and 5). After reduction, the heel should be in no more than 5° to 10° of valgus. Bone apposition is confirmed, and the need for bone graft is assessed.

A small stab wound is made in the heel. Guide wires for one or two 6.5-mm cannulated screws are introduced through the stab wound and then advanced through the calcaneus and into the talar body under fluoroscopic control. Proper pin placement must be confirmed on all three intraoperative views—that is, the lateral and AP views of the ankle and the axial view of the heel. The cannulated screws are then inserted in the usual manner. Stability of the construct is verified, and bone graft, if needed, is placed after thorough irrigation of the wound with saline solution. The addition of a flexor

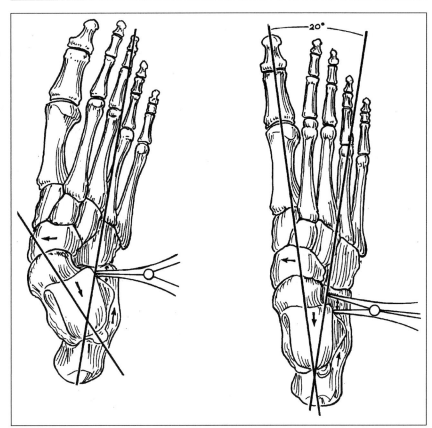

Figure 4   AP view of a reduction of a flatfoot deformity and forefoot abduction with use of a lamina spreader placed between the anterior aspect of the dorsal part of the calcaneus and the lateral shoulder of the talus. (Reproduced with permission from Hansen ST Jr: *Functional Reconstruction of the Foot and Ankle*. Philidelphia, PA, Lippincott Williams and Wilkins, 2000, p 302.)

digitorum longus tendon transfer to the navicular or the first cuneiform has been advocated to improve function and stabilize the talonavicular joint even when an isolated subtalar joint fusion is being performed.[9] The flexor digitorum longus tendon is pulled up through the hole in the navicular under moderate tension and is secured back on itself or to the surrounding periosteum with nonabsorbable sutures. Any tears in the spring ligament complex are also repaired.

Prior to wound closure, the extensor digitorum brevis is reapproximated with 2-0 Vicryl sutures. Postoperative care is as described above.

Outcomes and Complications

Outcomes of subtalar joint arthrodesis for the treatment of acquired adult flatfoot deformity have been described in the literature. Johnson and associates[20] reported on 17 feet treated with subtalar joint arthrodesis, reconstruction of the flexor digitorum longus, and repair of the spring ligament. At 2 years postoperatively, the results compared favorably with those of medial displacement calcaneal osteotomy and lateral column lengthening. Kitaoka and Patzer[21] reported 16 good or excellent results at 3 years following subtalar joint realignment and arthrodesis in 21 feet. Complications included symptomatic arthrosis of

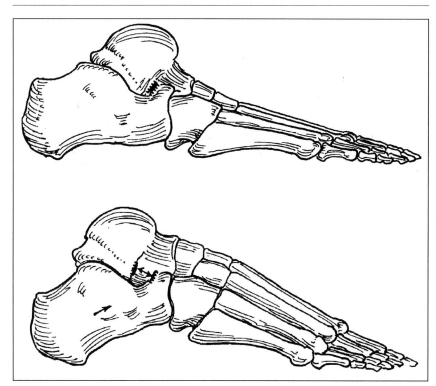

Figure 5 Lateral view showing flatfoot deformity and forefoot abduction deformity (top) and reduction of those deformities (bottom) with a lamina spreader placed between the anterior aspect of the calcaneus and the lateral shoulder of the talus. Cross-hatched locations on the talus and the calcaneus demonstrate proper placement of the lamina spreader. (Reproduced with permission from Hansen ST Jr: *Functional Reconstruction of the Foot and Ankle.* Philidelphia, PA, Lippincott Williams and Wilkins, 2000, pp 302.)

adjacent joints, malunion, and nonunion. Others have recommended the addition of a flexor digitorum longus transfer to the navicular to help stabilize the talonavicular joint when isolated subtalar arthrodesis is performed for stage II disease.[20] The addition of the flexor digitorum longus transfer in the treatment of stage II disease may also help to prevent the progressive development of valgus tilt of the ankle after triple arthrodesis, but it has not been widely used in that setting.

Double Arthrodesis (Calcaneocuboid and Talonavicular Joints)

A double arthrodesis involves fusion of the calcaneocuboid and talonavic-ular joints. It is indicated for a flexible moderate hindfoot deformity with a forefoot varus deformity. It has been stated that a double arthrodesis is indicated for a younger patient with a flexible hindfoot deformity and excessive forefoot varus, whereas an isolated talonavicular fusion is indicated for an older patient with that condition.[24] Given that the range of motion of the subtalar joint is essentially eliminated following double arthrodesis, a triple arthrodesis should be performed if there is tenderness or degenerative changes in the subtalar joint.[7]

Surgical Technique The approach to the talonavicular joint is performed as described above. The calcaneocuboid joint is approached in a

fashion similar to that described for a calcaneocuboid distraction arthrodesis. To correct a major forefoot varus deformity, care must be taken to débride enough of the talonavicular and calcaneocuboid joints to allow derotation of the forefoot and correction of forefoot varus. Because the talonavicular joint is at the apex of the deformity, most surgeons reduce and stabilize it first. Guide pins for the 4.5-mm cannulated screws can be used for provisional fixation. It is then verified that the talonavicular joint and the calcaneocuboid joint have been reduced simultaneously, and these joints are provisionally stabilized with either Steinmann pins or guide pins for the cannulated screws. The alignment of the foot and the position of the hardware are confirmed both clinically and fluoroscopically. The talonavicular joint is then fixed with two 4.5-mm cannulated screws; the calcaneocuboid joint is also fixed internally, either with a screw or staples. The skin is closed in the usual manner. Postoperative care is similar to that described above.

Outcomes and Complications Clain and Baxter[22] reported 4 excellent, 8 good, and 4 fair results at an average of 83 months after double arthrodeses performed on 16 feet with a variety of hindfoot disorders. There was one nonunion of the talonavicular joint, which remained asymptomatic. Progressive degenerative changes developed in the ankle of six patients and in the naviculocuneiform joints of seven. The authors concluded that double arthrodesis was better than isolated talonavicular fusion and a viable alternative to triple arthrodesis.

Mann and Beaman[8] reported the outcomes of 24 double arthrodeses at an average of 56 months. Sixteen of the double arthrodeses were performed for acquired adult flatfoot deformity because of posterior tibial tendon insufficiency, and eight were done for other diagnoses. Similar outcomes were observed in the two groups of patients, with 18 patients having a good or excellent result overall. Complications were more frequent in the patients who had flatfoot deformity. Talonavicular nonunion was the most frequent complication, occurring in four patients, three of whom required revision arthrodesis. The development of arthrosis in the surrounding joints was common but asymptomatic. For this reason, triple arthrodesis may be preferred for most patients.

Triple Arthrodesis

Triple arthrodesis is indicated for the treatment of acquired adult flatfoot deformity when the subtalar joint or transverse tarsal joint is not passively correctable, when there are degenerative changes at the subtalar joint or transverse tarsal joint, and for the salvage of a failed hindfoot reconstruction. The radiographic criteria for triple arthrodesis are controversial and are of limited value.[25] Myerson[1] recommended triple arthrodesis for a fixed hindfoot deformity with subfibular impingement. Others have stated that medial foot pain associated with dorsal peritalar subluxation should be corrected with triple arthrodesis.[26] The goal of triple arthrodesis is to fuse the subtalar, talonavicular, and calcaneocuboid joints with the hindfoot in 5° of valgus and to correct midfoot and forefoot deformities to neutral through repositional arthrodesis. A single extensile lateral or extensile medial incision could be used if needed for access to the joint in a triple arthrodesis, but a two-incision technique provides better exposure and allows

easier correction of the deformity.

Surgical Technique Two incisions are used for this procedure. The lateral incision is made obliquely from the tip of the distal part of the fibula to the base of the fourth metatarsal. Occasionally, branches of the intermediate branch of the superficial peroneal nerve may cross the surgical field near the anterior aspect of the calcaneus. If they do, these branches are identified and are retracted cephalad. The subcutaneous exposure involves creation of full-thickness flaps with meticulous soft-tissue handling. Care should be taken to identify and protect the sural nerve and any branches of the superficial peroneal nerve.

The peroneal tendons are identified and retracted. The extensor digitorum brevis is incised along its muscle fibers and is sharply raised from the calcaneal insertion. The subtalar joint is exposed as described above. The lateral talonavicular, calcaneocuboid, and naviculocuboid articulations are identified. A useful landmark for localizing the talonavicular joint is the insertion of the bifurcate ligament (ligament of Chopart). The bifurcate ligament consists of the lateral calcaneonavicular and medial calcaneocuboid ligaments and inserts into the calcaneonaviculocuboid region. The lateral aspect of the calcaneus is followed distally to the calcaneocuboid joint. The calcaneocuboid joint capsule is incised sharply both laterally and dorsally. The lateral aspect of the talonavicular joint may then be partially exposed and débrided through the lateral incision. The naviculocuboid articulation is débrided in a similar manner. Exposure of the calcaneocuboid joint can be facilitated by use of a small lamina spreader. The articular surfaces of the calcaneocuboid joint are then débrided.

The articular surfaces of the subtalar joint are prepared as described above.

The dorsomedial approach, as described above, is used to expose the remainder of the talonavicular joint and allow complete débridement of the talonavicular joint. The foot is placed into a plantigrade position. After the hindfoot is corrected to the "anatomic neutral" position, the necessity for adjunctive procedures should be assessed. Achilles tendon lengthening is almost always required and is usually performed at the outset of the procedure before the surgeon tries to reposition the foot. If there is residual heel valgus of > 5° to 10° after subtalar joint alignment has been reestablished, a medial displacement calcaneal osteotomy may be needed. Next, the position of the forefoot relative to the hindfoot needs to be considered because residual forefoot varus promotes a valgus thrust on the hindfoot with gait and may contribute to a poor outcome and late valgus deformity at the ankle secondary to insufficiency of the deltoid ligament. If the forefoot is abducted, distraction arthrodesis of the calcaneocuboid joint may be required. The medial column is evaluated for instability or any residual supination deformity that might require fusion of the first tarsometatarsal joint, plantar flexion cuneiform osteotomy, or naviculocuneiform fusion.

Intraoperatively, the decision to begin with reduction of the subtalar joint or the talonavicular joint is controversial.[6] Proponents of primary subtalar joint fusion cite the ability and importance of placing the hindfoot in slight valgus with subsequent reduction of the forefoot by lateral column lengthening or medial column arthrodesis.[23] Primary fixation of the talonavicular joint is favored by those who believe a multiplanar correction of the talonavicular joint will reduce the rest of the deformity.[22] We prefer correcting the deformity in a proximal to distal progression, beginning with the subtalar joint. Once the heel is in neutral, the midfoot is reduced at the talonavicular and calcaneocuboid joints.

After the subtalar joint is reduced in a position of 5° to 10° of valgus, inspection should confirm that the heel was not placed in varus. Several maneuvers to assist reduction have been described. A lamina spreader placed in the sinus tarsi between the calcaneus and the lateral talar process, or neck, can be used to push the forefoot out of abduction and effectively lengthen the lateral column, rather than distract the subtalar joint[23] (Figures 4 and 5). Alternatively, primary talonavicular reduction can be achieved by pushing the head of the talus laterally while adducting and pronating the forefoot.[27] Kirschner wire joysticks placed transversely across the midfoot may be helpful for elevating the lateral aspect of the forefoot and depressing the medial aspect of the forefoot during reduction of forefoot varus.

The reduction is confirmed fluoroscopically. Internal fixation with screws is used routinely at the subtalar, talonavicular, and calcaneocuboid joints. The guide pins for the cannulated screws can be used to provide provisional fixation. Staple fixation with or without a screw is commonly used at the calcaneocuboid joint.

A 6.5-mm cannulated screw can be inserted in either a retrograde fashion (as described above) or an antegrade fashion (from the dorsal aspect of the talar neck into the calcaneus) across the subtalar joint.

This screw is countersunk and is usually placed from the calcaneus to the talus to avoid the neurovascular bundle. The talonavicular joint is internally fixed with two cannulated 4.5-mm screws, approximately 40 to 50 mm long, from the navicular tuberosity into the head and neck of the talus. Technically, it is important to countersink the head of the screw in the navicular to minimize hardware prominence. The calcaneocuboid articulation is internally fixed with two 30 to 40-mm-long 4.5-mm cannulated screws or a staple device.

Postoperative care is similar to that following any arthrodesis of the hindfoot. Initially, a bulky compressive Robert Jones dressing and splint are applied. At 2 weeks, the foot is placed in a cast, which is worn for an additional 4 weeks. Protected weight bearing in a cast is begun at 6 weeks. At 10 weeks, a removable walker boot is applied, and the patient gradually resumes shoe wear at 12 to 14 weeks.

Outcomes and Complications Outcomes after triple arthrodesis have been well described.[25,27-34] Graves and associates[28] reported on a series of 18 feet in 17 patients who had undergone triple arthrodesis. At an average of 3.5 years, pain was decreased in all patients, although 11 feet were the source of residual discomfort. A substantial prevalence of degenerative changes in the ankle and foot was noted. The authors concluded that triple arthrodesis is a satisfactory salvage operation but is technically difficult and is associated with a relatively high complication rate. Fortin and Walling[27] and Haddad and associates[34] noted effective pain relief and improved function at four to six years following triple arthrodesis for deformity correction. Results from both studies con-

cluded that triple arthrodesis was an acceptable treatment of late-stage disease and noted a propensity for secondary degenerative changes to develop at the ankle joint. Similarly, in a report on the results 25 and 44 years after triple arthrodesis, Saltzman and associates[35] reported that 64 of 67 feet had a satisfactory result. Twenty feet had degenerative changes at the ankle at 25 years, and all had degenerative changes at 44 years. Interestingly, the radiographic appearance of the ankle did not correlate with symptoms.

Adjunctive Procedures

Adjunctive procedures may be necessary to fully correct a severe fixed flatfoot deformity. The need to perform these procedures is determined by careful preoperative and intraoperative assessment of the hindfoot alignment and the degree of fixed varus deformity of the forefoot. Achilles tendon lengthening or gastrocnemius-soleus lengthening is almost always necessary to correct the equinus contracture seen with acquired adult flatfoot deformity. These procedures are indicated when the patient lacks 10° of ankle dorsiflexion with the knee extended. Achilles tendon lengthening can be performed percutaneously or with an open technique, and gastrocnemius-soleus lengthening is performed in the midcalf through a small medial or midline incision. We prefer an open Z-lengthening of both the gastrocnemius and the soleus muscle at the myotendinous junction, as this allows a more controlled release of the gastrocnemius muscle either alone or in combination with the soleus, depending on which is tight. However, excellent results can be obtained with either method.

Medial displacement calcaneal

osteotomy is useful for correcting residual hindfoot valgus after initial realignment of the heel. Medial displacement calcaneal osteotomy helps to remove the deforming force of the Achilles tendon on the valgus heel by displacing its insertion medially. It may be used in conjunction with a lateral column lengthening by means of calcaneocuboid distraction arthrodesis if there is excessive residual hindfoot valgus along with excessive forefoot abduction. The need for a medial displacement calcaneal osteotomy can be assessed intraoperatively after provisional reduction and fixation of the calcaneus under the talus. The surgeon can then assess the hindfoot for any residual valgus deformity. If excessive hindfoot valgus is noted, either repeat repositioning of the subtalar joint can be performed if full correction was not obtained or a medial displacement calcaneal osteotomy can be used to correct the residual valgus.

A plantar flexion osteotomy through the medial cuneiform is useful for reducing residual varus forefoot deformity and restoring the weight-bearing tripod of the foot. The osteotomy is oriented in the coronal plane through the midportion of the medial cuneiform at the level of the second tarsometatarsal joint (Figure 6). The first ray is then plantar flexed through this osteotomy site by gently levering the site open with a small osteotome. The resulting gap in the cuneiform is measured once the first ray is plantar flexed to a neutral position. A wedge-shaped tricortical allograft bone block is then cut to this width. It is usually between 4 and 7 mm thick. The graft is impacted into the osteotomy site. The osteotomy site is secured with internal fixation with a 4.0-mm screw or a percutaneous

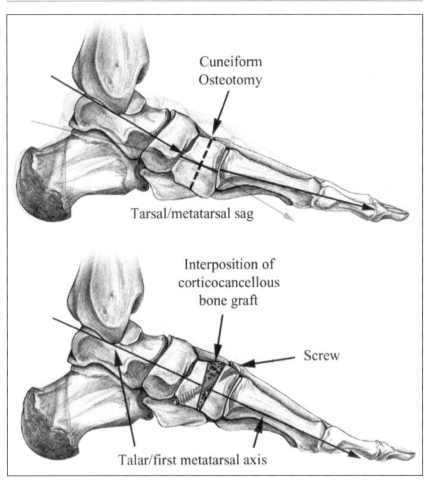

Figure 6 Schematic drawing of a completed plantar flexion osteotomy of the medial cuneiform with use of a corticocancellous bone graft and internal fixation. Note that the lateral talar-first metatarsal angle has been restored to normal. (Reproduced with permission from Johnson JE: Plantar flexion opening wedge cuneifrom-1 osteotomy for correction of fixed forefoot varus. *Tech Foot Ankle Surg* 2004;3:6.)

0.062-inch (1.575-mm) Kirschner wire. If the forefoot varus is secondary to instability, subluxation, or degenerative arthritis at the first tarsometatarsal joint, reduction and fusion of this joint is performed.

Summary

An accurate patient history, thorough physical examination, and accurate assessment of foot flexibility and localization of pain will aid in deciding on the best course of treatment for acquired adult flatfoot deformity. Nonsurgical management is the recommended initial treatment, but it

may not be successful for the treatment of advanced disease, particularly when there are degenerative changes. Surgical management of advanced acquired adult flatfoot deformity is indicated if nonsurgical management has failed. Adjunctive procedures, such as Achilles tendon lengthening, medial displacement calcaneal osteotomy, lateral column lengthening, stabilization of the first tarsometatarsal joint, and plantar flexion osteotomy of the medial column of the foot are useful for correcting residual deformities after hindfoot realignment intraoperatively.

References

1. Myerson MS: Adult acquired flatfoot deformity: Treatment of dysfunction of the posterior tibial tendon. *Instr Course Lect* 1997;46:393-405.

2. Johnson KA, Strom DE: Tibialis posterior tendon dysfunction. *Clin Orthop Relat Res* 1989;239:196-206.

3. Myerson MS, Corrigan J, Thompson F, Schon LC: Tendon transfer combined with calcaneal osteotomy for treatment of posterior tibial tendon insufficiency: A radiological investigation. *Foot Ankle Int* 1995;16:712-718.

4. Mosier-LaClair S, Pomeroy G, Manoli A II: Operative treatment of the difficult stage 2 adult acquired flatfoot deformity. *Foot Ankle Clin* 2001;6:95-119.

5. Mann RA: Rupture of the tibialis posterior tendon. *Instr Course Lect* 1984;33:302-309.

6. Pinney SJ, Van Bergeyk A: Controversies in surgical reconstruction of acquired adult flat foot deformity. *Foot Ankle Clin* 2003;8:595-604.

7. Astion DJ, Deland JT, Otis JC, Kenneally S: Motion of the hindfoot after simulated arthrodesis. *J Bone Joint Surg Am* 1997;79:241-246.

8. Mann RA, Beaman DN: Double arthrodesis in the adult. *Clin Orthop Relat Res* 1999;365:74-80.

9. Mann RA, Beaman DN, Horton GA: Isolated subtalar arthrodesis. *Foot Ankle Int* 1998;19:511-519.

10. Coetzee JC, Hansen ST: Surgical management of severe deformity resulting from posterior tibial tendon dysfunction. *Foot Ankle Int* 2001;22:944-949.

11. Mann RA: Talonavicular arthrodesis for the painful adult acquired flatfoot. *Foot Ankle Int* 1997;18:375-376.

12. Fortin PT: Posterior tibial tendon insufficiency: Isolated fusion of the talonavicular joint. *Foot Ankle Clin* 2001;6:137-151.

13. Harper MC: Talonavicular arthrodesis for the acquired flatfoot in the adult. *Clin Orthop Relat Res* 1999;365:65-68.

14. Gallina J, Sands AK: Lateral-sided bony procedures. *Foot Ankle Clin* 2003;8:563-567.

15. Toolan BC, Sangeorzan BJ, Hansen ST Jr: Complex reconstruction for the treatment of dorsolateral peritalar subluxation of the foot: Early results after distraction arthrodesis of the calcaneocuboid joint in conjunction with stabilization of, and transfer of the flexor digitorum longus tendon to, the midfoot to treat acquired pes planovalgus in adults. *J Bone Joint Surg Am* 1999;81:1545-1560.

16. Chi TD, Toolan BC, Sangeorzan BJ, Hansen ST Jr: The lateral column lengthening and medial column stabilization procedures. *Clin Orthop Relat Res* 1999;365:81-90.

17. Cooper PS, Nowak MD, Shaer J: Calcaneocuboid joint pressures with lateral column lengthening (Evans) procedure. *Foot Ankle Int* 1997;18:199-205.

18. Raines RA Jr, Brage ME: Evans osteotomy in the adult foot: An anatomic study of structures at risk. *Foot Ankle Int* 1998;19:743-747.

19. Neufeld SK, Myerson MS: Complications of surgical treatments for adult flatfoot deformities. *Foot Ankle Clin* 2001;6:179-191.

20. Johnson JE, Cohen BE, DiGiovanni BF, Lamdan R: Subtalar arthrodesis with flexor digitorum longus transfer and spring ligament repair for treatment of posterior tibial tendon insufficiency. *Foot Ankle Int* 2000;21:722-729.

21. Kitaoka HB, Patzer GL: Subtalar arthrodesis for posterior tibial tendon dysfunction and pes planus. *Clin Orthop Relat Res* 1997;345:187-194.

22. Clain MR, Baxter DE: Simultaneous calcaneocuboid and talonavicular fusion: Long-term follow-up study. *J Bone Joint Surg Br* 1994;76:133-136.

23. Hansen ST Jr: *Functional Reconstruction of the Foot and Ankle.* Philadelphia, PA, Lippincott Williams and Wilkins, 2000.

24. Coughlin MJ, Mann RA (eds): *Surgery of the Foot and Ankle*, ed 7. St. Louis, MO, Mosby, 1999.

25. Bednarz PA, Monroe MT, Manoli A II: Triple arthrodesis in adults using rigid internal fixation: An assessment of outcome. *Foot Ankle Int* 1999;20:356-363.

26. Maenpaa H, Lehto MU, Belt EA: What went wrong in triple arthrodesis: An analysis of failures in 21 patients. *Clin Orthop Relat Res* 2001;391:218-223.

27. Fortin PT, Walling AK: Triple arthrodesis. *Clin Orthop Relat Res* 1999;365:91-99.

28. Graves SC, Mann RA, Graves KO: Triple arthrodesis in older adults: Results after long-term follow-up. *J Bone Joint Surg Am* 1993;75:355-362.

29. Jayakumar S, Cowell HR: Rigid flatfoot. *Clin Orthop Relat Res* 1977;122:77-84.

30. Kadakia AR, Haddad SL: Hindfoot arthrodesis for the adult acquired flat foot. *Foot Ankle Clin* 2003;8:569-594.

31. Acosta R, Ushiba J, Cracchiolo A III: The results of a primary and staged pantalar arthrodesis and tibiotalocalcaneal arthrodesis in adult patients. *Foot Ankle Int* 2000;21:182-194.

32. Kelly IP, Easley ME: Treatment of stage 3 adult acquired flatfoot. *Foot Ankle Clin* 2001;6:153-166.

33. Laughlin TJ, Payette CR: Triple arthrodesis and subtalar joint arthrodesis: For the treatment of end-stage posterior tibial tendon dysfunction. *Clin Podiatr Med Surg* 1999;16:527-555.

34. Haddad SL, Myerson MS, Pell RF IV, Schon LC: Clinical and radiographic outcome of revision surgery for failed triple arthrodesis. *Foot Ankle Int* 1997;18:489-499.

35. Saltzman CL, Fehrle MJ, Cooper RR, Spencer EC, Ponseti IV: Triple arthrodesis: Twenty-five and forty-four-year average follow-up of the same patients. *J Bone Joint Surg Am* 1999;81:1391-1402.

Congenital Clubfoot

R. Jay Cummings, MD,
Richard S. Davidson, MD,
Peter F. Armstrong, MD, FRCSC, FAAP
Wallace B. Lehman, MD

Etiology

Genetic Factors

The incidence of clubfoot varies widely with respect to race and sex and increases with the number of affected relatives, suggesting that the etiology is at least partly influenced by genetic factors.[1] The incidence among different races ranges from 0.39 per 1,000 among the Chinese population to 1.2 per 1,000 among Caucasians to 6.8 per 1,000 among Polynesians.[2,3] Lochmiller and associates[4] recently reported a male-to-female ratio of 2.5:1. Siblings of affected individuals have up to a thirty-fold increase in the risk of clubfoot deformity. Clubfoot affects both siblings in 32.5% of monozygotic twins but only 2.9% of dizygotic twins.[5] Lochmiller and associates[4] reported that 24.4% of affected individuals have a family history of idiopathic talipes equinovarus.

Histologic Anomalies

Almost every tissue in the clubfoot has been described as being abnormal.[6] Ultrastructural muscle abnormalities were identified by Isaacs and associates.[7] Handelsman and Badalamente[8] demonstrated an increase in type I:II muscle fiber ratio from the normal 1:2 to 7:1, suggesting a possible link to a primary nerve abnormality. Conversely, Bill and Versfeld[9] were unable to demonstrate neuropathic or myopathic changes in

untreated clubfeet with electromyographic studies.

A primary germ plasm defect of bone resulting in deformity of the talus and navicular was suggested by Irani and Sherman in 1963.[10] Defects in the cartilage of clubfeet were demonstrated by Shapiro and Glimcher.[11] Ionasescu and associates[12] identified increased collagen synthesis in clubfeet. Ippolito[13] demonstrated deformity of the talus, with medial angulation of the neck and medial tilting and rotation of the body of the talus. Together with medial tilting and rotation of the calcaneus, these deformities accounted for the varus deformity of the hindfoot, which in turn accounted for the supination of the forefoot. In a study by Davidson and associates, MRI studies demonstrated plantar flexion and varus angular deformity of the talus, calcaneus, and cuboid in the infant's clubfoot (R Davidson, MD, M Hahn, MD, A Hubbard, MD, Amsterdam, The Netherlands, unpublished data, 1996).

Ippolito and Ponseti[6] proposed a theory of retraction fibrosis of the distal muscles of the calf and the supporting connective tissues. In a more recent anatomic and histologic study, Ippolito[13] demonstrated increased fibrosis of muscle tissue in four aborted fetuses with clubfoot. Dietz and associates[14] identified a reduction in cell number and cytoplasm in the posterior

tibial tendon sheath compared with that in the anterior tibial tendon sheath, suggesting a regional growth disturbance. Zimny and associates,[15] in an electron microscopic study of the fascia from the medial and lateral sides of clubfeet, suggested that myofibroblasts might contribute to contracture and deformity.

Sano and associates[16] performed immunohistochemical analyses and electron microscopic studies of 41 biopsy specimens from the clubfeet of patients 6 to 30 months old. Contractile proteins and a gradation of cells from fibroblasts to myofibroblasts were observed. The authors suggested that this pattern showed similarities to a healing process and that the presence of the proteins and cells indicated a cause both for the clubfoot deformity and for the common recurrence of the deformity after surgery.

Vascular Anomalies

Hootnick and associates[17] and Sodre and associates[18] observed that the majority of clubfoot deformities were associated with hypoplasia or absence of the anterior tibial artery. Hootnick and associates[17] suggested that vascular dysplasia might have a causal relationship to the clubfoot deformity. Muir and associates[19] found a substantially greater prevalence of the absence of the dorsalis pedis pulse in the parents of children with clubfoot.

Anomalous Muscles

Turco[3] identified anomalous muscles in about 15% of his patients with clubfoot. Porter[20] recently described an anomalous flexor muscle in the calf of five children with clubfoot. He also observed that patients with this anomalous muscle had a greater frequency of first-degree relatives with clubfoot. Chotigavanichaya and associates[21] reported a patient in whom clubfoot was corrected only after release of an accessory soleus muscle.

Intrauterine Factors

Hippocrates suggested that the foot is held in a position of equinovarus by external uterine compression and oligohydramnios.[3] However, Turco[3] suggested that it is unlikely that such increased pressure would repeatedly produce the same deformity, especially when there is sufficient room in the uterus at the time that a clubfoot forms (in the first trimester). In a review of the literature and of his own patients, Turco observed as many left as right clubfeet, despite the asymmetrical positioning of the fetus in the womb. This finding suggests that positioning is not a factor.

Bohm[22] described four stages of fetal development of the foot and suggested the possibility that clubfoot represents an interruption in the development of the normal foot. However, medial displacement of the navicular, which is common in clubfoot, is not seen at any stage in the normally developing foot. Kawashima and Uhthoff[23] studied the anatomy of the human foot from the 8th to the 21st intrauterine week in 147 specimens. Their results suggested that the normal foot appears to be similar to a clubfoot during the ninth week of gestation. They suggested that an interruption in development might be responsible for the deformity.

In recent studies of the complications of amniocentesis, an association has been observed between clubfoot and early amniocentesis (before the 11th week). Farrell and associates[24] reported that the rate of clubfoot after amniocentesis was 1.1%, approximately 10 times higher than the rate of 0.1% associated with all live births. The risk of bilateral deformity was noted to be about the same as that in the general population of patients with clubfoot. When early amniocentesis was associated with an amniotic fluid leak, the risk of clubfoot deformity increased to 15% from 1.1% when leakage did not occur. Farrell and associates[24] postulated that some event during early amniocentesis with fluid leakage stops the development of the foot at a time when the foot is in the clubfoot position. They observed that persistent oligohydramnios was not seen on subsequent ultrasound studies. Farrell and associates also postulated that altered pressure from the leak could alter the developmental process. The CEMAT (Canadian Early and Mid-Trimester Amniocentesis Trial) Group[24] did not find the same association with clubfoot and suggested that the amount of fluid removed at the time of amniocentesis might be responsible for the difference between their findings and those of Farrell and associates.

Robertson and Corbett[25] retrospectively reviewed the medical records of 330 children born with an uncomplicated clubfoot deformity and found that the mean month of conception of these children was June, a finding at variance with the peak months of conception for the overall population of the United States for the same period. They theorized that an intrauterine enterovirus infection with peak rates in the summer and fall could cause anterior horn-cell lesions at the appropriate stage of fetal development, leading to a deformity such as congenital clubfoot.

Physical Examination

It is important to examine the entire body of a patient with clubfoot. Associated anomalies of the upper extremities, back, and legs, as well as abnormal reflexes, can provide information about the etiology of the deformity and the likelihood of successful treatment.

A standardized examination of the clubfoot should be performed initially and after each interval of treatment with manipulation and a cast. A reference point, usually the knee in 90° of flexion, must be chosen for the examination of the foot. Torsional alignment, varus and valgus, and the overall size and shape of the leg, ankle, and foot should be assessed. Torsion is difficult to assess clinically in a patient with clubfoot because the medial malleolus is obscured by the navicular. The congenital clubfoot is generally shorter and wider than the normal foot. Transverse plantar creases or clefts at the midfoot and at the posterior part of the ankle should be noted.[26] Atrophy of the calf is an expected component of clubfoot, particularly in an older child with severe or residual deformity.

Equinus must be assessed with the knee both in extension and in flexion. The true contracture of the gastrocnemius-soleus muscle complex, which crosses the knee, is indicated by the equinus measured with the knee extended. The difference between the equinus measured with the knee flexed and that measured with it extended indicates the amount of stiffness in the ankle joint. The posterior aspect of the calcaneus must be palpated carefully when the equinus is measured because the bone may be pulled proximally away from the heel pad (Fig. 1).

The varus or valgus position of the heel at rest and in the position of best correction should be measured. Flexibility of the subtalar joint is difficult to measure but may give an indication about stiffness.

The lateral border of the foot should be held in the position of maximum correction and measured. Persistent varus, particularly after a trial of cast immobilization, may indicate varus deformity at the calcaneocuboid joint (medialization of the ossification center of the cuboid as

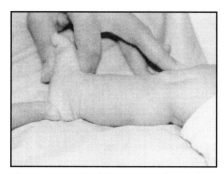

Fig. 1 Equinus should be measured with the knee extended, the subtalar rotation corrected, and the heel in neutral (as much valgus as possible). Although the heel pad may appear to be well positioned, the calcaneus may remain in equinus. Notice how the examiner's finger presses in the heel pad to the calcaneus in equinus position.

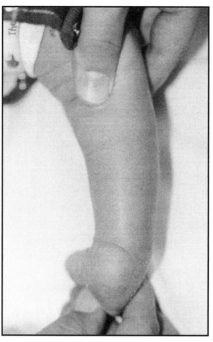

Fig. 2 In this foot, the heel is in varus position but the forefoot is well aligned with the heel. There is no supination of the forefoot on the hindfoot.

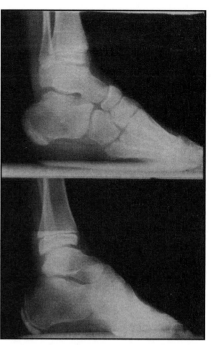

Fig. 3 Two radiographs of the same foot. **Top,** The x-ray beam is focused on the midfoot to demonstrate the talonavicular joint and the midtarsal bones. Note that the fibula is positioned posterior to the tibia and that the talar dome appears flattened. **Bottom,** The x-ray beam is focused on the hindfoot to demonstrate Kite's angle. Note that the fibula overlaps the posterior half of the tibia and that the talar dome is round and high.

described by Simons[27]) or varus deformity of the metatarsals.

The talar head should be palpated dorsolaterally at the midfoot. The talar head usually is lined up with the patella, although in plantar flexion. Manipulation to reduce the forefoot onto the talar head indicates the amount of midfoot stiffness.

Forefoot supination should be noted. All deformities should be assessed in relation to the next most proximal segment—ie, the forefoot on the midfoot, the midfoot on the hindfoot, and the hindfoot on the ankle. If the hindfoot is in 30° of varus and the forefoot (the line of the toes) is angulated 30° in relation to the tibia (Fig. 2), then the deformity is hindfoot varus and there is no forefoot supination. Errors in this assessment may lead the surgeon to overcorrect the forefoot in a cast or to surgically create a pronation deformity.[28]

Palpation of the lateral column with the foot in dorsiflexion can demonstrate overcorrection of the midfoot (iatrogenic rocker-bottom foot).

Radiographic Examination

Although radiographic examination has been used to demonstrate the deformities of the tarsal bones in clubfeet, the images

are hard to reproduce, evaluate, and measure. There are several reasons for this: (1) It is difficult to position the foot, particularly when it is very stiff and deformed, in a standard fashion in the x-ray beam. (2) The ossific nuclei do not represent the true shape of the mostly cartilaginous tarsal bones (R Davidson, MD, M Hahn, MD, A Hubbard, MD, Amsterdam, The Netherlands, unpublished data, 1996). (3) In the first year of life, only the talus, calcaneus, and metatarsals may be ossified (the cuboid is ossified at 6 months; the cuneiforms, after 1 year; and the navicular, after 3 years and even later).[29] (4) Rotation distorts the measured angles and makes the talar dome appear flattened (Fig. 3). (5) Failure to hold the foot in the position of best correction makes the foot look worse than it is on the radiograph.

To optimize the radiographic studies, the foot should be held in the position of best correction with weight bearing or, if

an infant is being examined, with simulated weight bearing. Because the AP and lateral talocalcaneal angles (Kite's angles[30]) are the most commonly measured angles, the x-ray beam should be focused on the hindfoot (about 30° from the vertical for the AP radiograph, and the lateral radiograph should be transmalleolar with the fibula overlapping the posterior half of the tibia, to avoid rotational distortion) (Fig. 3).

For an older child, it may be useful to focus the x-ray beam on the midfoot because this view allows assessment of dorsolateral subluxation and narrowing of the talonavicular joint. Lateral dorsiflexion and plantar flexion radiographs may be useful to assess ankle motion and hypermobility in the midfoot.

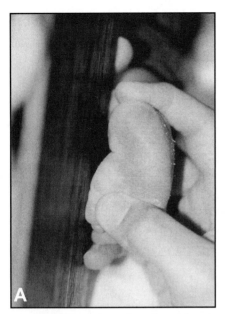
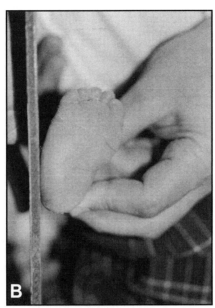

Fig. 4 A clubfoot is bean shaped. **A,** When the radiographic plate is placed against the medial part of the foot, the x-ray beam focuses on the midfoot with the hindfoot rotated, causing increased valgus measurement. **B,** The radiographic plate should be placed against the lateral aspect of the hindfoot so that the x-ray beam is perpendicular to the hindfoot.

Common Radiographic Measurements

Three measurements should be made on the AP radiograph:[30-32] (1) the AP talocalcaneal angle (usually less than 20° in a clubfoot), (2) the talar–first metatarsal angle (up to about 30° of valgus in a normal foot and mild-to-severe varus in a clubfoot), and (3) medial displacement of the cuboid ossification center on the axis of the calcaneus.[33-35] This apparent displacement may represent angular deformity of the calcaneus or medial subluxation of the cuboid on the calcaneus.

To make the lateral radiograph, the foot should be held in maximum dorsiflexion with lateral rotation but without pronation. The x-ray beam should be focused on the hindfoot. The foot should be positioned with the radiographic plate placed laterally against the posterior half of the foot. The clubfoot is bean shaped, and placement of the radiographic plate medially forces the foot to be rotated laterally in the x-ray beam (Fig. 4). Two measurements should be made: (1) the talocalcaneal angle (typically less than 25° in a clubfoot) and (2) the talar–first metatarsal angle. Plantar flexion of the forefoot on the hindfoot indicates contracted plantar soft tissues or midtarsal bone deformity (a triangular navicular).

Classification and Evaluation

Simons[27,32] distinguishes classification from evaluation. Classification involves typing the foot by etiology, such as neurologic, teratologic, or idiopathic. Evaluation involves measuring the foot—ie, the size, shape, range of motion of the joints, and radiographic angles. Both classification and evaluation are important to the understanding of comparative outcome studies and to the successful treatment of each clubfoot.

Clubfeet have been evaluated in many ways, yet there is little agreement on a standard and reproducible method. Cummings and Lovell[35] evaluated 85 parameters of history, physical examination, radiographs, and function in an interobserver study and found only 12 parameters that were reproducible at the 80% level. Watts[36] noted poor reproducibility in the interpretation and measurement of clubfoot radiographs. Flynn and associates[37] studied interobserver reliability in the evaluation of 55 feet with the use of two clubfoot grading systems described by Pirani and associates and by Dimeglio and associates. They found very good reliability after an initial learning curve but observed a lower correlation when therapists' scores were included.

Dimeglio and associates[38] divided clubfeet into four groups with use of a 20-point scale. Points were apportioned according to motion, with 4 points each for equinus, varus of the heel, internal torsion, and adduction. In addition, 1 point each was added for the presence of a posterior crease, a medial crease, cavus, and poor muscle condition. The points were then converted into four grades, each with implications for the success of treatment. Grade I indicated that the clubfoot was mild or postural, not requiring surgery; grade II, that there was considerable reducibility; grade III, that the clubfoot was resistant but partially reducible; and grade IV, that it was teratologic. They recommended that grade I feet be excluded from statistical analysis because they tended to improve results artificially. After excluding grade I feet from their own series, they found that 30% of the remaining deformities were grade II, 61% were grade III, and 9% were grade IV.

Other investigators have developed systems, some employing 100-point scales, for the classification and assessment of function in childhood and adulthood.[39-43] The reproducibility and reliability of these systems have not been established.

Nonsurgical Treatment

The first written record of clubfoot treatment is in the works of Hippocrates from around 400 BC. Hippocrates recommended gentle manipulation of the foot, followed by splinting.[44] The first advance in nonsurgical treatment occurred in 1836, when Guerin introduced the plaster-of-Paris cast.[45] Around the turn of the 20th century, devices such as the Thomas wrench, which allowed the foot to be "corrected" more rapidly through forceful manipulation, were introduced.[46] In 1932, Dr. Hiram Kite,[47] recognizing that forceful manipulation and extensive surgical releases were harmful, recommended a return to gentle manipulation and cast immobilization for the nonsurgical treatment of congenital clubfoot.

Principles of Nonsurgical Treatment
Stretching and Manipulation

The basis on which nonsurgical techniques rest is the correction of deformity through the production of plastic (permanent) deformation (lengthening) of the shortened ligaments and tendons in the involved foot. Serial manipulation and cast immobilization rely on the viscoelastic nature of connective tissue to produce plastic deformation through a process known as stress relaxation. Deformity is corrected as much as possible with gentle stretching, which places the shortened tissues under tension. As the foot is held in the maximally corrected position by the cast, the tension in the shortened tissues decreases over time. When the tension decreases sufficiently, more correction can be obtained by repeating the process.

Most, but not all, advocates of nonsurgical treatment of congenital clubfoot commence manipulative treatment with stretching of the foot. The specific viscoelastic properties of the tissues of the congenital clubfoot relative to those of other connective tissues do not appear to have been studied. Therefore, the duration for which the foot needs to be stretched, the amount of force that needs to be applied, and whether the force should be applied continuously or inter-

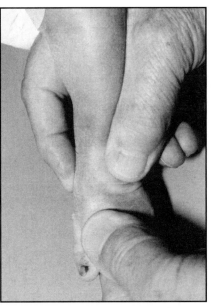

Fig. 5 The Kite and Lovell technique for reduction of the talonavicular joint, using the index finger to gently push the navicular onto the head of the talus.

mittently are unknown. Consequently, there is controversy regarding how much preliminary stretching of the foot should occur before manipulative correction of the deformity is attempted. However, all authors, seem to agree that treatment should be started as early as possible.

There are almost as many techniques for the manipulative treatment of congenital clubfoot as there are authors who write about congenital clubfoot. Many authors have reported success rates of less than 50% for nonsurgical treatment. The two methods that seem to be the most widely performed and that have the highest reported long-term success rates are the Kite and Lovell technique[48] and the Ponseti technique.[49]

The Kite and Lovell technique starts with stretching of the foot through longitudinal traction applied to the foot. Ponseti did not describe the use of preliminary stretching. In both the Kite and Lovell technique and the Ponseti technique, the manipulation starts with reduction of the talonavicular joint. In both

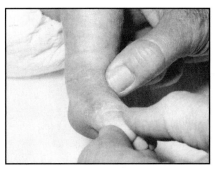

Fig. 6 The Ponseti technique of reduction of the talonavicular joint by pulling the forefoot laterally relative to the hindfoot. Note that the forefoot is aligned with the heel through supination of the forefoot relative to the leg.

techniques, a thumb is placed laterally in the sinus tarsi over the head of the talus. In the Kite and Lovell technique, the navicular is gently pushed onto the head of the talus with the index finger of the same hand (Fig. 5). In the Ponseti technique, the other hand is used to pull the forefoot, and the navicular along with it, laterally onto the head of the talus. Ponseti considered it very important to keep the forefoot supinated during this maneuver (in truth, the forefoot is kept in line with the hindfoot, which is initially in varus) (Fig. 6). Ponseti believed that failing to do so, or pronating the forefoot relative to the hindfoot, produces a cavus deformity. In the Kite and Lovell technique, a slipper cast is applied after the talonavicular joint is reduced. As the cast dries, the foot is molded on Plexiglas, with simultaneous pushing of the heel out of varus and flattening of the foot to prevent cavus.

The lateral pulling of the forefoot relative to the hindfoot in the Ponseti technique also corrects the forefoot adduction. The Kite and Lovell technique corrects forefoot adduction by abducting the forefoot on the hindfoot as the slipper cast dries. In this maneuver, a finger is placed laterally over the distal end of the calcaneus to act as a fulcrum. Ponseti termed this maneuver "Kite's error," con-

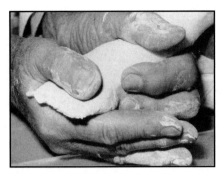

Fig. 7 Correction of the forefoot adduction by abducting the forefoot with counterpressure applied at the calcaneocuboid joint.

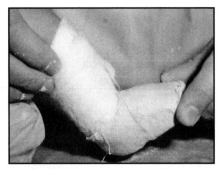

Fig. 8 The slipper cast is used to externally rotate the foot, correcting internal rotation or medial spin of the calcaneus beneath the talus.

tending that any force applied laterally to the distal part of the calcaneus to correct forefoot adduction prevents the distal end of the calcaneus from moving laterally as the calcaneus is externally rotated out from under the talus (Fig. 7). Kite and Lovell actually used the slipper cast to externally rotate the calcaneus and forefoot as a unit from beneath the talus (Fig. 8). In both techniques, the cast is then extended to the thigh while the foot is held in external rotation.

In both the Kite and Lovell technique and the Ponseti technique, no effort is made to correct equinus until forefoot adduction and heel varus are corrected because an attempt to correct equinus before correction of the other deformities leads to a rocker-bottom deformity. According to Ponseti,[49] when equinus persisted after the forefoot and hindfoot were corrected, a tenotomy of the Achilles tendon was performed percutaneously with the use of local anesthesia in the cast room, and then application of the cast was continued. Kite and Lovell preferred wedging the cast when equinus could not be corrected after the forefoot adduction and heel varus were corrected.[48]

Ponseti[49] reported that 89% of the feet in his study had a good or excellent result at 30-year follow-up. However, Achilles tenotomies were required in 70% of his patients. Ponseti reported a 50% rate of recurrence requiring addi-

tional cast treatment. Deformities that recurred frequently required lengthening of the Achilles tendon and transfer of the anterior tibial tendon to maintain correction.[49] Ponseti now reports that the recurrence rate in his patients is far lower (IV Ponseti, MD, personal communication, 2001). Kite and Lovell reported that up to 95% of feet can be completely corrected without any surgery. However, the average duration of cast treatment with their technique is 22 months compared with 2 to 4 months with the Ponseti technique (WW Lovell, MD, personal communication, 1998).

While the most common way to maintain the position of the foot after manipulation is with a plaster cast, other methods have been used. Shaw,[50] among others, favored the use of adhesive tape and reported a success rate of 70% with his technique.

How often the cycle of manipulation and immobilization is repeated varies. Most physicians change the cast and remanipulate the foot at weekly intervals. More rapid correction has been achieved with more frequent (daily) cast changes and manipulation.

After the foot has been corrected (usually as determined on radiographs), it is held in the corrected position for some period of time. The initial holding device is usually a cast, and after 2 to 4 weeks of

such treatment, the patient is frequently managed with braces. Kite used a Phelps splint, which was worn until the age of 10 years. Ponseti recommended that a Denis Browne bar be worn until the age of 2 to 4 years. Currently many surgeons discontinue splinting after the child is able to walk independently.

Newer Methods of Nonsurgical Treatment

For some time, there has been an interest in nonsurgical methods that emphasize motion and minimize immobilization. In 1937, Denis Browne[51] introduced a technique, modified in 1942 by Thomson,[52] in which the child's own "physiologic motions" were used to correct the foot through a dynamic mechanism. The technique consisted of the application of corrective shoes that were then attached to a bar. The attachment of the shoes to the bar allowed progressive external rotation of the feet. While the feet were in this apparatus, the constant kicking by the infant stretched the contracted tissues, thereby correcting the deformity. Recently, Yamamoto and Furuya[53] reported on a series of 91 clubfeet treated with a modified Denis Browne splint. Sixty feet were corrected without surgery, and good or excellent correction was maintained at an average of 6 years 3 months after treatment.

Bensahel and associates[54,55] developed a nonsurgical technique involving manipulation of the foot by a physical therapist. Each manipulative session lasts 30 minutes and is followed by taping of the foot to a wooden splint. This treatment is performed daily for up to 8 months. Bensahel and associates reported that 48% of their patients had a good result.

Dimeglio and associates[56] described what would seem to be the ultimate stretching treatment for congenital clubfoot, continuous passive motion. As with the method of Bensahel and associates, the foot is manipulated by a physical therapist for 30 minutes. After the manipulation, the foot is placed in a machine that performs stretching (continuous passive motion). Treatment is usually started at about 2 weeks of age. The machine is adjusted daily on the basis of an examination of the foot. The foot is maintained in the machine for up to 8 hours each day. After each session, a splint is applied to hold the foot in the maximally corrected position until the next day. Dimeglio and associates[56] reported that, in a series of 216 feet, 45 had to be excluded because the children's parents were "noncompliant" and 68% of the remaining feet were deemed to have a successful result. It is important to note that "success" did not necessarily mean that no surgery was required. Treatment was deemed to be successful when the required surgery proved to be less extensive than that predicted to be necessary on the basis of the examination of the foot before treatment was started. It was possible to avoid surgery on the lateral side of the foot in 32% of the feet that required surgery.

Johnston and Richards[57] recently reported their results with what they termed the French method. In their study, 48 feet were treated with a regimen of stretching exercises. A continuous passive motion machine was not used. Thirty-six feet were successfully treated without surgery, nine required minimal surgery, and three required a comprehensive soft-tissue release. In a follow-up study, Richards and associates found the French technique to be more effective than traditional manipulation and immobilization in a short-leg cast (BS Richards II, MD, CE Johnston II, MD, H Wilson, MD, Vancouver, BC, Canada, unpublished data, 2000). Ponseti, commenting on the later study, noted that short-leg casts, used by Richards and associates, were in his experience less effective than long-leg casts.

An interesting adjunct to the French technique, as described by Johnston and Richards, has recently been reported. Delgado and associates[58] injected botulinum toxin type A (Botox; Allergan, Irvine, CA) into the gastrocnemius-soleus and posterior tibial muscles of three infants with congenital clubfoot that had been incompletely corrected by the French method. After the injections, additional correction was obtained with continued nonsurgical treatment. The rationale for the use of Botox appears to be that a reduction of tone in the most contracted muscles might facilitate their lengthening by manipulative stretching. Determining whether such pharmacologic intervention is useful will require additional study.

Another process that can be used to produce plastic deformation of soft tissues is known as creep. Creep occurs when tendons and ligaments elongate as a result of a continuous stretching. Creep can be produced by dynamic splinting, which has been found to be helpful when used in conjunction with serial manipulation and cast treatment.[59] We have been unable to find reports on the use of dynamic splinting as a primary nonsurgical treatment modality. Skin irritation and, on occasion, skin breakdown may limit the usefulness of this technique.

Surgical Treatment
Despite our best efforts, some clubfeet cannot be completely corrected with nonsurgical treatment. In such feet, soft-tissue release is clearly indicated.

Preoperative Assessment
All clubfeet are not the same. Therefore, it is important to assess the foot carefully to determine the components of the deformity that remain. Once that has been done, the surgeon must think about which anatomic structures contribute to each component of the deformity. Obviously, those are the structures that need to be addressed at the time of surgery. A foot in which all components of the deformity are still present likely requires a full pos-

teromedial plantar lateral release. If the clinical examination indicates a flexible forefoot and midfoot with a straight lateral border and a palpable interval between the tuberosity of the navicular and the medial malleolus but a persistent equinus, then a posterior release may be all that is needed.

Radiographic assessment of the foot complements the clinical examination. Radiographs can be used to determine the relationship between the talus and the calcaneus in both the AP and lateral planes. The radiographs reveal whether there is subluxation of the talonavicular joint and the calcaneocuboid joint and whether the foot has a cavus component. The lateral radiograph can reveal the degree of persistent equinus in the ankle. We believe very strongly in the "à la carte" approach to the clubfoot as described by Bensahel and associates[60]—ie, do only what is necessary to get a good correction of the foot.

Age
Most surgeons have one of two opinions concerning the optimum age at which surgery should be performed. Advocates of "early" treatment perform the surgery when the patient is between 3 and 6 months old.[61] They argue that there is a great deal of growth in the foot and therefore a lot of remodeling potential during the first year of life. In contrast, advocates of "late" treatment prefer to wait until the child is 9 to 12 months old.[62] They believe that, because the components of the foot are larger, the pathoanatomy is more obvious, and the surgery is easier to perform. Also, because the child is by then old enough to walk, early weight bearing may help prevent the recurrence of deformity. Simons[63] recommended that the size of the foot rather than the age of the patient be used to determine the optimum time to perform the surgery. He stated that the foot should be 8 cm long or longer at the time of surgery.

Incisions

Incisions fall into one of three categories: the Turco oblique or hockey-stick posteromedial type of incision;[3] the circumferential incision, more commonly referred to as the Cincinnati incision;[64] and the two-incision or Carroll approach.[65] Each has its limitations. The Turco incision crosses the skin creases on the medial side of the foot and ankle. It is certainly more difficult to reach the posterolateral structures, such as the talofibular and calcaneofibular ligaments, through this incision. The origin of the plantar fascia also may be a challenge to expose and release. The Cincinnati incision has the potential for creating problems with the skin edges. It also has been criticized for its limited exposure of the Achilles tendon. The criticism of the Carroll approach is that it can limit the correction of the equinus and/or varus deformity because of the posteromedial skin tether. We prefer the Cincinnati incision.

Medial Plantar Release

The abductor hallucis muscle is the guide for the initial part of the procedure. As long as the surgeon cuts on top of the muscle, no vital structures will be damaged. It should be followed proximally to its origin from the calcaneus. As it is exposed proximally, some thickened fascia that crosses the muscle in a vertical direction may be encountered. The fascia is divided, and the abductor hallucis is released from the calcaneus. The part of the origin that passes between the medial and lateral neurovascular bundles and attaches to the sustentaculum tali also must be released. The muscle is then reflected distally. The motor branch from the medial plantar nerve can be cut without important consequences. Dividing the laciniate ligament then exposes the medial plantar neurovascular bundle. Careful dissection is continued distally to the forefoot. An artery and two small veins cross the nerve in the midfoot. They can be cauterized and divided. The

lateral plantar bundle is then identified. The main calcaneal branch is the most posterior structure. The bundle is protected by a 0.25-inch (0.64-cm) Penrose drain. The interval between the vein and the calcaneal branch is a safe area in which to approach the origin of the plantar fascia and the short toe flexors. Their origins are divided across the plantar aspect. Obviously, this release is done only when the deformity is thought to have a cavus component.[63]

The next structures to be identified are the tendons of the flexor digitorum longus and flexor hallucis longus. They are followed distally past the master knot of Henry and proximally above the ankle joint. As the flexor hallucis longus passes under the sustentaculum tali, there is a thick retinaculum to be divided. McKay[66] described preservation of the sheaths of these tendons. The dissection continues on the plantar aspect of the foot. The tendon of the peroneus longus is identified and is carefully released from its sheath as far as the lateral border of the foot. This tendon passes around the lateral border at the level of the calcaneocuboid joint. It must be carefully protected. Many surgeons make the mistake of looking for the calcaneocuboid joint too distally. Care must be taken because it is very easy to create a joint by cutting through cartilage. Once the joint definitely has been identified, it should be released medially and plantarly. A thin elevator such as a Freer elevator then can be used to fenestrate the lateral part of the capsule. The medial part of the capsule and the spring ligament are divided, which also helps to identify the medial-inferior portion of the talonavicular joint. By lifting the tendons and bundle, the medial portion of the talocalcaneal capsule can be identified and released. Care must be taken not to start the release too far posteriorly, where the ankle and subtalar joints are close together, because it is easy to mistake the subtalar joint for the ankle joint. The risk is that the deep deltoid ligament could be

divided completely. Care also should be taken not to damage the sustentaculum tali.

The tendon of the tibialis posterior muscle is then identified above the ankle joint. The sheath is carefully divided longitudinally. Some of the retinaculum is preserved as a bridge distally. A Z-plasty of the tendon is carried out, and the distal stump is pulled through the retinacular bridge. Finding the talonavicular joint can be somewhat challenging. It is critical to remember that the plane of this joint is parallel to the medial aspect of the talar neck. The inferior portion may be approached first. Distraction of the joint by pulling on the insertion of the tibialis posterior helps in the release. The dorsal structures, such as the tibialis anterior muscle, the extensor tendons, and the neurovascular structures, must be protected. As the capsule is released dorsally, care must be taken not to divide the deep deltoid ligament and to avoid the dorsum of the neck of the talus. Both of these areas contain important blood supplies to the talus. The talonavicular joint capsule should be fully divided dorsally, medially, and plantarly. The Freer elevator can be used to fenestrate the lateral aspect of the capsule. Carroll[67] also suggested division of the slips of the tibialis posterior that run forward to attach to the undersurfaces of the cuneiforms and the bases of the second, third, and fourth metatarsals. The medial plantar release should then be complete (Fig. 9).

Posterior Release

As the posterior part of the skin incision is made, it is important not to cut too deeply. The Achilles tendon is exposed as far proximally as possible. A Z-plasty is performed, detaching the medial end distally, to reduce the tendency of the tendon to pull the heel into varus. McKay[66] preferred to lengthen the Achilles tendon with a coronal Z-plasty.

The structures that pass behind the medial malleolus already have been iden-

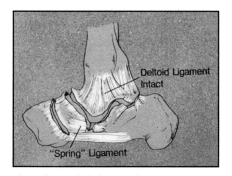

Fig. 9 The medial plantar release.

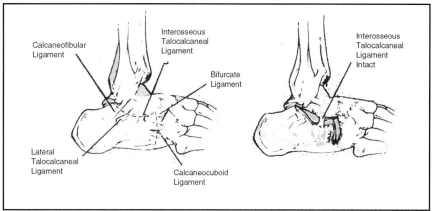

Fig. 10 The lateral release.

tified and protected. The lateral structures now need to be dissected. The sural nerve is found and protected. The peroneal tendons are exposed, and the sheath is divided distally, beginning at the tip of the lateral malleolus. The sheath should not be divided proximal to that level, if possible, to prevent later subluxation of the tendons anterior to the lateral malleolus. The talocalcaneal joint is opened first. The release already has been performed medially and is now continued posteriorly and laterally. With retraction of the lateral structures, the calcaneofibular ligament is divided. This is an important part of the procedure because this ligament tethers the calcaneus to the fibula. It would be impossible to rotate the calcaneus into the corrected position without this release. The lateral capsular release is continued as far as can be seen from the posterior perspective. Then the ankle joint is carefully approached. If the ankle is in substantial equinus, not much of the posterior part of the talar body is between the calcaneus and the tibial plafond. Care must be taken not to enter the distal tibial physis while looking for the ankle joint. The ankle joint capsule is released from the posteromedial corner of the body of the talus to the posterolateral corner. It is easy to mistake the lateral surface of the talus for the posterior surface and therefore carry out an extensive lateral release rather than a posterior release. The posterior talofibular ligament should be divided. Some

authors also have recommended the release of the posterior tibiofibular ligament to allow more room for the body of the talus when it is brought out of equinus.[48]

Lateral Release

The releases described allow for excellent correction of the deformity in many feet. In some feet, however, there will still be difficulty in rotating the calcaneus outwardly relative to the talus. In these cases, a more extensive lateral release needs to be performed (Fig. 10). During this dissection, the sural nerve and peroneal tendons are protected. Capsulotomies of the talonavicular and calcaneocuboid joints should be performed, if necessary. Also, as much of the interosseous ligament as necessary can be divided to spin the calcaneus on the talus. We usually try to preserve at least the medial portion of this ligament.

Reduction and Fixation

The talus should be inwardly rotated slightly, and the navicular should be reduced on the head of the talus. When the navicular is properly reduced, the medial tuberosity should be prominent. If it is flush with the medial aspect of the talar head and neck, it is overreduced laterally. It should, however, be flush with the dorsum of the talar head. According

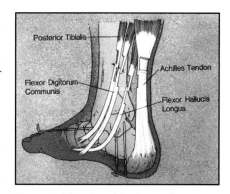

Fig. 11 Stabilization of the foot with pins.

to Simons,[63] the pin should be placed centrally in the head and drilled in a retrograde fashion until it emerges at the posterolateral ridge of the talus. The navicular is reduced, and the pin is then driven across the joint. In the sagittal plane, the pin should be in line with the first metatarsal. Often this is the only pin necessary to maintain the reduction. The calcaneus needs to be rotated such that the tuberosity moves medially away from the fibula. The cuboid needs to be reduced on the end of the calcaneus, and pinning may be required to stabilize this reduction. If the interosseous ligament has been completely released, the subtalar joint needs to be stabilized (Fig. 11). The pin is placed through the plantar surface of the calcaneus, across the subtalar joint and into the talus. It should not pass into the ankle joint. Care should be taken to ensure that the calcaneus is not tipped into varus or valgus.

Intraoperative Assessment

Once the reduction and pinning have been completed, the degree of tightness of the toe flexors should be assessed. If the toes cannot be brought easily to the neutral position, the flexor digitorum longus and/or the flexor hallucis longus should be lengthened. The position of the foot should be checked with the knee in 90° of flexion. It must be plantigrade without a varus, valgus, supination, or pronation deformity. The thigh-foot axis should be outwardly rotated 0° to 20°.

There is a difference of opinion about the value of intraoperative radiographs. Some surgeons use them, and others believe that radiographs are not necessary if the foot is carefully positioned and clinically assessed at the end of the procedure.[48] If there are any doubts about the quality of the reduction on clinical examination, radiographs can help determine the site of the problem. If the reduction is not satisfactory, the pins must be removed and the foot repositioned.

The distal stump of the tibialis posterior tendon is then pulled back under the bridge of the retinaculum. It is sutured under some tension to help to prevent the tendency for an overcorrected planovalgus foot to develop. If the flexor hallucis longus and flexor digitorum longus tendons have been lengthened, they are repaired without tension. The Achilles tendon is repaired with the ankle in 10° of plantar flexion so that there is some tension on it when the foot is in the neutral position.

Wound Closure

Some surgeons allow the foot to return to an equinovarus position and close the skin completely. A manipulation is planned for 1 to 3 weeks postoperatively to bring the foot up into the neutral position. Other surgeons position the foot in the neutral position, approximate the skin medially

and laterally, and leave a skin gap posteriorly. Gaps as large as 2 to 3 cm have been left with good healing and minimal scarring.[69] The wound is dressed, and some form of immobilization, which varies from a soft dressing to a full above-the-knee cast, is applied. Some surgeons bivalve the cast, and others do not.

Postoperative Management

We use either a continuous epidural block, begun after intubation, or a "one-shot" caudal block at the end of the procedure. We have been impressed with the comfort provided to the child, and, at the time of writing, there have not been any complications attributable to these blocks. At 1 week postoperatively, the child is sedated, the postoperative dressing is removed, and the wounds are inspected. The foot is held in the neutral, plantigrade position, and a cast is applied. The knee is held at 90° of flexion, the foot is outwardly rotated, and the cast is extended above the knee. The cast is worn for 4 to 6 weeks, after which the child returns to the clinic, the pin or pins are removed, and an ankle-foot orthosis is fitted. The orthosis is worn for 6 months, and the foot is then reevaluated.

Revision Surgery

The objective of clubfoot surgery is to obtain a complete and lasting correction with one operation. However, about 25% (range, 13% to 50%) of the feet have a recurrence.[69,70] The most common persistent deformities are forefoot adduction and supination. However, varus, equinus, cavus, and overcorrection of the heel all have been reported following clubfoot surgery.[71] Recurrence of one or more components of the clubfoot deformity may result from an incomplete correction, failure to maintain correction, tarsal bone remodeling, abnormal scar formation with tethering of tendons, and tarsal coalition that was either iatrogenic or missed during the surgical procedure.[70]

Preoperative Evaluation

A rating system has been developed to determine the need for revision surgery. S cores of less than 60 points (of a possible total of 100 points) indicate the need for revision (Fig. 12). The preoperative radiographic evaluation includes AP and lateral radiographs of the foot in maximum dorsiflexion, as previously described.[31,32] In addition, when the previously described radiographic angles are measured, the radiographs should be reviewed for other changes, including subluxation of the tarsal navicular, flattening of the trochlear surface of the talus, and shortening of the calcaneus. Once the clinical and radiographic evaluations are complete, attention is turned to correction of the residual deformity. An algorithm has been developed as a guide for the choice of which procedure or procedures to perform (Table 1).[72]

Treatment of Residual Deformity
Residual Forefoot Adduction

Residual adduction is usually found at the midfoot and occasionally at the forefoot. In patients younger than 2 years, forefoot adduction is treated with repeat complete soft-tissue releases.[73] In patients 2 to 4 years old, osteotomies are not recommended because of the immaturity of the foot. Excision of the calcaneocuboid joint cartilage or cuboid enucleation is a better option. These procedures must be combined with a medial soft-tissue release. Cuboid decancellation preserves the articular surface of the cuboid surface proximally and distally, while "crushing" of the bone shortens the lateral column and corrects adduction.[3]

For patients older than 4 years, many procedures have been described, including excision of the distal part of the calcaneus,[74] fusion of the calcaneocuboid joint,[75] opening wedge osteotomy of the first cuneiform, metatarsal osteotomies, and tarsometatarsal capsulotomies.[76] Lichtblau[77] in 1973 described a medial soft-tissue release and an osteotomy of the distal end of the calcaneus in which 1 cm of the distal lateral border and 2 mm of the distal medial border are removed. He claimed that the resected calcaneal articular surface was replaced by fibrocartilage, and he demonstrated mobility at the calcaneocuboid joint up to 6 years after surgery.

Evans[75] in 1961 described a procedure consisting of posteromedial releases in conjunction with lateral calcaneocuboid wedge resection and fusion. The procedure is not recommended for children younger than 4 years because of possible overcorrection. The correction of adduction occurs at the level of the midfoot, not distal to the navicular.[75,78,79] Accurate reduction of the navicular on the talus is essential because the position of the navicular is permanently stabilized by the procedure.[80] Only a narrow wedge from the calcaneocuboid joint should be removed; otherwise, overcorrection into valgus may occur.[75,78,79] The operation decreases growth of the lateral column of the foot. Satisfactory long-term functional results have been documented in 60% to 80% of the patients managed with the procedure.[75,78]

Fowler and associates[81] in 1959 described an opening wedge osteotomy of the medial cuneiform, and Hofmann and associates[82] in 1984 reported on this procedure for the treatment of residual adduction in clubfoot. The Fowler procedure includes an opening wedge osteotomy of the medial cuneiform, a radical plantar release, and a transfer of the tibialis anterior tendon to the dorsum of the first metatarsal. This procedure is reserved for children older than 8 years because a well-ossified first cuneiform is a prerequisite.[81] Supination of the midfoot is not addressed, and the degree of correction is limited by the intact lateral column complex of the calcaneocuboid joint.

McHale and Lenhart[83] described a procedure for an adducted forefoot and a supinated midfoot with hindfoot varus.

Functional Rating System for Clubfoot Surgery

Date _____

Patient: _____

Date of Birth: _____

Sex: Male / Female   MR #: _____

Clubfoot Side/Type:
Right _____   Left _____

FIRST SURGICAL INTERVENTION
Date: _____

By: _____

Type of Surgery: _____

Special Findings: _____

REVISION SURGERY
Date: _____

By: _____

Type of Surgery: _____

Special Findings: _____

TOTAL SCORE: _____

Points	Rating
85 – 100	Excellent
70 – 84	Good
60 – 69	Fair
≤59	Poor

*   Arc starting from neutral 90°
**   The *talocalcaneal index* is the sum of the talocalcaneal angles measured on lateral and anteroposterior radiographs

Category	Points
1. **Ankle motion (passive)**	
*Arc from neutral >20°	15
Arc from neutral >10°	5
Arc from neutral 0-5°	0
2. **Subtalar Joint Motion (passive motion)**	
≥15°	10
<15°	5
Stiff	0
3. **Position of Heel When Standing**	
0°-5° Valgus	10
>5° Valgus	5
Varus	0
4. **Forefoot (appearance)**	
Neutral	10
<5° Adduction/Abduction	5
>5° Adduction/Abduction	0
5. **Gait**	
Normal heel-toe gait	10
Cannot heel walk	6
Cannot toe walk	6
Flatfoot gait	5
6. **Radiographic Measurement**	
**Talocalcaneal Index	
≥40°	5
<40°	0
Talar-First Metatarsal Angle	
≤10°	5
>10°	0
7. **Shoes**	
Regular (no complaints)	5
Regular (with complaints)	3
Orthopaedic Shoes/ Inserts/Braces	0
8. **Function**	
Not limited	15
Occasionally limited	8
Usually limited	0
9. **Pain**	
Never	10
Occasionally	5
Usually	0
10. **Flexor Tendons**	
Full function	5
Partial function	2
No function	0

Fig. 12 Functional rating system for clubfoot surgery.

The procedure combines an opening wedge osteotomy of the medial cuneiform with a closing wedge osteotomy of the cuboid, treating both residual forefoot adduction and midfoot supination. The authors showed in a cadaver model that a cuboid osteotomy is necessary for correction of midfoot supination. Although hindfoot varus is not addressed, the procedure has gained popularity and good results have been reported.[84]

Köse and associates[85] in 1999 described transmidtarsal osteotomy. The procedure involves an opening wedge osteotomy of the medial cuneiform and

dorsal, truncated wedge osteotomies of the middle and lateral cuneiforms. Osteotomy of the middle and lateral cuneiforms allows better correction of rotational and cavus deformities. Again, the procedure requires well-formed tarsal bones and is most appropriate for patients older than 6 years.

Metatarsal osteotomies were described first by Steytler and Van der Walt[86] in 1966 and are indicated when the adduction deformity originates distal to the navicular. Care must be taken to avoid injury to the physis of the first metatarsal by osteotomy or by periosteal stripping;

Table 1
Algorithm for Surgical Reintervention in Clubfeet

Age of Patient at Time of Revision	Step	Method of Treatment
6 mo to 2 yr	1	Revision soft-tissue clubfoot release
	2	If prominent plantar crease, add plantar release
	3	If forefoot adductus is not corrected, add capsulotomies (navicular-first cuneiform or first cuneiform-first metatarsal), as needed
2 to 4 yr	4	If forefoot adductus is not fully corrected after steps 1, 2, and 3, add excision of cartilage of calcaneocuboid joint or decancellation of cuboid
4 to 8 yr	5	If forefoot adductus is not fully corrected after steps 1 through 4, add one of the following steps
	5A	Fusion of calcaneocuboid joint (Dillwyn Evans procedure)
	5B	Excision of distal part of calcaneus (Lichtblau procedure)
	5C	Cuboid decancellation
	5D	Opening wedge osteotomy of first cuneiform
	5E	Tarsometatarsal capsulotomies*
	5F	Metatarsal osteotomies (for patients > 5 yr old)
	6	If patient has overactive tibialis anterior tendon and weak peroneals, add tibialis anterior tendon transfer
	7	If varus angulation of heel remains uncorrected, add osteotomy of heel (Dwyer procedure)
8 to 10 yr†	8	Midtarsal osteotomy for persistent cavus
	9	Distraction osteogenesis (Ilizarov) as only procedure
>10 yr	10	Triple arthrodesis as only procedure

*Not recommended by authors of reports in the literature or by us.
†Note that in patients ≤ 10 years old, it is possible to start with steps 1 and 2, then proceed according to the deformity that remains—that is, proceed to step 7 if there is a deformity of the calcaneus or proceed to step 5A, 5B, 5C, or 5F if there is forefoot adductus.

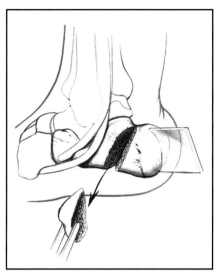

Fig. 13 Lateral closing wedge calcaneal osteotomy, as described by Dwyer.[89]

otherwise, shortening of the first metatarsal will result.[87] Heyman and associates[76] described release of the tarsometatarsal joints for correction of resistant metatarsus adductus or for treating residual clubfoot adduction deformity. Through a dorsal incision, complete capsulotomies and ligament releases were performed. Because of reports of frequent postoperative stiffness and pain, this procedure is not recommended.

Residual Cavus

Inadequate plantar release and muscle imbalance are both possible causes of residual cavus deformity. Soft-tissue release should be adequate in patients younger than 2 years. Steindler[88] in 1920 described release of the plantar fascia from its insertion at the calcaneus. Rigid cavus in children older than 8 years may require osteotomy of the tarsal bones or the calcaneus.[89] The Japas V-osteotomy, recommended for patients older than 6 years, allows correction at the midfoot without shortening the foot.[90] The Akron midtarsal osteotomy also allows correction at the midfoot but uses a so-called dome-type osteotomy to allow dorsoplantar and varus-valgus control.[91] A more distal osteotomy, at the level of the tarsometatarsal joints, was proposed by Jahss.[84] The wedge osteotomy of the tarsometatarsal joints is not intended for patients who have not reached skeletal maturity and requires normal vascular

and skin conditions. Arthrodesis at the hindfoot-midfoot region also has been described.[89]

Residual Varus or Valgus Angulation of the Heel

Dwyer[89] described a calcaneal osteotomy with either an opening or a closing wedge to treat varus and cavus angulation of the heel. Dwyer's lateral closing wedge osteotomy is recommended for children older than 4 years. The osteotomy does not correct the deformity at its apex, which is usually at the level of the midfoot (Fig. 13).

The extra-articular Grice procedure, originally developed for paralytic or spastic foot deformity, can be used to treat valgus angulation of the heel in younger patients because it does not interfere with subsequent growth.[92-94] It has been successful for flexible feet in children 4 to 10 years old. Rigid, overcorrected feet may require repeat soft-tissue releases, as well.[94]

Salvage Procedures

Triple arthrodesis has been used in children older than 10 years and is considered a salvage procedure (Fig. 14).[95] In a study of 15 patients with clubfoot deformity treated with this procedure, Adelaar and associates[96] noted that 11 had a good result and 2 each had a fair and a poor result. Angus and Cowell[97] noted that 65% of 26 feet with a rigid equinus foot deformity had a poor result at an average of 13 years after triple arthrodesis.

Wei and associates[98] and Fogel and associates[99] reported on limited talonavicular arthrodesis in patients who had had previous clubfoot surgery and had talonavicular osteoarthritis with dorsolateral subluxation and pain. The patients in the study by Wei and associates[98] were an average of 11 years old at the time of the surgery. Unlike adults who have undergone talonavicular arthrodesis, children have been noted to retain some subtalar motion. Fifteen of 16 patients reported satisfaction with the procedure after an average follow-up of 4 years.[98]

The Ilizarov apparatus has been combined with various osteotomies to provide distraction osteogenesis for the correction of residual deformity in the clubfoot and other foot deformities.[100,101] Equinus, varus angulation of the hindfoot, midfoot adductus, and cavus all may be addressed with the use of a circular frame and Kirschner wires. However, the potential complications are numerous.[100,101] Paley[101] reported that treatment of 25 various foot deformities with the Ilizarov apparatus resulted in 20 minor and major complications in 18 feet. The patient must understand that the final functional outcome will be a stiff but cosmetically improved plantigrade foot.

Dynamic Forefoot Supination

Transfer of the tibialis anterior tendon has a role in the treatment of a supple recurrent clubfoot (Fig. 15). Garceau[102] and Garceau and Palmer[103] mentioned several prerequisites for successful transfer of the tibialis anterior tendon for the treatment of recurrent varus and adductus. The patient must be younger than 6 years and have a passively correctable

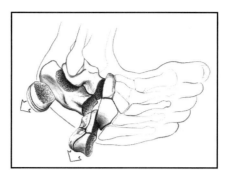

Fig. 14 Triple arthrodesis wedges removed for treatment of residual varus and forefoot adduction.

deformity, weak peroneals confirmed by electromyography, and no active abduction or eversion. Stiff joints or strong peroneals are contraindications. Gartland and Surgent[104] noted that recurrence after primary correction is more likely to respond to tibialis posterior transfer.

Residual Toeing-in

Two alternatives for a patient with a recurrent clubfoot with residual toeing-in are supramalleolar tibial osteotomy and talocalcaneal osteotomy. Hjelmstedt and Sahlstedt[105-107] recommended talocalcaneal wedge osteotomy through the talar neck and reported that 60% of 36 feet managed with the procedure had a good result, 20% had a fair result, and 20% had a poor result. Lloyd-Roberts and associates[108] and Swann and associates[109] reported on a supramalleolar tibial osteotomy with apex posterior angulation and medial rotation to correct equinus and adductus primarily. Neither of these osteotomy procedures is in wide use.

Dorsal Bunion

Dorsal bunion refers to a plantar flexion contracture of the first metatarsophalangeal joint with a dorsiflexion contracture of the first tarsometatarsal joint. It can be the result of imbalance between weak Achilles and peroneus longus tendons and strong flexor hallucis longus and tibialis anterior tendons. One proce-

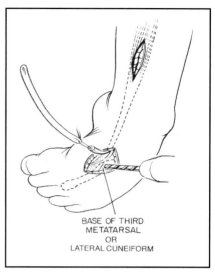

Fig. 15 Transfer of the tibialis anterior tendon to the base of the third metatarsal or lateral cuneiform.

dure described for its correction is the "reverse Jones" procedure,[110] which involves transfer of the flexor hallucis longus to the head of the first metatarsal. If necessary, a plantar flexion first metatarsal osteotomy and capsulorrhaphy can be included.

The Overcorrected Foot

Valgus position of the hindfoot and pronation of the forefoot characterize the overcorrected clubfoot deformity. Multiple factors may produce this deformity, including the release of the interosseous ligament at the subtalar joint and division of the deep deltoid ligament. The forefoot may be corrected nonsurgically by stretching and bracing and surgically by metatarsal and midfoot osteotomies. Treatment of the overcorrected clubfoot includes the use of orthoses for flexible deformity in children younger than 4 years and repeat soft-tissue release for rigid deformity. Subtalar or triple arthrodesis is recommended for a child older than 10 years. Combination medial and lateral column osteotomies of the calcaneus, cuboid, and cuneiforms also have been described.[111-114]

Skin Problems

Frequently, severe recurrent clubfoot deformities are associated with difficulty in skin closure. This problem is especially true of posteromedial wounds. Options to address the problem include tissue expanders;[115-117] free muscle flaps;[118] and partial wound closure, which allows secondary healing to close a wound to decrease the risk of necrosis.[119] Free muscle flaps such as gracilis flaps require microvascular techniques, but no debulking is required because shrinkage is expected. Other techniques that may assist in wound closure are lateral skin release and Z-plasty of the skin.[116]

Summary

Although the etiology of congenital clubfoot remains unknown, reproducible pretreatment grading now seems possible. However, the lack of an agreed-on and reproducible posttreatment evaluation system still hinders outcome studies of the treatment of clubfoot.

The literature from about 1970 to 1990[3,66,120] contains enthusiastic reports on the correction of congenital clubfoot through extensive surgical release procedures. Over time, we have come to recognize the complications of such surgery, including recurrence, overcorrection, stiffness, and pain (WJ Shaughnessy, MD, P Dechet, MD, HB Kitaoka, MD, Vancouver, BC, Canada, unpublished data, 2000). Perhaps because of these findings, there is a renewed interest in nonsurgical techniques for the correction of congenital clubfoot. Recent studies have documented the effectiveness of the two leading techniques involving serial manipulation and cast treatment. The Ponseti technique[49] appears to be effective and requires only a reasonable amount of time out of the lives of the patient and his or her parents. The technique frequently includes some minimally invasive surgery. The Kite and Lovell technique[48] requires minimally invasive surgery less often but is more time consuming.

French investigators and others have introduced new ideas that may reduce the need to immobilize the foot. The French approach requires fairly extensive physical therapy and demands substantial parental time and attention.[56] It is not yet clear that the French technique is more successful in obviating the need for surgery than is expertly applied serial manipulation and cast immobilization. It also has not been proved that the long-term results of the French technique are better than those of serial manipulation and cast immobilization. It is probably that unless the French technique is found to substantially decrease the need for surgery, it will prove to be less cost effective than serial manipulation and cast immobilization.

It is likely that a small number of clubfeet will require surgery even after expertly applied nonsurgical treatment. However, it is hoped that such surgery will be less extensive than procedures commonly performed in the recent past.

References

1. Wynne-Davies R: Family studies and the cause of congenital club foot: Talipes equinovarus, talipes calcaneo-valgus, and metatarsus varus. *J Bone Joint Surg Br* 1964;46:445-463.

2. Shimizu N, Hamada S, Mitta M, Hiroshima K, Ono K: Etiological considerations of congenital clubfoot deformity, in Simons GW (ed): *The Clubfoot: The Present and a View of the Future.* New York, NY, Springer-Verlag, 1994, pp 31-38.

3. Turco VJ: Surgical correction of the resistant club foot: One-stage posteromedial release with internal fixation: A preliminary report. *J Bone Joint Surg Am* 1971;53:477-497.

4. Lochmiller C, Johnston D, Scott A, Risman M, Hecht JT: Genetic epidemiology study of idiopathic talipes equinovarus. *Am J Med Genet* 1998;79:90-96.

5. The foot and leg, in Tachdjian MO (ed): *Pediatric Orthopedics,* ed 2. Philadelphia, PA, WB Saunders, 1990, pp 2405-3012.

6. Ippolito E, Ponseti IV: Congenital club foot in the human fetus: A histological study. *J Bone Joint Surg Am* 1980;62:8-22.

7. Isaacs H, Handelsman JE, Badenhorst M, Pickering A: The muscles in club foot: A histological histochemical and electron microscopic study. *J Bone Joint Surg Br* 1977;59:465-472.

8. Handelsman JE, Badalamente MA: Neuromuscular studies in clubfoot. *J Pediatr Orthop* 1981;1:23-32.

9. Bill PL, Versfeld GA: Congenital clubfoot: An electromyographic study. *J Pediatr Orthop* 1982;2:139-142.

10. Irani RN, Sherman MS: The pathological anatomy of club foot. *J Bone Joint Surg Am* 1963;45:45-52.

11. Shapiro F, Glimcher MJ: Gross and histological abnormalities of the talus in congenital club foot. *J Bone Joint Surg Am* 1979;61:522-530.

12. Ionasescu V, Maynard JA, Ponseti IV, Zellweger H: The role of collagen in the pathogenesis of idiopathic clubfoot: Biochemical and electron microscopic correlations. *Helv Paediatr Acta* 1974;29:305-314.

13. Ippolito E: Update on pathologic anatomy of clubfoot. *J Pediatr Orthop B* 1995;4:17-24.

14. Dietz FR, Ponseti IV, Buckwalter JA: Morphometric study of clubfoot tendon sheaths. *J Pediatr Orthop* 1983;3:311-318.

15. Zimny ML, Willig SJ, Roberts JM, D'Ambrosia RD: An electron microscopic study of the fascia from the medial and lateral sides of clubfoot. *J Pediatr Orthop* 1985;5:577-581.

16. Sano H, Uhthoff HK, Jarvis JG, Mansingh A, Wenckebach GF: Pathogenesis of soft-tissue contracture in club foot. *J Bone Joint Surg Br* 1998;80:641-644.

17. Hootnick DR, Levinsohn EM, Crider RJ, Packard DS Jr: Congenital arterial malformations associated with clubfoot: A report of two cases. *Clin Orthop* 1982;167:160-163.

18. Sodre H, Bruschini S, Mestriner LA, et al: Arterial abnormalities in talipes equinovarus as assessed by angiography and the Doppler technique. *J Pediatr Orthop* 1990;10:101-104.

19. Muir L, Laliotis N, Kutty S, Klenerman L: Absence of the dorsalis pedis pulse in the parents of children with club foot. *J Bone Joint Surg Br* 1995;77:114-116.

20. Porter RW: An anomalous muscle in children with congenital talipes. *Clin Anat* 1996;9:25-27.

21. Chotigavanichaya C, Scaduto AA, Jadhav A, Otsuka NY: Accessory soleus muscle as a cause of resistance to correction in congenital club foot: A case report. *Foot Ankle Int* 2000;21:948-950.

22. Böhm M: The embryologic origin of club-foot. *J Bone Joint Surg* 1929;11:229-259.

23. Kawashima T, Uhthoff HK: Development of the foot in prenatal life in relation to idiopathic club foot. *J Pediatr Orthop* 1990;10:232-237.

24. Farrell SA, Summers AM, Dallaire L, Singer J, Johnson JA, Wilson RD: Club foot, an adverse outcome of early amniocentesis: Disruption or deformation? CEMAT: Canadian Early and Mid-Trimester Amniocentesis Trial. *J Med Genet* 1999;36:843-846.

25. Robertson WW Jr, Corbett D: Congenital clubfoot: Month of conception. *Clin Orthop* 1997;338:14-18.

26. Carroll NC: Pathoanatomy and surgical treatment of the resistant clubfoot. *Instr Course Lect* 1988;37:93-106.

27. Simons GW: Calcaneocuboid joint deformity in talipes equinovarus: An overview and

update. *J Pediatr Orthop B* 1995;4:25-35.

28. Ponseti IV (ed): *Congenital Clubfoot: Fundamentals of Treatment*. Oxford, England, Oxford University Press, 1996, p 55.

29. Howard CB, Benson MK: The ossific nuclei and the cartilage anlage of the talus and calcaneum. *J Bone Joint Surg Br* 1992;74:620-623.

30. Kite JH: Non-operative treatment of congenital clubfeet: A review of one hundred cases. *South Med J* 1930;23:337-345.

31. Simons GW: Analytical radiography of club feet. *J Bone Joint Surg Br* 1977;59:485-489.

32. Simons GW: A standardized method for the radiographic evaluation of clubfeet. *Clin Orthop* 1978;135:107-118.

33. McKay DW: New concept of and approach to clubfoot treatment: Section III. Evaluation and results. *J Pediatr Orthop* 1983;3:141-148.

34. Vanderwilde R, Staheli LT, Chew DE, Malagon V: Measurements on radiographs of the foot in normal infants and children. *J Bone Joint Surg Am* 1988;70:407-415.

35. Cummings RJ, Lovell WW: Operative treatment of congenital idiopathic club foot. *J Bone Joint Surg Am* 1988;70:1108-1112.

36. Watts H: Reproducability of reading club foot x-rays. *Orthop Trans* 1991;15:105.

37. Flynn JM, Donohoe M, Mackenzie WG: An independent assessment of two clubfoot-classification systems. *J Pediatr Orthop* 1998;18:323-327.

38. Dimeglio A, Bensahel H, Souchet P, Mazeau P, Bonnet F: Classification of clubfoot. *J Pediatr Orthop* 1995;4:129-136.

39. Bensahel H, Catterall A, Dimeglio A: Practical applications in idiopathic clubfoot: A retrospective multicentric study in EPOS. *J Pediatr Orthop* 1990;10:186-188.

40. Bensahel H, Dimeglio A, Souchet P: Final evaluation of clubfoot. *J Pediatr Orthop B* 1995;4:137-141.

41. Berenshtein SS: Classification of congenital clubfoot. [Russian] *Ortop Travmatol Protez* 1983;5:32-35.

42. Catterall A: A method of assessment of the clubfoot deformity. *Clin Orthop* 1991;264:48-53.

43. Goldner JL: Congenital talipes equinovarus. *Foot Ankle* 1981;2:123-125.

44. Withington ET (trans): *Hippocrates*. Loeb Classical Library. London, England, Heinemann, 1927, vol 3.

45. Guerin M: Division of the tendon Achilles in clubfoot. *Lancet* 1935;2:648.

46. Preston ET, Fell TW: Congenital idiopathic clubfoot. *Clin Orthop* 1977;122:102-109.

47. Kite JH: The treatment of congenital clubfeet: A study of the results in two hundred cases. *JAMA* 1932;99:1156-1162.

48. Kite JH (ed): *The Clubfoot*. New York, NY, Grune and Stratton, 1964.

49. Ponseti IV: Treatment of congenital club foot. *J Bone Joint Surg Am* 1992;74:448-454.

50. Shaw NE: The early management of clubfoot. *Clin Orthop* 1972;84:39-43.

51. Browne D: Modern methods of treatment of club-foot. *Br Med J* 1937;2:570-572.

52. Thomson SA: Treatment of congenital talipes equinovarus with a modification of the Denis Browne method and splint. *J Bone Joint Surg* 1942;24:291-298.

53. Yamamoto H, Furuya K: Treatment of congenital club foot with a modified Denis Browne splint. *J Bone Joint Surg Br* 1990;72:460-463.

54. Bensahel H, Guillaume A, Czukonyi Z, Desgrippes Y: Results of physical therapy for idiopathic clubfoot: A long-term follow-up study. *J Pediatr Orthop* 1990;10:189-192.

55. Bensahel H, Guillaume A, Czukonyi Z, Themar-Noel C: The intimacy of clubfoot: The ways of functional treatment. *J Pediatr Orthop B* 1994;3:155-160.

56. Dimeglio A, Bonnet F, Mazeau P, De Rosa V: Orthopaedic treatment and passive motion machine: Consequences for the surgical treatment of clubfoot. *J Pediatr Orthop B* 1996;5:173-180.

57. Johnston WH, Richards BS: Abstract: Non-operative treatment of clubfoot: The French technique. *Proceedings of the 1999 Annual Meeting, Pediatric Orthopaedic Society of North America*. Lake Buena Vista, FL, Pediatric Orthopaedic Society of North America, 1999, p 25.

58. Delgado MR, Wilson H, Johnston C, Richards S, Karol L: A preliminary report of the use of botulinum toxin type A in infants with clubfoot: Four case studies. *J Pediatr Orthop* 2000; 20:533-538.

59. Reimann I, Lyquist E: Dynamic splint used in the treatment of club foot. *Acta Orthop Scand* 1969;40:817-824.

60. Bensahel H, Csukonyi Z, Desgrippes Y, Chaumien JP: Surgery in residual clubfoot: One-stage medioposterior release "a la carte." *J Pediatr Orthop* 1987;7:145-148.

61. Osterman K, Merikanto J: Critical aspects of neonatal surgery in clubfoot. *J Pediatr Orthop B* 1996;5:55-56.

62. Turco VJ: Resistant congenital club foot: One-stage posteromedial release with internal fixation: A follow-up report of a fifteen-year experience. *J Bone Joint Surg Am* 1979;61:805-814.

63. Simons GW: Complete subtalar release in club feet: Part II. Comparison with less extensive procedures. *J Bone Joint Surg Am* 1985; 67:1056-1065.

64. Crawford AH, Marxen JL, Osterfeld DL: The Cincinnati incision: A comprehensive approach for surgical procedures of the foot and ankle in childhood. *J Bone Joint Surg Am* 1982;64:1355-1358.

65. Henry AK: *Extensile Exposure*, ed 2. Baltimore, MD, Williams and Wilkins, 1970.

66. McKay DW: New concept of and approach to clubfoot treatment: II. Correction of the clubfoot. *J Pediatr Orthop* 1983;3:10-21.

67. Carroll NC: Controversies in the surgical

management of clubfoot. *Instr Course Lect* 1996;45:331-337.

68. Mountney J, Khan T, Davies AG, Smith TW: Scar quality from partial or complete wound closure using the Cincinnati incision for clubfoot surgery. *J Pediatr Orthop B* 1998;7:223-225.

69. Crawford AH, Gupta AK: Clubfoot controversies: Complications and causes for failure. *Instr Course Lect* 1996;45:339-346.

70. Vizkelety T, Szepesi K: Reoperation in treatment of clubfoot. *J Pediatr Orthop* 1989;9:144-147.

71. Tarraf YN, Carroll NC: Analysis of the components of residual deformity in clubfeet presenting for reoperation. *J Pediatr Orthop* 1992;12: 207-216.

72. Lehman WB, Atar D, Grant AD, Strongwater AM: Re-do clubfoot: Surgical approach and long-term results. *Bull NY Acad Med* 1990;66: 601-617.

73. Lichtblau S: Section of the abductor hallucis tendon for correction of metatarsus varus deformity. *Clin Orthop* 1975;110:227-232.

74. Toohey JS, Campbell P: Distal calcaneal osteotomy in resistant talipes equinovarus. *Clin Orthop* 1985;197:224-230.

75. Evans D: Relapsed club foot. *J Bone Joint Surg Br* 1961;43:722-733.

76. Heyman CH, Herndon CH, Strong JM: Mobilization of the tarsometatarsal and inter-metatarsal joints for the correction of resistant adduction of the fore part of the foot in congenital club-foot or congenital metatarsus varus. *J Bone Joint Surg Am* 1958;40:299-310.

77. Lichtblau S: A medial and lateral release operation for club foot: A preliminary report. *J Bone Joint Surg Am* 1973;55:1377-1384.

78. Addison A, Fixsen JA, Lloyd-Roberts GC: A review of the Dillwyn Evans type collateral operation in severe club feet. *J Bone Joint Surg Br* 1983;65:12-14.

79. Graham GP, Dent CM: Dillwyn Evans operation for relapsed club foot: Long-term results. *J Bone Joint Surg Br* 1992;74:445-448.

80. Abrams RC: Relapsed club foot: The early results of an evaluation of Dillwyn Evans' operation. *J Bone Joint Surg Am* 1969;51:270-282.

81. Fowler SB, Brooks AL, Parrish TF: The cavovarus foot. *J Bone Joint Surg Am* 1959;41:757.

82. Hofmann AA, Constine RM, McBride GG, Coleman SS: Osteotomy of the first cuneiform as treatment of residual adduction of the fore part of the foot in club foot. *J Bone Joint Surg Am* 1984;66:985-990.

83. McHale KA, Lenhart MK: Treatment of residual clubfoot deformity—the "bean-shaped" foot—by opening wedge medial cuneiform osteotomy and closing wedge cuboid osteotomy: Clinical review and cadaver correlations. *J Pediatr Orthop* 1991;11:374-381.

84. Jahss MH: Tarsometatarsal truncated-wedge arthrodesis for pes cavus and equinovarus deformity of the fore part of the foot. *J Bone Joint Surg Am* 1980;62:713-722.

85. Köse N, Günal I, Gökturk E, Seber S: Treatment of severe residual clubfoot deformity by trans-midtarsal osteotomy. *J Pediatr Orthop B* 1999;8:251-256.

86. Steytler JC, Van der Walt ID: Correction of resistant adduction of the forefoot in congenital clubfoot and congenital metatarsus varus by metatarsal osteotomy. *Br J Surg* 1966; 53:558-560.

87. Holden D, Siff S, Butler J, Cain T: Shortening of the first metatarsal as a complication of metatarsal osteotomies. *J Bone Joint Surg Am* 1984;66:582-587.

88. Steindler A: Stripping of the os calcis. *J Orthop Surg* 1920;2:8-12.

89. Dwyer FC: Osteotomy of the calcaneum for pes cavus. *J Bone Joint Surg Br* 1959;41:80-86.

90. Japas LM: Surgical treatment of pes cavus by tarsal V-osteotomy: Preliminary report. *J Bone Joint Surg Am* 1968;50:927-944.

91. Wilcox PG, Weiner DS: The Akron midtarsal dome osteotomy in the treatment of rigid pes cavus: A preliminary review. *J Pediatr Orthop* 1985;5:333-338.

92. Grice DS: Further experience with extra-articular arthrodesis of the subtalar joint. *J Bone Joint Surg Am* 1955;37:246-259, 365.

93. Grice DS: An extra-articular arthrodesis of the subastragalar joint for correction of paralytic flat feet in children. *J Bone Joint Surg Am* 1952;34:927-940.

94. Scott SM, Janes PC, Stevens PM: Grice subtalar arthrodesis followed to skeletal maturity. *J Pediatr Orthop* 1988;8:176-183.

95. Galindo MJ, Siff SJ, Butler JE, Cain TE: Triple arthrodesis in young children: A salvage procedure after failed releases in severely affected feet. *Foot Ankle* 1987;7:319-325.

96. Adelaar RS, Dannelly EA, Meunier PA, Stelling FH, Goldner JL, Colvard DF: A long term study of triple arthrodesis in children. *Orthop Clin North Am* 1976;7:895-908.

97. Angus PD, Cowell HR: Triple arthrodesis: A critical long-term review. *J Bone Joint Surg Br* 1986;68:260-265.

98. Wei SY, Sullivan RJ, Davidson RS: Talo-navicular arthrodesis for residual midfoot deformities of a previously corrected clubfoot. *Foot Ankle Int* 2000;21:482-485.

99. Fogel GR, Katoh Y, Rand JA, Chao EY: Talonavicular arthrodesis for isolated arthrosis: 9.5-year results and gait analysis. *Foot Ankle* 1982;3:105-113.

100. Lehman WB, Grant AD, Atar D: The use of distraction osteogenesis (Ilizarov) in complex foot deformities, in Jahss MH (ed): *Disorders of the Foot and Ankle: Medical and Surgical Management*, ed 2. Philadelphia, PA, WB Saunders, 1991, pp 2735-2744.

101. Paley D: The correction of complex foot deformities using Ilizarov's distraction osteotomies. *Clin Orthop* 1993;293:97-111.

102. Garceau GJ: Anterior tibial tendon transfer for recurrent clubfoot. *Clin Orthop* 1972;84:61-65.

103. Garceau GJ, Palmer RM: Transfer of the anterior tibial tendon for recurrent club foot: A long-term follow-up. *J Bone Joint Surg Am* 1967;49:207-231.

104. Gartland JJ, Surgent RE: Posterior tibial transplant in the surgical treatment of recurrent clubfoot. *Clin Orthop* 1972;84:66-70.

105. Hjelmstedt A, Sahlstedt B: Talo-calcaneal osteotomy and soft-tissue procedures in the treatment of clubfeet: I. Indications, principles and technique. *Acta Orthop Scand* 1980;51:335-347.

106. Hjelmstedt A, Sahlstedt B: Talo-calcaneal osteotomy and soft-tissue procedures in the treatment of clubfeet: II. Results in 36 surgically treated feet. *Acta Orthop Scand* 1980; 51:349-357.

107. Hjelmstedt A, Sahlstedt B: Role of talocalcaneal osteotomy in clubfoot surgery: Results in 31 surgically treated feet. *J Pediatr Orthop* 1990; 10:193-197.

108. Lloyd-Roberts GC, Swann M, Catterall A: Medial rotational osteotomy for severe residual deformity in club foot: A preliminary report on a new method of treatment. *J Bone Joint Surg Br* 1974;56:37-43.

109. Swann M, Lloyd-Roberts GC, Catterall A: The anatomy of uncorrected club feet: A study of rotation deformity. *J Bone Joint Surg Br* 1969; 51:263-269.

110. Kuo KN, Jansen LD: Rotatory dorsal subluxation of the navicular: A complication of clubfoot surgery. *J Pediatr Orthop* 1998;18:770-774.

111. Rathjen KE, Mubarak SJ: Calcaneal-cuboid-cuneiform osteotomy for the correction of valgus foot deformities in children. *J Pediatr Orthop* 1998;18:775-782.

112. Mosca VS: Calcaneal lengthening for valgus deformity of the hindfoot: Results in children who had severe, symptomatic flatfoot and skewfoot. *J Bone Joint Surg Am* 1995;77:500-512.

113. Evans D: Calcaneo-valgus deformity. *J Bone Joint Surg Br* 1975;57:270-278.

114. Phillips GE: A review of elongation of os calcis for flat feet. *J Bone Joint Surg Br* 1983;65:15-18.

115. Atar D, Grant AD, Silver L, Lehman WB, Strongwater AM: The use of a tissue expander in club-foot surgery: A case report and review. *J Bone Joint Surg Br* 1990;72:574-577.

116. Lehman WB, Atar D: Complications in the management of talipes equinovarus, in Drennan JC (ed): *The Child's Foot and Ankle*. New York, NY, Raven Press, 1992, pp 135-153.

117. Grant AD, Atar D, Lehman WB, Strongwater AM: The use of tissue expanders in clubfoot surgery, in Simons GW (ed): *The Clubfoot: The Present and a View of the Future*. New York, NY, Springer-Verlag, 1994, pp 235-241.

118. Haasbeek JF, Zuker RM, Wright JG: Free gracilis muscle transfer for coverage of severe foot deformities. *J Pediatr Orthop* 1995;15:608-612.

119. Ferlic RJ, Breed AL, Mann DC, Cherney JJ: Partial wound closure after surgical correction of equinovarus foot deformity. *J Pediatr Orthop* 1997;17:486-489.

120. Simons GW: Complete subtalar release in club feet: Part I. A preliminary report. *J Bone Joint Surg Am* 1985;67:1044-1055.

38

Treatment of a Recurrent Clubfoot Deformity After Initial Correction With the Ponseti Technique

Frederick R. Dietz, MD

Abstract

Early recognition and appropriate treatment of recurrent deformity (relapse) is an important component of the Ponseti technique of clubfoot correction. After correction of a clubfoot deformity by the Ponseti technique, relapse usually involves equinus and varus of the hindfoot. Cavus and adductus rarely recur to a clinically significant degree. Clubfoot recurs most frequently and quickly while the foot is rapidly growing—during the first several years of life. Recurrence of deformity will almost always occur, even after complete correction with the Ponseti technique, if appropriate bracing is not used.

Treatment of clubfoot relapse in infants and toddlers is identical to the original correction maneuver. In a patient approximately 2.5 years of age, a relapse can be treated with anterior tibial tendon transfer to the third cuneiform with or without Achilles tendon lengthening. The indication for anterior tibial tendon transfer is the presence of dynamic supination during gait. After tendon transfer, bracing is no longer required because the eversion force of the transferred tendon maintains the correction. In a long-term follow-up study of patients treated by the Ponseti technique, the necessity for anterior tibial tendon transfer did not compromise the outcome with respect to level of pain and functional limitations. Because anterior tibial tendon transfer is joint sparing, the foot retains maximal strength and suppleness. Good long-term results can be anticipated despite clubfoot relapse.

Recurrence of deformity or relapse is the development of one or more of the original deformities of equinus, varus, adduction, and cavus after full correction of an idiopathic clubfoot. After correction of clubfoot by the Ponseti technique, relapse usually involves equinus and varus of the hindfoot.[1] Cavus and adductus rarely recur to a clinically significant degree. Worsening of incompletely corrected foot deformities is expected; appropriate initial treatment achieves full and complete correction. The cause of a relapse in a foot that had been completely corrected by the Ponseti technique is unknown, but would logically result from the same pathology that initially caused the clubfoot. Unfortunately, this pathology remains incompletely understood despite more than a century of investigation.

One striking characteristic of clubfoot is its tendency to recur most frequently and most quickly while the foot is rapidly growing—during the first several years of life. Relapses are most common in the first through third years of life. Relapse is less common after age 3 years, rare after age 5 years, and almost never occurs in patients older than 7 years of age. These findings suggest that the pathologic process is most active during the most rapid growing period of the foot or is in some way dependent on rapid growth to create the deformity. Identifying genes that may predispose some people to clubfoot appears to be the most promising avenue for discovering the causes of idiopathic clubfoot.

Bracing

Almost all clubfeet will relapse after full correction if appropriate bracing is not used. Simple abduction bracing can prevent most relapses. Because part-time bracing used during sleeping hours can prevent relapse, it is believed that the pathologic process must be subtle. However, the pathology is also persistent because bracing is required for 3 to 4 years to prevent most relapses. A study by

Morcuende and associates[2] clearly showed the importance of using a foot abduction orthosis to prevent relapse after clubfoot correction. The authors reviewed the outcomes of 157 patients (256 feet) who were treated between 1991 and 2001 using the Ponseti method. Seventeen patients (11%) had a relapse. They found that 2 of 140 patients (approximately 1%) whose parents reported compliance with the bracing regimen had a relapse, compared with the occurrence of a relapse in 15 of 17 patients (89%) whose parents were not compliant with the bracing regimen. Dobbs and associates[3] evaluated recurrence risk in 51 consecutive infants with 86 idiopathic clubfeet and found that brace wear compliance was the factor that was most strongly related to relapse with an odds ratio of 183 ($P < 0.00001$).

Neither study found a correlation between the initial severity of the deformity, place of prior treatment, number of casts required for initial correction, or patient age at initiation of treatment. Therefore, ensuring parent and patient compliance with the bracing regimen is the most effective method for avoiding relapse. The author's approach to achieving this goal is to emphasize the importance of the brace at every office visit, especially at the prenatal visit and during every cast change; to state with conviction that if the brace is not used the clubfoot deformity will return and that further casting and even surgical intervention will then be necessary; and to recommend the use of the brace whenever the child is put in the crib or bed to sleep. Children are much less likely to resist brace wear if the brace is used in a completely consistent manner. Most children will become unwilling to wear the brace sometime between 3 and 4 years of

age. Because this is past the peak time for relapse, discontinued use of the brace is acceptable. If the patient and the family are not resistant to brace wear, the author recommends use of the brace until the child is 5 years old because relapse after that age is extremely rare.

Presentation of Relapse

Clubfoot relapses will occur and are more effectively and easily treated if recognized promptly. Most relapses that occur before walking age are attributable to failure to wear the abduction foot orthosis. The parents will often describe a history of difficulty in applying the braces as prescribed. As a relapse occurs, bracing becomes more difficult. Equinus recurs first and makes it difficult to place the patient's heel completely "down" into the heel of the orthotic shoe. Therefore, the heel slips up and often completely out of the shoe. The parents report having to reposition the foot in the shoe multiple times or that the brace is not on the patient's foot in the morning. Physical examination will show less dorsiflexion than on previous examinations. If the foot cannot be dorsiflexed past neutral, and usually at least 5° to 10°, treatment for a relapse should begin.

Treatment

Treatment for recurrent clubfoot is identical to the original corrective maneuver. The foot is abducted using the head of the talus as the fulcrum. In most feet, in which complete correction had been obtained, the foot will again abduct and dorsiflex into full correction. Two or three castings are usually required and are applied at 2-week intervals in these older infants. If the foot corrects except for the equinus, a percutaneous Achilles tenotomy should

be repeated. The upper patient age limit for a percutaneous Achilles tenotomy as opposed to an open Achilles tendon lengthening has not been established. The author has performed a percutaneous tenotomy in an 18-month-old patient, although traditionally open lengthening has been performed in patients older than 1 year of age.

Clubfoot relapse in children of walking age who are younger than 2.5 years of age will usually have the same history and static physical findings. In addition, the treating physician can observe the recurrent equinus and varus during gait. Most commonly, relapse in patients in this age group consists of recurrent equinus with or without recurrent varus. Mild adductus may be present in a small percentage of such patients. Recurrence of cavus is rare. Treatment is needed for these patients because the relapse will not "walk itself out." Treatment consists of manipulation and casting, which can be challenging in children of walking age if they are uncooperative. With patience, correction can be regained in most children. Occasionally, the patient's history will reveal no difficulties with brace wear and the static examination will show a fully corrected foot; however, the child ambulates in a supinated position. These feet should be treated with abduction/dorsiflexion manipulation and two or three castings at 2-week intervals. These feet have an incomplete reduction of the navicular resulting in a supinating force of the anterior tibial tendon. Because patients younger than 2.5 years of age are too young for an anterior tibial tendon transfer to the third cuneiform, manipulation and casting are appropriate. In the author's experience, most feet that relapse after walking age will require an anterior tibial tendon transfer when the patient is old enough for the procedure. This situation probably occurs because families who were noncompliant with brace wear after the initial treatment for clubfoot remain noncompliant with brace wear even after treatment for the first relapse.

Relapses in infants or toddlers may occur more than once. Each time a relapse is identified, it is treated in the same manner. Abduction manipulation is performed. The foot usually will dorsiflex as the calcaneus moves into a more valgus position. If equinus is persistent, the Achilles tendon must be relengthened, either percutaneously or by an open lengthening, depending on the age of the child.

Tendon Transfer

When a patient is approximately 2.5 years of age, a relapse can be treated by anterior tibial tendon transfer to the third cuneiform with or without Achilles tendon lengthening. At age 2.5 years, the ossific nucleus of the third cuneiform is sufficiently large that the anterior tibial tendon can be transferred into the ossific nucleus, ensuring tendon healing to bone and avoiding damage to the growth cartilage of the third cuneiform.

The necessity of anchoring the transferred tendon into bone has been questioned. Huang and associates[4] reported on anterior tibial tendon transfer as the principal corrective procedure after initial manipulation and casting in 159 feet in 111 patients. Sixty-seven transfers were made to the third cuneiform, 88 transfers were made to the medial cuboid, and 2 were made to the second cuneiform. Additional procedures consisted mainly of percutaneous or open lengthening of the Achilles tendon. Thirty-three transfers were performed on 6- to 12-

month-old patients and 35 procedures were done on children 1 to 3 years of age. All patients in this study were at least 13 years of age at follow-up. No complications with tendon pullout or cuneiform growth disturbance from anchoring the anterior tibial tendon into the cartilage anlagen of the cuneiform were found (L Zhao, MD, personal communication, 2000). Huang and associates reported 91.8% good and excellent results using a rating system that combined satisfaction, function, and anatomic criteria. Outcomes were best when surgery was performed before the children were 5 years old. Huang and associates[4] concluded that the optimal time for tendon transfer was when patients were between 6 and 12 months old.

The author has not used anterior tendon transfer into the cartilage of the third cuneiform because of concerns regarding tendon pull-out, growth disturbance, or overcorrection of deformity. The approach of using an anterior tibial tendon transfer to treat infants is intriguing, especially as an alternative to repeated casting for patients who are noncompliant with brace wear.

At the author's institution, an anterior tibial tendon transfer is not performed until the ossific nucleus of the third cuneiform is large enough to accept the entire tendon. Based on the results of a 30-year follow-up study[5] on Ponseti's early patients, tendon transfer is a recommended procedure. In this study, 45 patients with 71 clubfeet who were an average of 34 years old at follow-up answered questions about pain and function to measure outcome satisfaction. These patients were compared with a control group of patients who had no congenital foot deformity. Fifty-three percent of the feet with clubfoot deformity had

undergone anterior tibial tendon transfer and had outcomes, with respect to pain and function, that were comparable with feet that did not require the transfer. Outcomes were not significantly different in the control group without clubfoot. The high percentage of feet requiring anterior tibial tendon transfer in this cohort study resulted from Ponseti's developing recognition of the importance of overcorrection of the deformity and the necessity of abduction bracing of the feet for a prolonged period of time (IV Ponsetti, MD, Iowa City, IA, personal communication).

The indication for anterior tibial tendon transfer is the presence of dynamic supination during gait. The entire foot supinates during the swing phase and is supinated to some degree in the stance phase such that weight bearing is placed excessively on the lateral border of the foot. This condition usually results from an incomplete correction of the medial displacement of the navicular, which may occur in severe clubfoot deformities despite optimal manipulation and casting. As with all tendon transfers, the deformity observed during gait must be passively correctable. If the equinus and varus are not passively correctable, two or three manipulation and casting sessions are necessary until the static deformity is completely corrected. If 10° of dorsiflexion is not obtained, Achilles tendon lengthening should be performed at the time of anterior tibial tendon transfer. After tendon transfer, bracing is no longer required because the eversion force of the transferred tendon maintains the correction.

Techniques for Anterior Tendon Transfer

To perform an anterior tendon transfer (Figure 1), a 3- to 4-cm incision is made over the medial as-

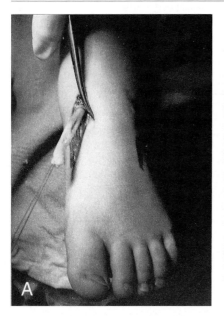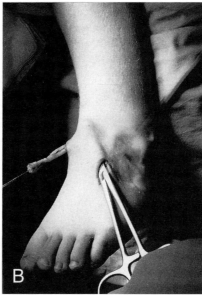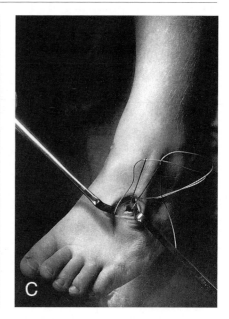

Figure 1 **A,** The anterior tibial tendon is released from its insertion on the base of the first metatarsal and freed of all peritendinous attachments proximally to the extensor retinaculum of the ankle. **B,** The third cuneiform is identified through a small, separate lateral incision. A large hemostat is passed subcutaneously from the lateral wound into the medial wound, thereby creating a tunnel for the redirection of the anterior tibial tendon. **C,** The anterior tibial tendon is anchored into a drill hole in the ossific nucleus of the third cuneiform.

pect of the foot in line with the anterior tibial tendon. The tendon is released from its insertion on the base of the first metatarsal maintaining maximum length. Attachments to the tendon that would tether it during transfer are released up to the inferior ankle retinaculum using scissors. A Bunnell stitch is placed in the tendon using a heavy nonabsorbable suture. A second 3-cm incision is made over the third cuneiform. In younger children (age 2.5 to 5 years), the author uses Fluoro-Scan (FluoroScan Imaging Systems, Northbrook, IL) and a Keith needle to identify the center of the ossific nucleus of the third cuneiform. A hand drill is used to make a hole larger than the tendon (so no binding of the tendon in the bone tunnel will occur) in the center of the ossific nucleus. A large hemostat is introduced through the incision over the third cuneiform. The hemostat is pushed under the subcutaneous tis-

sue in a proximal-medial direction to the center of the inferior ankle retinaculum. The hemostat is then directed medially into the wound over the anterior tibial tendon. The sutures in the tendon are grasped and the tendon is brought into the wound over the third cuneiform. The tendon is drawn into the bone tunnel using Keith needles and the suture is tied over a padded button on the sole of the foot. The foot should lie with the calcaneus in neutral varus-valgus and should lie in 10° or less of plantar flexion. If 10° to 15° of dorsiflexion were not present prior to surgery, Achilles tendon lengthening should be performed before the anterior tibial tendon transfer is sutured. The author performs a coronal Z-lengthening with the tendon cuts performed anteriorly in the distal tendon and posteriorly in the proximal tendon. This technique ensures that there is no raw tendon surface distally where

the tendon is most subcutaneous and therefore avoids the risk of scarring of the tendon to the overlying tissues. An above-knee cast is placed with the knee flexed 90° to ensure that weight bearing does not occur for 6 weeks. For children younger than 5 years of age, the cast and button are removed at 6 weeks and unrestricted weight bearing is permitted. Older children have the cast changed at 6 weeks. The button and suture are removed and a below-knee walking cast is applied for 3 weeks to ensure complete healing of the transferred tendon to the bone.

Summary

To prevent clubfoot relapse it is important to encourage compliance with brace wear. Even with proper compliance, relapses will occur and should be recognized early for optimal outcomes. A small amount of heel varus or equinus will not resolve spontaneously. Treatment should be done with repeat manipulations and castings. In children older than 2.5 years of age with dynamic supination, treatment is performed by an anterior tibial tendon transfer to the third cuneiform with Achilles tendon lengthening as needed. Because this approach is joint sparing, the foot retains maximal strength and suppleness. Good long-term results can be anticipated despite the occurrence of clubfoot relapse.

References

1. Ponseti IV: *Congenital Clubfoot: Fundamentals of Treatment.* New York, NY, Oxford University Press, 1996.

2. Morcuende JA, Dolan L, Dietz FR, Ponseti IV: Radical reduction in the rate of extensive corrective surgery for clubfoot using the Ponseti Method. *Pediatrics* 2004;113:376-380.

3. Dobbs MB, Rudzki JR, Purcell DB, et al: Factors predictive of outcome after use of the Ponseti method for treatment of idiopathic clubfeet. *J Bone Joint Surg Am* 2004;86-A:22-27.

4. Huang YT, Lei W, Zhao L, et al: The treatment of congenital club foot by operation to correct deformity and achieve dynamic muscle balance. *J Bone Joint Surg Br* 1999,81:858-862.

5. Cooper DM, Dietz FR: Treatment of idiopathic clubfoot: A thirty-year follow-up note. *J Bone Joint Surg Am* 1995;77:1477-1489.

Index

D